Spine Imaging

Guest Editor

TIMOTHY P. MAUS, MD

RADIOLOGIC CLINICS OF NORTH AMERICA

www.radiologic.theclinics.com

Consulting Editor
FRANK H. MILLER, MD

July 2012 • Volume 50 • Number 4

SAUNDERS an imprint of ELSEVIER, Inc.

W.B. SAUNDERS COMPANY
A Division of Elsevier Inc.

1600 John F. Kennedy Boulevard • Suite 1800 • Philadelphia, Pennsylvania 19103-2899

http://www.theclinics.com

RADIOLOGIC CLINICS OF NORTH AMERICA Volume 50, Number 4
July 2012 ISSN 0033-8389, ISBN 13: 978-1-4557-3928-8

Editor: Sarah Barth
Developmental Editor: Donald Mumford

Radiologic Clinics of North America (ISSN 0033-8389) is published bimonthly by Elsevier Inc., 360 Park Avenue South, New York, NY 10010-1710. Months of issue are January, March, May, July, September, and November. Periodicals postage paid at New York, NY and additional mailing offices. Subscription prices are USD 421 per year for US individuals, USD 659 per year for US institutions, USD 202 per year for US students and residents, USD 491 per year for Canadian individuals, USD 827 per year for Canadian institutions, USD 606 per year for international individuals, USD 827 per year for international institutions, and USD 290 per year for Canadian and foreign students/residents. To receive student and resident rate, orders must be accompanied by name of affiliated institution, date of term and the signature of program/residency coordinatior on institution letterhead. Orders will be billed at individual rate until proof of status is received. Foreign air speed delivery is included in all *Clinics* subscription prices. All prices are subject to change without notice. **POSTMASTER:** Send address changes to *Radiologic Clinics of North America*, Elsevier Health Sciences Division, Subscription Customer Service, 3251 Riverport Lane, Maryland Heights, MO63043. **Customer Service: Telephone: 1-800-654-2452** (U.S. and Canada); **1-314-447-8871** (outside U.S. and Canada). **Fax: 1-314-447-8029. E-mail: journalscustomerservice-usa@elsevier.com** (for print support); **journalsonlinesupport-usa@elsevier.com** (for online support).

Reprints. For copies of 100 or more of articles in this publication, please contact the Commercial Reprints Department, Elsevier Inc., 360 Park Avenue South, New York, New York 10010-1710. Tel.: (+1) 212-633-3812; Fax: (+1) 212-462-1935; E-mail: reprints@elsevier.com.

Radiologic Clinics of North America also published in Greek Paschalidis Medical Publications, Athens, Greece.

Radiologic Clinics of North America is covered in *MEDLINE/PubMed (Index Medicus), EMBASE/Excerpta Medica, Current Contents/Life Sciences, Current Contents/Clinical Medicine, RSNA Index to Imaging Literature, BIOSIS, Science Citation Index,* and *ISI/BIOMED*.

Printed in the United States of America.

Contributors

CONSULTING EDITOR

FRANK H. MILLER, MD
Professor of Radiology; Chief, Body Imaging Section and Fellowship Program and GI Radiology; Medical Director MRI, Department of Radiology, Northwestern University Feinberg School of Medicine, Chicago, Illinois

GUEST EDITOR

TIMOTHY P. MAUS, MD
Assistant Professor of Radiology, Department of Radiology, Mayo Clinic, Rochester, Minnesota

AUTHORS

KIMBERLY K. AMRAMI, MD
Professor of Radiology, Department of Radiology, Mayo Clinic, Rochester, Minnesota

CHARLES N. APRILL, MD
Clinical Professor, Departments of Radiology and Physical Medicine and Rehabilitation, Louisiana State University Health Sciences Center, New Orleans; Private Practice, Interventional Spine Specialists, Kenner, Louisiana

NIKOLAI BOGDUK, BSc(Med), MB, BS, PhD, MD, DSc, MMed, Dip Anat, FAFMM, FAFRM, FFPM(ANZCA)
Conjoint Professor of Pain Medicine, University of Newcastle, Callaghan; Director of Clinical Research, Newcastle Bone and Joint Institute, Royal Newcastle Centre, Newcastle, New South Wales, Australia

JOHN A. CARRINO, MD, MPH
Section Chief, Musculoskeletal Radiology, Russell H. Morgan Department of Radiology and Radiological Science, Associate Professor of Radiology and Orthopaedic Surgery, The Johns Hopkins University School of Medicine, Baltimore, Maryland

AVNEESH CHHABRA, MD
The Russell H. Morgan Department of Radiology and Radiological Science, Johns Hopkins Hospital, Baltimore, Maryland

ROGER CHOU, MD
Associate Professor, Departments of Medicine, Medical Informatics, and Clinical Epidemiology, Oregon Health & Science University, Portland, Oregon

FILIPPO DEL GRANDE, MD, MBA, MHEM
Research Fellow of Radiology, Section of Musculoskeletal Radiology, The Johns Hopkins Medical Institutions, Russell H. Morgan Department of Radiology and Radiological Science, Baltimore, Maryland

RICHARD A. DEYO, MD, MPH
Professor, Departments of Family Medicine, Medicine, Public Health, and Preventive Medicine, Center for Research on Occupational and Environmental Toxicology, Oregon Health & Science University; Kaiser Permanente Center for Health Research, Portland, Oregon

FELIX E. DIEHN, MD
Assistant Professor of Radiology, Division of Neuroradiology, Department of Radiology, Mayo Clinic, Rochester, Minnesota

JEFFREY G. JARVIK, MD, MPH
Professor, Departments of Radiology, Neurological Surgery, and Health Services, Harborview Medical Center, University of Washington, Seattle, Washington

JAD G. KHALIL, MD
Chief Resident, Department of Orthopedic Surgery, Henry Ford Hospital, Detroit, Michigan

A. JAY KHANNA, MD, MBA
Associate Professor of Orthopaedic Surgery and Biomedical Engineering, Department of Orthopaedic Surgery, The Johns Hopkins University School of Medicine, Bethesda, Maryland

AMY L. KOTSENAS, MD
Assistant Professor of Radiology, Division of Neuroradiology, Department of Radiology, Mayo Clinic, Rochester, Minnesota

JOHN P. MALLOY IV, DO
Spine Surgeon, Alexander Orthopaedic Associates, Largo, Florida

TIMOTHY P. MAUS, MD
Assistant Professor of Radiology, Department of Radiology, Mayo Clinic, Rochester, Minnesota

JONATHAN M. MORRIS, MD
Associate Professor of Radiology, Department of Radiology, Mayo Clinic, Rochester, Minnesota

NAVEEN S. MURTHY, MD
Assistant Professor of Radiology, Division of Musculoskeletal Radiology, Department of Radiology, Mayo Clinic, Rochester, Minnesota

AHMAD NASSR, MD
Assistant Professor and Consultant, Department of Orthopedic Surgery, Mayo Clinic, Rochester, Minnesota

RASHMI S. THAKKAR, MD
Postdoctoral Research Fellow, The Russell H. Morgan Department of Radiology and Radiological Science, The Johns Hopkins University School of Medicine, Baltimore, Maryland

SAVYASACHI C. THAKKAR, MD
Resident, Department of Orthopaedic Surgery, The Johns Hopkins University School of Medicine, Baltimore, Maryland

GAURAV K. THAWAIT, MD
The Russell H. Morgan Department of Radiology and Radiological Science, Johns Hopkins Hospital, Baltimore, Maryland

JOHN T. WALD, MD
Assistant Professor of Medicine, Department of Radiology, Division of Neuroradiology, Mayo Clinic, Rochester, Minnesota

Contents

Imaging the Intervertebral Disk: Age-Related Changes, Herniations, and Radicular Pain 629

Filippo Del Grande, Timothy P. Maus, and John A. Carrino

The articulations of the spinal motion segment, the intervertebral disk, and the zygapophyseal joints, inevitably undergo age-related changes. This article focuses on the intervertebral disk, specifically when fissures sufficiently weaken the posterior annulus so as to allow herniation of nuclear material into the outer annular structure as a contained protrusion or breach the annulus and pass into the epidural space as an extrusion. This article examines the imaging of the age-related changes of the disk and disk herniation: nomenclature, the reliability and relative merits of imaging modalities, the imaging natural history of disk herniations, and, most importantly, the clinical significance.

Imaging of Spinal Stenosis: Neurogenic Intermittent Claudication and Cervical Spondylotic Myelopathy 651

Timothy P. Maus

Spinal stenosis in either the cervical or lumbar spinal segments is one of the most common indications for spine imaging and intervention, particularly among the elderly. This article examines the pathophysiology and imaging of the corresponding clinical syndromes, cervical spondylotic myelopathy or neurogenic intermittent claudication. The specificity fault of spine imaging is readily evident in evaluation of spinal stenosis, as many patients with anatomic cervical or lumbar central canal narrowing are asymptomatic. Imaging also may be insensitive to dynamic lesions. Those imaging features that identify symptomatic patients, or predict response to interventions, are emphasized.

Lumbar Diskogenic Pain, Provocation Diskography, and Imaging Correlates 681

Timothy P. Maus and Charles N. Aprill

Diskogenic pain refers to pain mediated by the intrinsic innervation of the intervertebral disk. It is experienced as pain centered at the symptomatic spine segment (axial pain) without radicular features or radiculopathy. There is no pathoanatomic gold standard; histologic examination cannot identify a painful disk. The current reference standard for diskogenic pain is provocation diskography. This article reviews diskogenic pain, the history of provocation diskography, and its current use in the diagnosis of lumbar diskogenic pain. The extensive literature describing imaging features which may predict a positive diskogram, and allow non-invasive diagnosis of diskogenic pain, is examined.

Imaging of Posterior Element Axial Pain Generators: Facet Joints, Pedicles, Spinous Processes, Sacroiliac Joints, and Transitional Segments 705

Amy L. Kotsenas

The role of the posterior elements in generating axial back and neck pain is well established; the imaging detection of posterior element pain generators remains problematic. Morphologic imaging findings have proved to be nonspecific and are frequently present in asymptomatic patients. Edema, inflammation, and hypervascularity are more specific for sites of pain generation, but are often overlooked by imagers if physiologic imaging techniques such as fat-suppressed T2 or contrast-enhanced T1-weighted magnetic resonance imaging, radionuclide bone scanning with single-photon emission computed tomography (CT), or ^{18}F-fluorodeoxyglucose positron emission tomography combined with CT are not used.

Imaging the Postoperative Spine 731

Rashmi S. Thakkar, John P. Malloy IV, Savyasachi C. Thakkar, John A. Carrino, and A. Jay Khanna

Imaging assessment of the postoperative spine is complex and depends on many factors. Postoperative imaging studies evaluate the position of implants, adequacy of decompression, fusion status, and potential complications. This article provides a review of various imaging techniques, with their advantages and disadvantages, for the evaluation of the postoperative spine. It also gives an overview of normal and abnormal postoperative appearances of the spine as seen via various modalities, with an emphasis on postoperative complications.

Imaging of Spine Neoplasm 749

John T. Wald

Although most often back pain is of benign origin, it can occasionally be a harbinger of a more serious spinal condition, including spine neoplasm. Knowledge of the typical clinical history of spinal tumors and an understanding of the innervation of the spine and surrounding supporting structures may allow us to better understand when to pursue advanced imaging in the evaluation of spinal pain syndromes. Many radiologists have divided the differential diagnosis of neoplasms of the spine into compartments. These compartments include the extradural compartment, intradural/extramedullary compartment, and the intramedullary compartment.

Imaging of Spine Infection 777

Felix E. Diehn

This article reviews the imaging and relevant clinical details of infection of the extradural spine. Spine infections are increasing in incidence and in frequency of diagnosis. They are clinically important despite their relative rarity, because they may be life-threatening, and because early diagnosis leads to improved outcomes. The focus is on pyogenic spondylodiscitis. The also typically pyogenic conditions of epidural and subdural abscess, facet joint infection, and pyomyositis are discussed. Nonpyogenic, granulomatous infections are also addressed. Magnetic resonance imaging is emphasized. The radiologist's role in performing minimally invasive sampling procedures is highlighted.

Imaging of Stress Fractures of the Spine 799

Naveen S. Murthy

Back pain caused by stress fractures, fatigue, or insufficiency, affects varied patient populations based on the level of physical activity and bone mineral density. Stress fractures may involve the vertebral body, pars interarticularis, and the pedicle; often overlooked are stress fractures of the sacrum or bony pelvis, which can mimic pain of spinal origin and delay diagnosis. The choice of optimal imaging (radiographs, nuclear medicine, magnetic resonance imaging, and computed tomography) also depends on the patient population under study and the clinically suspected diagnosis. The diagnosis typically determines which imaging modality is best to follow healing or progression.

Imaging of Dural Arteriovenous Fistula 823

Jonathan M. Morris

Spinal dural arterial venous fistulas (SDAVFs) are the most common vascular malformation of the spine. They typically present in elderly men with slowly progressive

myelopathic symptoms. They often go undiagnosed because of the similar clinical presentation of more common entities in this age group. Radiologists should be familiar with the imaging features of this entity, with the surgical and angiographic interventions, and with the expected postprocedural radiographic appearance. This article reviews spinal vascular anatomy, the radiographic appearances of SDAVF, techniques for finding the SDAVF, clinical presentations, treatment options, and postprocedural radiographic appearances of the spinal cord.

Imaging of the Seronegative Spondyloarthopathies **841**

Kimberly K. Amrami

The seronegative spondyloarthropathies are a diverse group of conditions most commonly affecting the axial spine, often presenting with back pain of an inflammatory nature. The primary unifying feature of these disorders is sacroiliitis. The distinction between subtypes of spondyloarthritis is based on genotype (HLA-B27 positivity as in ankylosing spondylitis), peripheral manifestations of disease (psoriatic and reactive arthritis), and factors such as age, gender, and comorbidity. Although radiography has long been used to diagnose the spondyloarthropathies, advanced imaging with magnetic resonance is better able to diagnose these disorders at their earliest stages and monitor disease-modifying therapies.

Index **855**

GOAL STATEMENT

The goal of the *Radiologic Clinics of North America* is to keep practicing radiologists and radiology residents up to date with current clinical practice in radiology by providing timely articles reviewing the state of the art in patient care.

ACCREDITATION

The *Radiologic Clinics of North America* is planned and implemented in accordance with the Essential Areas and Policies of the Accreditation Council for Continuing Medical Education (ACCME) through the joint sponsorship of the University of Virginia School of Medicine and Elsevier. The University of Virginia School of Medicine is accredited by the ACCME to provide continuing medical education for physicians.

The University of Virginia School of Medicine designates this enduring material activity for a maximum of 15 *AMA PRA Category 1 Credit*(s)™ for each issue, 90 credits per year. Physicians should only claim credit commensurate with the extent of their participation in the activity.

The American Medical Association has determined that physicians not licensed in the US who participate in this CME enduring material activity are eligible for a maximum of 15 *AMA PRA Category 1 Credit*(s)™for each issue, 90 credits per year.

Credit can be earned by reading the text material, taking the CME examination online at http://www.theclinics.com/home/cme, and completing the evaluation. After taking the test, you will be required to review any and all incorrect answers. Following completion of the test and evaluation, your credit will be awarded and you may print your certificate.

FACULTY DISCLOSURE/CONFLICT OF INTEREST

The University of Virginia School of Medicine, as an ACCME accredited provider, endorses and strives to comply with the Accreditation Council for Continuing Medical Education (ACCME) Standards of Commercial Support, Commonwealth of Virginia statutes, University of Virginia policies and procedures, and associated federal and private regulations and guidelines on the need for disclosure and monitoring of proprietary and financial interests that may affect the scientific integrity and balance of content delivered in continuing medical education activities under our auspices.

The University of Virginia School of Medicine requires that all CME activities accredited through this institution be developed independently and be scientifically rigorous, balanced and objective in the presentation/discussion of its content, theories and practices.

All authors/editors participating in an accredited CME activity are expected to disclose to the readers relevant financial relationships with commercial entities occurring within the past 12 months (such as grants or research support, employee, consultant, stock holder, member of speakers bureau, etc.). The University of Virginia School of Medicine will employ appropriate mechanisms to resolve potential conflicts of interest to maintain the standards of fair and balanced education to the reader. Questions about specific strategies can be directed to the Office of Continuing Medical Education, University of Virginia School of Medicine, Charlottesville, Virginia.

The faculty and staff of the University of Virginia Office of Continuing Medical Education have no financial affiliations to disclose.

The authors/editors listed below have identified no financial or professional relationships for themselves or their spouse/partner:

Kimberly K. Amrami, MD; Charles N. Aprill, MD; Nikolai Bogduk, BSc(Med), MB, BS, PhD, MD, DSc, MMed, Dip Anat, FAFMM, FAFRM, FFPM(ANZCA); Sarah Barth, (Acquisitions Editor); Richard A. Deyo, MD, MPH; Felix E. Diehn, MD; Jad G. Khalil, MD; Amy L. Kotsenas, MD; John P. Malloy, IV, DO; Frank H. Miller, MD (Consulting Editor); Jonathan M. Morris, MD; Naveen S. Murthy, MD; Ahmad Nassr, MD; Rashmi S. Thakkar, MD; Savyasachi C. Thakkar, MD; Gaurav K. Thawait, MD; and John T. Wald, MD.

The authors/editors listed below have identified the following financial or professional relationships for themselves or their spouse/partner:

John A. Carrino, MD, MPH receives research funding from Siemens, Toshiba, and Carestream; is a consultant for Quality Medical Metrics, GE, and Vital, and owns stock in Merge.

Avneesh Chhabra, MD is a consultant for Siemens Medical Solutions.

Roger Chou, MD receives research funding from the American Pain Society, and is a consultant for Wellpoint Inc., Blue Cross Blue Shield Association, and Palladian Health.

Filippo Del Grande, MD, MBA, MHEM has an institutional grant from Siemens, and owns stock in General Electric.

Klaus D. Hagspiel, MD (Test Author) is an industry funded research/investigator for Siemens Medical Solutions.

Jeffrey G. Jarvik, MD, MPH is a consultant and is on the Advisory Board for GE Healthcare, owns stock and is a patent holder for PhysioSonics, and is a consultant for HealthHelp.

A. Jay Khanna, MD, MBA receives book royalties from Thieme Medical Publishers, is a consultant for Orthofix, Inc. and the American Academy of Orthopaedic Surgeons, and owns stock in New Era Orthopaedics, Cortical Concepts and Boss Medical.

Timothy P. Maus, MD (Guest Editor) is on the Advisory Board for the International Spine Intervention Society.

Disclosure of Discussion of Non-FDA Approved Uses for Pharmaceutical Products and/or Medical Devices

The University of Virginia School of Medicine, as an ACCME provider, requires that all faculty presenters identify and disclose any off-label uses for pharmaceutical and medical device products. The University of Virginia School of Medicine recommends that each physician fully review all the available data on new products or procedures prior to clinical use.

TO ENROLL

To enroll in the Radiologic Clinics of North America Continuing Medical Education program, call customer service at 1-800-654-2452 or sign up online at http://www.theclinics.com/home/cme. The CME program is available to subscribers for an additional annual fee USD 245.

RADIOLOGIC CLINICS OF NORTH AMERICA

FORTHCOMING ISSUES

September 2012
Imaging of Lung Cancer
Ella Kazerooni, MD, and
Baskaran Sundaram, MD, *Guest Editors*

November 2012
Athletic Injuries of the Upper Extremity
Martin Lazarus, MD, *Guest Editor*

January 2013
PET/CT
Yong Bradley, MD, *Guest Editor*

RECENT ISSUES

May 2012
Pancreatic Imaging
Desiree E. Morgan, MD, and
Koenraad J. Mortele, MD, *Guest Editors*

March 2012
Genitourinary Imaging
Paul Nikolaidis, MD, and
Nancy A. Hammond, MD, *Guest Editors*

January 2012
Emergency Radiology
Jorge A. Soto, MD, *Guest Editor*

RELATED INTERESTS

PET Clinics, Vol. 7, No. 2 (April 2012)
PET Imaging of Infection and Inflammation
Abass Alavi, MD, PhD (Hon), DSc (Hon), and Hongming Zhuang, MD, PhD, *Guest Editors*

PET Clinics, Vol. 7, No. 3 (July 2012)
Clinical Utility of 18F NaF PET/CT in Benign and Malignant Disorders
Mohsen Beheshti, MD, *Guest Editor*

Preface
Spine Imaging

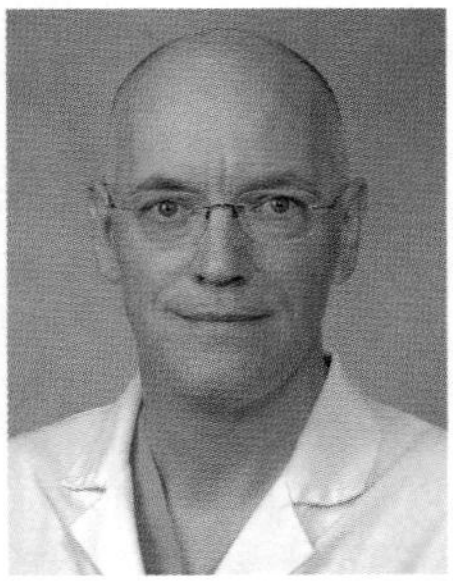

Timothy P. Maus, MD
Guest Editor

Back and limb pain are the second most common reasons for physician office visits in the United States, and health care expenditures to treat these maladies are certainly in excess of $100 billion annually. Imaging is brought to bear in evaluating back and limb pain with ever-increasing frequency. Despite the increasing use of imaging, and the increasing surgical and minimally invasive interventions which flow from that imaging, back pain remains the single greatest cause of work disability in the United States. There is no evidence of improved patient outcomes despite this intensity of care.

This issue attempts to summarize the current literature addressing the appropriate use and interpretation of imaging in the evaluation of the patient with back or limb pain. The lumbar spine receives primary emphasis. Spine imaging has advanced remarkably in recent decades, with the evolution of multi-detector CT, high field strength MRI, SPECT/CT, and PET/CT. What is most important, however, is whether this exquisite depiction of anatomy and pathology can identify the source of pain, assist in the selection of therapies, and ultimately result in improved patient outcomes: diminished pain, functional recovery, and no further need for health care consumption.

The primary goal in imaging the spine or limb pain patient is the identification of systemic disease as the cause of the patient's pain or functional impairment. It is known that this is a rare circumstance; systemic disease is responsible for <5% of the back or limb pain that precipitates a primary care physician visit. In several articles in this issue, my Mayo Radiology colleagues will address the imaging features of spine neoplasm (Dr Wald), infection (Dr Diehn), seronegative spondyloarthropathy (Dr Amrami), stress fractures (Dr Murthy), and dural arteriovenous fistulas (Dr Morris), which may present with pain and neurologic dysfunction.

The vast majority of spine imaging studies will exclude systemic disease as a cause of back or limb pain. Most imaging studies will reveal age-related changes, including alterations in disc signal, height, or contour, facet arthrosis, alteration in ligamentum flavum contour, and compromise of the cross-sectional area of the central canal, lateral recesses, or neural foramina. The evolution of these changes, their frequent presence in asymptomatic subjects, and their lack of association with pain constitute a major specificity fault in all spine imaging; Dr Bogduk will elaborate on this topic. There is also a sensitivity fault in advanced spine imaging: dynamic lesions may only be apparent with weight-bearing and assumption of physiologic spinal alignment. Drs Khalil and Naasr address physiologic imaging.

As a physician considers whether to initiate an imaging evaluation of the spine in a back pain patient, a risk/benefit judgment must occur, as it should for all medical procedures. Certainly there are benefits to be derived from spine imaging, including the rare identification of systemic disease as the cause of the patient's pain. The exclusion of sinister disease should result in reassurance. Spine lesions of a "degenerative" nature (internal disc disruption, disc herniation, central canal stenosis) may be implicated as causal of the patient's pain, and a therapeutic plan based

Radiol Clin N Am 50 (2012) xi–xii
doi:10.1016/j.rcl.2012.04.015
0033-8389/12/$ – see front matter

on that causation may evolve. There are, however, risks associated with imaging: labeling the patient as suffering from a degenerative disease, radiation exposure, enormous individual and societal monetary costs, and the risk of precipitating invasive procedures of uncertain merit. Drs Chou, Deyo, and Jarvik have provided an excellent distillation of current literature addressing these possible harms of imaging, as well as commentary on the most significant question: does the use of imaging improve patient outcomes, and if so, under what circumstances? It is the burden of spine imaging professionals to be cognizant of the documented risks and benefits of imaging and guide its responsible use.

In the younger patient who presents with radicular pain, the most likely imaging correlate will be a disc herniation. Dr Carrino and colleagues discuss spine enumeration, imaging of disc herniations, and the postoperative spine. In the older patient, radicular or neuroclaudicatory pain is most likely due to fixed, stenotic lesions. The pain syndromes of neurogenic intermittent claudication and cervical spondylotic myelopathy, their pathologic underpinning, and imaging expression are considered. In the elaboration of these topics, the emphasis is on the underlying pathophysiology, and the impact of imaging on patient therapy and outcomes, not simply imaging observations.

Axial pain may arise from either the anterior or the posterior columns of the spine. Dr Bogduk describes the pathogenesis of anterior column pain in internal disc disruption; the literature detailing the challenges of the imaging diagnosis of discogenic pain is reviewed. Dr Aprill discusses its diagnosis by provocation discography. The posterior column of the spine also harbors structures causal of axial pain; Dr Kotsenas reviews the literature on zygapophyseal (facet) and sacroiliac joint imaging.

Several themes emerge as we journey through this review of spine imaging. The lack of a pathological-anatomic gold standard confounds attempts to correlate imaging with pain generators; we cannot examine a sample of excised disc or facet cartilage and conclude the joint was painful. Hence it is very difficult to construct studies to validate imaging findings. Purely structural or morphologic deviations from normal are not helpful. Age-related "degenerative" changes are ubiquitous and unrelated to pain syndromes. Imaging findings that suggest the presence of the physiologic phenomena of edema, inflammation, and hypervascularity are more likely to be related to a clinical complaint, although confirmatory studies are often lacking or inadequate. The future of spine imaging is rooted in the biochemistry of inflammation, and the complexities of physiologic motion, not static structural evaluation.

The major specificity fault of spine imaging, the widespread presence of asymptomatic age-related changes, also implies that the imager must know the nature of the patient's pain syndrome to suggest a causal relationship with imaging observations. The overused maxim "the answer is on the film" is not helpful in the spine; rather, the answer will generally emerge from the patient's historical description of the location and character of the index pain. The imager must be privy to this information, by either a robust medical record, an intake document, or an actual interaction with the patient. Only then can the imager filter out the asymptomatic age-related changes and focus on imaging findings likely to be causal of the individual patient's pain or neurologic dysfunction. Treatment decisions must always be directed to the patient, not the images.

The sensitivity fault of spine imaging, the inability of advanced imaging to display the dynamic nature of spine anatomy and pathology in physiologic positions, will surface repeatedly. This is no longer a conceptual challenge, as there is ample literature describing the phenomena; rather, it is an innovation and engineering challenge, as we develop techniques to realize dynamic imaging. It is the responsibility of the imaging community to advocate for such innovation, but also restrain its use until it is validated with sound studies in the peer-reviewed literature. We need technological advancements that demonstrably improve patient outcomes at reasonable cost, not marketing tools.

It is my hope that the subsequent articles are both enjoyable and instructive. My thanks to all my colleagues, who have provided excellent contributions to this effort. I also wish to thank my secretary, Deb Berg, for her assistance and patience, and Ms Sarah Barth at Elsevier, for her effort and support.

Timothy P. Maus, MD
Department of Radiology
Mayo Clinic
200 First Street SW
Rochester, MN 55905, USA

E-mail address:
Maus.Timothy@mayo.edu

Appropriate Use of Lumbar Imaging for Evaluation of Low Back Pain

Roger Chou, MD[a,b,*], Richard A. Deyo, MD, MPH[a,c,d,e,f,g],
Jeffrey G. Jarvik, MD, MPH[h,i,j]

KEYWORDS

• Low back pain • Radiography • MRI • CT

KEY POINTS

- Strong evidence shows that routine back imaging does not improve patient outcomes, exposes patients to unnecessary harms, and increases costs.
- Diagnostic imaging studies should only be performed in patients who have severe or progressive neurologic deficits or with features suggesting a serious or specific underlying condition.
- Advanced imaging with MRI or CT should be reserved for patients with a suspected serious underlying condition or neurologic deficits or who are candidates for invasive interventions.
- To be effective, efforts to reduce imaging overuse should be multifactorial and address clinician behaviors, patient expectations and education, and financial incentives.
- Radiologists can help reduce imaging overuse by accurately reporting and providing consultative expertise regarding the prevalence and potential clinical significance (or insignificance) of imaging findings.

Funding statement: No funding was received for this manuscript.
Disclosures: Roger Chou was the lead author on guidelines developed by the American Pain Society and American College of Physicians on diagnosis and management of low back pain, including recommendations on imaging, and has consulted with Wellpoint Inc, Blue Cross Blue Shield Association, and Palladian Health on implementing low back pain guidelines.
Jeffrey G. Jarvik is a consultant to General Electric Healthcare serving on their Comparative Effectiveness Advisory Board. He also consults with HealthHelp, a radiology benefits management company. He is a cofounder of PhysioSonics, a company that uses high-intensity focused ultrasound for diagnostic purposes, is a stockholder, and receives royalties for intellectual property.
[a] Department of Medicine, Oregon Health & Science University, 3181 Southwest Sam Jackson Park Road, Portland, OR 97239, USA; [b] Department of Medical Informatics and Clinical Epidemiology, Oregon Health & Science University, 3181 Southwest Sam Jackson Park Road, Portland, OR 97239, USA; [c] Department of Family Medicine, Oregon Health & Science University, 3181 Southwest Sam Jackson Park Road, Portland, OR 97234, USA; [d] Department of Public Health, Oregon Health & Science University, 3181 Southwest Sam Jackson Park Road, Portland, OR 97234, USA; [e] Department of Preventive Medicine, Oregon Health & Science University, 3181 Southwest Sam Jackson Park Road, Portland, OR 97234, USA; [f] Center for Research on Occupational and Environmental Toxicology, Oregon Health & Science University, 3181 Southwest Sam Jackson Park Road, Portland, OR 97234, USA; [g] Kaiser Permanente Center for Health Research, 3800 North Interstate Avenue, Portland, OR 97227-1078, USA; [h] Department of Radiology, Harborview Medical Center, University of Washington, 325 Ninth Avenue, Box 359728, Seattle, WA 98104, USA; [i] Department of Neurological Surgery, Harborview Medical Center, University of Washington, 325 Ninth Avenue, Box 359728, Seattle, WA 98104, USA; [j] Department of Health Services, Harborview Medical Center, University of Washington, 325 Ninth Avenue, Box 359728, Seattle, WA 98104, USA
* Corresponding author. Department of Medicine, Oregon Health & Science University, 3181 Southwest Sam Jackson Park Road, Portland, OR 97239.
E-mail address: chour@ohsu.edu

Radiol Clin N Am 50 (2012) 569–585
doi:10.1016/j.rcl.2012.04.005

radiologic.theclinics.com

Low back pain is extremely common, ranking as the second most common symptomatic reason for office visits in the United States.[1,2] About one-third of adults in the United States report back pain during the past 3 months,[1] and nearly three-quarters of adults report at least one episode of low back pain during their lifetime.[3]

Low back pain is also very costly. In 1998, total health care expenditures for individuals with back pain in the United States were estimated at $90 billion,[4] and costs have since risen. The inflation-adjusted increase (in 2005 U.S. dollars) in average total health expenditures for people with back and neck problems was 65% ($4795 per year in 1997 to $6096 per year in 2005).[5] Low back pain also results in high indirect costs from disability, lost time from work, and decreased productivity while at work,[6] and is the most common cause for activity limitations in younger adults. In the United States, 14% of workers lose at least 1 day of work each year because of low back pain.[7]

Lumbar spine imaging (plain radiography, CT, and MRI) is often performed in patients with low back pain. Although clinical practice guidelines recommend imaging only in the presence of progressive neurologic deficits or signs or symptoms suggesting a serious or specific underlying condition (the so-called red flags of low back pain),[8] imaging is often performed in the absence of a clear clinical indication for it.[9] This fact is concerning, because routine imaging does not seem to improve clinical outcomes, exposes patients to unnecessary harms, and contributes to the rising costs associated with low back pain.[10–12]

Eliminating unnecessary tests would help rein in costs associated with low back pain while maintaining high-quality care.[13] Overuse of low back imaging has long been noted as a problem,[14] yet the use of imaging (particularly advanced imaging) continues to increase rapidly.[15] This article reviews costs associated with spinal imaging, current imaging practice patterns and trends, evidence on benefits and harms associated with spinal imaging, factors that promote or are permissive of imaging overuse, and potential strategies for improving imaging practices.

COSTS

Direct Costs

Direct costs of imaging include costs of equipment and facilities, radiologic department staff, professional fees for interpreting the test, and other overhead. Because direct costs are often difficult to measure, reimbursement rates or charges are often used as surrogate measures. Although estimates vary substantially depending on geographic location, insurance status, and other factors, reimbursement rates and charges for lumbar spine CT generally run 5 to 10 times higher than lumbosacral spine plain radiography, and MRI 10 to 15 times higher (**Table 1**). Despite its relatively lower cost, lumbosacral spine radiography is a major contributor to costs because of its frequent use. In 2004, an estimated 66 million lumbar radiographs were performed in the United States.[16]

Downstream Costs

In addition to direct costs, imaging can also lead to downstream cascade effects, referring to the subsequent tests, referrals, and interventions performed as a result of imaging.[17] In some cases, the end result can be an invasive and expensive operation or other procedure of limited or

Table 1
Costs of spine imaging and fusion surgery

Intervention	Cost
Lumbar spine radiography (two or three views)[a]	$54
Lumbar spine CT scan[a]	$344 (without contrast) $426 (with contrast)
Lumbar spine MRI[a]	$645 (without contrast) $794 (with contrast)
Fusion surgery[b]	Without bone morphogenetic proteins: median, $57,393 (interquartile range, $39,660–$83,608) With bone morphogenetic proteins: median, $74,254 (interquartile range, $54,737–$102,663)

[a] Medicare reimbursement for San Francisco area, in 2011 dollars, calculated at http://www.trailblazerhealth.com/Tools/Fee%20Schedule/MedicareFeeSchedule.aspx.
[b] Total charge for hospitalization, excluding professional fees, based on 2006 Nationwide Inpatient Sample data.
Data from Cahill KS, Chi JH, Day A, et al. Prevalence, complications, and hospital charges associated with use of bone-morphogenetic proteins in spinal fusion procedures. JAMA 2009;302(1):58–66.

questionable benefit. In 2006, according to the Nationwide Inpatient Sample, the median total cost for fusion surgery without bone morphogenetic proteins was nearly $60,000, excluding professional fees.[18] Although the increased number of unnecessary operations that occur from unneeded imaging tests is difficult to estimate, data show that rates of spine MRIs increased sharply at the same time as back surgeries.[11,19] Similarly, over about a 10-year period starting in the mid-90s, rates of interventional procedures such as epidural steroid and facet joint injections more than tripled,[20] a pattern that roughly parallels trends in increased use of MRI tests.

Increased use of surgery and interventional procedures would not necessarily be a problem if the procedures resulted in important clinical benefits. However, even though rates of surgery are two to five times higher in the United States than in other developed countries,[21] no evidence shows that patients with low back pain fare better in the United States than in other countries, and randomized trials suggest that surgery and interventional procedures are associated with limited or unclear benefit in patients with nonradicular low back pain.[22–24] In the case of spinal fusion, the widespread use of expensive add-ons, such as instrumentation and bone-morphogenetic proteins, have further increased costs, despite little evidence of improved patient outcomes, and in some cases emerging evidence of harms.[18,25–27] In fact, despite spending more on low back pain and performing more invasive procedures, clinical progress is difficult to discern. In adults with back or neck problems in the United States, self-reported measures of mental health, physical functioning, work or school limitations, and social limitations were all similar or poorer in 2005 compared with 1997.[5] Some data suggest the situation may be getting even worse. In North Carolina, the proportion of adults reporting chronic low back pain that impaired activity more than doubled between 1992 and 2006, from 3.9% to 10.2%.[28]

IMAGING PRACTICES

Practice Variations

Clinicians vary substantially in how frequently they obtain low back pain imaging. One study found that Medicare beneficiaries living in high-use geographic areas in the United States were more than five times more likely to undergo lumbar spine MRI and CT than if they lived in low-use areas.[11] In addition, wide variations in diagnostic testing rates have been observed between, and within, medical specialties.[29–32] One survey found internists almost evenly divided regarding whether they would obtain imaging for uncomplicated low back pain.[30]

Why are practice variations a cause for concern? If they occur in otherwise similar populations and settings, variations may indicate inequalities in resource use or areas in which care is haphazard or arbitrary.[33] In addition, research on regional variations in the United States suggests that high-use areas are generally not associated with better clinical outcomes but contribute significantly to overall health care costs.[34,35] This finding often signifies inefficiencies in medical care, which can be caused by clinical uncertainty or a failure to implement evidence-based practice.

Imaging Rates

A study based on a national database of private insurance claims (covering 8 million beneficiaries) found that more than 40% of patients with acute low back pain underwent imaging.[36] The median time to imaging was the same day as the index diagnosis. Data indicate that imaging rates continue to increase, despite efforts to curb overuse. An Australian study showed that imaging rates for new low back pain problems in patients seen in general practice increased slightly despite the publication of guidelines recommending against routine imaging.[37]

Routine Imaging

In one survey, approximately 40% of family practice and 13% of internal medicine physicians reported ordering routine diagnostic imaging for acute low back pain.[31] Another survey of physicians found that in the absence of any worrisome features, approximately one-quarter would order a lumbosacral spine radiograph for acute low back pain without sciatica, and about two-thirds for low back pain with sciatica.[38] Data on actual imaging practices are consistent with the survey results. One study found that among 35,000 Medicare beneficiaries with acute low back pain and no diagnostic code indicating a serious underlying condition, nearly 30% underwent imaging (lumbar radiography or advanced imaging) within 28 days.[9]

Advanced Imaging

Use of advanced spinal imaging is increasing rapidly. Among Medicare part B beneficiaries, the number of lumbar MRI scans performed increased approximately fourfold between 1994 and 2005 (**Fig. 1**).[15] Similarly, in a large health care organization, the rate of MRIs tripled between 1997 and 2006.[39] In North Carolina, more than one-third of patients with chronic low back pain underwent lumbar spine MRI or CT within the

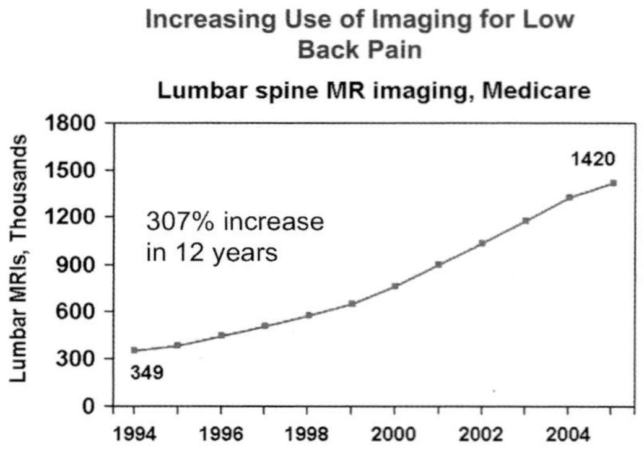

Fig. 1. Number of lumbar spine MRIs among Medicare beneficiaries, from Part B claims. (*From* Deyo RA, Mirza SK, Turner JA, et al. Overtreating Chronic Back Pain: Time to Back Off? J Am Board Fam Med 2009;22:62–8. Reproduced by permission of the American Board of Family Medicine).

past year,[40] and other studies show even higher rates.[41] In the emergency department setting, one recent study found that use of CT or MRI for low back pain tripled from 2002 to 2006 (3.2% vs 9.6%; *P*<.01 for trend).[42] MRIs are often ordered in patients who have not undergone any treatments, despite recommendations for a trial of therapy before imaging in patients without red flags. According to Medicare's Hospital Compare Web site, approximately one-third of Medicare patients with low back pain who underwent an outpatient lumbar spine MRI had not received any prior conservative treatment.[43]

EFFECTIVENESS

The ultimate goal of any diagnostic test is to improve clinical outcomes. Most studies of diagnostic tests estimate how accurately they can identify a disease or condition, or how well the test provides prognostic information. However, even accurate tests do not necessarily result in improved patient outcomes. The ultimate effects of diagnostic testing depend on how clinicians and patients use the test results, the effectiveness of subsequent treatments, and harms related to the diagnostic test and subsequent tests and treatments. Well-conducted randomized trials are at the top of the diagnostic evidence hierarchy because they provide the most direct information about the clinical benefits and harms of alternative testing strategies.[44–46] In the case of low back pain, these studies are particularly important because no adequate reference standard exists to distinguish symptomatic from asymptomatic common degenerative or age-related findings, which would be required to estimate the diagnostic accuracy of the tests for symptomatic low back pain.

Spine imaging is one of the few areas of diagnostic imaging in which multiple randomized trials reporting clinical outcomes are available. A meta-analysis of six randomized trials (n = 1804) of patients with primarily acute or subacute low back pain and no red flags found no differences between routine lumbar imaging (plain radiography, MRI, or CT) and usual care without routine imaging on measures of pain, function, quality of life, or overall patient-rated improvement (**Table 2**).[10] In fact, for short-term pain, function, and quality of life, trends slightly favored usual care without routine imaging. Despite the perception that routine imaging can help alleviate patient anxiety about back pain,[47] routine imaging also was not associated with better psychological outcomes.[10] Patient satisfaction was reported in only a few trials and effects were mixed, with some trials showing no effect and others showing

Table 2
Results from meta-analysis of randomized controlled trials of routine imaging versus usual care without routine imaging

Outcome	Short-Term (<3 mo) SMD	Long-Term (>6 mo to ≤1 y) SMD
Pain	0.19 (−0.01–0.39), three trials	−0.04 (−0.15–0.07), four trials
Function	0.11 (−0.29–0.50), three trials	0.01 (−0.17–0.19), four trials
Quality of life	−0.10 (−0.53–0.34), two trials	−0.15 (−0.33–0.04), three trials
Mental health	0.12 (−0.37–0.62), two trials	0.01 (−0.32–0.34), three trials
Overall improvement	RR, 0.83 (0.65–1.06), four trials	RR, 0.82 (0.64–1.05), one trial

Abbreviations: RR, relative risk; SMD, standardized mean difference.

Data are mean SMD or point estimate for RR (95% CI). A negative SMD favors routine imaging for pain and function, whereas a positive SMD favors routine imaging for quality of life and mental health. For overall improvement, an RR <1 favors routine imaging.

Data from Chou R, Fu R, Carrino JA, et al. Imaging strategies for low-back pain: systematic review and meta-analysis. Lancet 2009;373(9662):463–72.

that routine imaging was associated with higher satisfaction.[10] Three of the trials restricted enrollment to patients older than 50 or 55 years, and most of the trials enrolled at least some patients with radiculopathy. The conclusions of the meta-analysis did not seem affected by whether radiography or advanced imaging (MRI or CT) was evaluated.

COST-EFFECTIVENESS

A prerequisite to evaluating the cost-effectiveness of a clinical service is to understand its clinical effectiveness.[13] In this case, for patients with no red flags, routine imaging is no more effective than usual care without routine imaging. Performing imaging is also more expensive. Services that are more costly than the alternative, yet offer no clear clinical advantages (or do more harm than good), cannot be cost-effective, because they will always be associated with higher (or negative) cost-effectiveness ratios (in this case, the incremental cost of routine imaging compared with no routine imaging divided by the incremental clinical benefit of routine imaging compared with no routine imaging).[13,48]

WHY DOESN'T ROUTINE IMAGING LEAD TO BETTER CLINICAL OUTCOMES?

Favorable Natural History

In most patients with acute back pain, with or without radiculopathy, substantial improvement in pain and function occurs in the first 4 weeks, regardless of whether and how patients are treated.[49,50] Routine imaging is unlikely to improve on this already favorable prognosis. Thus, the natural history of low back pain helps explain why routine imaging does not result in better clinical outcomes.

Low Prevalence of Serious Underlying Conditions

Another reason routine imaging is not beneficial is that the frequency of conditions that require urgent identification (eg, because of the potential for permanent neurologic sequelae with delayed diagnosis) is low. In patients with low back pain in primary care settings, approximately 0.7% have metastatic cancer, 0.01% spinal infection, and 0.04% cauda equina syndrome.[51,52] Although vertebral compression fractures (4%) and inflammatory back disease (<1%) are more common, the diagnostic urgency for these conditions is not as great, because they are not generally associated with progressive or irreversible neurologic impairment.[52,53]

Studies also show that of the small proportion of patients with a serious or specific underlying condition, almost everyone will have an identifiable risk factor. In a retrospective study of 963 patients with acute low back pain, all 8 with tumors or fractures had clinical risk factors.[54] A prospective study found no cases of cancer in 1170 patients younger than 50 years with acute low back pain and no history of cancer, weight loss, other sign of systemic illness, or failure to improve.[55] Similarly, four trials (n = 399) that enrolled patients without risk factors and obtained imaging in all participants or recorded diagnoses through at least 6 months of clinical follow-up found that no serious conditions were missed.[10]

Weak Correlation Between Imaging Findings and Symptoms

Another reason that routine imaging is not beneficial is that most lumbar imaging findings are common in people without low back pain. In fact, these imaging findings are only weakly associated with back symptoms. A systematic review reported odds ratios that ranged from 1.2 to 3.3 for the association between low back pain and disc degeneration on plain radiography, and no association with spondylosis or spondylolisthesis (**Fig. 2**).[56]

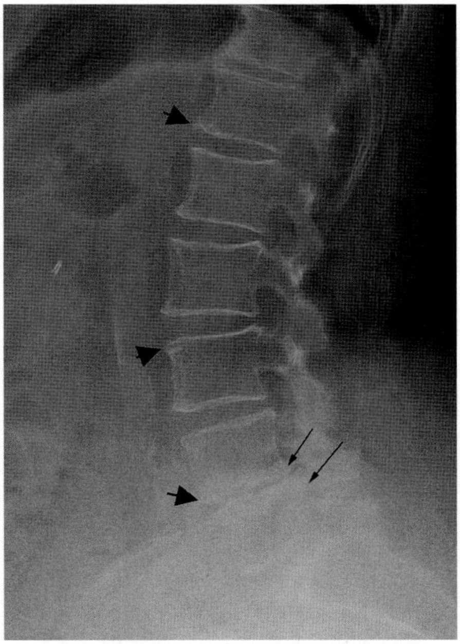

Fig. 2. Lateral radiograph of the lumbar spine shows several common findings: (1) spondylolisthesis: grade 1 (<25%) anterolisthesis of L4 on L5 (*arrows*); (2) marked disc space narrowing at L4/5; (3) sclerosis of inferior end plate of L4 and superior end plate of L5; and (4) multilevel spondylosis deformans (*arrowheads*).

Although advanced imaging provides both increased contrast and spatial resolution compared with plain radiography, resulting in greater anatomic detail, detection of many of the findings seen on advanced imaging usually does not provide additional clinically important information. A systematic review[57] reported odds ratios that ranged from 1.8 to 2.8 for the association between chronic low back pain and disc degeneration on MRI (**Figs. 3–5**), similar to the risk estimates observed in studies of plain radiography. Consistent with these findings, a randomized trial failed to show any incremental value of rapid MRI over radiography for evaluating low back pain in patients referred for imaging by their primary care physician.[58]

In fact, most of the findings on advanced imaging are so common in asymptomatic adults that they could be viewed as normal signs of aging. In one cross-sectional study of asymptomatic persons aged 60 years or older, 36% had a herniated disc, 21% had spinal stenosis, and more than 90% had a degenerated or bulging disc.[59] Other studies have reported similar results.[60–62] Recently published studies indicate that imaging findings frequently precede symptoms, and changes on imaging do not correlate well with the clinical course. One of the few prospective studies found that among patients with documented lumbar imaging findings before the onset of low back pain, 84% had unchanged or even improved findings after symptoms developed.[63] Another prospective study found that presence of disc protrusion on baseline MRI was a negative predictor of subsequent back pain (hazard ratio [HR], 0.5; 95% CI, 0.3–0.9) and presence of disc extrusion was not predictive (HR, 1.2; 95% CI, 0.4–3.4).[64] Although nerve root contact and central stenosis were associated with trends

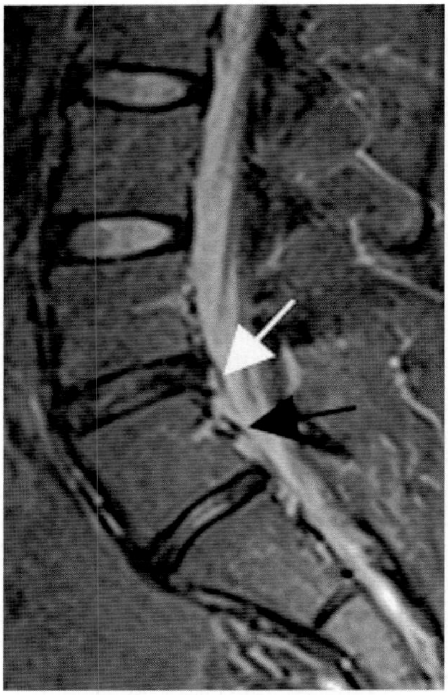

Fig. 4. Sagittal T2-weighted MR image of the lumbar spine. White arrow points to an annular fissure at L4/5. Black arrow points to a sequestered disc fragment behind the L5 vertebral body.

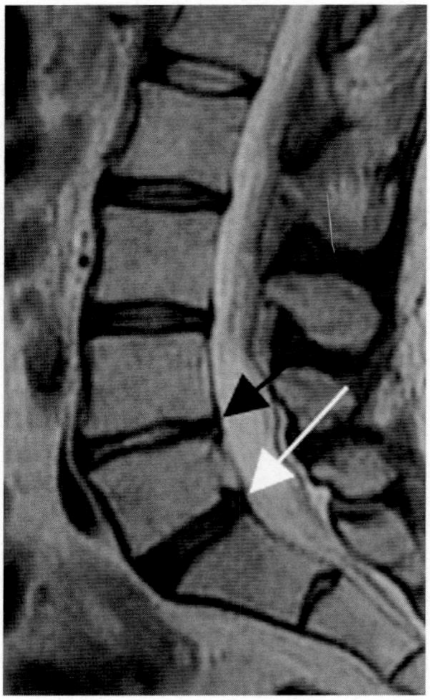

Fig. 3. Sagittal T2-weighted MR image of the lumbar spine. Black arrow at L4/5 shows disc height loss and a mild bulge. White arrow points to the L5/S1 disc, which has low signal, indicating desiccation.

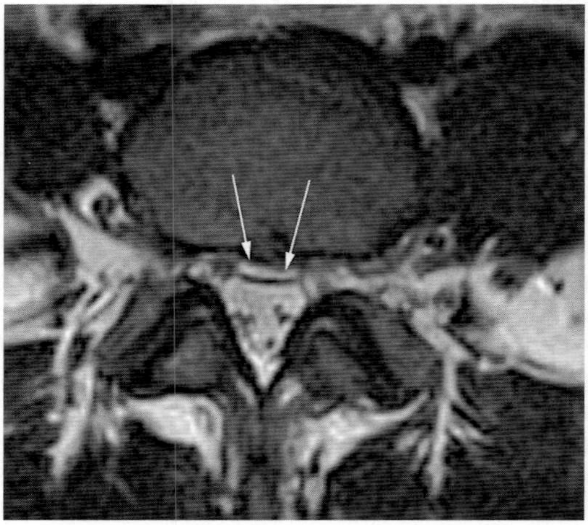

Fig. 5. Axial T2-weighted MR image of the lumbar spine. Arrows point to an annular fissure associated with a focal disc protrusion.

toward increased risk of future back pain (HR, 2.2; 95% CI, 0.6–8.0 and HR, 1.9; 95% CI, 0.8–4.8, respectively), the associations were not statistically significant. In fact, the only statistically significant predictor was not an imaging finding, but rather presence of depression (HR, 2.3; 95% CI, 1.2–4.4).

Minimal Impact on Clinical Decision Making

Back imaging also may not affect patient outcomes because results typically have no important impact on clinical decision making. Imaging studies rarely reveal unexpected findings. One review of 68,000 lumbar radiographic examinations in persons 20 to 50 years of age with low back pain estimated clinically unsuspected findings in 1 out of approximately every 2500 patients.[65] In two studies of patients who underwent lumbar radiography (sample size approximately 100 in each), imaging affected the management plan in only 1 or 2 patients each.[66,67] Similarly, a randomized trial found no differences between patients who underwent routine advanced imaging and those who did not undergo imaging in diagnosis and treatment plans.[68] The limited therapeutic impact of routine imaging could be because the clinical significance of most imaging findings, and therefore what to do about them, is largely unknown. In fact, no evidence shows that selecting therapies based on the presence of the most common imaging findings (eg, presence of degenerative discs, facet joint arthritis, or bulging discs without nerve root compression) improves outcomes compared with a more generalized approach.[8] Imaging findings are also a poor predictor of prognosis or response to treatment. One study found no association between the presence of common degenerative changes on MRI and outcomes after therapy.[69]

HARMS

Direct Harms

Radiation exposure

Lumbar plain radiography and CT contributes to an individual's cumulative low-level radiation exposure, which could promote carcinogenesis (**Table 3**). Lumbar spine CT is associated with an average effective radiation dose of 6 millisieverts (mSv).[70] Based on the 2.2 million lumbar CT scans performed in the United States in 2007, one study projected 1200 additional future cancers.[71] Another study estimated that cancer would be expected to occur as a result of radiation exposure in approximately 1 of every 270 women aged 40 years who underwent coronary angiography,[39] a procedure associated with a similar average effective radiation dose compared with lumbar spine CT.[70] In a 20-year-old woman, the estimated risk was about twice as high. Lumbar CT may also involve use of iodinated contrast, which is associated with nephropathy and hypersensitivity reactions.

Table 3
Average effective radiation doses

Imaging Procedure	Average Radiation Dose (millisieverts)
Chest radiograph (posterior-anterior view)	0.02
Lumbar spine plain radiography	1.5
Lumbar spine CT	6
Diagnostic cardiac catheterization	7

Data from Fazel R, Krumholz HM, Wang Y, et al. Exposure to low-dose ionizing radiation from medical imaging procedures. N Engl J Med 2009;361:849–57.

Because lumbar plain radiography is performed much more frequently than lumbar CT, it accounts for a greater proportion of the total radiation dose from medical imaging procedures in the United States (3.3% vs 0.7% for lumbar CT), despite a lower average effective radiation dose (1.5 mSv).[70] The average radiation exposure from lumbar radiography is 75 times higher than from chest radiography.[70] This fact is of particular concern for women of child-bearing age, because of the proximity of lumbar radiography to the gonads, which are difficult to effectively shield. According to some estimates, the amount of female gonadal irradiation from lumbar radiography is equivalent to the exposure from a daily chest radiograph for several years.[52]

Labeling

Spine imaging could result in unintended harms from labeling effects, which occur when patients are told that they have a condition of which they were not previously aware.[72] A classic example of labeling was a study of blood pressure screening in steel workers in Canada, which found increased rates of absenteeism 1 year later in persons diagnosed with hypertension, particularly in persons previously unaware of their diagnosis.[73] The authors concluded that labeling causes patients to adopt a "sick role" and treat themselves as more fragile. Similar effects may occur in patients who learn that they have findings, often described as abnormalities, on lumbar imaging. In one acute low back pain trial that performed lumbar spine MRI in all patients, those randomized to routinely receive their results reported smaller improvements in self-rated general health than those who were blinded to the results.[74] In another trial, patients with subacute or chronic back pain who underwent routine radiography reported more pain and worse overall health status after 3 months and were more likely to seek follow-up care than those who did not undergo radiography.[75] Knowledge of clinically irrelevant imaging findings might hinder recovery by causing patients to worry more, focus excessively on minor back symptoms, or avoid exercise and other recommended activities because of fears that they could cause more structural damage, a pattern of maladaptive coping referred to as *fear avoidance*.[76] These behaviors are associated with the development of chronic low back pain,[77] can be difficult to change, and may be insidious, affecting patients even when they are not consciously aware of them. These potential harms emphasize the need for imaging professionals to choose descriptive language with care, and to recognize their obligation to educate referring physicians and patients regarding the insignificance of age-related imaging findings.

Downstream Harms

Association between imaging and surgery

Despite all of the uncertainties related to the interpretation of imaging tests, patients and clinicians frequently view findings on imaging as targets for surgery or other procedures.[78] In fact, the association between rates of advanced spine imaging and rates of spine surgery is strong.[19] One study showed that variation in rates of spine MRI use accounted for 22% of the variability in overall spine surgery rates in Medicare beneficiaries, or more than double the variability accounted for by differences in patient characteristics.[11] In one study, patients randomized to rapid MRI had twice the number of lumbar operations as those receiving plain radiographs, although small numbers made the difference only marginally statistically significant.[58] Another study found that for work-related acute low back pain, MRI within the first month was associated with a more than eightfold increase in risk for surgery and more than a fivefold increase in subsequent total medical costs compared with propensity-matched controls who did not undergo early MRI.[12]

WHY ISN'T CURRENT PRACTICE CONSISTENT WITH THE EVIDENCE?

Patient Expectations

One reason that current practice is not consistent with the evidence is patient expectations.[79] Patients want a specific diagnosis to explain their symptoms. In addition, patients may equate a decision to not obtain imaging or provide a precise diagnosis with low-quality or suboptimal care, or interpret the decision to not perform imaging as implying that their pain is not legitimate or important.[78] In patients with chronic back pain, the desire for diagnostic tests is a frequent reason for repeat office visits.[80]

Patient preferences about diagnostic testing seem to be communicated to physicians, who frequently accede to patient desires or requests for imaging.[47] In one study, an increased likelihood of obtaining low back pain imaging was strongly associated with how intensely patients believed imaging was necessary.[81] A survey of physicians in the United States showed that over one-third would order a lumbar MRI for uncomplicated acute low back pain if a patient insisted on it, even after explaining that it was unnecessary.[82]

Imaging decisions may themselves affect patient expectations, because those who undergo imaging for one episode of low back pain may come to expect it for future episodes. One trial showed that patients randomized to routine imaging became more likely to believe it was necessary compared with those randomized to an educational intervention without routine imaging, despite no beneficial effects on clinical outcomes.[83]

Financial Incentives

Financial incentives can influence imaging decisions. For example, performance incentives may be linked to markers of patient satisfaction. At the same time, performing more imaging tends to be associated with higher patient satisfaction. Randomized trials show that patients express more satisfaction with their care when they undergo routine lumbar imaging compared with no routine imaging,[75] and when they undergo advanced imaging instead of radiography,[58] even when their clinical outcomes are no better. A study of Medicare beneficiaries found earlier use of imaging and more advanced imaging when clinician incentives were based on patient satisfaction.[9] Therefore, financial incentives based on patient satisfaction can encourage overuse of imaging.

From a health systems perspective, financial incentives may exist for using imaging units. A top-of-the-line MRI unit can cost $2 million or more to purchase, and approximately $800,000 a year to operate.[84,85] At the same time, advanced imaging offers a high profit margin. Relative to actual costs, Medicare provides far greater reimbursement for MRI (reimbursement-to-cost ratio, 2.3) than for conventional radiography (reimbursement-to-cost ratio, 0.9).[86]

Research shows that greater availability of imaging units seems to correlate with increased use. The number of MRI scanners in the United States more than tripled from 2000 to 2005, from 7.6 to 26.6 per million people.[84] In 2006, about 7000 sites in the United States offered MRI studies,[87] which translates into a number of MRIs per capita almost twice as high as in any other industrialized country, and more than four times as high as in Canada or the United Kingdom.[87] In 2006, estimates showed that almost as many MRI machines were available in western Pennsylvania (N = 140) as in all of Canada (N = 151).[85] One study found that each new MRI unit added within a geographic area was associated with approximately 40 additional lumbar MRIs over a 5-year period.[84]

Imaging self-referral, or acquisition of imaging equipment and billing for imaging tests by non-radiologist physicians, is also associated with increased imaging use. A 2009 report from the Medicare Payment Advisory Commission found physician ownership or investment in imaging facilities associated with higher use rates after adjustment for potential confounders.[88] A study of Medicare claims found that acquisition of MRI equipment by primary care physicians increased MRI use rates from 11% to 17% (P<.001) in the following 180 days.[84] In orthopedic surgery practices, the MRI rates increased from 22% to 27% (P<.001). An earlier study of workman's compensation cases found more inappropriate imaging requests when physicians self-referred.[89]

Defensive Medicine

Overuse of back imaging could also be related to perceived liability risks of missing a serious diagnosis. "Defensive medicine" refers to the alteration of clinical behavior because of concerns over malpractice liability. Inappropriate imaging seems to be a very common form of defensive medicine. In one study, more than 90% of physicians from six specialties in Pennsylvania reported defensive medicine practices.[90] Almost half of those with positive responses reported use of imaging in clinically unnecessary circumstances as their most recent defensive act. Defensive medicine practices are probably more likely when there is a higher likelihood (or a perceived higher likelihood) of a legal claim related to the back pain, or when patients express dissatisfaction. Low back pain imaging is often a routine part of the evaluation in workman's compensation and disability cases, despite the absence of evidence that it improves outcomes in these settings.

Time

Another reason that back imaging is overused may be that clinicians are frequently overworked and pressed for time, and ordering an imaging test seems more expedient than explaining why imaging is not necessary.[47,91] In patients who have strong notions about the need for back imaging, the perceived (or real) time savings may be particularly high.

RECOMMENDATIONS ON IMAGING USE

When to Image

Routine imaging in low-risk patients does not improve patient outcomes but increases costs and exposes patient to harms, including unnecessary radiation exposure and invasive treatments, and the deleterious effect of likely labeling that person as a patient with a degenerative spinal disorder. Several professional societies have issued practice guidelines and standards to help address overuse of low back imaging. In 2007, the American College of Physicians (ACP) and the American Pain Society (APS) published a joint clinical practice guideline on diagnosis and treatment of low back pain.[8] The key recommendations regarding diagnostic imaging were:

- Do not routinely obtain imaging or other diagnostic tests in patients with nonspecific low-back pain
- Perform diagnostic imaging and testing when severe or progressive neurologic deficits are present or when serious underlying conditions are suspected
- Evaluate patients with persistent low back pain and signs or symptoms of radiculopathy or spinal stenosis who are candidates for surgery or epidural steroid injection.

In 2009, the American College of Radiology published consensus-based criteria on appropriateness of imaging for various low back pain scenarios that were largely consistent with the ACP/APS guidelines.[92] For uncomplicated low back pain with or without radiculopathy, imaging was deemed inappropriate in the absence of the following red flags:

- Recent significant trauma or milder trauma at age older than 50 years
- Unexplained weight loss
- Unexplained fever
- Immunosuppression
- History of cancer
- Intravenous drug use
- Prolonged use of corticosteroids or osteoporosis

- Age older than 70 years
- Focal neurologic deficit with progressive or disabling symptoms
- Duration longer than 6 weeks.

Subsequently, the ACP published more detailed guidance on use of lumbar imaging (**Table 4**).[93] All of the guidelines are consistent in recommending immediate imaging in patients with signs, symptoms, or risk factors for cauda equina syndrome or vertebral infection. Although these conditions are rare, the prevalence of suggestive findings or risk factors for them is low,[94] and timely diagnosis and treatment may prevent serious sequelae related to compression of the spinal cord (which typically ends at the L1 or L2 level) or cauda equina. Clinical findings for cauda equina syndrome or vertebral infection include new

Table 4
Suggestions for imaging in patients with acute low back pain

Imaging Action	Suggestions for Initial Imaging
Immediate imaging	
Radiography (with erythrocyte sedimentation rate)	Major risk factors for cancer (new onset of low back pain with history of cancer, multiple risk factors for cancer, or strong clinical suspicion for cancer)
MRI	Risk factors for spinal infection (new onset of low back pain with fever and history of intravenous drug use or recent infection) Risk factors for or signs of cauda equina syndrome (new urinary retention, fecal incontinence, or saddle anesthesia) Severe neurologic deficits (progressive motor weakness or motor deficits at multiple neurologic levels)
Defer imaging after a trial of therapy	
Radiography (with or without erythrocyte sedimentation rate)	Weaker risk factors for cancer (unexplained weight loss or age >50 y)
Radiography	Risk factors for or signs of ankylosing spondylitis (morning stiffness that improves with exercise, alternating buttock pain, awakening because of back pain during the second part of the night, or younger age [20–40 y]) Risk factors for vertebral compression fracture (history of osteoporosis, use of corticosteroids, significant trauma, or older age [>75 y for men or >65 y for women])
MRI	Signs and symptoms of radiculopathy (back pain with leg pain in an L4, L5, or S1 nerve root distribution or positive result on straight leg raise or crossed straight leg raise test) in patients who are candidates for surgery or epidural steroid injection Risk factors for or symptoms of spinal stenosis (radiating leg pain, older age, or pseudoclaudication) in patients who are candidates for surgery
No imaging	No criteria for immediate imaging and back pain improved or resolved after a 1-month trial of therapy Previous spinal imaging with no change in clinical status

Reproduced from Chou R, Qaseem A, Owens DK, et al. Diagnostic imaging for low back pain: advice for high-value health care from the American College of Physicians. Ann Intern Med 2011;154:181–9; with permission.

urinary retention, saddle anesthesia, fecal incontinence, or fever (especially in patients with risk factors for bacteremia). Urinary retention is the most common finding for cauda equina syndrome. Without urinary retention, the likelihood of cauda equina syndrome is on the order of 1 in 10,000.[51] Imaging is also recommended for patients with severe or progressive neurologic deficits, defined as objective motor weakness at a single level, or deficits at multiple spinal levels.

In patients with findings or risk factors for other specific conditions, such as cancer (age >50 years, failure to improve after 1 month, weight loss), vertebral compression fracture (older age, history of or risk factors for osteoporosis, significant trauma), ankylosing spondylitis (morning stiffness, improvement with exercise, younger age, chronic symptoms), herniated disc (radiculopathy, positive straight leg raise), or symptomatic spinal stenosis (older age, leg pain, pseudoclaudication), optimal diagnostic strategies are less clear. The traditional recommendation has been to act on all risk factors by obtaining imaging. However, the low frequency of these conditions and the low specificity of most risk factors would result in high imaging rates with low positive predictive values.[54,95] For example, one study of 1172 consecutive patients with acute back pain presenting to primary care found that approximately one-quarter were older than 55 years, approximately one-quarter had morning back stiffness, and approximately one-third had pain that improved with exercise.[95] All of these are considered risk factors for cancer or inflammatory back pain, but no cases of cancer and only two inflammatory conditions were identified in this cohort.

A more efficient strategy proposed by the ACP is to perform imaging based on the estimated prevalence of the condition before risk factor assessment (the pretest probability) and how strongly the risk factors predict the condition (**Table 5**).[93] For instance, the prevalence of cancer in a primary care population is approximately 0.7%.[55] A previous history of cancer (not including nonmelanoma skin cancer) is the strongest risk factor for spinal tumor (positive likelihood ratio, 15).[55] Unexplained weight loss, failure to improve after 1 month, and age older than 50 years are weaker risk factors (positive likelihood ratio, 2.7–3.0). Based on these likelihood ratios, the probability of cancer if a history of prior cancer is present would increase to approximately 9%, or high

Table 5
Using likelihood ratios to update estimated probabilities of spinal tumor in patients with low back pain

Step	Example: 57-Year-Old Man Presents to Primary Care Clinic with 3 Days of Acute Low Back Pain
1. Estimate the pretest probability of persistent low back pain (the probability before assessing for risk factors)	A study of patients seen in a primary care clinic estimated an overall prevalence of low back pain of 0.7%[55]
2. Convert the pretest probability to pretest odds	Pretest probability for cancer = 0.7% or 7/1000; pretest odds = 7/(1000−7)[a] = 7/993
3. Determine which risk factors for cancer are present, and the associated likelihood ratio	Example A: assume that the patient has a personal history of prostate cancer; the likelihood ratio for spinal tumor in persons with such a history is 15[55] Example B: assume that the patient has a no risk factors for cancer other than age >50 y; the likelihood ratio for spinal tumor in patients aged >50 years is 2.7[55]
4. Multiple the pretest odds by the likelihood ratio to determine the posttest odds	Example A: posttest odds for spinal tumor = 7/993 × 15 or 105/993 Example B: posttest odds for spinal tumor = 7/993 × 2.7 or 19/993
5. Convert the posttest odds to posttest probability	Example A: posttest probability for spinal tumor = 105/(105 + 993)[b] = 105/1098 = 9.6% Example B: Posttest probability for spinal tumor = 19/(19+993) = 19/1012 = 1.9%

[a] Converting probability to odds: probability x/y = odds x/(y − x).
[b] Converting odds to probability: odds x/y = probability x/(x + y).

enough to warrant immediate imaging (a strong clinical suspicion for cancer would give a similar result).[94] In patients with any one of the other three risk factors, the posttest probability only increases marginally, to 1% to 2%.[55] Deferring imaging would be reasonable in most cases, unless symptoms fail to improve after several weeks.[54,96] For patients without signs of neurologic compromise but with minor risk factors for vertebral compression fracture, ankylosing spondylitis, herniated disc, or spinal stenosis, a trial of therapy before imaging is also warranted according to the ACP criteria, because delaying imaging in these circumstances is unlikely to result in missed therapeutic opportunities. For herniated disc or spinal stenosis, none of the trials showing benefits of surgery have enrolled patients with fewer than 6 to 12 weeks of symptoms, and no serious neurologic complications were seen among patients not randomized to immediate surgery.[97–100]

Diagnostic rules based on the evaluation of multiple risk factors could help better inform imaging decisions but require further development. For vertebral compression fracture, one study evaluated a diagnostic rule based on four risk factors (female sex, age >70 years, significant trauma, or prolonged use of corticosteroids).[94] It found a likelihood ratio of 1.8 (95% CI, 1.1–2.0) if one of four risk factors was present, and 15 (95% CI, 7.2–25) if two or more were present. However, these rules require more external validation before they can be recommended for general use.

Choice of Imaging Procedure

The ACR appropriateness criteria recommend lumbar plain radiography for the initial evaluation of low back pain in patients with recent trauma or history of osteoporosis, and in persons aged 70 years or older,[92] which is consistent with ACP recommendations[93] on imaging. Both societies recommend lumbar spine and pelvis plain radiography for evaluation of suspected ankylosing spondylitis.[92,93] Both also recommend that advanced imaging be reserved for situations in which findings are more likely to influence clinical decision making, as in patients with major trauma or severe neurologic compromise (objective or progressive motor weakness, deficits at multiple levels, or suspected cauda equina syndrome) and in those with risk factors for vertebral infection.[93] When cancer is not strongly suspected and in the absence of neurologic signs, obtaining initial imaging with lumbar radiography plus an erythrocyte sedimentation rate is a reasonable approach,[96] although advanced imaging may be appropriate when high clinical suspicion persists despite initial negative tests. For persistent radicular symptoms or spinal stenosis without severe neurologic compromise, advanced imaging should be performed after at least a 1-month trial of therapy if patients are interested in and candidates for surgery or an epidural steroid injection.[8]

Repeat Imaging

Repeat back imaging is common. In one study of patients with low back pain in North Carolina who had received an MRI or CT of the back, more than half reported a second advanced imaging test within the previous year.[40] Although evidence on the effects of repeat imaging on patient outcomes is not available, prospective studies of repeat imaging indicate that new MRI findings are uncommon.[60,63] Rather, typical findings are progression of already identified degenerative changes and, in some cases, improvement and regression over time. Therefore, periodically performing repeat imaging on a routine basis is extremely unlikely to be an effective or informative approach. Rather, repeat imaging should only be performed for new or changed clinical features, such as acute or progressive neurologic symptoms or recent trauma.

Patient Education

Patient expectations regarding back imaging are frequently discordant with the evidence.[79] However, most patients do not want tests that are unnecessary, costly, or potentially harmful. The ACP guidelines recommend education to help bring patient expectations more in line with the evidence.[93] Explaining that risk factor assessment is sensitive for identifying worrisome conditions such as cancer or infection, acute low back pain is highly likely to improve in the first 4 weeks, and imaging can be performed later if symptoms fail to improve may help reassure some patients that they have been appropriately assessed and that the problem is not being simply dismissed. In fact, effective education may be less burdensome than often assumed. One randomized trial found that a brief educational intervention regarding back imaging took less than 5 minutes and resulted in similar patient satisfaction with overall care (and similar clinical outcomes) compared with routinely performing lumbar spine plain radiography.[83] Supplementing face-to-face information with patient handouts, self-care education books,[101] online materials,[93] or other methods could be an efficient strategy to reinforce or expand on key educational points.

Effecting Change

Changing clinician behaviors is challenging. In general, research suggests that active and individualized methods are more effective for changing clinician behaviors than passive ones, such as simply providing guidelines.[102] Similarly, a systematic review of interventions for increasing appropriate low back pain imaging found varying effects from distribution of educational materials.[103] Prior authorization requirements for advanced spine imaging have been imposed by many health insurers and are more effective at reducing inappropriate imaging than more passive approaches, but are often viewed as onerous by physicians.[87] As a potentially more acceptable alternative, one randomized trial found that an intervention consisting of an educational session by local clinical leaders followed by clinician audit and feedback was more effective than no intervention for reducing inappropriate lumbar imaging.[104] Another promising method is computer-based decision support that provides information at the time of ordering, such as whether the patient has undergone a recent imaging study, and compares ordering patterns to those of peers.[87] Radiologists could play an important role in making decision support effective through providing mandatory consultation when provider requests for imaging are inconsistent with guidelines.[105] One retrospective study showed that one-quarter of imaging requests for MRI or CT were inappropriate and could have potentially been avoided with decision support, including radiology consultation.[106] A prerequisite, of course, is that radiologists must be familiar with and able to discuss guideline recommendations with referring physicians.

The most effective interventions for reducing inappropriate imaging may be multifactorial. One study found that implementing an intervention that included a requirement for providers to identify an approved lumbar imaging indication before ordering an advanced imaging study, institutional education programs on appropriate imaging, periodic audits and feedback for providers who ordered imaging tests inconsistent with the criteria, and availability of same- or next-day physical therapy and consultation for patients in whom imaging was not indicated reduced the rate of lumbar MRI for low back pain by 23% (relative risk, 0.77; 95% CI, 0.67–0.87).[107]

When imaging tests are performed, radiologists play an important role in how findings are communicated. For example, describing uncomplicated degenerative findings as common or incidental age-related phenomena rather than as abnormalities could potentially reduce labeling effects and unnecessary downstream testing and treatments.[108] Conversely, the liberal application of terms such as *herniation* to small or trivial intervertebral disc findings that are unlikely to be clinically relevant may imply a diagnosis that supports surgical interventions.[108] One study found inclusion of an epidemiologic statement in lumbar imaging reports describing the prevalence of common findings on lumbar spine MRI in asymptomatic adults was associated with a trend toward decreased likelihood of repeat imaging (odds ratio [OR], 0.21; 95% CI, 0.03–1.7) and decreased the likelihood of opioid prescription use (OR, 0.29; 95% CI, 0.11–0.77), although no difference was seen in the rate of surgical consultations or surgeries.[109] Studies show that primary care clinicians prefer a more active role from radiologists in interpreting imaging findings, such as radiology reports that include management recommendations, such as suggestions for potential treatments and referrals.[110,111] Additional research is needed to understand effective methods for accurately describing imaging findings, their potential clinical significance, and appropriate management options.

Efforts to decrease inappropriate imaging must also address financial incentives that influence overuse. For example, clinician incentive programs that are based on patient satisfaction may have a tendency to reward unnecessary testing and therefore be counterproductive.[9] Rather, financial incentives should be based on how well clinicians adhere to guidelines. Other efforts to curb overuse include payment reductions by Medicare to limit rewards for imaging self-referral, and federal legislation mandating disclosure of physician ownership interests.[87,88,112,113]

SUMMARY

Strong evidence shows that routine back imaging does not improve patient outcomes, exposes patients to unnecessary harms, and increases costs. However, imaging practices remain inconsistent with evidence-based guidelines and use continues to rise. Diagnostic imaging studies should only be performed in selected higher-risk patients who have severe or progressive neurologic deficits or are suspected of having a serious or specific underlying condition, and advanced imaging with MRI or CT should be reserved for patients with a suspected serious underlying condition or neurologic deficits, or who are candidates for invasive interventions. To be most effective, efforts to reign in imaging should be multifactorial and address clinician behaviors,

patient expectations and education, and financial incentives. Radiologists can play a critical role in these efforts through providing consultative expertise in decision support programs related to appropriateness of imaging requests, and accurately reporting the prevalence and potential clinical significance (or insignificance) of imaging findings.

REFERENCES

1. Deyo RA, Mirza SK, Martin BI. Back pain prevalence and visit rates. Spine 2006;31:2724–7.
2. Hart LG, Deyo RA, Cherkin DC. Physician office visits for low back pain: Frequency, clinical evaluation, and treatment patterns from a U.S. national survey. Spine 1995;20:11–9.
3. Koes BW, van Tulder MW, Thomas S. Diagnosis and treatment of low back pain. BMJ 2006; 332(7555):1430–4.
4. Luo X, Pietrobon R, Sun SX, et al. Estimates and patterns of direct health care expenditures among individuals with back pain in the United States. Spine 2004;29(1):79–86.
5. Martin BI, Deyo RA, Mirza SK, et al. Expenditures and health status among adults with back and neck problems. JAMA 2008;299:656–64.
6. Stewart WF, Ricci JA, Chee E, et al. Lost productive time and cost due to common pain conditions in the US workforce. JAMA 2003;290:2443–54.
7. Loeser JD, Volinn E. Epidemiology of low back pain. Neurosurg Clin N Am 1991;2:713–25.
8. Chou R, Qaseem A, Snow V, et al. Diagnosis and treatment of low back pain: a joint clinical practice guideline from the American College of Physicians and the American Pain Society. Ann Intern Med 2007;147:478–91.
9. Pham HH, Landon BE, Reschovsky JD, et al. Rapidity and modality of imaging for acute low back pain in elderly patients. Arch Intern Med 2009;169:972–81.
10. Chou R, Fu R, Carrino JA, et al. Imaging strategies for low-back pain: systematic review and meta-analysis. Lancet 2009;373(9662):463–72.
11. Lurie JD, Birkmeyer NJ, Weinstein JN. Rates of advanced spinal imaging and spine surgery. Spine 2003;28(6):616–20.
12. Webster BS, Cifuentes M. Relationship of early magnetic resonance imaging for work-related acute low back pain with disability and medical utilization outcomes. J Occup Environ Med 2010; 52:900–7.
13. Owens DK, Qaseem A, Snow V, et al. High-value, cost conscious care: concepts for clinicians to evaluate benefits, harms, and costs of medical interventions. Ann Intern Med 2010;154: 174–80.
14. Hall FM. Overutilization of radiological examinations. Radiology 1976;120:443–8.
15. Deyo RA, Mirza SK, Turner JA, et al. Overtreating chronic back pain: time to back off? J Am Board Fam Med 2009;22:62–8.
16. Spelic DC, Kaczmarek RV, Hilohi MC, et al. Nationwide surveys of chest, abdomen, lumbosacral spine radiography, and upper gastrointestinal fluoroscopy: a summary of findings. Health Phys 2010;98:498–514.
17. Deyo RA. Cascade effects of medical technology. Annu Rev Public Health 2002;23:23–44.
18. Cahill KS, Chi JH, Day A, et al. Prevalence, complications, and hospital charges associated with use of bone-morphogenetic proteins in spinal fusion procedures. JAMA 2009;302(1):58–66.
19. Verrilli D, Welch HG. The impact of diagnostic testing on therapeutic interventions. JAMA 1996; 275:1189–91.
20. Friedly J, Chan L, Deyo R. Increases in lumbosacral injections in the Medicare population. Spine 2007;32:1754–60.
21. Cherkin DC, Deyo RA, Loeser JD, et al. An international comparison of back surgery rates. Spine 1994;19:1201–6.
22. Brox JI, Sorensen R, Friis A, et al. Randomized clinical trial of lumbar instrumented fusion and cognitive intervention and exercises in patients with chronic low back pain and disc degeneration. Spine 2003;28(17):1913–21.
23. Fairbank J, Frost H, Wilson-MacDonald J, et al. Randomised controlled trial to compare surgical stabilisation of the lumbar spine with an intensive rehabilitation programme for patients with chronic low back pain: the MRC spine stabilisation trial. BMJ 2005;330(7502):1233.
24. Fritzell P, Hagg O, Wessberg P, et al. 2001 Volvo award winner in clinical studies: Lumbar fusion versus nonsurgical treatment for chronic low back pain: a multicenter randomized controlled trial from the Swedish Lumbar Spine Study Group. Spine 2001;26(23):2521–32.
25. Carragee EJ, Hurwitz EL, Weiner BK. A critical review of recombinant human bone morphogenetic protein-2 trials in spinal surgery: emerging safety concerns and lessons learned. Spine J 2011; 116(6):471–91.
26. Gibson J, Waddell G. Surgery for degenerative lumbar spondylosis: updated Cochrane review. Spine 2005;30(20):2312–20.
27. Maghout-Juratli S, Franklin GM, Mirza SK, et al. Lumbar fusion outcomes in Washington state workers' compensation. Spine 2006;31(23):2715–23.
28. Freburger JK, Holmes GM, Agans RP, et al. The rising prevalence of chronic low back pain. Arch Intern Med 2009;169:251–8.
29. Carey TS, Garrett J. Patterns of ordering diagnostic tests for patients with acute low back pain. The

North Carolina Back Pain Project. Ann Intern Med 1996;125:807–14.
30. Cherkin DC, Deyo RA, Wheeler K, et al. Physician variation in diagnostic testing for low back pain. Who you see is what you get. Arthritis Rheum 1994;37:15–22.
31. Di Iorio D, Henley E, Doughty A. A survey of primary care physician practice patterns and adherence to acute low back problem guidelines. Arch Fam Med 2000;9:1015–21.
32. Webster BS, Courtney TK, Huang YH, et al. Survey of acute low back pain management by specialty group and practice experience. J Occup Environ Med 2006;48:723–32.
33. Wennberg DE. Variation in the delivery of health care: the stakes are high. Ann Intern Med 1998; 128:866–8.
34. Fisher ES, Bynum JP, Skinner JS. Slowing the growth of health care costs—lessons from regional variation. N Engl J Med 2009;360:849–52.
35. Fisher ES, Wennberg DE, Stukel TA, et al. The implications of regional variations in Medicare spending. Part 2: health outcomes and satisfaction with care. Ann Intern Med 2003;138:288–98.
36. Ivanova JI, Birnbaum HG, Schiller M, et al. Real-world practice patterns, health-care utilization, and costs in patients with low back pain: the long road to guideline-concordant care. Spine J 2011;11: 622–32.
37. Williams CM, Maher CG, Hancock MJ, et al. Low back pain and best practice care. A survey of general practice physicians. Arch Intern Med 2010;170:271–7.
38. Webster BS, Courtney TK, Huang YH, et al. Brief report: physicians' initial management of acute low back pain versus evidence-based guidelines. J Gen Intern Med 2005;20:1132–5.
39. Smith-Bindman R, Miglioretti DL, Larson EB. Rising use of diagnostic medical imaging in a large integrated health system. Health Aff 2008;27: 1491–502.
40. Carey TS, Freburger JK, Holmes GM, et al. A long way to go. Practice patterns and evidence in chronic low back pain care. Spine 2009;34:718–24.
41. Weiner DK, Kim YS, Bonino P, et al. Low back pain in older adults? are we utilizing healthcare resources wisely? Pain Med 2006;7:143–50.
42. Friedman BW, Chilstrom M, Bijur PE, et al. Diagnostic testing and treatment of low back pain in United States emergency departments. Spine 2010;35:E1406–11.
43. U.S. Department of Health and Human Services. Hospital compare. Available at: http://www.hospitalcompare.hhs.gov/hospital-search.aspx. Accessed April 22, 2012.
44. Fryback DG, Thornbury JR. The efficacy of diagnostic imaging. Med Decis Making 1991;11:88–94.
45. Guyatt GH, Tugwell PX, Feeny DH, et al. A framework for clinical evaluation of diagnostic technologies. Can Med Assoc J 1986;134:587–94.
46. Sackett DL, Haynes RB. The architecture of diagnostic research. BMJ 2002;324:539–41.
47. Schers H, Wensing M, Huijsmans Z, et al. Implementation barriers for general practice guidelines on low back pain. Spine 2001;26:E348–53.
48. Department of Clinical Epidemiology, and Biostatistics, McMaster University Health Sciences Centre. How to read clinical journals: VII. To understand an economic evaluation. Can Med Assoc J 1984;130:1542–9.
49. Pengel LH, Herbert RD, Maher CG, et al. Acute low back pain: systematic review of its prognosis. BMJ 2003;327:323–7.
50. Vroomen P, de Krom M, Knottnerus J. Predicting the outcome of sciatica at short-term follow-up. Br J Gen Pract 2002;52:119–23.
51. Deyo RA, Rainville J, Kent DL. What can the history and physical examination tell us about low back pain? JAMA 1992;268:760–5.
52. Jarvik JG, Deyo RA. Diagnostic evaluation of low back pain with emphasis on imaging. Ann Intern Med 2002;137:586–97.
53. Underwood MR, Dawes P. Inflammatory back pain in primary care. Br J Rheumatol 1995;34:1074–7.
54. Suarez-Almazor ME, Belseck E, Russell AS, et al. Use of lumbar radiographs for the early diagnosis of low back pain. JAMA 1997;277:1782–6.
55. Deyo R, Diehl A. Cancer as a cause of back pain: frequency, clinical presentation, and diagnostic strategies. J Gen Intern Med 1988;3:230–8.
56. van Tulder MW, Assendelft WJ, Koes BW, et al. Spinal radiographic findings and nonspecific low back pain: a systematic review of observational studies. Spine 1997;22(4):427–34.
57. Chou D, Samartzis D, Bellabarba C, et al. Degenerative magnetic resonance imaging changes in patients with chronic low back pain. Spine 2011; 36:543–53.
58. Jarvik JG, Hollingworth W, Martin B, et al. Rapid magnetic resonance imaging vs radiographs for patients with low back pain: a randomized controlled trial. JAMA 2003;289:2810–8.
59. Boden SD, David DO, Dina TS, et al. Abnormal magnetic-resonance scans of the lumbar spine in asymptomatic subjects. J Bone Joint Surg 1990; 72:403–8.
60. Jarvik JJ, Hollingworth W, Heagerty P, et al. The longitudinal assessment of imaging and disability of the back (LAIDBACK) study. Spine 2001;26: 1158–66.
61. Jensen MC, Brant-Zawadzki MN, Obuchowski N, et al. Magnetic resonance imaging of the lumbar spine in people without back pain. N Engl J Med 1994;331:69–73.

62. Wiesel SW, Tsourmas N, Feffer HL, et al. 1984 Volvo Award in clinical sciences. A study of computer-assisted tomography. I. The incidence of positive CAT scans in an asymptomatic group of patients. Spine 1984;9:549–51.
63. Carragee E, Alamin T, Cheng I, et al. Are first-time episodes of serious LBP associated with new MRI findings? Spine J 2006;6:624–35.
64. Jarvik JG, Hollingworth W, Heagerty PJ, et al. Three-year incidence of low back pain in an initially asymptomatic cohort. Spine 2005;30:1541–8.
65. Nachemson A. The lumbar spine: an orthopaedic challenge. Spine 1975;1:59–71.
66. Halpin SF, Yeoman L, Dundas DD. Radiographic examination of the lumbar spine in a community hospital: an audit of current practice. BMJ 1991; 303:813–5.
67. Rockey P, Tompkins R, Wood R, et al. The usefulness of x-ray examinations in the evaluation of patients with back pain. J Fam Pract 1978;7: 455–65.
68. Gillan MG, Gilbert FJ, Andrew JE, et al. Influence of imaging on clinical decision making in the treatment of lower back pain. Radiology 2001;220: 393–9.
69. Kleinstuck F, Dvorak J, Mannion AF. Are "structural abnormalities" on magnetic resonance imaging a contraindication to the successful conservative treatment of chronic nonspecific low back pain? Spine 2006;31:2250–7.
70. Fazel R, Krumholz HM, Wang Y, et al. Exposure to low-dose ionizing radiation from medical imaging procedures. N Engl J Med 2009;361: 849–57.
71. Berrington de Gonzalez A, Mahesh M, Kim KP, et al. Projected cancer risks from computed tomographic scans performed in the United States in 2007. Arch Intern Med 2009;169:2071–7.
72. Fisher ES, Welch HG. Avoiding the unintended consequences of growth in medical care. JAMA 1999;281:446–53.
73. Haynes RB, Sackett DL, Taylor DW, et al. Increased absenteeism from work after detection and labeling of hypertensive patients. N Engl J Med 1978;299: 741–4.
74. Gilbert FJ, Grant AM, Gillan MG, et al. Low back pain: influence of early MR imaging or CT on treatment and outcome—multicenter randomized trial. Radiology 2004;231:343–51.
75. Kendrick D, Fielding K, Bentley E, et al. Radiography of the lumbar spine in primary care patients with low back pain: randomised controlled trial. BMJ 2001;322:400–5.
76. Leeuw M, Goossens ME, Linton SJ, et al. The fear-avoidance model of musculoskeletal pain: current state of scientific evidence. J Behav Med 2007; 30:77–94.
77. Chou R, Shekelle P. Will this patient develop persistent disabling low back pain? JAMA 2010;303: 1295–302.
78. Rhodes LA, McPhillips-Tangum CA, Markham C, et al. The power of the visible: the meaning of diagnostic tests in chronic back pain. Soc Sci Med 1999;48:1189–203.
79. Verbeek J, Sengers M, Riemens L, et al. Patient expectations of treatment for back pain. Spine 2004;29:2309–18.
80. McPhillips-Tangum CA, Cherkin DC, Rhodes LA, et al. Reasons for repeated medical visits among patients with chronic back pain. J Gen Intern Med 1998;13:289–95.
81. Wilson IB, Dukes K, Greenfield S, et al. Patients' role in the use of radiology testing for common office practice complaints. Arch Intern Med 2001; 161:256–63.
82. Campbell EG, Regan S, Gruen RL, et al. Professionalism in medicine: results of a national survey of physicians. Ann Intern Med 2007;147:795–802.
83. Deyo RA, Diehl AK, Rosenthal M. Reducing roentgenography use. Can patient expectations be altered? Arch Intern Med 1987;147:141–5.
84. Baras JD, Baker LC. Magnetic resonance imaging and low back pain care for Medicare patients. Health Aff 2009;28:w1133–40.
85. Snowbeck C. Region still rich with MRI machines. Pittsburgh: Pittsburgh Post-Gazette; 2005.
86. Gray DT, Deyo RA, Kreuter W, et al. Population-based trends in volumes and rates of ambulatory lumbar spine surgery. Spine 2006;31:1957–63.
87. Iglehart JK. Health insurers and medical-imaging policy—a work in progress. N Engl J Med 2009; 360:1030–7.
88. Medicare Payment Advisory Commission. Report to the congress: aligning incentives in the Medicare program. Available at: http://www.medpac.gov/documents/Jun09_EntireReport.pdf. Accessed April 6, 2012.
89. Swedlow A, Johnson G, Smithline N, et al. Increased costs and rates of use in the California workers' compensation system as a result of self-referral by physicians. N Engl J Med 1992;327: 1502–6.
90. Studdert DM, Mello MM, Sage WM, et al. Defensive medicine among high-risk specialist physicians in a volatile malpractice environment. JAMA 2005; 293:2609–17.
91. Anonymous Is time management an important cause of excessive imaging?. Backletter 2009; 24:50.
92. Davis PC, Wippold FJ II, Brunberg JA, et al. ACR appropriateness criteria on low back pain. J Am Coll Radiol 2009;6:401–7.
93. Chou R, Qaseem A, Owens DK, et al. Diagnostic imaging for low back pain: advice for high-value

health care from the American College of Physicians. Ann Intern Med 2011;154:181–9.
94. Henschke N, Maher CG, Refshauge KM. Screening for malignancy in low back pain patients: a systematic review. Eur Spine J 2007;16:1673–9.
95. Henschke N, Maher CG, Refshauge KM, et al. Prevalence of and screening for serious spinal pathology in patients presenting to primary care settings with acute low back pain. Arthritis Rheum 2009;60:3072–80.
96. Joines JD, McNutt RA, Carey TS, et al. Finding cancer in primary care outpatients with low back pain: a comparison of diagnostic strategies. J Gen Intern Med 2001;16:14–23.
97. Peul W, van den Hout W, Brand R, et al. Prolonged conservative care versus early surgery in patients with sciatica caused by lumbar disc herniation: two year results of a randomised controlled trial. BMJ 2008;336:1355–8.
98. Weinstein J, Tosteson T, Lurie J, et al. Surgical versus nonsurgical therapy for lumbar spinal stenosis. N Engl J Med 2008;358(8):794–810.
99. Weinstein JN, Lurie JD, Tosteson TD, et al. Surgical versus nonsurgical treatment for lumbar degenerative spondylolisthesis. N Engl J Med 2007;356(22): 2257–70.
100. Weinstein JN, Lurie JD, Tosteson TD, et al. Surgical vs nonoperative treatment for lumbar disk herniation: the Spine Patient Outcomes Research Trial (SPORT) observational cohort. JAMA 2006; 296(20):2451–9.
101. Burton AK, Waddell G, Tillotson KM, et al. Information and advice to patients with back pain can have a positive effect. A randomized controlled trial of a novel educational booklet in primary care. Spine 1999;24:2484–91.
102. Grimshaw JM, Shirran L, Thomas R, et al. Changing provider behavior: an overview of systematic reviews of interventions. Med Care 2001; 39(Suppl 2):II2–45.
103. French SD, Green S, Buchbinder R, et al. Interventions for improving the appropriate use of imaging in people with musculoskeletal conditions. Cochrane Database Syst Rev 2010;1:CD006094.
104. Schectman JM, Schroth WS, Verme D, et al. Randomized controlled trial of education and feedback for implementation of guidelines for acute low back pain. J Gen Intern Med 2003;18: 773–80.
105. Khorasani R. Can radiology professional society guidelines be converted to effective decision support? J Am Coll Radiol 2010;7:561–2.
106. Lehnert BE, Bree RL. Analysis of appropriateness of outpatient CT and MRI referred from primary care clinics at an academic medical center: how critical is the need for improved decision support? J Am Coll Radiol 2010;7:192–7.
107. Blackmore CC, Mecklenburg RS, Kaplan GS. Effectiveness of clinical decision support in controlling inappropriate imaging. J Am Coll Radiol 2011; 8:19–25.
108. Breslau J, Seidenwurm D. Socioeconomic aspects of spinal imaging: impact of radiological diagnosis on lumbar spine-related disability. Top Magn Reson Imaging 2000;11:218–23.
109. McCullough BJ, Johnson GR, Martin BI, et al. Lumbar spine MR imaging and reporting: do epidemiological data in reports affect clinical management? Radiology 2012;262(3):941–6.
110. Eskander MG, Leung A, Lee D. Style and content of CT and MR imaging lumbar spine reports: radiologist and clinician preferences. Am J Neuroradiol 2010;31:1842–7.
111. Grieve FM, Plumb AA, Khan SH. Radiology reporting: a general practitioner's perspective. Br J Radiol 2010;83:17–22.
112. Hillman BJ, Goldsmith J. Imaging: the self-referral boom and the ongoing search for effective policies to contain it. Health Aff 2010;29: 2231–6.
113. Report to Congressional Requesters. Medicare part B imaging services. Rapid spending growth and shift to physician offices indicate need for CMS to consider additional management practices, GAO-08-452. Washington, DC: United States Government Accountability Office; 2008. Available at: http://www.gao.gov/new.items/d08452.pdf. Accessed April 6, 2012.

Spine Segmentation and Enumeration and Normal Variants

Gaurav K. Thawait, MD*, Avneesh Chhabra, MD,
John A. Carrino, MD, MPH

KEYWORDS

• Spine variation • Vertebral enumeration • Spine congenital variants • Transitional vertebra

KEY POINTS

- Various spinal variants such as cervical ribs, transitional vertebrae, block vertebrae, and Schmorl nodes are frequently encountered in clinical practice, and a thorough understanding of these variations is required.
- Accurate vertebral enumeration is essential to avoid wrong-level spinal procedures.
- Imaging of the whole spine should be encouraged and incorporated into routine clinical practice for spine pathologies.
- This article provides a review of the commonly found spinal variants along with the pertinent embryology and classification to help the reader develop a better understanding of the normal variants of spine along with their imaging appearances.

INTRODUCTION

The spine is one of the most frequently imaged body areas in all age categories. The spectrum of imaging indications is broad but dominated by the evaluation of pain. The application of cross-sectional imaging techniques, computed tomography (CT) and magnetic resonance (MR) imaging, to complement or replace radiography in the study of the painful spine is widely accepted in routine clinical practice.

The most common morphologic pattern of the spine consists of 24 presacral (cephalad to the sacrum) mobile segments distributed as 7 non–rib-bearing cervical, 12 rib-bearing thoracic, and 5 non–rib-bearing lumbar vertebrae. However, there is significant variation in the number of thoracic and lumbar segments. The cervical spine exhibits relative morphologic stability, with a fixed vertebral count of 7, which may be confounded by the presence of congenital osseous anomalies in the cervical spine. These range from occipitoatlantal fusion and atlantoaxial anomalies to Klippel-Feil syndrome.[1] Frequently encountered spinal abnormalities bearing relevant clinical implications include cervical ribs, thoracolumbar transitional segments, and lumbosacral transitional vertebrae (LSTVs). The prevalence of cervical ribs has been reported as ranging from 0.05% to 6.10%.[2,3] LSTVs have been documented in 4% to 30% of the population in various studies; the prevalence of thoracolumbar transitional vertebra (TLTV) is not known.

Disclosures: Avneesh Chhabra acknowledges the support of research grants from Siemens AG and Integra Life Sciences as well as the support of a GE-AUR Fellowship. John A. Carrino acknowledges grant from Siemens Medical Systems to study MR neurography.
The authors report no conflicts of interest.
Musculoskeletal Radiology, The Russell H. Morgan Department of Radiology and Radiological Science, Johns Hopkins Hospital, 601 North Caroline Street, Baltimore, JHOC 5165, MD 21287, USA
* Corresponding author.
E-mail address: gthawai1@jhmi.edu

Radiol Clin N Am 50 (2012) 587–598
doi:10.1016/j.rcl.2012.04.003
0033-8389/12/$ – see front matter

Deviation from the typical vertebral anatomy may confuse the clinician, potentially leading to significant clinical errors. The presence of a transitional vertebra can create confusion in the correspondence of nerve and segment, either at the time of injection or surgery. Cervical ribs or extra rib-bearing lumbar segments may also lead to confusion and inaccurate numbering of the vertebral segments, which might have serious implications in an interventional procedure. There is a relative paucity of literature on the prevalence of these developmental variations, as these have not been assessed systematically on whole spine imaging. Determining the prevalence of spinal variations in a systematic manner provides valuable clarity for spine imagers and clinicians, ensuring appropriate patient care during various spine interventional procedures. The principal aim of this article is to help the reader develop a better understanding of the normal variants of the spine and their imaging appearances with emphasis on their prevalence within the spinal column. We review the normal anatomy of the spine with essential and clinically relevant spinal segment variants and their effect on spinal enumeration. For better understanding of the topic, we also touch upon the embryology and development of the spine.

NORMAL EMBRYOLOGY AND DEVELOPMENT

The spinal column is a complex structure, the majority of which is formed during a short period. This renders the spine vulnerable to frequent variations during the rapid formation of this intricate structure.

Formation of the Vertebral Column

The embryologic precursors of the spine appear in the third week of gestation during gastrulation when the primitive streak forms on the bilaminar embryonic disc. It precedes the migration of epiblastic cells through the streak to form a new layer of mesodermal cells distributed between the layers of the bilaminar disc, thus forming the trilaminar embryonic disc.[4] Along the cranial end of the primitive streak is the Hensen node through which the cells migrate to give rise to the prechordal plate and the notochordal process. The notochordal process eventually becomes the notochord, the embryonic structure most directly responsible for vertebral development. The notochord itself consists of a mucoid matrix with sparse polygonal cells and acts as a frame upon which mesodermal cells organize to give rise to the vertebral column.[5]

On either side of the notochord, the mesoderm differentiates into 3 parts, one of which is called the paraxial mesoderm, which forms the somites, also called the primitive segments. These are masses of bilaterally symmetric regularly spaced cells. The somites are composed of a sclerotome consisting of cells that will form the vertebral column and a dermatome consisting of cells that will eventually form the overlying muscles and skin. The cells along the ectodermal side of the notochord undergo the process of neurulation at this time. The neural plate invaginates and closes to form the neural tube, which forms the precursor of the central nervous system comprising the brain and the spinal cord.[4]

During the fourth week of gestation, the sclerotomes migrate and surround the notochord and the overlying neural tube, with each sclerotome separating into 2 distinct layers. One of them forms a cranial area of loosely packed cells and the other a caudal area of densely packed cells. Between these 2 areas is a cell-free space that eventually becomes the site of the intervertebral disk as some mesenchymal cells later migrate into this space to form the outer annulus fibrosis, leaving the remnants of the notochord to form the inner nuclear pulposus.[6] The vertebral body is formed by the centrum, which is in turn formed by the cranial, dense area of one somite fusing with the caudal loose area of the somite immediately cranial to it. Thus, the formation of a normal vertebral body is the result of a cohesive intersegmental union between portions of 2 adjacent somites.[6] The portions of the sclerotomes that surrounded the neural tube go on to form the neural arches, which form the posterior bony elements of the spinal column.

During the sixth week of gestation, signals from the notochord and neural tube lead to chondrification, which ultimately leads to ossification, at which point the notochord disintegrates.[7] There are 3 main ossification centers within each vertebra, one in the centrum and one on each side of the neural arch, which can be identified on prenatal ultrasonography. The fusion of the 2 portions of the posterior elements is not complete until 6 years of age, whereas fusion of the vertebral body with the posterior elements is usually not complete until 5 to 8 years of age. After birth, there is formation of 5 additional secondary ossification centers, one for each transverse process, one for the spinous process, and one each for the superior and inferior vertebral body end plates.[8]

Several notable exceptions to the classical segmentation pattern occur at the occipitocervical junction. The cranial portion of the first cervical sclerotome, sometimes called the proatlas, undergoes complex and unique segmentation and contributes to the occipital condyles, the dorsal cranial articular processes of C1, and the tip of the odontoid process.[9] The caudal portion of the C1 sclerotome forms the anterior and posterior arches of C1 and contributes to the odontoid process. The C1 anterior ossification center typically does not ossify until 1 year of age, and fusion of the anterior and posterior arch to form the C1 ring is not complete until 7 years of life.[10] The axis contains 6 ossification centers in utero derived from 2 sclerotomes; 3 are derived from the C2 sclerotome, a bilaterally symmetric pair that corresponds to the centrum of C1 and the apex of the odontoid, which is derived from the proatlas. The odontoid process fuses with the body of C2 between ages 3 and 6 years, although a remnant of the apophyseal fusion line can persist up to age 11 years. A secondary ossification center cranial to the odontoid process termed the ossiculum terminale appears at age 3 years and does not fuse until age 12 years or so.

The spinal curvature also evolves developmentally with age. The normal curvature of the fetal and newborn spine is kyphotic. The cervical and lumbar lordoses emerge after birth and are thought to be functional in origin, the cervical curvature resulting primarily due to the infant holding its head upright and the lumbar lordosis emerging later in development as the infant/toddler assumes an erect posture.[4]

Formation of the Spinal Cord

Formation of the spinal cord is classically divided into 2 main movements: primary and secondary neurulation. Primary neurulation begins in week 3 when the newly formed notochord induces the formation of the neural tube, which ultimately gives rise to the brain and spinal cord. Fusion begins at or near the fourth somite and proceeds in both directions, typically complete by day 26.[11]

The process of secondary neurulation refers to the formation of the most caudal elements of the spinal cord and is further divided into canalization and retrogressive differentiation. During the process of canalization, a group of undifferentiated cells at the caudal end of the neural tube develops cysts and vacuoles, which merge with one another and eventually with the central canal of the caudal end of the cord that originated from primary neurulation to further elongate the neural tube. Retrogressive differentiation refers to the process whereby the caudal cell mass regresses, eventually leaving only the conus medullaris, ventricular laminalis, and the filum terminale. The process of primary neurulation accounts for structures as caudal as somite 31 or the vertebral level of S2. Vertebral bodies cephalad to S2 are thus derived from the notochord where those caudal to S2 derive from the caudal cell mass.[12]

Genetic Factors

Homeobox, or Hox, genes are a family of genes that regulate the differentiation processes of the axial and appendicular skeletons.[13,14] These genes regulate the embryonic differentiation and segmentation of the craniocaudal axis by activation and repression of DNA sequences that encode the transcription factors and proteins affecting the order and direction of development of the axial skeleton.[15] Mutations of the homeobox genes may be responsible for congenital/developmental anomalies of the cervical spine.[16] Some studies have shown that the normal patterns of lumbar and sacral vertebrae as well as the changes in the axial pattern, such as LSTV, result from mutations in the Hox-10 and Hox-11 paralogous genes.[17,18]

VARIANT ANATOMY

The variations in the vertebral column can be broadly classified as failure of formation, failure of segmentation, or the occurrence of neural tube defects during embryologic development. However, these variations often present as a combination of developmental errors of multifactorial etiology.

VARIANTS OF FORMATION

As the name suggests, variants of formation occur as a result of failure of formation of any anatomic component of the vertebra. Most common defects include hemivertebrae (**Fig. 1**) and wedge vertebrae. Hemivertebrae are manifest when there is failure of development of part of the vertebral body. The prognosis of patients with hemivertebrae depends on the extent of the failure of development and their laterality in cases of multiple hemivertebrae.[4]

VARIANTS OF SEGMENTATION

The variants of segmentation occur when there is failure of separation of 2 adjacent vertebrae because of a segmentation defect in 2 contiguous somites. These include block vertebrae, unilateral bar vertebrae, and atlanto-occipital fusion.

Block vertebrae result when there is failure of intervertebral disk formation between 2 contiguous vertebrae resulting in total fusion. Block vertebrae can be complete or incomplete and may lead to congenital kyphosis or lordosis. Congenital block vertebrae show waist formation

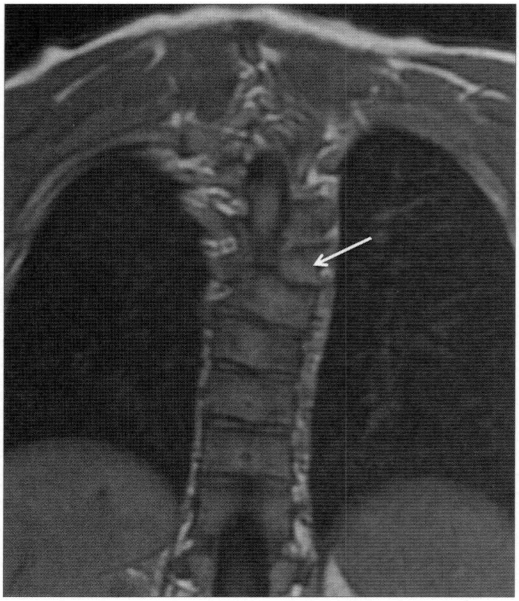

Fig. 1. Coronal T1-weighted MR image in a 10-year-old boy evaluated for scoliosis showing hemivertebra at T6 level (*arrow*).

at the site of fusion, not seen with acquired fusion from previous infection or inflammation. They occur most commonly within the cervical spine.[19] Vertebral fusion at 4 or more levels raises suspicion for Klippel-Feil syndrome; a search should then be made for involvement of any other organ system, such as the thyroid and kidney.

Unilateral bar vertebrae occur when a part of intervertebral disk fails to form, resulting in partial fusion of the adjacent vertebral bodies.

Atlanto-occipital fusion is a type of block vertebra, except that it involves the failure of segmentation of the proatlas and/or the sclerotome.[20]

MISCELLANEOUS VARIANTS

Butterfly vertebrae (anterior spina bifida) are vertebral bodies with a dysplastic or absent center and 2 large lateral masses. They arise due to failure of fusion of bilaterally symmetric chondrification centers to fuse in the midline (**Fig. 2**).[21]

Limbus vertebrae occur when there is an early intravertebral disk herniation and the disk material extends beneath the ring apophysis, thus preventing its fusion with the vertebral body (**Fig. 3**).

Schmorl nodes are the result of herniation of the intervertebral disk into and through the central portion of the vertebral end plate (see **Fig. 3**).[22] These may be associated with adjacent bone marrow edema. Multilevel Schmorl nodes in a young patient raise the suspicion of underlying end plate weakness/osteochondrosis (Scheuermann disease).

SPINAL SEGMENT VARIANTS

Cervical Ribs

Cervical ribs are implicated in the pathoetiology of thoracic outlet syndrome; for the most part, these are normal variants that only predispose to the clinical syndrome under specific circumstances. A cervical rib can either articulate with the first rib just posterior to the scalene tubercle or end freely in the soft tissues of the neck (often referred to as a cervical rib variant). In cases in which the rib ends in soft tissue, there is usually a fibrous band connecting the tip of the cervical rib to the first rib. As a cervical rib variant, an elongated C7 transverse process (transverse apophysomegaly or transverse mega-apophysis) is fused with the C7 vertebra and may also connect to the first rib by a fibrous band. It probably represents an incomplete cervical rib.[23]

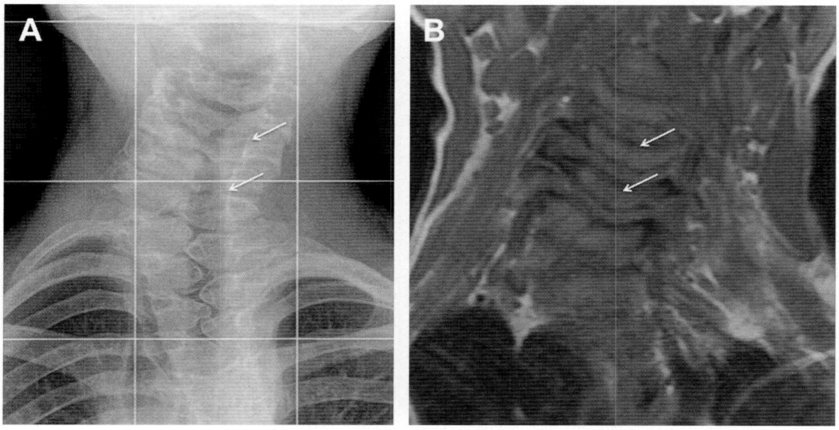

Fig. 2. Frontal radiograph (*A*) and corresponding T1-weighted MR image (*B*) in a 10-year-old boy evaluated for scoliosis showing multiple butterfly vertebrae in cervical and upper thoracic spine (*arrows*).

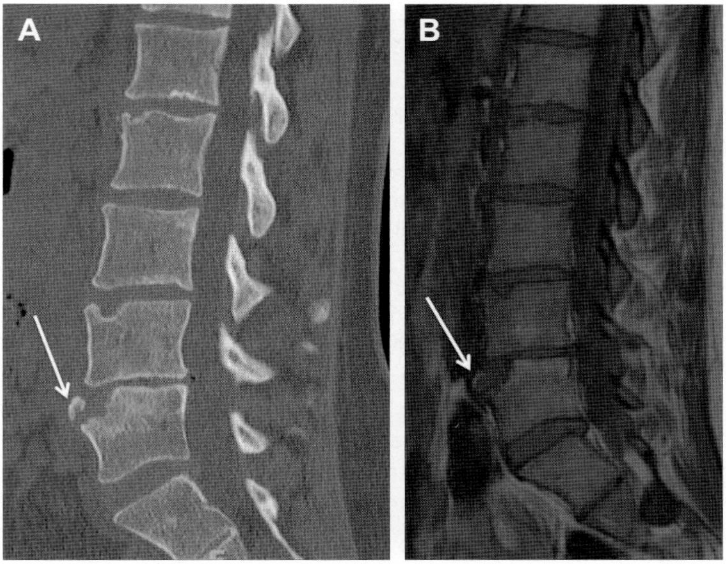

Fig. 3. Sagittal CT (*A*) and corresponding T1-weighted MR image (*B*) in a 30-year-old man evaluated for back pain showing limbus vertebra at L5 level (*arrow*). Also note, multilevel Schmorl nodes suggesting underlying end plate weakness.

Cervical ribs are the source of origin of neurogenic and/or vascular symptoms in about 10% of patients; they may also result in confusion in enumeration of vertebra with potentially serious surgical and clinical implications. The spine imager or the clinician must be able to define and identify a cervical rib. The cervical rib is best seen on radiography or CT (**Fig. 4**). A rib articulating with an inferiorly directed transverse process represents a cervical rib and can be differentiated from the first rib, which arises from a superiorly directed transverse process. However, the presence of a fibrous band can be better appreciated on MR imaging.

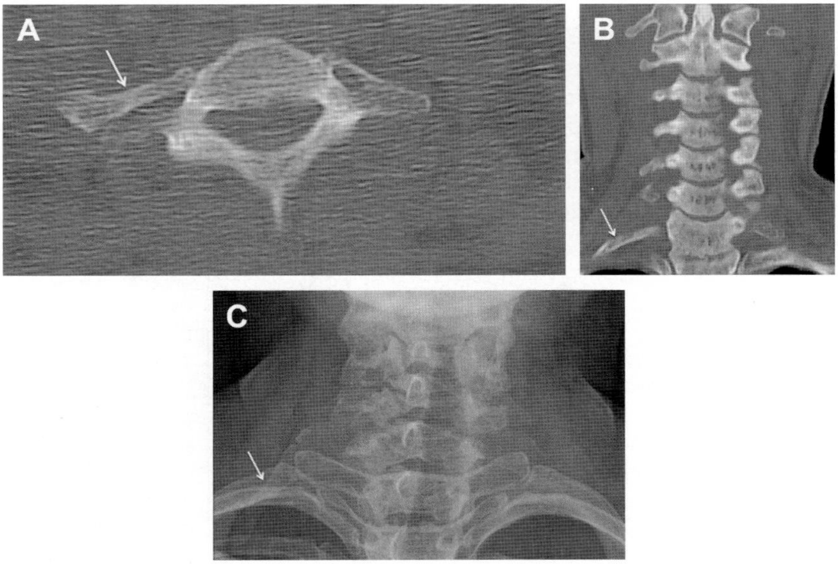

Fig. 4. Axial (*A*) and coronal (*B*) CT images with an anteroposterior radiograph (*C*) in a 35-year-old woman showing a cervical rib on the right side (*arrow*).

The cervical rib has been variously defined in the literature; most currently, Brewin and colleagues[2] defined it by the following criteria:

1. The cervical rib must adjoin the seventh cervical vertebral transverse process.
2. It must have no connection with the manubrium sternum, although it may form a synostosis with the first rib (thus differentiating it from a rudimentary first rib).
3. The cervical rib must be separate from, but articulate with, the transverse process of C7. (If fused with the vertebra, it is classified as an elongated cervical transverse process.)

The length of a C7 transverse process necessary to designate it as a cervical rib variant was interpreted by Erken and colleagues[3] as more than 30 mm.

Transitional Vertebrae

A transitional vertebra retains partial features of the segment above it and the segment below it.[24] Variability in the thoracolumbar spine may arise when there is a shift from the typical distribution of 12 thoracic and 5 lumbar segments. It can also result from the presence of an anomalous total number of vertebrae or when there are TLTVs or LSTVs.

The most common spinal morphology is that of 24 presacral mobile segments. However, some individuals have 23 or 25 presacral segments rather than 24, which causes an alteration in the thoracolumbar segmental distribution. Carrino and colleagues,[25] in their study of 147 subjects with complete spine radiographs, noted that 91.8% had 24 presacral segments, 4.8% had 23 segments, and 3.4% had 25 segments. In another study, Hanson and colleagues[26] performed spine MR imaging, including total spine sagittal localizer images, in 750 consecutive patients. They assumed 7 cervical vertebrae and 12 thoracic vertebrae. Their data demonstrated 24 presacral segments in 80%, 23 segments in 5.3%, and 25 segments in 14.5%. One case of 22 presacral segments was noted. Stratified by gender, the data revealed that two-thirds of the patients with 4 lumbar vertebrae were women, whereas two-thirds of the subjects with 6 lumbar vertebrae were men. The disparity from Carrino and colleagues' data, particularly in the frequency of 25 presacral segments, may arise in the identification of the first sacral segment; Carrino and colleagues were able to examine frontal radiographs, whereas Hanson and colleagues' study relied on limited coronal MR imaging sections. A third recent study by Akbar and associates,[27] using full spine sagittal MR imaging localizers in 207 subjects, noted 23 mobile presacral segments in 3.3% and 25 mobile presacral segments also in 3.3%, much closer to the findings by Carrino and colleagues. LSTVs were seen on the sagittal images in 1%; the exclusive use of sagittal images underestimates LSTV. Significantly, 69% of the anomalies of segmentation or transitional segments were not noted in the radiology reports in the study by Akbar and colleagues.[27]

Additional variations have been reported in the distribution of thoracolumbar anatomy, such as the presence of 13 rib-bearing thoracic vertebrae with 4 lumbar-type vertebrae and the presence of 12 rib-bearing thoracic vertebrae with 6 lumbar-type vertebrae.[28] In Carrino and colleagues' study, when 24 presacral segments were present, 97% had 12 thoracic and 5 lumbar vertebrae; 13 thoracic rib-bearing and 4 lumbar-type vertebrae were more common than 11 thoracic and 6 lumbar bodies in the remainder.[25] A total of 10.9% of subjects had an anomalous number or distribution of thoracolumbar segments.

The TLTV

The TLTV was defined by Wigh[24] as the presence of hypoplastic ribs, less than 3.8 cm in length, on the lowest rib-bearing segment (**Fig. 5**). In Carrino

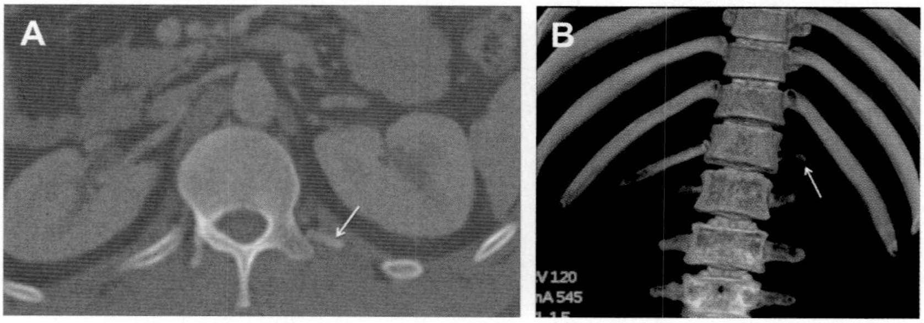

Fig. 5. TLTV. Axial CT (*A*) and 3-dimensional volume-rendered (*B*) images in a 29-year-old man showing transitional thoracic segment with a short rib (<3.8 cm) on the left side (*arrow*).

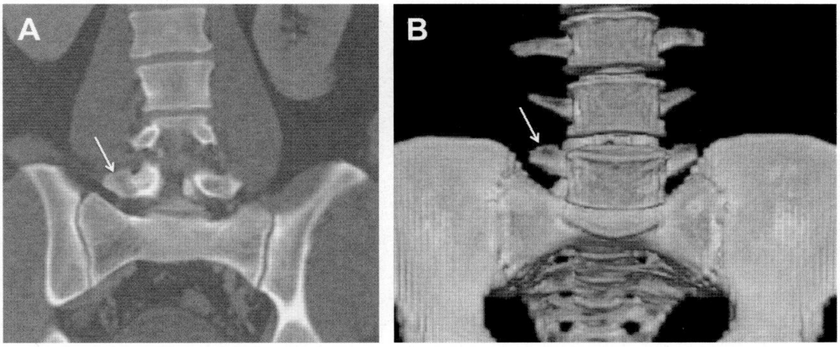

Fig. 6. Castellvi type Ia. Coronal CT (*A*) and 3-dimensional volume-rendered (*B*) images in a 28-year-old man showing enlarged L5 transverse process on the right side (*arrow*).

and colleagues' study, 4.1% of subjects had transitional thoracolumbar segments; two-thirds of those also had transitional lumbosacral segments.[25]

The LSTV

LSTVs have a prevalence ranging anywhere from 4% to 30%.[28–33] Morphologically, in LSTV, either the fifth lumbar vertebra may show assimilation to the sacrum (sacralization), or the first sacral vertebra may show transition to a lumbar configuration (lumbarization). Castellvi and colleagues[30] defined LSTV by the relationship of the enlarged lumbar transverse process to the sacrum: type I: unilateral (Ia) or bilateral (Ib) dysplastic transverse process, measuring at least 19 mm in craniocaudal dimension (**Figs. 6** and **7**); type II: unilateral (IIa) or bilateral (IIb) lumbarization/sacralization with an enlarged transverse process that has a diarthrodial joint with the sacrum (**Figs. 8** and **9**); type III: unilateral (IIIa) or bilateral (IIIb) lumbarization/sacralization with complete osseous fusion of the transverse process to the sacrum (**Figs. 10** and **11**); type IV: unilateral type II transition with a type III transition on the contralateral side (**Fig. 12**) (**Table 1**).

O'Driscoll and colleagues[34] developed a 4-type classification system to enhance identification of LSTV on MR images. The system is based predominantly on the S1-2 disk morphology as seen on sagittal MR images, depending on the presence or absence of disk material and the anteroposterior (AP) length of the disk. Type 1 exhibits no disk material and is seen in patients without transitional segments. Type 2 consists of a small residual disk with an AP length less than that of the sacrum. This type is also most often seen in patients without transitional segments. Type 3 is a well-formed disk extending the entire AP length of the sacrum and can be seen in normal spines as well as in those with LSTVs. Type 4 is similar to type 3 but with the addition of squaring of the presumed upper sacral segment (**Table 2**). Good correlation was found between a type 4 S1-2 disk and an S1 LSTV (Castellvi type III or IV).[34] There have been several other studies describing the morphology of LSTV; Nicholson and colleagues[35] described a decreased height on radiographs of the disk between a lumbar

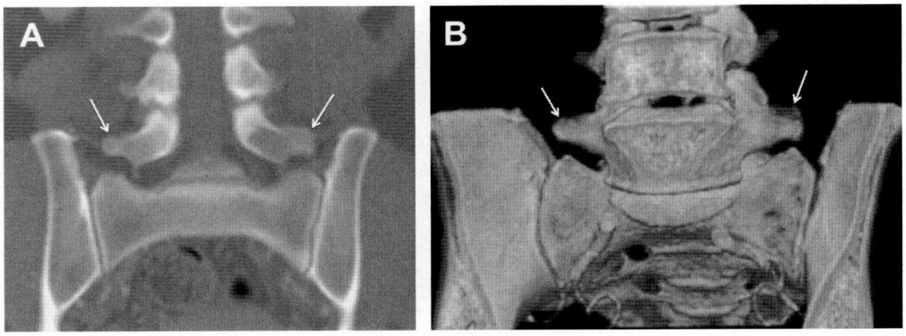

Fig. 7. Castellvi type Ib. Coronal CT (*A*) and 3-dimensional volume-rendered (*B*) images in a 46-year-old woman showing enlarged transverse process on both sides of L5 vertebra (*arrows*).

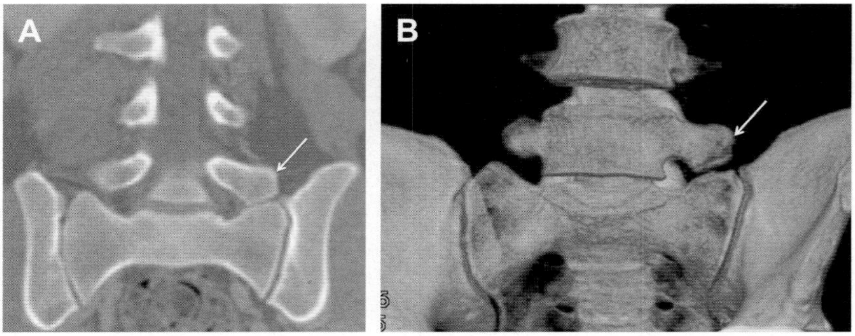

Fig. 8. Castellvi type IIa. Coronal CT (*A*) and 3-dimensional volume-rendered (*B*) images in a 36-year-old woman showing enlarged right L5 transverse process forming a diarthrodial joint with sacrum on the right side (*arrow*).

transitional segment and the sacrum in comparison with the normal disk height between L5 and S1; Wigh and Anthony[36] described squaring of the upper sacral segment when it is lumbarized and wedging of the lowest lumbar segment when it is sacralized.

Along with the morphologic characterization, it is also imperative to know the accurate numbering of an LSTV for precise clinical and surgical decision making. The presence of a transitional lumbosacral segment greatly increased the likelihood (7-fold) of an anomalous number of presacral segments in Carrino and colleagues' study.[25] Many studies have proposed the use of an anatomic marker to identify the corresponding vertebra, including the aortic bifurcation, right renal artery, conus medullaris, and the iliolumbar ligaments. However, these markers have all been proved to be significantly unreliable. An LSTV can be accurately characterized on AP radiographs or coronal CT or MR imaging sections because of their clear illustration of the relationship of the enlarged transverse processes of the lowest lumbar vertebra with the superior sacrum and, sometimes, inclusion of the thoracic ribs. Methodical identification of the correct vertebral level is critical; wrong-level spine surgeries are attributable to variant spine anatomy in some cases.[37] Carrino and colleagues[25] suggest that the identification of an LSTV should prompt additional imaging to verify spine enumeration before spine interventions. Counting of vertebrae from C2 is the only certain method of completely documenting spinal enumeration.

It has become common to omit radiographs and proceed directly to MR imaging to evaluate pain syndromes thought to be of spinal origin. Typical MR imaging protocols may not include coronal images, and accurate identification of LSTV may be challenging. Intraoperative spinal localization may consist only of lateral radiographs, often of modest quality. This sets the stage for errors of localization. Radiologists should actively encourage and assist preoperative correlation of radiographs with pathologic conditions identified on MR imaging. This correlation becomes critical in cases in which an LSTV is present or suspected and in thoracic lesions for which intraoperative localization is particularly difficult. This may require radiographs of the entire spine or correlation of

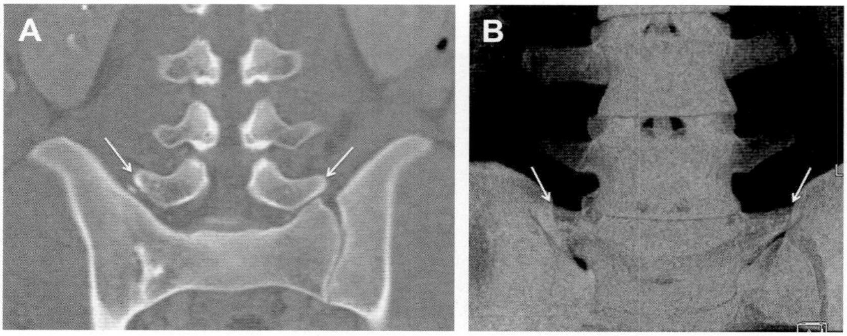

Fig. 9. Castellvi type IIb. Coronal CT (*A*) and 3-dimensional volume-rendered (*B*) images in a 28-year-old man showing enlarged transverse processes of L5 vertebra with diarthrodial joint formation with sacrum on both sides (*arrows*).

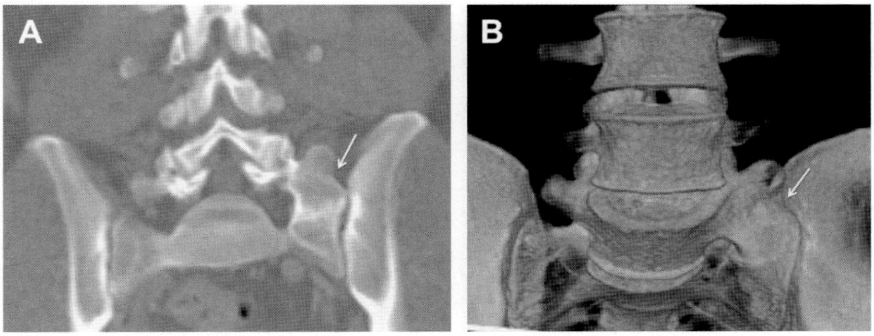

Fig. 10. Castellvi type IIIa. Coronal CT (*A*) and 3-dimensional volume-rendered (*B*) images in a 38-year-old man showing enlarged left transverse process of L5 vertebra with complete osseous fusion with sacrum on the left side (*arrow*).

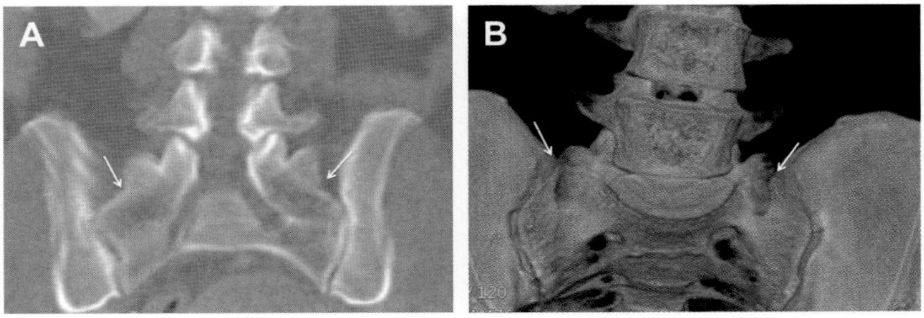

Fig. 11. Castellvi type IIIb. Coronal CT (*A*) and 3-dimensional volume-rendered (*B*) images in a 28-year-old woman showing enlarged transverse processes of L5 vertebra with complete osseous fusion with sacrum on both sides (*arrows*).

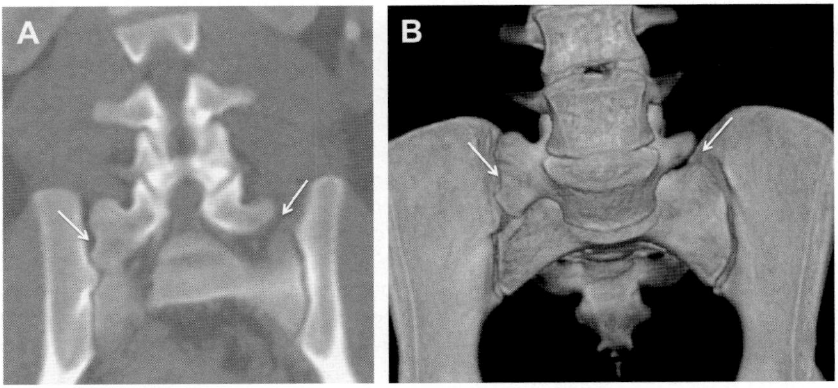

Fig. 12. Castellvi type IV. Coronal CT (*A*) and 3-dimensiona volume-rendered (*B*) images in a 21-year-old woman showing enlarged bilateral L5 transverse processes with a type II transition on the left side and a type III transition on the right side (*arrows*).

Table 1
Classification of LSTV

Type	Description
I	Dysplastic transverse process (unilateral, Ia; bilateral, Ib)
II	Incomplete lumbarization/sacralization showing enlarged transverse processes with unilateral (IIa) or bilateral (IIb) pseudarthrosis with the adjacent sacral ala
III	Complete lumbarization/sacralization showing enlarged transverse processes with unilateral (IIIa) or bilateral (IIIb) fusion with the adjacent sacral ala
IV	Mixed (eg, type IIa on one side and type IIIa on the other)

Data from Castellvi AE, Goldstein LA, Chan DP. Lumbosacral transitional vertebrae and their relationship with lumbar extradural defects. Spine (Phila Pa 1976) 1984; 9(5):493–5.

radiographs of the index spine segment with whole spine MR imaging localizer images. Enumeration of all segments from the C2 to the sacrum is necessary.

The localization concern is further confounded by studies that have shown patients with LSTVs also have variation in segmental innervation[38] and alteration in function of the lumbosacral nerve roots, which leads to a poor correlation with clinical symptoms.[39] Typically the L4 nerve supplies the vastus medialis and lateralis, the L5 nerve the tibialis anterior and extensor hallucis longus, and the S1 nerve the medial head of the gastrocnemius and soleus. This provided the basis for the typical radicular pain patterns of L4 (anterior thigh), L5 (lateral thigh, anterolateral calf, dorsum of foot), and S1 (posterior thigh, calf, plantar foot). McCulloch and Waddell[40] studied cadavers and patients with LSTV and concluded that the nerve exiting at the most caudal mobile segment was functionally L5 in its innervation pattern. This study did not account for the number of presacral segments. Kim and colleagues[39] studied 32 patients with LSTV using stimulation of the L4, L5, and S1 roots. They counted vertebrae caudally from T1 to establish the level of T12. The functional innervation of a lumbarized S1 (L6) nerve was most commonly that of a typical S1 nerve. However, in patients with a sacralized L5 segment, the L4 nerve frequently supplied a typical L5 distribution. Several patients in both groups showed overlap of typical distributions. The imager, clinician, and surgeon must all be cognizant of such variation in the selection of patients with radicular pain syndromes for interventional procedures. Disk herniations or apparent compromise of the central canal, lateral recess, or neural foramen detected by imaging are often asymptomatic. Only careful correlation of a pain syndrome with the spinal anatomy depicted by imaging, including accounting for segmental enumeration, can suggest a causal relationship.

In patients with radicular pain syndromes and an LSTV, the imager must also be aware of the possibility of an extraforaminal nerve root entrapment between the enlarged transverse process of the LSTV and the sacral ala; this is best identified on coronal images.[41] The disk above the LSTV has an increased likelihood of herniation; there is also an increased likelihood of central canal compromise at the disk level above an LSTV.[41]

The relationship between LSTV and axial pain, Bertolotti syndrome, is controversial. In a large study of 4000 patients, Tini and colleagues[41] found no evidence of an association between back pain and the presence of an LSTV. The presence of an LSTV may alter the biomechanics of the lumbosacral junction. The diminished mobility of an LSTV protects this disk from age-related "degenerative" changes but may lead to hypermobility at the disk level above, at an anomalous pseudoarticulation, or at a normally formed facet contralateral to the anomalous articulation. Either the pseudoarticulation or the contralateral facet is a potential axial pain generator. As noted earlier, the disk above an LSTV is prone to age-related change and herniation. The Bertolotti syndrome is discussed elsewhere in this issue by Kotsenas.

Table 2
Classification of first sacral intervertebral disk morphology

Type	Description
1	No disk material between S1 and the sacrum
2	A small residual disk between S1 and the sacrum
3	A well-formed residual disk between S1 and the sacrum
4	A well-formed disk between S1 and the remainder of the sacrum, in addition to an abnormal sagittal outline to the sacrum ("squaring" of the first sacral element)

Data from O'Driscoll CM, Irwin A, Saifuddin A. Variations in morphology of the lumbosacral junction on sagittal MRI: correlation with plain radiography. Skeletal Radiol 1996;25:225–30

SUMMARY: VERTEBRAL ENUMERATION

Variants in vertebral enumeration are common; 11% to 20% of patients exhibit alteration in the number or distribution of thoracolumbar vertebra.[25–27] Anatomic landmarks for vertebral enumeration could be related to any structures that are typically included in view of routine spine imaging. Intradural spinal landmarks such as the conus medullaris or dural sac termination along with nonspinal anatomic landmarks such as the abdominal vasculature are problematic because of their variable location and potential changes in location with age.[42] The use of musculoskeletal-related spinal landmarks such as the iliolumbar ligament has also been found to be insufficiently accurate to denote the L5 vertebra.[25]

Imaging of the entire spine, either by radiographs or a combination of radiographs and entire spine localizers, allows the physician to enumerate the vertebrae by counting caudally from C2 and also for differentiating hypoplastic ribs from lumbar transverse processes, which helps in accurate assignment of an LSTV segmental level. As the identification and accurate labeling of vertebral segments is critical before a surgical or percutaneous procedure to avoid wrong-level exposure or injection, additional preprocedure imaging to verify the spinal anatomy should be encouraged. In radiology reporting of spine imaging studies, it would be prudent to initially specifically state the spinal enumeration in the study being reported and its correlation with other spine imaging studies present in the medical record.

REFERENCES

1. Guille JT, Sherk HH. Congenital osseous anomalies of the upper and lower cervical spine in children. J Bone Joint Surg Am 2002;84(2):277–88.
2. Brewin J, Hill M, Ellis H. The prevalence of cervical ribs in a London population. Clin Anat 2009;22(3): 331–6.
3. Erken E, Ozer HT, Gulek B, et al. The association between cervical rib and sacralization. Spine (Phila Pa 1976) 2002;27(15):1659–64.
4. Kaplan KM, Spivak JM, Bendo MD. Embryology of the spine and associated congenital abnormalities. Spine J 2005;5:564–76.
5. Christopherson LR, Rabin BM, Hallam DK, et al. Persistence of the notochordal canal: MR and plain film appearance. Am J Neuroradiol 1999;20: 33–6.
6. O'Rahilly R. Human embryology and teratology. New York: John Wiley & Sons; 1996.
7. Nolting D, Hansen B, Keeling J, et al. Prenatal development of the normal human vertebral corpora in different segments of the spine. Spine 1998;23(21): 2265–71.
8. Moore K, Persaud TVN. The developing human: clinically oriented embryology. 6th edition. Philadelphia: W.B. Saunders Company; 1998.
9. O'Rahilly O, Muller F, Meyer DB. The vertebral column at the end of the embryonic period proper; 2. The occipitocervical junction. J Anat 1983;136: 181–95.
10. Lustrin ES, Karakas SP, Ortiz AI, et al. Pediatric cervical spine: normal anatomy, variants, and trauma. Radiographics 2003;23:539–60.
11. Rossi A, Cama A, Piatelli G, et al. Spinal dysraphism: MR imaging rationale. J Neuroradiol 2004; 31:3–24.
12. Muller F, O'Rahilly R. The development of the human brain, the closure of the caudal neuropore, and the beginning of secondary neurulation at stage 12. Anat Embryol (Berl) 1987;176:413–30.
13. Galis F. Why do almost all mammals have seven cervical vertebrae? Developmental constraints, Hox genes, and cancer. J Exp Zool 1999;285(1): 19–26.
14. McGinnis W, Krumlauf R. Homeobox genes and axial patterning. Cell 1992;68(2):283–302.
15. Manak JR, Scott MP. A class act: conservation of homeodomain protein functions. Dev Suppl 1994; 61–77.
16. Subramanian V, Meyer BI, Gruss P. Disruption of the murine homeobox gene Cdx1 affects axial skeletal identities by altering the mesodermal expression domains of Hox genes. Cell 1995;83(4):641–53.
17. Carapuço M, Nóvoa A, Bobola N, et al. Hox genes specify vertebral types in the presomitic mesoderm. Genes Dev 2005;19(18):2116–21.
18. Wellik DM, Capecchi MR. Hox10 and Hox11 genes are required to globally pattern the mammalian skeleton. Science 2003;301(5631):363–7.
19. Leivseth G, Frobin W, Brinchmann P. Congenital block vertebrae are associated with caudally adjacent discs. Clin Biomech 2005;20:669–74.
20. Richetti ET, States L, Hosalker HS, et al. Radiographic study of the upper cervical spine in the 22q11.2 deletion syndrome. J Bone Joint Surg Am 2004;86:1751–60.
21. Muller F, O'Rahilly R, Benson DR. The early origin of vertebral anomalies, as illustrated by a "butterfly vertebra". J Anat 1986;149:157–69.
22. Saluja G, Fitzpatrick K, Bruce M, et al. Schmorl's nodes (intravertebral herniations of intervertebral disc tissue) in two historic British populations. J Anat 1986;145:87–96.
23. Redenbach DM, Nelems B. A comparative study of structures comprising the thoracic outlet in 250 human cadavers and 72 surgical cases of thoracic outlet syndrome. Eur J Cardiothorac Surg 1998; 13(4):353–60.

24. Wigh RE. The thoracolumbar and lumbosacral transitional junctions. Spine (Phila Pa 1976) 1980;5(3):215–22.
25. Carrino JA, Campbell PD Jr, Lin DC, et al. Effect of spinal segment variants on numbering vertebral levels at lumbar MR imaging. Radiology 2011;259(1):196–202.
26. Hanson EH, Mishra RK, Chang DS, et al. Sagittal whole-spine magnetic resonance imaging in 750 consecutive outpatients: accurate determination of the number of lumbar vertebral bodies. J Neurosurg Spine 2010;12(1):47–55.
27. Akbar JJ, Weiss KL, Saafir MA, et al. Rapid MRI detection of vertebral numeric variation. AJR Am J Roentgenol 2010;195(2):465–6.
28. Kier EL. Some developmental and evolutionary aspects of the lumbosacral spine. In: Gouaze A, Salamon G, editors. Brain anatomy and magnetic resonance imaging. Berlin: Springer-Verlag; 1988. p. 116–39.
29. Bron JL, van Royen BJ, Wuisman PI. The clinical significance of lumbosacral transitional anomalies. Acta Orthop Belg 2007;73(6):687–95.
30. Castellvi AE, Goldstein LA, Chan DP. Lumbosacral transitional vertebrae and their relationship with lumbar extradural defects. Spine (Phila Pa 1976) 1984;9(5):493–5.
31. Delport EG, Cucuzzella TR, Kim N, et al. Lumbosacral transitional vertebrae: incidence in a consecutive patient series. Pain Physician 2006;9(1):53–6.
32. Hahn PY, Strobel JJ, Hahn FJ. Verification of lumbosacral segments on MR images: identification of transitional vertebrae. Radiology 1992;182(2):580–1.
33. Taskaynatan MA, Izci Y, Ozgul A, et al. Clinical significance of congenital lumbosacral malformations in young male population with prolonged low back pain. Spine (Phila Pa 1976) 2005;30(8):E210–3.
34. O'Driscoll CM, Irwin A, Saifuddin A. Variations in morphology of the lumbosacral junction on sagittal MRI: correlation with plain radiography. Skeletal Radiol 1996;25:225–30.
35. Nicholson AA, Roberts GM, Williams LA. The measured height of the lumbosacral disc in patients with and without transitional vertebrae. Br J Radiol 1988;61(726):454–5.
36. Wigh RE, Anthony HF Jr. Transitional lumbosacral discs. probability of herniation. Spine (Phila Pa 1976) 1981;6(2):168–71.
37. Malanga GA, Cooke PM. Segmental anomaly leading to wrong level disc surgery in cauda equina syndrome. Pain Physician 2004;7(1):107–10.
38. Seyfert S. Dermatome variations in patients with transitional vertebrae. J Neurol Neurosurg Psychiatry 1997;63(6):801–3.
39. Kim YH, Lee PB, Lee CJ, et al. Dermatome variation of lumbosacral nerve roots in patients with transitional lumbosacral vertebrae. Anesth Analg 2008;106(4):1279–83, Table of Contents.
40. McCulloch JA, Waddell G. Variation of the lumbosacral myotomes with bony segmental anomalies. J Bone Joint Surg Br 1962;62:475–80.
41. Tini PG, Wieser C, Zinn WM. The transitional vertebra of the lumbosacral spine: its radiological classification, incidence, prevalence, and clinical significance. Rheumatol Rehabil 1977;16:180–5.
42. Kornreich L, Hadar H, Sulkes J, et al. Effect of normal ageing on the sites of aortic bifurcation and inferior vena cava confluence: a CT study. Surg Radiol Anat 1998;20(1):63–8.

Physiologic Imaging of the Spine

Jad G. Khalil, MD[a,*], Ahmad Nassr, MD[b],
Timothy P. Maus, MD[c]

KEYWORDS

• Physiologic imaging • Dynamic imaging • Spine • Lumbar stenosis • Radiculopathy • EOS
• Upright MRI

KEY POINTS

- Static and unloaded spine imaging may not always reveal relevant spinal pathology.
- Dynamic imaging allows for positioning more reflective of the patient's symptoms, and may reveal occult pathology not seen on more traditional tests.
- The use of some dynamic imaging modalities (such as upright magnetic resonance imaging) as routine examinations is not advisable because of their poor resolution and high false-positive rate.
- New imaging modalities, such as EOS, may help us understand more complex spinal deformity and its relationship with pelvic parameters.

INTRODUCTION

Imaging of the spine poses particular challenges, both to the radiologist and to the clinician. The dynamic nature of the spine and its mobility across multiple segments is difficult to depict with any single imaging modality. Supine imaging, which is often used for advanced imaging studies, fails to provide an understanding of the physiologic changes that are seen with weight bearing or change of position.[1–3]

The vast majority of symptoms in patients with spinal disorders occur in axially loaded positions, such as sitting or standing. This is unaccounted for in supine radiographs, computed tomography (CT), and magnetic resonance imaging (MRI). Numerous studies have shown that changes occur in the seated and erect posture in relation to the disc space, sagittal alignment of the spine, dynamic stenosis, and segmental stability. These anatomic changes are a composite of the effects of axial load and physiologic extension.

In the lumbar spine, intradiscal pressures are significantly higher when sitting or standing than in a recumbent position.[4] In a cadaver study, Inufusa and colleagues[5] demonstrated that the cross-sectional area of the lumbar central canal and lateral recesses diminished with extension positioning, and increased in flexion, relative to neutral positioning. There were also pronounced effects on the neural foramina, with a significant reduction in cross-sectional area in extension and an increase in flexion. Neural compression within the foramen was more common in extension than in neutral position; compression was least common in flexion. In another cadaveric study focused on the lumbar neural foramina, Fujiwara and colleagues[6] observed the neural foraminal area to increase significantly with flexion and side bending or rotation away from the index foramen. Extension or side bending or rotation toward the measured foramen diminished its area relative to neutral positioning.

Schmid and colleagues[7] studied healthy volunteers with an open-configuration MRI and noted a 40-mm^2 reduction in cross-sectional area of the dural sac at the L3–L4 level in moving from flexion to extension. The neural foraminal

[a] Department of Orthopedic Surgery, Henry Ford Hospital, Detroit, MI, USA; [b] Department of Orthopedic Surgery, Mayo Clinic, Rochester, MN, USA; [c] Department of Radiology, Mayo Clinic, 200 First Street SW Rochester, MN 55905, USA
* Corresponding author.
E-mail address: jadkhalil@gmail.com

Radiol Clin N Am 50 (2012) 599–611
doi:10.1016/j.rcl.2012.04.004

cross-sectional area was reduced by 23% in moving from an upright neutral to an upright extended position. Danielson and Willen[8] noted a significant decrease in the dural sac cross-sectional area with axial loading in 56% of subjects, most commonly at L4–L5, and more common with increasing age. Dynamic reduction in dural sac area with loading was less frequent in healthy volunteers than in a population of patients with neurogenic intermittent claudication. The ligamentum flavum was implicated as the most important structure resulting in dynamic reduction in the lumbar central canal area under physiologic loading by Hansson and colleagues.[9] The work of Madsen and colleagues[10] would suggest that physiologic extension positioning of the lumbar spine is more significant than axial load in the dynamic reduction in dural cross-sectional area seen in the upright lumbar spine.

Similar dynamic changes are evident in the cervical spine. In a cadaveric study, Chen and colleagues[11] demonstrated an increase in disc bulging and central ligamentum flavum buckling in the movement from flexion to extension; the effect of the ligamentum flavum on central canal dimensions was dominant. In an MRI study of patients, Muhle and colleagues[12] observed an increase in central canal stenosis in the movement from neutral positioning to either flexion or extension. Increasing central canal stenosis was significantly more common in extension, with contributions from either the anterior column (disc, disc-osteophyte complex) or posterior column (ligamentum flavum, facet hypertrophy), or both. Increasing stenosis was less common in flexion; when present it was primarily caused by anterior column impingement. Muhle and colleagues[12] observed cervical neural foraminal area to decrease in extension and increase slightly in flexion. Similarly, Zhang and colleagues[13] noted that the cross-sectional area of the cervical central canal was greatest in the neutral position; it was reduced more in extension than flexion. Kitagawa and colleagues[14] used CT to study the cervical foramina of healthy volunteers. Flexion significantly increased foraminal height, width, and cross-sectional area; extension significantly reduced all these parameters over the neutral position.

It is thus well established that all compartments of the spinal canal undergo significant dimensional change with assumption of axial load and upright positioning, and in physiologic flexion and extension motion. In the lumbar spine, extension and axial load reduce the area of all spine compartments; these are increased in flexion. In the cervical spine, the central canal area is diminished in both extension and flexion; the deleterious effect is greater in extension. Cervical neural foramina, like their lumbar counterparts, narrow in extension and enlarge in flexion. This constitutes the greatest sensitivity challenge faced by spine imaging: conventional static or unloaded imaging may fail to reveal a lesion that is causal of the patient's symptoms when that lesion is expressed only in physiologic postures. It is postulated that imaging in a position that is more physiologic may unmask such abnormalities. Numerous methods have been devised that allow for more physiologic spine imaging. Many are variations of conventional modalities; others have been uniquely designed for this purpose.

RADIOGRAPHS

Standing and Supine Radiographs

The simplest form of dynamic imaging is the standing radiograph. In a comparison of 50 patients with low back pain with matched asymptomatic volunteers, Wood and colleagues[15] found that both groups exhibited an increase in thoracic kyphosis and lumbar lordosis when imaged in the standing versus supine position. Increased lumbar lordosis (extension) will narrow all lumbar spine compartments. Instability, most commonly manifested as degenerative spondylolisthesis at the L4–L5 lumbar level, may not be evident on supine radiographs, but can be detected on standing films.[16] Standing frontal and lateral radiographs are the typical initial radiographic evaluation of the patient with back or limb pain; specialized views may complement this evaluation in specific circumstances.[17,18] Although changes are usually subtle in patients without overt pathology, they can be remarkable when deformity exists (**Fig. 1**).

Flexion and Extension Radiographs

Functional radiography, using dynamic flexion-extension (F/E) views of the spine, may provide information that is occult to static views. F/E views are routinely used by spine practitioners looking for subtle instability, which may affect treatment decisions. In a study by Hammouri and colleagues,[19] 43% of practicing spine surgeons stated that they obtained these views as part of the initial radiographic assessment. The clinical implications, however, were less clear. A retrospective analysis by the same authors revealed that only 2 of 342 evaluated patients were found to have new findings on F/E views that were not appreciated on the anteroposterior and lateral films.[19] They concluded that F/E films added little to the information obtained on static upright radiographs. This cost and radiation exposure is best

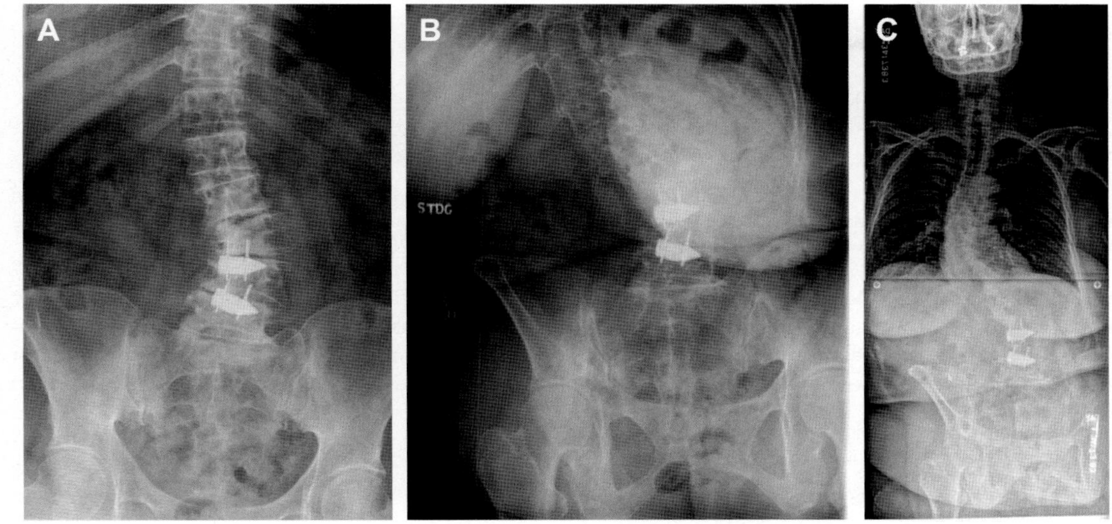

Fig. 1. A 65-year-old woman initially evaluated for low back pain and progressive deformity with supine (*A*) imaging. Standing lumbar (*B*) and scoliosis (*C*) images demonstrate an uncompensated coronal deformity that is underwhelming on the supine film.

deferred to a presurgical setting, not during an initial evaluation of the patient with back pain.

More advanced methods of evaluating spinal instability on dynamic radiographs may add precision to classical modalities of instability measurement. Lee and associates validated a method of evaluating spinal instability using electrogoniometers and video fluoroscopy. They concluded that lumbar motion segments flexed in descending order during lumbar flexion, with the greatest amount of flexion observed at L1 and the least at L5.[20] Wong and colleagues[21] used videofluoroscopy with an auto-tracking system and focused on continuous dynamic F/E assessment. They also concluded that lumbar flexion is contributed by spinal segments in decreasing order. The authors found that extension was evenly distributed; there was also a steady increase in lumbar lordosis with extension.

The role of F/E imaging of the cervical spine is well established in trauma[22] as a means of assessing ligamentous integrity and detecting instability. The use of dynamic x-ray imaging in degenerative cervical conditions is more controversial. In a retrospective cohort of 258 consecutive patients, only 2 patients (<1%) were found to have spondylolisthesis not detected on neutral lateral radiographs. None of these patients' clinical management was changed based on these findings, leading the investigators to abandon F/E cervical radiographs as part of the initial evaluation of degenerative cervical conditions.[23]

Similarly, the routine use of oblique radiographs of the lumbar or cervical spine is not to be condoned. Lumbar oblique radiographs double the gonadal dose without measurable benefit to the patient.[24] Cervical oblique views will add radiation to sensitive thyroid tissue to no benefit. Scoliosis series may reasonably include both recumbent and upright views, as recumbent views may assist in the preoperative assessment of expected surgical correction.[25] Care must be used in serial radiation exposure.

In summary, standing or weight-bearing frontal and lateral radiographs are an appropriate initial imaging study of the patient with spine or limb pain. Routine use of F/E or oblique radiographs is not justified except in specific presurgical circumstances.

AXIALLY LOADED IMAGING OF THE SPINE

Physiologic imaging would ideally include standing or seated imaging; this is not always possible with current advanced imaging technologies. Axial loading of the spine in the supine position has been one of the methods used to achieve a simulated weight-bearing posture during imaging. As detailed previously, axial loading of the spine, particularly when combined with extension positioning, diminishes all canal dimensions in the lumbar spine. Devices exist that allow performing CT and MRI scans of the lumbar spine in an axially loaded position with mild extension. One example is the Dyna Well (DynaMed AB, Stockholm, Sweden) (**Fig. 2**); this apparatus is nonmagnetic and consists of a harness that is applied to the patient with balanced loads. The harness is

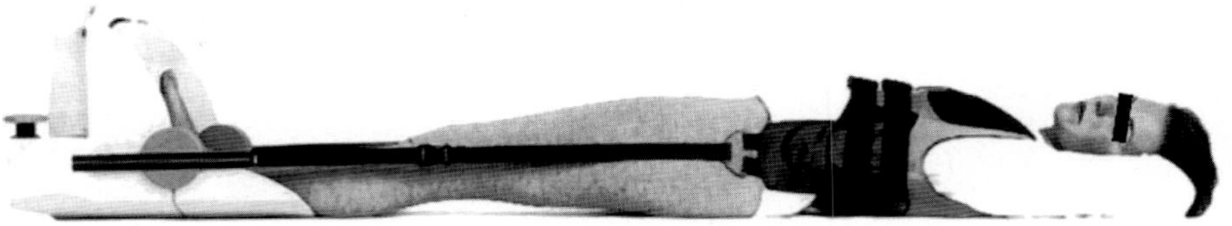

Fig. 2. The DynaWell: a nonmagnetic device that consists of a harness and straps that allow the application of an evenly distributed axial load. (*Reproduced from* Danielson B, Willen J. Axially loaded magnetic resonance image of the lumbar spine in asymptomatic individuals. Spine (Phila Pa 1976) 2001;26(23):2601–6; with permission.)

not fixed to the CT or MRI table. The goal is to apply an even axial load that would reproduce the effects of weight bearing; when the axis of compression is appropriately adjusted, it will also create lumbar extension.[8,26]

Willen and colleagues[26] compared the results of CT myelograms and MRI scans done with the patient in a psoas-relaxed position and those in a supine, axially loaded, slightly extended position. Their results showed that axial loading significantly increased the sensitivity and specificity of both modalities in the diagnosis of lumbar spinal stenosis. The investigators therefore recommended an axial-loading study in patients with canal diameters smaller than 130 mm^2. This recommendation has been carried forward in the 2011 North American Spine Society's evidence-based guidelines on evaluation and treatment of spinal stenosis[27]; axially loaded imaging is suggested with suspected neurogenic intermittent claudication and stenosis unconfirmed by conventional imaging, with a canal diameter smaller than 110 mm^2. The use of axial loading in the identification of spinal stenosis that is not detectable on recumbent studies has been frequently cited in the literature. Choi and associates[28] reported on cases where the pathology was not evident on conventional MRI but detected on an axially loaded study. Willen and colleagues[29] demonstrated that surgical results of cases of occult lumbar spinal stenosis detected only by axially loaded MRI were comparable with those of stenosis seen by unloaded MRI examinations.

ROTATIONAL CT SCANNING

CT can also be used in maximally rotated positions of the spine to identify findings that are subtle or simply not evident in a static, neutral spine. This is exemplified in the diagnosis of nontraumatic atlantoaxial rotatory subluxation (AARS), also known as Grisel syndrome.[30] Patients usually present with a fixed deformity known as the "cock-robin" posture. Traditionally, the diagnosis had relied on radiographic criteria, such as the odontoid-lateral mass interspace asymmetry.[31] More recently, CT scanning has been widely used in this diagnosis.[32] Diagnostic criteria include displacement of facets at the atlantoaxial joint and persistent displacement of the dens between the lateral masses. It is sometimes unclear whether displacement in a rotated position is the result of a pathologic condition or an artifact of the positioning. A dynamic CT study on healthy adult subjects showed that images obtained in maximal rotation could be erroneously interpreted as abnormal.[33] Been and colleagues[34] presented a series of patients, all referred with a presumed diagnosis of AARS after CT scans were obtained in the "cock-robin" position. The investigators then conducted CT examinations under anesthesia that showed no abnormality; imaging in a fixed neck position only may lead to an erroneous diagnosis. Additionally, dynamic CT scanning of patients with confirmed AARS provides information about the severity of the condition and may affect treatment and prognosis. McGuire and associates[35] noted that the stage of the disease (as measured by the degree of motion limitation on dynamic CT evaluation) directly correlated with the duration of symptoms and intensity of treatment. In a cooperative patient, CT should be performed in maximally right-rotated and left-rotated head positions; this evaluates for rotation of the axis and atlas to confirm the diagnosis.

DYNAMIC MRI OF THE SPINE

Background

MRI has been well established as the imaging modality of choice for most spinal conditions and is routinely used in the assessment of radicular pain, radiculopathy, and somatic referred axial pain in all spine segments. Its utility is restricted both by the specificity fault common to all spine imaging (high prevalence of asymptomatic age-related changes) and a sensitivity fault in the detection of dynamic lesions evident only under axial load and with physiologic positioning. The specificity fault is discussed elsewhere in this issue. The sensitivity fault is implicit in imaging studies obtained in the supine position. The supine position negates the effect of gravity and abdominal musculature on the spine[2] and allows a more uniform weight distribution on the vertebrae. Additionally, in the supine position, the spine is in a position of relative flexion because of hip and knee flexion; this may mask the magnitude of stenosis in the central canal, lateral recesses, or neural foramina.[36]

Back and limb pain is most clinically evident when sitting or standing. It is intuitive to perform the MRI study in the position that typically reproduces the patient's symptoms. This may include flexion, extension, side bending, or rotation, performed while standing, sitting, or kneeling. This is achievable, although with important compromises. A commonly used upright MRI is a product of Fonar (Upright MRI, Fonar Corporation, Melville, NY) (**Fig. 3**). It consists of a tilting table positioned between the 2 resistive magnets producing a 0.6-T magnetic field. This allows the patient to achieve positions between −20° and 90°(vertical); it also allows for flexion and extension.[36] The open configuration may be beneficial with claustrophobic patients; the upright position may also benefit those with cardiopulmonary disease who cannot tolerate the supine position.

Following early reports showing the capabilities of dynamic MRI, a number of centers have incorporated this technique into their practice.[37–39] Conditions in which dynamic MRI may play an important role in clinical management are summarized in the following section.

Dynamic MRI of the Cervical Spine

Early reports by Epstein and colleagues[40] in 1987 described the utility of F/E MRI in diagnosing

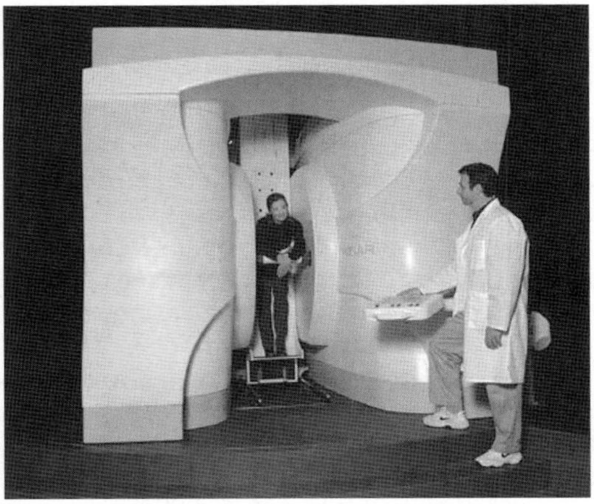

Fig. 3. The upright MRI unit allows the patient to be scanned recumbent, standing and at various degrees of flexion and extension. (*Reproduced from* Jinkins JR, Dworkin JS, Damadian RV. Upright, weight-bearing, dynamic-kinetic MRI of the spine: initial results. Eur Radiol 2005;15(9):1815–25; with permission.)

ventral and dorsal cord compression that was not apparent on static images. They also described this technique as useful in surgical planning and postoperative assessment. Case reports have subsequently described cervical disc protrusions that were unmasked by performing MRI with the head tilted to the side of the lesion.[38]

Similarly, Jinkins and associates[2] reported on a patient with cervical central canal stenosis that was not visible on recumbent MRIs, but became apparent on images obtained with neck extension (**Fig. 4**).

Schlamann and associates[41] reported on their experience using the Neuroswing system (Hightech electronic GmbH, Geldersheim, Germany), which allows positioning of the neck over a continuous spectrum of flexion and extension (**Fig. 5**). This device is compatible with a conventional closed MRI scanner. Twenty patients with symptomatic cervical spondylotic myelopathy were evaluated in neutral, flexion, and extension positions. In 5 of the patients, a previously known stenosis became more significant during movement (**Fig. 6**).

Dynamic MRI of the Lumbar Spine

Lumbar spine MRI is a commonly ordered imaging study in the workup of axial low back pain, radicular pain, or radiculopathy. It may be insensitive to dynamic lesions.[42] Traditional supine MRI images in the unloaded state are often not representative of patient postural complaints; the images on which we base our assessment may not reflect the pathology that the patient experiences. Axially loaded supine MRI provides some simulation of the upright position[43] but may fail to reproduce the postural effects of gravity and core muscle activation.[36] The effects of posture and loading on the intervertebral disk, central canal, lateral recess, foramen, and overall spinal alignment are discussed.

Intervertebral disk

Several studies have shown increased lumbar disc bulging on upright imaging.[2,44] Weishaupt and colleagues[45] noted that most discs demonstrated an increased bulge in upright extension and decreased bulge in upright flexion compared with supine imaging. Similarly, Zamani and associates[37] observed that 41.0% of disks showed increased bulging in extension, 2.2% decreased bulging in flexion, and 57.0% did not change relative to the neutral upright position. Zou and colleagues[44] studied intervertebral disk bulging as a function of the degree of disc age-related ("degenerative") changes on axially loaded MRI in flexion and extension. They noted that advancing disc age-related

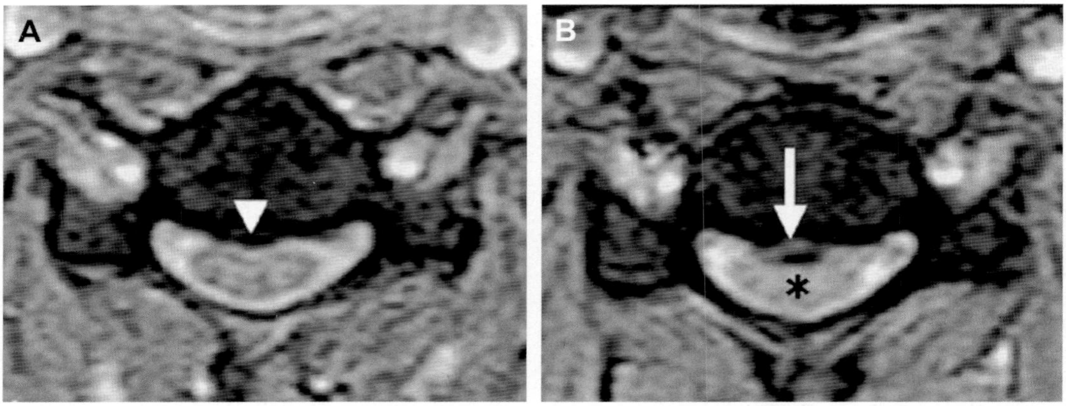

Fig. 4. Axial images in (*A*) neutral position of a patient with clinical symptoms of cervical spinal stenosis; cord compromise is not evident. Arrowhead denotes a posterior osteophyte extending into the spinal canal. Similar image in cervical extension (*B*) shows posterior disc herniation. Asterisk denotes spinal cord indentation. (*Reproduced from* Jinkins JR, Dworkin JS, Damadian RV. Upright, weight-bearing, dynamic-kinetic MRI of the spine: initial results. Eur Radiol 2005;15(9):1815–25; with permission.)

change was associated with increased bulging, typically at the L4–L5 and L5–S1 segments. In its clinical application, dynamic MRI can unmask a symptomatic disk herniation that is occult on recumbent imaging (**Fig. 7**).[2,36] It is important to correlate these findings with the patient's symptoms, as most abnormalities detected with MRI are asymptomatic.

Lumbar spinal stenosis

Acquired lumbar spinal stenosis typically affects patients older than 50; it is of increasing prevalence and poses specific diagnostic challenges.[46]

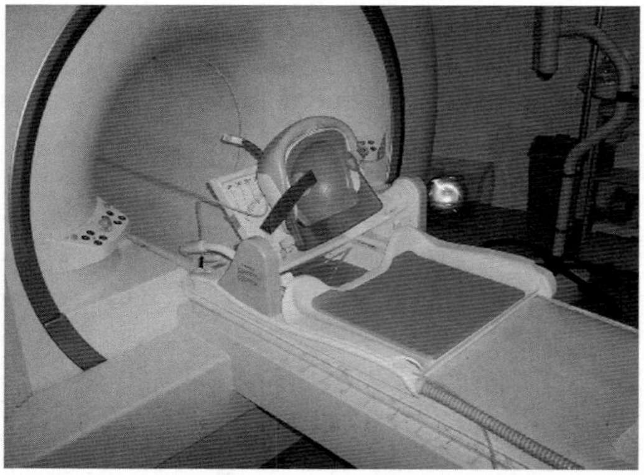

Fig. 5. The NeuroSwing system is compatible for use with a conventional closed MRI system; shown here with a Siemens Sonata 1.5 T system (Siemens Medical Solutions, Erlangen, Germany). (*Reproduced from* Schlamann M, Reischke L, Klassen D, et al. Dynamic magnetic resonance imaging of the cervical spine using the NeuroSwing System. Spine (Phila Pa 1976) 2007;32(21):2398–401; with permission.)

Its presentation as neurogenic intermittent claudication is a positional entity by definition. MRI is the imaging modality of choice in the diagnosis and preoperative planning of this condition.[27] The typical patient is asymptomatic at rest, in the supine position, or in an upright flexed position; recumbent MRI scans may not demonstrate the pathology that is responsible for the symptoms, or underestimate its severity. Several of the studies documenting reduction in central canal, lateral recess, and foraminal area in an upright extended posture have been described previously. The literature contains numerous clinical examples in which MRI in an upright, extended posture can unmask a significant stenosis not apparent on supine imaging.[2,36,47,48] It could thus be a valuable tool when selectively applied to this subset of patients (**Fig. 8**).

Assessment of spinal instability

Early stages of lumbar instability can be difficult to detect on static imaging. The use of F/E radiography has been used to identify unstable motion segments in surgical planning. Indirect signs of instability evident on supine imaging include facet degeneration, effusions, hypertrophy, and ligament attenuation.[49,50] Facet joint effusions particularly may warrant further imaging, as even subtle instability may affect treatment options.[3] Upright, dynamic MRI can directly demonstrate such instability and show evidence of vertebral segmental motion. Similarly, vertebral segments below a degenerative level may exhibit increased motion; this can be directly visualized.[49] Jinkins and associates[2] demonstrated that even minor sagittal instability (anterolisthesis or retrolisthesis) can be

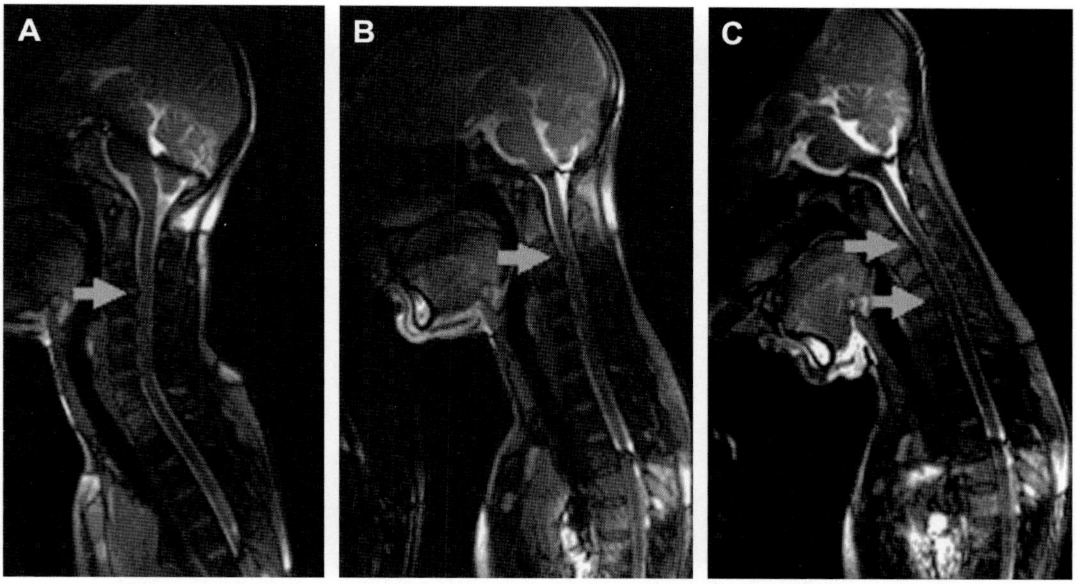

Fig. 6. Sagittal MRI images of a patient scanned at various degrees of neck motion: 25.8° of extension (*A*), neutral (*B*), and 31.8° of flexion (*C*) showing worsening of a known disk protrusion at C3–C4 and newly detected protrusion at C5–C6 with flexion. (*Reproduced from* Schlamann M, Reischke L, Klassen D, et al. Dynamic magnetic resonance imaging of the cervical spine using the NeuroSwing System. Spine (Phila Pa 1976) 2007;32(21):2398–401; with permission.)

unmasked and quantified using direct region-of-interest measurements. This obviates the effects of image magnification and patient positioning errors, which may confound F/E radiographs. In patients with unexplained axial pain on static imaging, dynamic MRI can reveal occult instability.[51] Treatment implications in this circumstance are unclear.

In a group of patients with isthmic spondylolysis and spondylolisthesis, Niggemann and colleagues[48] have shown that dynamic MRI can further characterize the instability into 1 of 3 types: anterior instability evidenced by unstable slips (**Fig. 9**), angular instability, which is characterized by increased angular movement (**Fig. 10**), and a much rarer posterior instability. Although the

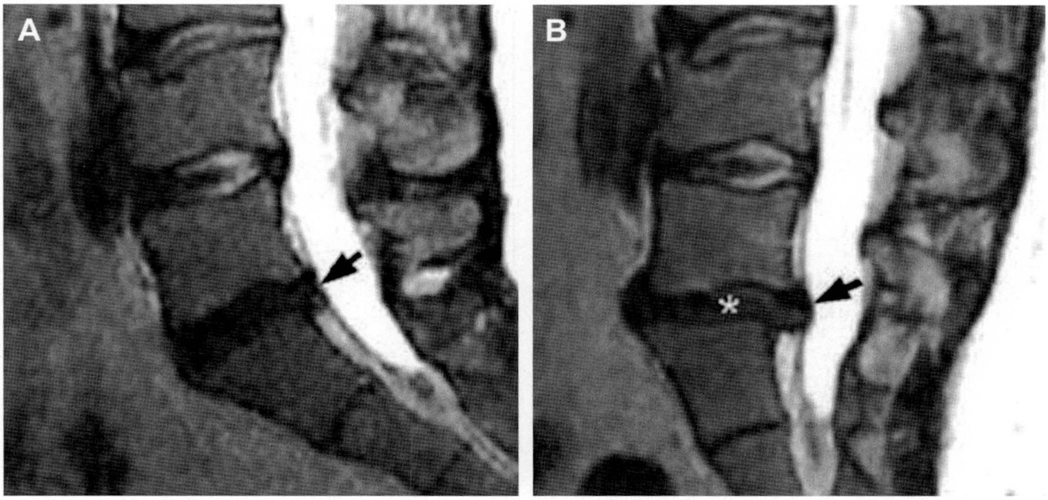

Fig. 7. A patient with an occult disk herniation (*arrow*) at L5–S1 that is insignificant on recumbent MRI (*A*). Upright MRI (*B*) clearly reveals the L5–S1 disk herniation along with a minor component of retrolisthesis (*arrow*). Asterisk denotes L5-S1 nucleus pulposus. (*Reproduced from* Jinkins JR, Dworkin JS, Damadian RV. Upright, weight-bearing, dynamic-kinetic MRI of the spine: initial results. Eur Radiol 2005;15(9):1815–25; with permission.)

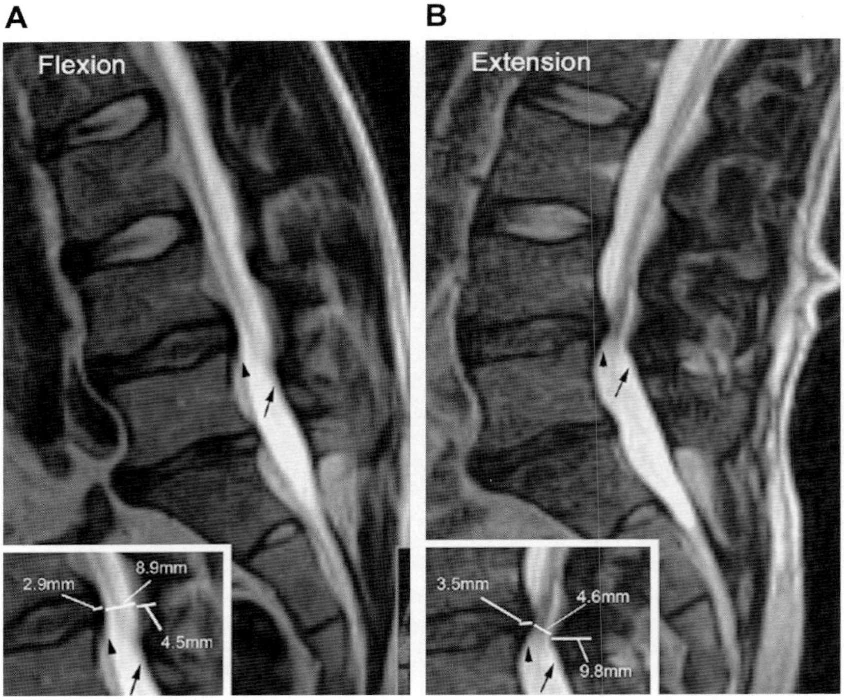

Fig. 8. Mid-sagittal T2 images in seated flexion (*A*) and extension (*B*) of a patient with nonspecific back pain. The extension views demonstrate an increase in posterior disk bulging at L4–L5 (*arrowheads*). Also demonstrated is significant ligamentum flavum infolding (*arrows*). Both of these contribute to reduction of the central canal diameter. (*Reproduced from* Alyas F, Connell D, Saifuddin A. Upright positional MRI of the lumbar spine. Clin Radiol 2008;63(9):1035–48; with permission.)

clinical implications are still unclear, this information may provide important clinical clues to the etiology of radicular pain associated with spinal instability; it might also help direct treatment when surgical intervention is contemplated.[51]

It seems unquestionable that dynamic MRI imaging in functional postures has important advantages in understanding clinical pain and dysfunction syndromes. The practical challenge is that currently available systems are of low field strength, with an unavoidable reduction in image quality. This reduction in image quality can have important consequences for clinical image interpretation. If current low field strength dynamic systems were applied selectively to cases where conventional imaging fails to demonstrate a correlative lesion causal of the patient's pain, the patient would likely benefit. All too often, however, the cost of these systems results in their routine use, or even promotion as the best available imaging

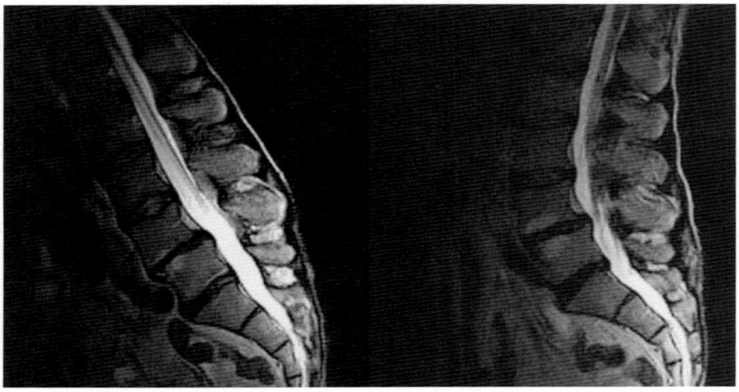

Fig. 9. T2-weighted MRI scans of the lumbar spine in flexion (*left*) and extension (*right*) demonstrating anterior instability at the L4/L5 level, which reduces in extension and contributes to greater central canal compromise in flexion. (*Reproduced from* Niggemann P, Kuchta J, et al. Spondylolysis and spondylolisthesis: prevalence of different forms of instability and clinical implications. Spine (Phila Pa 1976) 2011;36(22):E1463–8; with permission.)

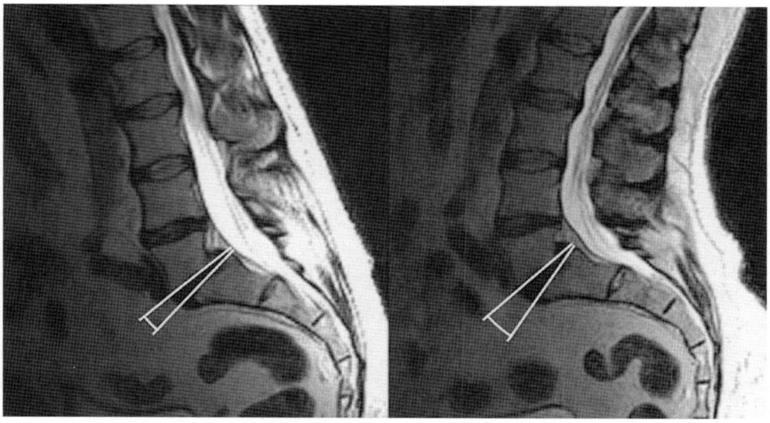

Fig. 10. T2-weighted MRI scans of the lumbar spine in flexion (*left*) and extension (*right*). The angle subtended by the L5 and S1 end plates increases by 8° with lumbar extension, consistent with the diagnosis of angular instability. (*Reproduced from* Niggemann P, Kuchta J, Beyer HK, et al. Spondylolysis and spondylolisthesis: prevalence of different forms of instability and clinical implications. Spine (Phila Pa 1976) 2011;36(22): E1463–8; with permission.)

tool for all spine conditions. This could result in patient harm, as diminished image quality reduces sensitivity to the detection of sinister lesions, which is the primary goal of imaging the patient with back pain (**Fig. 11**).

Biplanar stereoradiography and 3-dimensional imaging

Three-dimensional spine imaging is uniquely suited to the study of spinal deformities. Virtual reconstruction of objects in 3 dimensions can be accomplished using CT,[52] MRI,[53,54] and MRI myelography.[55] Spine stereoradiography using biplanar imaging is an evolving technique showing promise in the evaluation of spinal deformities.

Georges Charpak received the Nobel prize in physics in 1992 for inventing and developing particle detectors and the multiwire proportional chamber.[56] This technique led to radiographic applications that produce high-quality images with a substantial reduction in radiation dose as compared with conventional radiography.[57] Within the past decade, collaboration among physicists, biomechanical engineers, and physicians led to the creation of a low-dose imaging system that generates 3-dimensional spine images in a seated or standing position at low radiation doses.[58,59] EOS (Coll. LBM, Paris; LIO, Montreal; Saint-Vincent de Paul Hospital, Paris; Biospace Instruments, Paris, France) uses 2 tightly collimated horizontal fan beams and linked proprietary detector systems that simultaneously scan the standing or seated patient in frontal and lateral projections; the system can use these data to generate 2-dimensional or 3-dimensional images. Validation studies have shown EOS to have an anatomic reliability comparable with 3-dimensional spine reconstructions obtained via conventional CT scanning, at significantly lower radiation doses.[60] One major advantage of this new technology is the ability to image not only the spine, but also the entire axial and appendicular skeleton on one image in a functional position. It remains primarily a bone-imaging technique.

The EOS system is initially seeing utility in the study of spinal deformity. Deschenes and colleagues[59] used the system in the study and surgical planning of spinal deformity and scoliosis cases; EOS provided overall better-quality images while reducing radiation over conventional computed radiography. The impact of 3-dimensional imaging on the study of scoliosis is only beginning to be appreciated. Illes and colleagues[61] recently used EOS in their description of the concept of vertebra vectors, suggesting a new classification of scoliosis reflective of the rotational deformities of vertebral segments.

Morvan and associates[62] used EOS in identifying pelvic parameters related to spinal sagittal balance; this new modality could serve an important role in the study of sagittal balance with reduced radiation exposure. Increasing understanding of the importance and impact of the anatomy of the pelvis and lower extremities on lumbar deformity will be a driving force in more widespread adoption of this technology.

DISCUSSION

Most spinal complaints are reported by patients to occur during standing, sitting, or active motion; it is intuitive that physiologic imaging of the spine in such positions would provide superior information to that obtained in a recumbent position. This intuition is supported by ample anatomic evidence that all compartments of the spine undergo significant dimensional changes under axial load; in physiologic lordotic positioning; and

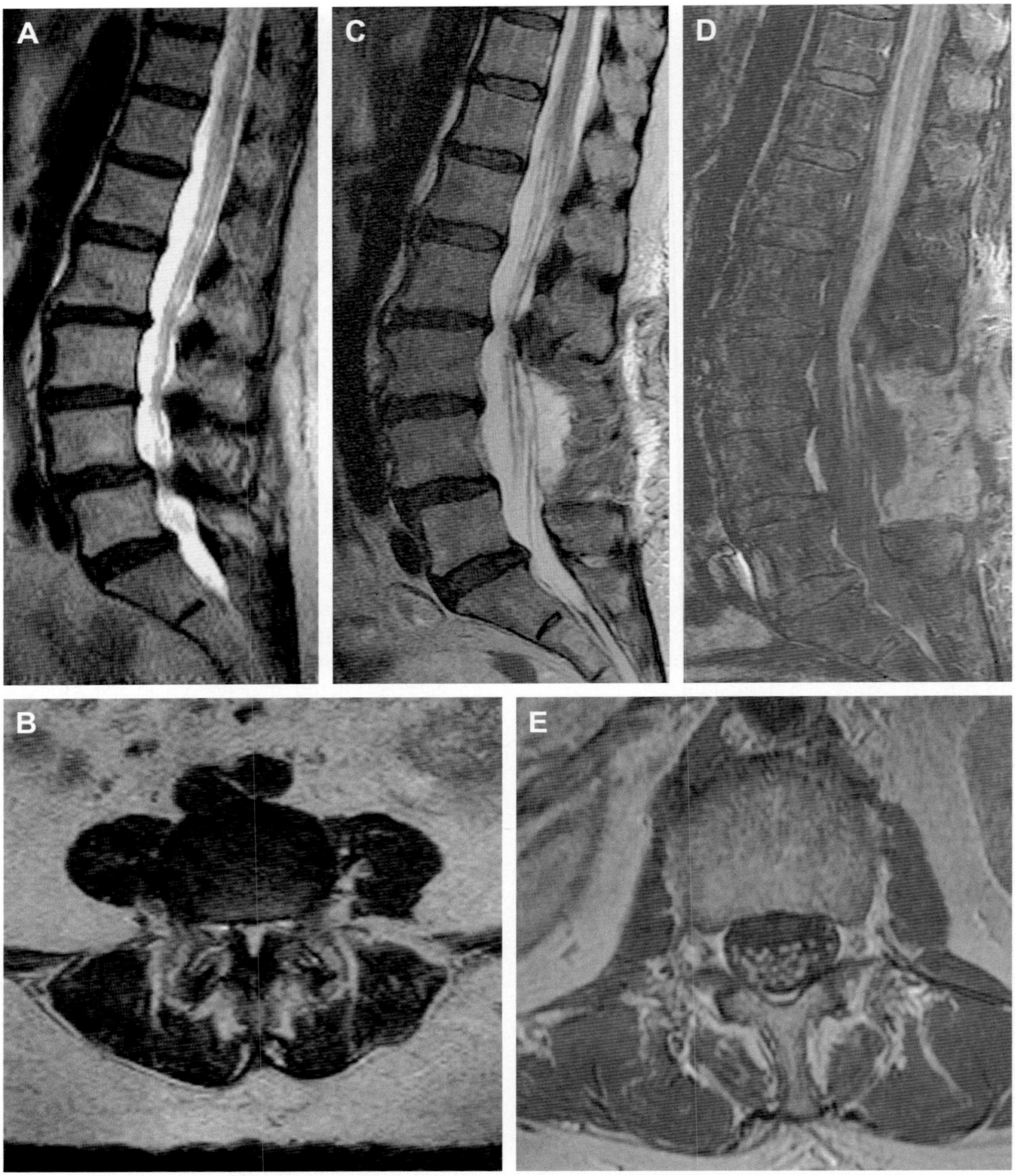

Fig. 11. A 74-year-old woman presented with bilateral lower extremity weakness and pain with a low field strength MRI from another institution. Sagittal T2 image (*A*) and axial T2 image (*B*) at the L4 level show degenerative spondylolisthesis at L4 with central canal compromise. She underwent an L3–L5 decompression without change in symptoms. A 1.5-T MRI performed 3 weeks postoperatively demonstrated nodularity in the cauda equina on a T2 sagittal image (*C*). Gadolinium-enhanced fat-saturated T1 sagittal (*D*) and axial (*E*) images demonstrate diffuse leptomeningeal metastases from breast cancer. She died in 2 months. A high-quality preoperative MRI would have likely led to the diagnosis and avoided an unnecessary operation.

in active flexion, extension, rotational, and lateral bending motions.

Upright radiographs and F/E views of the cervical and lumbar spine display spine architecture and alignment in a position of function. The role of upright radiography for the degenerative spine is well established, and should be the initial screening imaging study. F/E radiographs of either the cervical or lumbar spine may unmask instability in a very small percentage of patients; they are best applied selectively, not routinely.

Axially loaded images, obtained in a recumbent position on conventional CT or MRI scanners are able to replicate many of the changes seen in erect loading of the spine. The available literature suggests this technique may reveal central canal compromise not evident on standard recumbent imaging, and may be effective in the selection of patients for surgical intervention. This modality seems best applied to cases of clinical neurogenic intermittent claudication where recumbent imaging does not demonstrate a correlative stenosis, or in whom the symptoms are disproportionate to the imaging findings.

Upright or postural MRI is conceptually the modality of choice for dynamic imaging of the spine. It combines the superior contrast resolution of MRI with the advantages of imaging the spine in a truly functional position. Even in the immature state of upright MRI, the literature has demonstrated its potential usefulness in cases of occult stenosis, dynamic disc herniations, and spinal instability. It is not without controversy and pitfalls. It may reveal dynamic lesions that are asymptomatic, and hence exacerbate the imaging specificity fault. Current scanners are 0.6 T; limited image quality may reduce the sensitivity to the detection of systemic disease underlying the back or limb pain complaint. It is best used selectively, despite economic pressures for routine use. As engineering advances allow higher field strength scanners in this configuration, it will see more widespread utility.

Three-dimensional bony imaging via horizontal fan beam techniques, such as the EOS system, offer great promise in increasing our understanding of spinal deformities. The 3-dimensional modeling capabilities at reduced radiation exposure will also assist in planning and following complex surgical interventions in these challenging patients.

As technology improves, clinical correlation becomes more important than ever. Patients with specific, reproducible, and meaningful clinical pain and dysfunction syndromes but with unrevealing conventional imaging studies will be the best candidates for these new techniques. The clinical acumen to establish correlates between imaging and clinical picture will play an ever-increasing and important role.

REFERENCES

1. Wilke HJ, Neef P, Caimi M, et al. New in vivo measurements of pressure in the intervertebral disc in daily life. Spine (Phila Pa 1976) 1999;24:755–62.
2. Jinkins JR, Dworkin JS, Damadian RV. Upright, weight-bearing, dynamic-kinetic MRI of the spine: initial results. Eur Radiol 2005;15(9):1815–25.
3. Rihn JA, Lee JY, Khan M, et al. Does lumbar facet fluid detected on magnetic resonance imaging correlate with radiographic instability in patients with degenerative lumbar disease? Spine 2007; 32(14):1555–60.
4. Nachemson AL. Disc pressure measurements. Spine (Phila Pa 1976) 1981;6(1):93–7.
5. Inufusa A, An HS, Lim TH, et al. Anatomic changes of the spinal canal and intervertebral foramen associated with flexion-extension movement. Spine (Phila Pa 1976) 1996;21(21):2412–20.
6. Fujiwara A, An HS, Lim TH, et al. Morphologic changes in the lumbar intervertebral foramen due to flexion-extension, lateral bending, and axial rotation: an in vitro anatomic and biomechanical study. Spine (Phila Pa 1976) 2001;26(8): 876–82.
7. Schmid MR, Stucki G, Duewell S, et al. Changes in cross-sectional measurements of the spinal canal and intervertebral foramina as a function of body position: in vivo studies on an open-configuration MR system. AJR Am J Roentgenol 1999;172(4): 1095–102.
8. Danielson B, Willen J. Axially loaded magnetic resonance image of the lumbar spine in asymptomatic individuals. Spine (Phila Pa 1976) 2001;26(23): 2601–6.
9. Hansson T, Suzuki N, Hebelka H, et al. The narrowing of the lumbar spinal canal during loaded MRI: the effects of the disc and ligamentum flavum. Eur Spine J 2009;18:679–86.
10. Madsen R, Jensen TS, Pope M, et al. The effect of body position and axial load on spinal canal morphology: an MRI study of central spinal stenosis. Spine (Phila Pa 1976) 2008;33(1):617.
11. Chen IH, Vasavada A, Panjabi M. Kinematics of the cervical spine canal: changes with sagittal plane loads. J Spinal Disord 1994;7(2):93–101.
12. Muhle C, Weinert D, Falliner A, et al. Dynamic changes of the spinal canal in patients with cervical spondylosis at flexion and extension using magnetic resonance imaging. Invest Radiol 1998;33(8): 444–9.
13. Zhang L, Zeitoun D, Rangel A, et al. Preoperative evaluation of the cervical spondylotic myelopathy with flexion-extension magnetic resonance imaging: about a prospective study of fifty patients. Spine (Phila Pa 1976) 2011;36(17):E1134–9.
14. Kitagawa T, Fujiwara A, Kobayashi N, et al. Morphologic changes in the cervical neural foramen due to flexion and extension: in vivo imaging study. Spine (Phila Pa 1976) 2004;29(24):2821–5.

15. Wood KB, Kos P, et al. Effect of patient position on the sagittal-plane profile of the thoracolumbar spine. J Spinal Disord 1996;9(2):165–9.
16. Bendo JA, Ong B. Importance of correlating static and dynamic imaging studies in diagnosing degenerative lumbar spondylolisthesis. Am J Orthop 2001; 30(3):247–50.
17. Torgerson WR, Dotter WE. Comparative roentgenographic study of the asymptomatic and symptomatic lumbar spine. J Bone Joint Surg Am 1976; 58(6):850–3.
18. Simmons ED Jr, Guyer RD, et al. Radiographic assessment for patients with low back pain. Spine (Phila Pa 1976) 1995;20(16):1839–41.
19. Hammouri QM, Haims AH, et al. The utility of dynamic flexion-extension radiographs in the initial evaluation of the degenerative lumbar spine. Spine (Phila Pa 1976) 2007;32(21):2361–4.
20. Lee SW, Wong KW, et al. Development and validation of a new technique for assessing lumbar spine motion. Spine 2002;27(8):E215–20.
21. Wong KW, Luk KD, et al. Continuous dynamic spinal motion analysis. Spine 2006;31(4):414–9.
22. Harris MB, Kronlage SC, et al. Evaluation of the cervical spine in the polytrauma patient. Spine 2000;25(22):2884–91 [discussion: 2892].
23. White AP, Biswas D, et al. Utility of flexion-extension radiographs in evaluating the degenerative cervical spine. Spine 2007;32(9):975–9.
24. Hall FM. Back pain and the radiologist. Radiology 1980;137(3):861–3.
25. Cheh G, Lenke LG, Lehman RA, et al. The reliability of preoperative supine radiographs to predict the amount of curve flexibility in adolescent idiopathic scoliosis. Spine (Phila Pa 1976) 2007; 32(24):2668–72.
26. Willen J, Danielson B, et al. Dynamic effects on the lumbar spinal canal: axially loaded CT-myelography and MRI in patients with sciatica and/or neurogenic claudication. Spine (Phila Pa 1976) 1997;22(24): 2968–76.
27. North American Spine Society. Evidence-based clinical guidelines for multidisciplinary spine care, diagnosis and treatment of degenerative lumbar spinal stenosis. Burr Ridge (IL): North American Spine Society; 2011.
28. Choi KC, Kim JS, et al. Dynamic lumbar spinal stenosis: the usefulness of axial loaded MRI in preoperative evaluation. J Korean Neurosurg Soc 2009;46(3):265–8.
29. Willen J, Wessberg PJ, et al. Surgical results in hidden lumbar spinal stenosis detected by axial loaded computed tomography and magnetic resonance imaging: an outcome study. Spine (Phila Pa 1976) 2008;33(4):E109–15.
30. Wurm G, Aichholzer M, et al. Acquired torticollis due to Grisel's syndrome: case report and follow-up of non-traumatic atlantoaxial rotatory subluxation. Neuropediatrics 2004;35(2):134–8.
31. Lee S, Joyce S, et al. Asymmetry of the odontoid-lateral mass interspaces: a radiographic finding of questionable clinical significance. Ann Emerg Med 1986;15(10):1173–6.
32. Subach BR, McLaughlin MR, et al. Current management of pediatric atlantoaxial rotatory subluxation. Spine 1998;23(20):2174–9.
33. Monckeberg JE, Tome CV, et al. CT scan study of atlantoaxial rotatory mobility in asymptomatic adult subjects: a basis for better understanding C1-C2 rotatory fixation and subluxation. Spine 2009; 34(12):1292–5.
34. Been HD, Kerkhoffs GM, et al. Suspected atlantoaxial rotatory fixation-subluxation: the value of multidetector computed tomography scanning under general anesthesia. Spine 2007;32(5):E163–7.
35. McGuire KJ, Silber J, et al. Torticollis in children: can dynamic computed tomography help determine severity and treatment. J Pediatr Orthop 2002; 22(6):766–70.
36. Alyas F, Connell D, et al. Upright positional MRI of the lumbar spine. Clin Radiol 2008;63(9):1035–48.
37. Zamani AA, Moriarty T, et al. Functional MRI of the lumbar spine in erect position in a superconducting open-configuration MR system: preliminary results. J Magn Reson Imaging 1998;8(6): 1329–33.
38. Gilbert JW, Wheeler GR, et al. Imaging in the position that causes pain. Surg Neurol 2008;69(5): 463–5 [discussion: 465].
39. Gilbert JW, Wheeler GR, et al. Open stand-up MRI: a new instrument for positional neuroimaging. J Spinal Disord Tech 2006;19(2):151–4.
40. Epstein NE, Hyman RA, et al. "Dynamic" MRI scanning of the cervical spine. Spine (Phila Pa 1976) 1988;13(8):937–8.
41. Schlamann M, Reischke L, et al. Dynamic magnetic resonance imaging of the cervical spine using the NeuroSwing System. Spine (Phila Pa 1976) 2007; 32(21):2398–401.
42. Berthelot JM, Maugars Y, et al. Magnetic resonance imaging for lumbar disk pathology. incidence of false negatives. Presse Med 1995;24(29):1329–31 [in French].
43. Saifuddin A, Blease S, et al. Axial loaded MRI of the lumbar spine. Clin Radiol 2003;58(9):661–71.
44. Zou J, Yang H, et al. Dynamic bulging of intervertebral discs in the degenerative lumbar spine. Spine (Phila Pa 1976) 2009;34(23):2545–50.
45. Weishaupt D, Schmid MR, et al. Positional MR imaging of the lumbar spine: does it demonstrate nerve root compromise not visible at conventional MR imaging? Radiology 2000;215(1):247–53.
46. Arbit E, Pannullo S. Lumbar stenosis: a clinical review. Clin Orthop Relat Res 2001;(384):137–43.

47. Vitzthum HE, Konig A, et al. Dynamic examination of the lumbar spine by using vertical, open magnetic resonance imaging. J Neurosurg 2000;93(Suppl 1):58–64.
48. Niggemann P, Kuchta J, et al. Spondylolysis and spondylolisthesis: prevalence of different forms of instability and clinical implications. Spine (Phila Pa 1976) 2011;36(22):E1463–8.
49. Karadimas EJ, Siddiqui M, et al. Positional MRI changes in supine versus sitting postures in patients with degenerative lumbar spine. J Spinal Disord Tech 2006;19(7):495–500.
50. Kong MH, Morishita Y, et al. Lumbar segmental mobility according to the grade of the disc, the facet joint, the muscle, and the ligament pathology by using kinetic magnetic resonance imaging. Spine (Phila Pa 1976) 2009;34(23):2537–44.
51. Kong MH, Hymanson HJ, et al. Kinetic magnetic resonance imaging analysis of abnormal segmental motion of the functional spine unit. J Neurosurg Spine 2009;10(4):357–65.
52. Penning L, Wilmink JT. Rotation of the cervical spine. A CT study in normal subjects. Spine 1987;12(8):732–8.
53. Ishii T, Mukai Y, et al. Kinematics of the cervical spine in lateral bending: in vivo three-dimensional analysis. Spine 2006;31(2):155–60.
54. Ishii T, Mukai Y, et al. Kinematics of the subaxial cervical spine in rotation in vivo three-dimensional analysis. Spine 2004;29(24):2826–31.
55. Crispino M, Gasparotti R, et al. Magnetic resonance myelography. Preliminary experience. Radiol Med 1995;89(1–2):42–8.
56. Charpak G. La detection des particules. Recherche 1981;128:1384–96.
57. Kalifa G, Charpak Y, et al. Evaluation of a new low-dose digital x-ray device: first dosimetric and clinical results in children. Pediatr Radiol 1998;28(7): 557–61.
58. Le Bras A, Laporte S, et al. 3D detailed reconstruction of vertebrae with low dose digital stereoradiography. Stud Health Technol Inform 2002;91:286–90.
59. Deschenes S, Charron G, et al. Diagnostic imaging of spinal deformities: reducing patients' radiation dose with a new slot-scanning X-ray imager. Spine (Phila Pa 1976) 2010;35(9):989–94.
60. Rousseau MA, Laporte S, et al. Reproducibility of measuring the shape and three-dimensional position of cervical vertebrae in upright position using the EOS stereoradiography system. Spine (Phila Pa 1976) 2007;32(23):2569–72.
61. Illes T, Tunyogi-Csapo M, et al. Breakthrough in three-dimensional scoliosis diagnosis: significance of horizontal plane view and vertebra vectors. Eur Spine J 2011;20(1):135–43.
62. Morvan G, Mathieu P, et al. Standardized way for imaging of the sagittal spinal balance. Eur Spine J 2011;20(Suppl 5):602–8.

Degenerative Joint Disease of the Spine

Nikolai Bogduk, BSc(Med), MB, BS, PhD, MD, DSc, MMed, Dip Anat, FAFMM, FAFRM, FFPM(ANZCA)[a,b,*]

KEYWORDS

• Lumbar • Cervical • Degeneration • Disk • Zygapophysial joint

KEY POINTS

- Degenerative changes are an expression of metabolic stress in spinal joints.
- Genetic factors predispose to degenerative changes, but age is the strongest correlate.
- Degenerative changes do not constitute a diagnosis because there is little, if any, correlation with pain.
- In contrast, the morphologic and biophysical features of internal disk disruption correlate strongly with back pain, as do certain magnetic resonance features.

INTRODUCTION

Throughout the vertebral column, consecutive vertebrae are connected by a triad of joints: an intervertebral disk and a pair of zygapophysial joints. These joints can show changes that have attracted various labels, each using the adjective degenerative. These labels include degenerative disk disease, disk degeneration, and degenerative joint disease. This is an unfortunate adjective because it can imply a hostile process, a noxious process, or a condition that qualifies as a diagnosis for spinal pain. Each of these implications is wrong.

The word degeneration implies falling apart or decaying, with the further implication that the process is inexorable and incurable. This meaning might not be what radiologists intend, but it is what many patients perceive the word to mean.[1–3] Moreover, patients explicitly associate it with poorer prognosis.[3] Yet the biologic evidence shows that the changes in question are neither destructive nor malevolent. What is destructive is the fear that a rubric such as degenerative evokes in patients. It tells them that they have an incurable disease when, in truth, they do not.

> Degenerative joint disease is a disturbing label that patients associate with a poor prognosis.

The most common reason why patients undergo imaging of the spine is pain. In the past, degenerative disk disease, or degenerative joint disease, was invoked as the diagnosis for that pain. It is still maintained in some circles, particularly in medicolegal disputes, that the patient's pain can be attributed to preexisting degenerative changes. Yet there is no known mechanism whereby degenerative changes can be painful, and the epidemiologic evidence shows that they are not. This evidence precludes degeneration from being used as a diagnosis for spinal pain.

DEFINITION

There is no universally accepted, comprehensive definition of degeneration. It means different things to different experts, depending on what they look at and the tools with which they look. To a biochemist, degeneration means changes in proteoglycans,

[a] University of Newcastle, Callaghan, New South Wales, Australia; [b] Newcastle Bone and Joint Institute, Royal Newcastle Centre, PO Box 664J, Newcastle, New South Wales 2300, Australia
* Newcastle Bone and Joint Institute, Royal Newcastle Centre, PO Box 664J, Newcastle, New South Wales 2300, Australia.
E-mail address: vickin.caesar@hnehealth.nsw.gov.au

Radiol Clin N Am 50 (2012) 613–628
doi:10.1016/j.rcl.2012.04.012
0033-8389/12/$ – see front matter

radiologic.theclinics.com

changes in the relative proportions of different proteoglycans, changes in the type of collagen, and changes in water concentration. To a pathologist, degeneration means osteophytes, desiccation, fragmentation, and fissures. To a radiologist, degeneration can mean osteophytes, loss of disk height or loss of joint space, subchondral sclerosis, or reduced signal intensity on magnetic resonance (MR) imaging, or altered shape of the disk.

Nevertheless, it is possible to unify this spectrum. Degeneration is not a disease; it is the way that joints express themselves in response to insults. Moreover, connective tissues are limited in how they might express themselves, and degeneration may be the only available means by which a joint might respond to an insult. The clinical significance of degenerative changes lies not in the changes themselves but in what precipitates them. Sometimes the causes are clinically significant; sometimes they are not. Clinical significance arises if and when the changes are a manifestation of a systemic, metabolic disorder. Clinical significance evaporates when the changes are no more than a correlate of age. The responsibility of physicians lies not in simply recognizing degenerative changes, but in determining why they have arisen.

BIOLOGY

At a molecular level, intervertebral disks and synovial joints are essentially similar. The nucleus pulposus is homologous to articular cartilage; the anulus fibrosus is homologous to the joint capsule; and the vertebral end plate is homologous to subchondral bone. The nucleus pulposus and articular cartilage both contain water held by proteoglycans, which, in turn, are bound by collagen. They differ only with respect to the exact type of proteoglycans and the size of the aggregates that they form. Consequently, descriptions of the molecular biology of synovial joints effectively apply to intervertebral disks, and vice versa.

In disks and in articular cartilage, homeostasis is maintained by chondrocytes (**Fig. 1**).[4] Fibroblasts are responsible in joint capsules, and fibroblasts or chondrocytes are responsible in the anulus fibrosus. The chondrocytes exercise both synthesis and degradation. They synthesize the proteoglycans that form the matrix of the nucleus or articular cartilage, and the collagen that binds the matrix or forms the anulus fibrosus or joint capsule. Once formed, the matrix attracts and holds water. The matrix components are in slow, but constant turnover. To make way for refreshed components, old components must be removed. This goal is achieved by metalloproteases than can degrade proteoglycans and collagen. Chemical agents that promote synthesis include transforming growth factor, basic fibroblast growth factor, and insulinlike growth factor. Cytokines that promote degradation are tumor necrosis factor α and interleukin-1. Degradation is also promoted by superoxide radicals and nitric oxide.

If, for whatever reason, the balance between synthesis and degradation is disturbed to favor degradation, so-called degenerative changes occur (see **Fig. 1**). These changes are expressed at the molecular level by changes in the nature and concentration of various proteoglycans, and their ability to hold water; cross-linking occurs in the collagen both in the matrix and in the capsule or anulus fibrosus. At the microscopic level, the components fibrose, and can crack or tear. Macroscopically, the matrix can thin and fragment. Cross-linking of collagen stiffens it, which can be detected biomechanically or expressed clinically as reduced range of movement. Dehydration depressurizes the matrix, and is reflected as reduced signal intensity on MR imaging.

> Degenerative changes are the expression of an imbalance between synthesis and degradation of the matrix of intervertebral disks or articular cartilage.

These changes occur as a final common pathway, essentially irrespective of what triggers it. Triggers could act on the chondrocyte, or directly on the matrix or the enzymes that degrade it. The chondrocyte might be impaired genetically, by metabolic factors, or by physical factors. Toxins might accumulate in the matrix. Cytokines, superoxide, or nitric oxide could be released into the matrix by exogenous inflammatory cells, such as macrophages, that invade the matrix in response to injury. Each of these triggers results in the same consequences, but the appearance of those consequences does not reflect the trigger.

Perplexing, as a feature of degeneration, are osteophytes. They do not share the negative properties of other features. They are not breaches of integrity as are cracks and tears; they are not deficiencies as are dehydration and thinning. Rather, they are new, and have to be synthesized (as opposed to degraded). Teleologically, osteophytes are easier to view as adaptive remodeling. They are attempts to increase the surface area of the joint so as to reduce the point pressure throughout a joint that is suffering excessive compression loads. That remodeling might occur in a relatively normal joint that is exposed to excessive external loads, or it might occur as a response in a joint in which the

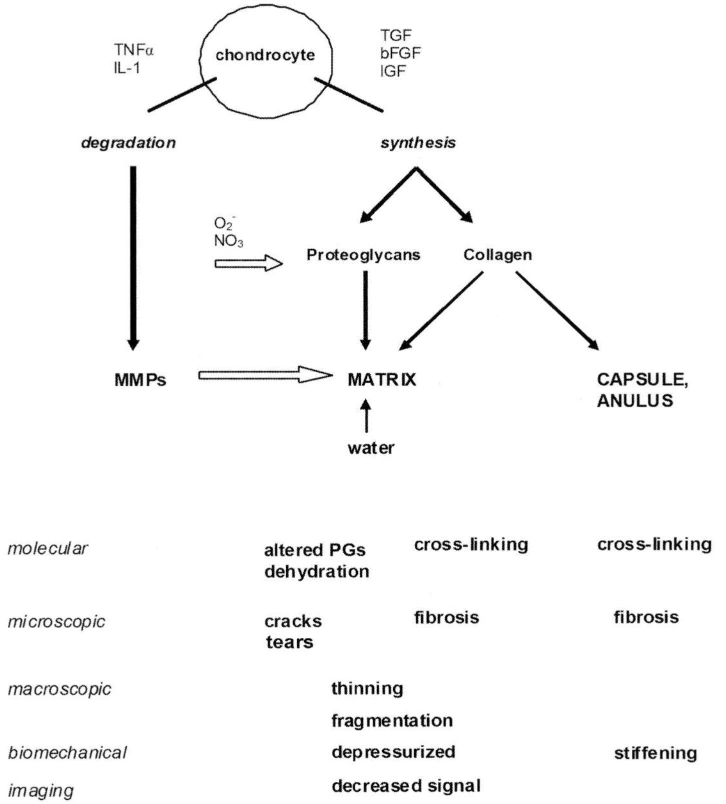

Fig. 1. The biology of degenerative changes in the disk and synovial joints. In a normal joint, the chondrocytes maintain a balance between the synthesis and degradation of the matrix and the collagen of the joint capsule or anulus fibrosus. Synthesis is promoted by growth factors such as transforming growth factor (TGF), basic fibroblast growth factor (bFGF), and insulinlike growth factor (IGF). Degradation is achieved by the action of metalloproteases, whose synthesis is activated by tumor necrosis factor α (TNFα) and interleukin-1 (IL-1). Other molecules that can degrade the matrix are superoxide (O_2^-) and nitric oxide (NO_3). Degradation of the matrix, and associated changes in the joint capsule, can be expressed by various molecular, microscopic, macroscopic, and biomechanical features, and some can be shown by medical imaging.

capacity to bear loads has been compromised by degradation of the matrix.

REGIONAL DIFFERENCES

At a macroscopic level, the structure and biomechanics of joints in the cervical spine and lumbar spine differ. These differences modify the expression of degenerative changes at different sites in the vertebral column, and their potential causes.

> Cervical disks differ from lumbar disks in their anatomic structure and their expression of degenerative changes.

Cervical disks differ in structure from lumbar disks.[5] Cervical disks lack a concentric anulus fibrosus; the anulus is well developed only anteriorly, where it serves more as an interosseous ligament, and not as a circumferential constraint around the nucleus.[5] The nucleus pulposus is relatively small at birth and persists until the second decade of life, but thereafter it gradually disappears,[6] leaving a firm, dry plate of fibrocartilage. As a result, cervical disk changes are harder, drier, and more physical in nature than those of lumbar disks. They tend to express themselves as internal cracks and fissures, and slowly developing, fibrocartilaginous bulges and osteophytes.[7] Transverse fissures across the posterior segments of cervical disks are normal.[7,8] They appear in childhood and are fully established by the third decade.

They are essential for allowing axial rotation of the typical cervical spinal segments.[9] In contrast, degenerative changes in lumbar disks are more chemical in nature: expressed as changes in the proteoglycans and hydration of the nucleus, which are reflected by demonstrable changes in the internal structure and signal intensity of these disks, when viewed with MR imaging.

The cervical zygapophysial joints face upwards as well as backward and, therefore, share equally with the intervertebral disks in bearing axial, compression loads. Therefore, mechanical insults affecting these joints are most likely to arise from weight bearing. Degenerative chances in the cervical zygapophysial joints occur at all segmental levels but more commonly in the joints of the C3 and C4 vertebrae.[7]

The lumbar zygapophysial joints face posteriorly and laterally, and share little of the axial load, which is borne almost entirely by the intervertebral disks. The zygapophysial joints resist axial rotation, and their anterior ends resist anterior translation (listhesis). Consonant with the latter, degenerative changes arise earlier, and are more advanced, in the anteromedial regions of the joints, which resist translation.[10] Degenerative changes are more common in the joints of the L4 and L5 vertebrae.[11]

> Cervical and lumbar zygapophysial joints differ in their biomechanics and the factors that might initiate degenerative changes.

CAUSE

Specific metabolic causes of degenerative disk disease are rare. They are limited to diabetes mellitus and ochronosis.[4] The disks of patients with diabetes mellitus have reduced hexosamine content, deficiencies of proteoglycan synthesis, and reduced concentrations of keratosulfate, which is a critical component of proteoglycans.[4] Ochronosis produces deposits of a black pigment derived from homogentisic acid, which ostensibly impedes the normal metabolism of the disk matrix.[4]

Impaired nutrition has been promoted as a cause of disk degeneration, largely from laboratory studies, but incriminating, epidemiologic evidence is lacking. Measurable parameters of impaired nutrition, such as vascular disease and smoking, correlate only weakly with degenerative changes.[4]

Low-grade infection has been explored as a cause of disk degeneration, but studies to date have not yielded consistent results. Whereas some have incriminated certain organisms, others have not been able to confirm the findings.[4]

> Specific metabolic causes of degenerative changes are rare, and the evidence is weak for nutrition or infection as a cause.

The strongest relationship with degenerative changes (both in intervertebral disks and in zygapophysial joints) is with age. The prevalence of disk degeneration clearly increases with age, both in the cervical spine[12–14] and in the lumbar spine,[15–17] as does the prevalence of osteoarthritis of cervical[18] and lumbar[19] zygapophysial joints (**Tables 1–4**). This relationship implies a variety of possible, causative factors acting alone or in combination.

> Age is the strongest correlate of degenerative changes.
>
> Degenerative changes are normal age changes.

Chondrocytes might be subject to an innate senescence. With the passage of time they become less able to maintain the homeostasis of the matrix. They might have genetic abnormalities that affect the quality of the matrix that they produce, or the function of otherwise normal cells might become impaired by the accumulation over time of toxins or mechanical stresses.

In this regard, the zygapophysial joints have not been explicitly studied, but it seems reasonable to include these joints under the umbrella of synovial joints in general. The prevailing view is that osteoarthrosis is the result of various combinations of factors such as genetic predisposition, obesity, previous injury, abnormal biomechanics, and overload on the joint.[20]

For lumbar disk degeneration, the evidence is more explicit. Studies of twins have provided major insights into the cause of lumbar disk degeneration. Studies of twins have the advantage of providing natural controls for demographic, anthropometric, and social factors, which allows other factors of interest to be brought into relief. Such studies have examined the determinants of certain signs of disk degeneration such as signal intensity on MR imaging, disk height, and disk bulging. They have shown that biomechanical factors, such as lifting heavy loads or heavy leisure activities, account for only some of the variance between presence and absence of degenerative changes. Larger proportions are explained by genetic factors.

At upper lumbar levels, age, occupational, and environmental factors account for only 16% of the variance, whereas genetic factors account for

Table 1
The number of asymptomatic individuals who show features of spondylosis, by gender and age

Feature	20–25	30–35	40–45	50–55	60–65
Men by Age Group (y) (N = 20 in each group)					
Narrowing	0	1	4	13	15
Sclerosis	0	1	1	10	13
Anterior osteophytes	1	5	7	16	19
Posterior osteophytes	0	1	4	10	14
Any of the above	1	5	7	16	19
Women by Age Group (y) (N = 20 in each group)					
Narrowing	0	2	6	9	13
Sclerosis	0	0	5	7	6
Anterior osteophytes	0	3	6	13	11
Posterior osteophytes	0	1	5	8	12
Any of the above	0	4	7	14	14
Men and Women by Age Group (y) (N = 40 in each group)					
Narrowing	0	1	4	13	15
Sclerosis	0	1	1	10	13
Anterior osteophytes	1	5	7	16	19
Posterior osteophytes	0	1	4	10	14
Any of the above	1	5	7	16	19

Data from Gore DR, Sepic SB, Gardner GM. Roentgenographic findings of the cervical spine in asymptomatic people. Spine 1986;1:521–4.

61%.[21] At lower lumbar levels, age and physical loading account for 11% of the variance, and genetic factors account for 32%.[21] The remaining 57% of the variance remains unexplained.[21] Genetic factors may be more influential in women.[22]

Genetic factors constitute a predisposition to degenerative changes, but are not the sole cause.

The relationship to genetic factors is complex. Candidate genes include variants of the genes for proteoglycans, different types of collagen, various interleukins, metalloprotease-3, and the vitamin D receptor.[23,24] Each variant creates a difference in the molecular composition of the structure that it produces, which in turn compromises the function of that structure. Although statistically more common, individual variants occur in only a few individuals affected by disk degeneration,[21] and their prevalence differs in different ethnic populations.[4] Whereas some are common in Scandinavian populations, they are uncommon or absent in Chinese populations; other genes have a converse relative prevalence.[4] However, no single gene is responsible. Rather, the effects of various genes seem to be summative. Certain variants affect signal intensity, whereas other variants affect disk height; and whereas certain variants affect all segmental levels, others affect only lower lumbar levels.[25] Consequently, the phenotype expressed depends on how many and which variants occur in the genotype.

Multiple genetic factors interact in a summative manner, but the prevalence of different genetic aberrations differs in different populations.

However, disk degeneration is not a congenital disease. The evidence does not show that genetic factors cause disk degeneration. Rather, it shows that genetic factors predispose individuals, or render them susceptible, to developing degenerative changes. What those factors are has yet to be determined. However, although an explanation for degenerative changes remains an intellectual puzzle, for clinical purposes an explanation

Table 2
The prevalence of radiologic features of the cervical spine in asymptomatic individuals

Feature	Number of Subjects by Age (y) <30	30–40	40–50	>50
Normal	24	18	18	2
Osteophytes	0	3	7	14
Narrowing of disk space	0	0	7	18
Sclerosis of articular surface	0	0	0	7
Osteoporosis	0	0	0	4
Calcification of anterior ligament	0	0	0	4
Loss of lordosis	0	0	0	4
Number of patients	24	21	32	25
Males	5	7	20	18
Females	19	14	12	7

Data from Elias F. Roentgen findings in the asymptomatic cervical spine. N Y State J Med 1958;58:3300–3.

Table 4
The prevalence of lumbar disk degeneration in asymptomatic individuals of various ages

Source (Ref.)	Degeneration	Age Group (y) 18–29	30–39	40–49	≥50
17	Severe	0.28	0.31	0.35	0.59
	Mild	0.14	0.17	0.35	0.29
	Total	0.42	0.48	0.70	0.88
15	Any	0.34		0.59	0.93
		20–39		40–59	60–80
		Age Group (y)			

Data from Boden SD, Davis DO, Dina TS, et al. Abnormal magnetic-resonance scans of the lumbar spine in asymptomatic subjects. A prospective investigation. J Bone Joint Surg Am 1990;72:403–8; and Cheung KM, Karpinnen J, Chan D, et al. Prevalence and pattern of lumbar magnetic resonance imaging changes in a population study of one thousand forty-three individuals. Spine 2009;34:934–40.

becomes effectively irrelevant, because degenerative changes are not symptomatic.

CORRELATIONS

One method of determining if a morphologic feature is responsible for pain is to compare its prevalence in people who have pain and people who do not have pain. If the prevalence is significantly higher in those with pain, an association is established and a search for the mechanism that links the 2 features can be undertaken. On the other hand, if the prevalence is not significantly higher, the morphologic feature is refuted as having any association with pain. Such studies have been conducted in the context of degenerative changes of joints of the spine. The literature is most abundant for the lumbar spine, but is not lacking for the cervical spine. The thoracic spine has not been studied in the same way.

Another method is to anesthetize joints that express degenerative changes, in patients with spinal pain. If the pain is relieved, then the target joint is implicated as the source of pain, and the degenerative changes might be responsible. On the other hand, if anesthetizing the joint does not relieve the pain, then the joint and the degenerative changes are refuted as being responsible for the pain.

For the cervical spine, a study conducted in a hospital radiology department matched patients presenting with neck pain with control patients who had cervical spine radiographs for other reasons, such as barium swallows.[26] Across all ages, there were no statistically significant differences between cases and controls in the prevalence of spondylosis, severe disk changes, or degenerative changes in the synovial joints (**Table 5**).

A similar study found a significantly higher prevalence of degenerative changes in the C5-6 disk of symptomatic patients, but not at any other level

Table 3
The prevalence of abnormalities on MR imaging of the cervical spine in asymptomatic individuals

Feature	Prevalence (%) Age <40 y N = 167 Major	Minor	Age >40 y N = 97 Major	Minor
Herniated disk	3	4	1	4
Bulging disk	0	5	1	5
Foraminal stenosis	3	4	9	14
Disk narrowing	2	11	16	22
Degenerated disk	8	—	37	—
Spondylosis	3	14	6	34
Cord impingement	9	9	1	18

Data from Boden SD, McCowin PR, Davis DG, et al. Abnormal magnetic-resonance scans of the cervical spine in asymptomatic subjects: a prospective investigation. J Bone Joint Surg Am 1990;72:1178–84.

Table 5
The prevalence of spondylosis and associated features in patients with and without neck symptoms attending a hospital radiology department over a 12-month period

	N		Spondylosis (%)		Severe Disk Changes (%)		Severe Joint Changes (%)	
Age (y)	Case	Control	Case	Control	Case	Control	Case	Control
Men								
<40	63	29	21	10	6	3		
40–59	98	64	65	58	41	39	1	8
>60	93	54	90	89	88	62	28	21
Women								
<40	127	31	14	13	6	3		
40–59	166	98	58	56	39	29	7	5
>60	106	89	85	88	79	61	16	21

Data from Heller CA, Stanley P, Lewis-Jones B, et al. Value of x-ray examinations of the cervical spine. Br Med J 1983;287:1276–8.

(**Fig. 2**).[27] That study also showed no significant differences in the prevalence of degenerative changes in the cervical zygapophysial joints at any segmental level; the prevalence tended to be higher in asymptomatic individuals (see **Fig. 2**).

Degenerative changes in the cervical intervertebral disks or zygapophysial joints do not correlate with neck pain.

Two lines of evidence have refuted osteoarthrosis of the lumbar zygapophysial joints (facet arthropathy) as a cause of back pain. A large population study using plain radiography[28] and a smaller one using computed tomography (CT)[19] found osteoarthrosis to be equally prevalent in individuals with no pain as in patients with back pain (**Tables 6** and **7**). Osteoarthrosis was more common in older patients, irrespective of pain (see **Table 7**).[19] A third study graded the severity of arthropathy, as seen on CT, of joints that were anesthetized using placebo-controlled intra-articular blocks.[29] It found no difference in the grade of arthropathy between joints that were painful and those that were not.

Many studies have studied the prevalence of disk degeneration in individuals with and without back pain. A systematic review rated these as either low-quality or high-quality studies.[30] Using only the data from high-quality studies, no clinically significant association between degenerative changes and low back pain emerges (**Table 8**). The association is even less if all studies are included.

The statistics associated with these data reveal clinically insignificant correlations. A specificity of 0.58 means that 42% of the population have asymptomatic degenerative changes. A sensitivity

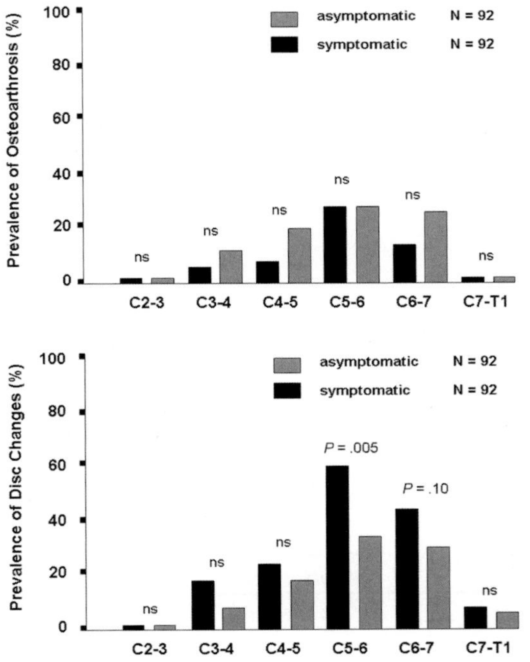

Fig. 2. Histograms showing the relative prevalence of degenerative changes in the cervical intervertebral disks and cervical zygapophysial joints in individuals with and without neck pain. (*Data from* Fridenberg ZB, Miller WT. Degenerative disc disease of the cervical spine. A comparative study of asymptomatic and symptomatic patients. J Bone Joint Surg Am 1963;45:1171–8.)

Table 6
A contingency table showing lack of association between various grades of osteoarthrosis of the lumbar spine and back pain in a large population study

	Osteoarthrosis		
	Grade 0–1	Grade 2	Grade 3
Pain	398	82	19
No pain	403	60	15

($\chi^2 = 3.46$, $P = .177$).

Data from Lawrence JS, Bremner JM, Bier F. Osteoarthrosis. Prevalence in the population and relationship between symptoms and x-ray changes. Ann Rheum Dis 1966;25:1–24.

of 0.56 means that 56% of the population with back pain have degenerative changes. Combining the 2 figures reveals that 42 of the 56% of patients with back pain and degenerative changes (ie, 75%; 42/56) have degenerative changes that are not symptomatic. Therefore, in a given patient, the odds are overwhelmingly in favor of the degenerative changes being not relevant to the pain. Under those conditions, the 25% whose pain might be caused by degeneration cannot be distinguished from the 75% in whom it is not.

> Degenerative changes in the lumbar intervertebral disks or zygapophysial joints do not correlate with back pain.

Table 7
A contingency table showing lack of association between osteoarthrosis of the lumbar zygapophysial joints and back pain across various ages.[19] None of the proportions is significantly different from another, using a Fisher exact test

	Age Group (y)					
	<40	40–49	50–59	60–69	>70	All
Back pain	1	3	11	8	1	24
Proportion	0.25	0.75	0.61	1.00	0.50	0.65
No back pain	5	18	38	25	8	94
Proportion	0.25	0.42	0.83	0.89	0.70	0.64

Data from Kalichman L, Li L, Kim DH, et al. Facet joint osteoarthritis and low back pain in the community-based population. Spine 2008;33:2560–5.

Similar results arise from studies that used MR imaging.[17,41–43] Features such as reduced signal intensity, altered shape of the nucleus pulposus, reduced disk height, and anular tears are only marginally more common in individuals who report a history of back pain, with odds ratios only in the range between 1.5 and 2.6.[42] A systematic review[44] concluded that the evidence was insufficient to implicate degenerative changes as the cause of back pain.

INTERNAL DISK DISRUPTION

Internal disk disruption is a condition that affects lumbar intervertebral disks. It has been interpreted and misrepresented as representing degenerative changes, but it does not. Moreover, it is a condition that does correlate with pain.

Definition

Internal disk disruption is characterized by the presence of isolated, radial fissures penetrating from the nucleus pulposus into the anulus fibrosus but without breaching the outer anulus. The presence of a fissure distinguishes an affected disk from a normal disk, and the presence of a single fissure distinguishes the disk from those affected by widespread degenerative changes.

> Internal disk disruption is characterized by isolated radial fissures through the anulus fibrosus of lumbar intervertebral disks.

The fissures can be graded according to the extent to which they penetrate the anulus (**Fig. 3**). Grade I, II, and III fissures reach the inner, middle, and outer third of the anulus, respectively.[45] If a grade III fissure spreads circumferentially around the annulus, it is promoted to grade IV.[46]

Diagnosis

The conventional means of diagnosing internal disk disruption is postdiskography CT scanning. The diskography places contrast medium into the nucleus and into any fissures that may be present, whereas CT scanning shows the radial and circumferential nature of the fissure.

Cause

Internal disk disruption arises as a result of injury to the overlying vertebral end plate. This condition can occur as a result of a sudden, severe

Table 8
The validity of finding degenerative changes on plain radiographs as a diagnosis of low back pain

Source (Ref.)	Degenerative Changes	Back Pain Present	Back Pain Absent	Sensitivity	Specificity
31,32	Present	130	92	0.55	0.61
	Absent	106	142		
31,32	Present	170	135	0.72	0.44
	Absent	66	106		
33	Present	90	61	0.46	0.68
	Absent	105	127		
34	Present	45	19	0.23	0.80
	Absent	151	77		
35	Present	115	71	0.32	0.77
	Absent	243	237		
36	Present	39	42	0.58	0.70
	Absent	28	100		
37	Present	462	360	0.59	0.52
	Absent	320	390		
38	Present	55	77	0.75	0.37
	Absent	18	45		
39	Present	139	51	0.80	0.45
	Absent	35	41		
40	Present	177	35	0.81	0.36
	Absent	41	20		
Pooled	Present	1422	943	0.56	0.58
	Absent	1113	1285		

compression injury, or it can occur as a result of fatigue failure of the end plate.

Biomechanics studies have shown that vertebral end plates are susceptible to fatigue failure.[47] When subjected to repeated compression loads as small as 50% to 60% of the ultimate tensile strength of the end plate, the end plate can fracture after as few as 100 repetitions.[48,49]

The end-plate fracture constitutes an insult to the underlying disk, and precipitates degradation of the matrix. The mechanism remains uncertain. The injury might trigger an inflammatory response in the matrix, or the trigger might be more subtle: a reduction in pH in the region of the injury that increases the activity of metalloproteases that degrade the matrix. Nevertheless, it has now been shown in animal studies that deliberately fracturing the end plate results in chemical changes in the matrix akin to those of degeneration, namely changes in proteoglycans and glycosaminoglycans, and progressive dehydration of the nucleus.[50–52]

> Biomechanics studies and animal studies implicate end-plate injury as the cause of internal disk disruption.

How radial fissures develop has not been established, but a possible explanation is that once the matrix is degraded it no longer braces the anulus from buckling inwards. Continued normal activities of daily living might then progressively tear elements of the unsupported anulus.

Once the nuclear matrix has been degraded, the ability of the nucleus to sustain compression loads is compromised. This situation is evident from the internal biomechanics of the affected disk.

Biomechanics

Internal stresses within a disk can be measured using stress profilometry.[47,53] If a transducer

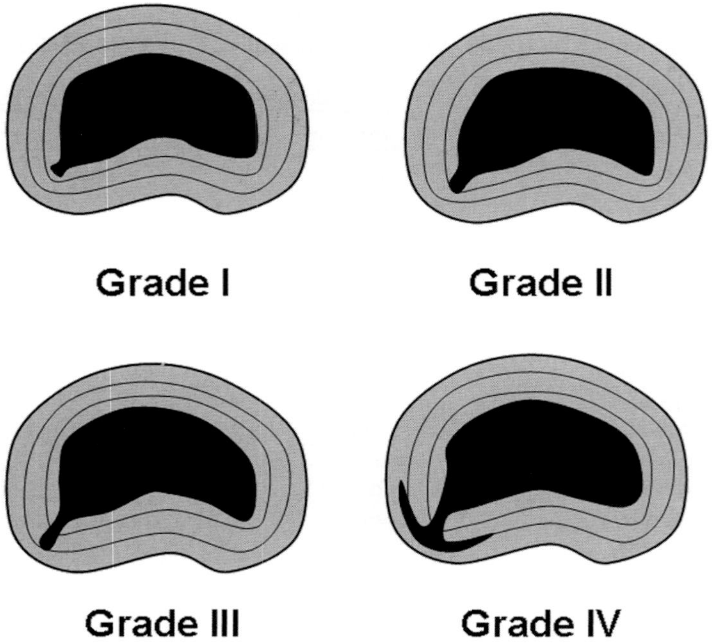

Fig. 3. The appearance of various grades of radial fissures in lumbar intervertebral disks.

probe is inserted into a disk and progressively withdrawn, it can be used to measure ambient stresses across the diameter (profile) of the disk.

In a normal disk, internal stresses are uniform. The outer, ligamentous anulus shows no compression stresses, but the inner anulus and the nucleus show compression stresses that are uniform across the nucleus but with a small peak in the posterior anulus (**Fig. 4**).[47,53]

> Internally disrupted disks show distinctly abnormal distributions of stress in the nucleus pulposus and posterior anulus.

In a disk with internal disruption, the internal stresses are irregular and reduced in magnitude, in some disks and in some regions reducing to zero.[47,53] This observation means that the nucleus is not bearing compression loads normally. As a result, the posterior anulus comes to bear more than its accustomed share of the axial load, and shows increased stresses (see **Fig. 4**). In laboratory experiments using cadaver disks, these biophysical features are precipitated immediately after the end plate fails.[47]

Correlations

Radial fissures are neither degenerative nor age changes. They occur independently of age or degenerative changes.[54] However, they are strongly associated with the affected disk being painful on diskography (**Tables 9** and **10**).

The biophysical features of internal disk disruption also correlate with the disk being painful. Decreased nuclear stress and increased stress in the posterior anulus each, independently, correlate with reproduction of pain (**Table 11**).[58]

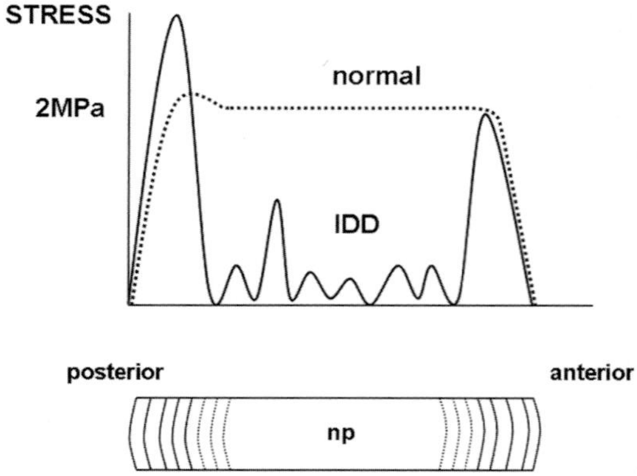

Fig. 4. The features of a normal disk and one affected by internal disk disruption (IDD) under stress profilometry. The graph shows the magnitude of the stresses within the disk across a diameter that pass from the anterior anulus to the posterior anulus. In a normal disk, the stresses are uniform. In a disk with IDD, the stresses in the nucleus pulposus (np) are irregular, decreased, and may be zero, but the stress in the posterior anulus is increased substantially more than normal.

Table 9
The association between the grade of anular disruption and reproduction of pain by disk stimulation. The numbers refer to the number of patients showing the features tabulated

	Anulus Disruption			
Pain Reproduction	Grade III	Grade II	Grade I	Grade 0
Exact	43	29	6	4
Similar	32	36	21	8
Dissimilar	9	11	6	2
None	16	24	67	86

$\chi^2 = 148$; $P<.001$.
Data from Moneta GB, Videman T, Kaivanto K, et al. Reported pain during lumbar discography as a function of anular ruptures and disc degeneration. A re-analysis of 833 discograms. Spine 1994;17:1968–74.

> Radial fissures correlate strongly with the disk being painful.
>
> Decreased nucleus stress and increased posterior anulus stress each correlate with the disk being painful.

Two features evident on MR imaging are signs of internal disk disruption. Modic changes reflect current or past inflammatory responses around the end plate, whereas high-intensity zones reflect circumferential tears. Each of these MR imaging features independently correlates with the affected disk being painful. Not all studies agree on this conclusion but most are consistent (**Tables 12** and **13**). Studies have differed on the sensitivity of these signs (ie, how well and how often they can be detected), but all studies agree that the signs are highly specific (ie, when present, they are unlikely to be false-positive signs that the affected disk is painful).

> High-intensity zones and Modic changes correlate with the disk being painful.

Mechanisms of Pain

For understandable reasons, the mechanisms by which internal disk disruption evokes pain have not been directly studied. Patients have not volunteered to have their disks explored with microelectrodes to sample or deliver potentially noxious chemicals, or with probes that might mechanically stress selected zones of the disk. Nevertheless, the circumstantial evidence allows for 2 models or a combination thereof.

Two features of internal disk disruption are pivotal to explaining how it becomes painful. First, the clinical data indicate that grade III and IV fissures are most likely to be painful. This finding suggests that nuclear material must have access to the outer third of the anulus, which is where the nociceptive apparatus of the disk is located. In turn, this finding suggests that noxious chemicals, such as nitric oxide, might stimulate nociceptors to produce chemical nociception.

The second feature is the increased stress in the posterior anulus seen on stress profilometry. This finding suggests that the posterior anulus is being excessively stressed mechanically, which allows for mechanical nociception from the nociceptors in the posterior anulus.

Table 10
The association between grades of anulus disruption and reproduction of pain on disk stimulation, as found in 4 studies. A, Aprill and Bogduk[46]; B, Smith et al[55]; C, Lim et al[56]; D, Kokkonen et al.[57]

	Anulus Disruption	
A	Grade III, IV	Grade 0–II
Pain	38	0
Not pain	37	31
$P = .000$		

	Anulus Disruption	
B	Grade III, IV	Grade 0–II
Pain	39	5
Not pain	67	51
$P = .000$		

	Anulus Disruption	
C	Grade III, IV	Grade 0–II
Pain	33	27
Not pain	1	36
$P = .000$		

	Anulus Disruption	
D	Grade III, IV	Grade 0–II
Pain	16	31
Not pain	11	54
$P = .003$		

Table 11
The correlation between abnormal stress profiles and pain on stimulation of a lumbar intervertebral disk

Biophysical Properties	Disk	
	Painful	Not Painful
Nuclear Stress		
Depressurized	11	0
Normal	7	13
	Fisher exact test; $P = .017$	
Anular Stress		
Stressed	17	2
Normal	1	11
	Fisher exact test; $P = .001$	

Data from McNally DS, Shackleford IM, Goodship AE, et al. In vivo stress measurement can predict pain on discography. Spine 1996;21:2500–87.

Table 12
The sensitivity, specificity, and likelihood ratio of Modic changes as predictors of the affected disk being painful, as reported by 12 studies

Sample	Sensitivity	Specificity	Likelihood Ratio	95% Confidence Interval	Source (Ref.)
2457	0.25	0.94	4.2	3.3–5.2	59
152	0.23	0.97	7.7	1.9–31.6	60
101	0.22	0.95	4.4	1.3–15.0	61
255	0.18	0.90	1.8	0.9–3.5	62
178	0.14	0.87	1.1	0.5–2.6	63
97	0.09	0.83	0.52	0.2–1.8	56
3240	0.24	0.83	3.4	2.8–4.1	All

Table 13
The sensitivity, specificity, and likelihood ratio of the high-intensity zone as a predictor of the affected disk being painful, as reported by 12 studies

Sample	Sensitivity	Specificity	Likelihood Ratio	95% Confidence Intervals	Source (Ref.)
142	0.37	1.00	∞		64
120	0.82	0.89	7.5	4.0–14.1	46
256	0.45	0.94	7.5	3.7–15.1	65
152	0.27	0.95	5.4	1.7–17.1	66
101	0.52	0.90	5.2	2.4–11.2	61
155	0.81	0.79	3.9	2.5–6.0	67
178	0.57	0.84	3.6	2.2–5.7	63
109	0.45	0.84	2.8	1.4–5.5	68
152	0.26	0.90	2.6	1.2–5.8	55
97	0.56	0.70	1.9	1.2–3.0	56
116	0.27	0.85	1.8	0.9–3.8	69
80	0.09	0.93	1.3	0.3–5.4	70
1658	0.45	0.88	3.8	3.1–4.5	All

Both chemical nociception and mechanical nociception might be combined. Chemical factors might sensitize the nociceptors, rendering them more susceptible to mechanical nociception.

This model can be elaborated by adding the ingrowth of nerve fibers along radial fissures.[71–76] This neoinnervation increases the susceptibility of the anulus to nociception beyond that of which it is capable from its normal innervation.

Prevalence

Internal disk disruption is common amongst patients with chronic back pain who undergo invasive investigations. The original study found a prevalence of 39% (29%–49%) in 92 consecutive patients.[77] Two subsequent studies reported prevalences of 26% (18%–34%)[78] and 42% (34%–49%).[79] Although the estimates are not the same, their 95% confidence intervals overlap and are, therefore, compatible.

> Internal disk disruption is a common cause of pain in patients with chronic back pain.

Summary

Internal disk disruption is the most thoroughly studied, putative source of chronic back pain. The condition has a cause, and has been produced in biomechanics studies and induced in experimental animals. Its morphologic features can be clearly defined and can be detected on postdiskography CT. The condition has internal biophysical features. The morphologic features and the biophysical features each correlate with the disk being painful. The condition is strongly associated with characteristic signs on MR imaging. The condition is common.

DISCUSSION

As conventionally understood, so-called degenerative changes are irrelevant to spinal pain. They might become relevant if osteophytes compromise nerve roots and cause radicular pain, but they are not relevant for neck pain or back pain.

The causes of degenerative changes remain elusive, but the available evidence indicates that they amount to no more than normal age changes. Only exceptionally do degenerative changes reflect systemic metabolic disorders.

Clinically, degenerative changes have no correlation with neck pain, and no useful correlation with back pain. Therefore, they do not constitute valid diagnoses of the cause of pain.

Whereas radiologists have a legitimate responsibility to report what they see, they also have a responsibility to use appropriate terminology. The term degenerative is unnecessarily emotive and compromises the management of patients with pain. It is unnecessary and counterproductive. For that reason, it can be expunged from the radiologic lexicon. A simpler and accurate term is normal age changes.

Entirely different is the entity internal disk disruption. This entity is a genuine and well-studied cause of back pain, but it is not synonymous with degeneration. It shares some of the processes and features of degenerative changes in the disk, but is a response to injury. It cannot be seen and diagnosed on plain radiographs or conventional CT scans, because it shows no external features. For diagnosis in full form, internal disk disruption requires postdiskography CT scanning. However, some patients with this condition show Modic changes or high-intensity zones on MR imaging, each of which strongly, but not absolutely, implicates the affected disk as the source of pain.

Zygapophysial joints in any spine segment may also be a source of axial pain, but there is no correlation between radiologically observed zygapophysial joint osteoarthrosis and pain. Diagnosis of zygapophysial joint pain demands relief of the index pain with controlled anesthetic blocks of the joint innervation. There are suggestions in the literature that physiologic imaging parameters (T2 hyperintensity, gadolinium enhancement) may reveal painful zygapophysial joint synovitis, but definitive studies have yet to be performed.

REFERENCES

1. Bogduk N. What's in a name? The labelling of back pain. Med J Aust 2000;173:400–1.
2. Bogduk N, McGuirk B. Appendix 2. How to label back pain. In: Bogduk N, McGuirk B, editors. Medical management of acute and chronic low back pain. An evidence-based approach. Amsterdam: Elsevier; 2002. p. 215–8.
3. Sloan TJ, Walsh DA. Explanatory and diagnostic labels and perceived prognosis in chronic low back pain. Spine 2010;35:E1120–5.
4. Hadjipavlou AG, Tzermiadianos MN, Bogduk N, et al. The pathophysiology of disc degeneration: a critical review. J Bone Joint Surg Br 2008;90:1261–70.
5. Mercer S, Bogduk N. The ligaments and anulus fibrosus of human adult cervical intervertebral discs. Spine 1999;24:619–26.

6. Bland JH, Boushey DR. Anatomy and physiology of the cervical spine. Semin Arthritis Rheum 1990;20: 1–20.
7. Holt S, Yates PO. Cervical spondylosis and nerve root lesions. Incidence at routine necropsy. J Bone Joint Surg Br 1966;48:407–23.
8. Oda J, Tanaka H, Tsuzuki N. Intervertebral disc changes with aging of human cervical vertebra. Spine 1988;11:1205–11.
9. Bogduk N, Mercer SR. Biomechanics of the cervical spine. I: Normal kinematics. Clin Biomech 2000;15: 633–48.
10. Taylor JR, Twomey LT. Age changes in lumbar zygapophyseal joints. Spine 1986;11:739–45.
11. Magora A, Schwartz A. Relation between the low back pain syndrome and x-ray findings I. Degenerative osteoarthritis. Scand J Rehabil Med 1976;8: 115–25.
12. Gore DR, Sepic SB, Gardner GM. Roentgenographic findings of the cervical spine in asymptomatic people. Spine 1986;1:521–4.
13. Elias F. Roentgen findings in the asymptomatic cervical spine. N Y State J Med 1958;58:3300–3.
14. Boden SD, McCowin PR, Davis DG, et al. Abnormal magnetic-resonance scans of the cervical spine in asymptomatic subjects: a prospective investigation. J Bone Joint Surg Am 1990;72:1178–84.
15. Boden SD, Davis DO, Dina TS, et al. Abnormal magnetic-resonance scans of the lumbar spine in asymptomatic subjects. A prospective investigation. J Bone Joint Surg Am 1990;72:403–8.
16. Videman T, Battié MC, Gill K, et al. Magnetic resonance imaging findings and their relationships in the thoracic and lumbar spine. Insights into the etiopathogenesis of spinal degeneration. Spine 1995;2:928–35.
17. Cheung KM, Karpinnen J, Chan D, et al. Prevalence and pattern of lumbar magnetic resonance imaging changes in a population study of one thousand forty-three individuals. Spine 2009;34:934–40.
18. Lee MJ, Riew DK. The prevalence cervical facet arthrosis: an osseous study in a cadaveric population. Spine J 2009;9:711–4.
19. Kalichman L, Li L, Kim DH, et al. Facet joint osteoarthritis and low back pain in the community-based population. Spine 2008;33:2560–5.
20. Wollheim FA, Lohmander LS. Pathogenesis and pathology of osteoarthritis. In: Hochberg MC, Silman AJ, Smolen JS, et al, editors. Rheumatology. 4th edition. Philadelphia: Mosby Elsevier; 2007. p. 1711–28.
21. Battié MC, Videman T, Kaprio J, et al. The Twin Study: contributions to a changing view of disc degeneration. Spine J 2009;2:47–59.
22. McGregor AHJ, Andrew T, Sambrook PN, et al. Structural, psychological, and genetic influences on low back and neck pain: a study of adult female twins. Arthritis Rheum 2004;51:160–7.
23. Videman T, Saarela J, Kaprio J, et al. Associations of 25 structural, degradative, and inflammatory candidate genes with lumbar disc desiccation, bulging and height narrowing. Arthritis Rheum 2009;60:470–81.
24. Kalichman L, Hunter DJ. The genetics of intervertebral disc degeneration. Associated genes. Joint Bone Spine 2008;75:388–96.
25. Battié MC, Videman T, Levälahti E, et al. Genetic and environmental effects on disc degeneration by phenotype and spinal level. A multivariate study. Spine 2008;33(25):2801–8.
26. Heller CA, Stanley P, Lewis-Jones B, et al. Value of x-ray examinations of the cervical spine. Br Med J 1983;287:1276–8.
27. Fridenberg ZB, Miller WT. Degenerative disc disease of the cervical spine. A comparative study of asymptomatic and symptomatic patients. J Bone Joint Surg Am 1963;45:1171–8.
28. Lawrence JS, Bremner JM, Bier F. Osteo-arthrosis. Prevalence in the population and relationship between symptoms and x-ray changes. Ann Rheum Dis 1966;25:1–24.
29. Schwarzer AC, Wang S, O'Driscoll D, et al. The ability of computed tomography to identify a painful zygapophysial joint in patients with chronic low back pain. Spine 1995;20:907–12.
30. van Tulder MW, Assendelft WJ, Koes BW, et al. Spinal radiographic findings and nonspecific low back pain. A systematic review of observational studies. Spine 1997;22:427–34.
31. Symmons DP, van Hemert AM, Vandenbroucke JP, et al. A longitudinal study of back pain and radiological changes in the lumbar spines of middle aged women: I. Clinical findings. Ann Rheum Dis 1991;50:158–61.
32. Symmons DP, van Hemert AM, Vandenbroucke JP, et al. A longitudinal study of back pain and radiological changes in the lumbar spines of middle aged women: II. Radiographic findings. Ann Rheum Dis 1991;50:162–6.
33. Horal J. The clinical appearance of low back disorders in the city of Gothenburg, Sweden: comparison of incapacitated probands with matched controls. Acta Orthop Scand Suppl 1969;118:1–73.
34. Frymoyer JW, Newberg A, Pope MH, et al. Spine radiographs in patients with low-back pain. J Bone Joint Surg Am 1984;66:1048–55.
35. Biering-Sorensen F, Hansen FR, Schroll M, et al. The relation of spinal X-ray to low-back pain and physical activity among 60-year old men and women. Spine 1985;10:445–51.
36. Wiikeri M, Nummi J, Riihimaki H, et al. Radiologically detectable lumbar disc degeneration in concrete reinforcement workers. Scand J Work Environ Health 1978;4(Supp 1):47–53.
37. Lawrence JS. Disc degeneration: its frequency and relationship to symptoms. Ann Rheum Dis 1969;28: 121–37.

38. Kellgren JH, Lawrence JS. Rheumatism in miners: part II. X-ray study. Br J Ind Med 1952;9:197–207.
39. Sairanen E, Brushhaber L, Kaskinen M. Felling work, low back pain and osteoarthritis. Scand J Work Environ Health 1981;7:18–30.
40. Hult L. The Munkfors investigation. Acta Orthop Scand Suppl 1954;16:1–75.
41. Savage RA, Whitehouse GH, Roberts N. The relationship between the magnetic resonance imaging appearance of the lumbar spine and low back pain, age and occupation in males. Eur Spine J 1997;6:106–14.
42. Kjaer P, Leboeuf C, Korsholm L, et al. Magnetic resonance imaging and low back pain in adults: a diagnostic imaging study of 40-year-old men and women. Spine 2005;30:1173–80.
43. Bendix T, Kjaer P, Korsholm L. Burned-out discs stop hurting. Fact or fiction? Spine 2008;33:E962–7.
44. Chou D, Samartzis D, Bellabarba C, et al. Degenerative magnetic resonance imaging changes in patients with chronic low back pain. Spine 2011;36:S43–53.
45. Vanharanta H, Sachs BL, Spivey MA, et al. The relationship of pain provocation to lumbar disc deterioration as seen by CT/discography. Spine 1987;12:295–8.
46. Aprill C, Bogduk N. High-intensity zone: a diagnostic sign of painful lumbar disc on magnetic resonance imaging. Br J Radiol 1992;65:361–9.
47. Adams MA, McNally DS, Wagstaff J, et al. Abnormal stress concentrations in lumbar intervertebral discs following damage to the vertebral bodies: a cause of disc failure? Eur Spine J 1993;1:214–21.
48. Hansson TH, Keller TS, Spengler DM. Mechanical behaviour of the human lumbar spine. II. Fatigue strength during dynamic compressive loading. J Orthop Res 1987;5:479–87.
49. Liu YK, Njus G, Buckwalter J, et al. Fatigue response of lumbar intervertebral joints under axial cyclic loading. Spine 1983;8:857–65.
50. Holm S, Kaigle-Holm A, Ekstrom L, et al. Experimental disc degeneration due to endplate injury. J Spinal Disord Tech 2004;17:64–71.
51. Cinotti G, Della Rocca C, Romeo S, et al. Degenerative changes of porcine intervertebral disc induced by vertebral endplate injury. Spine (Phila Pa 1976) 2005;30:174–80.
52. Haschtmann D, Stoyanov JV, Gédet P, et al. Vertebral endplate trauma induces disc cell apoptosis and promotes organ degeneration in vitro. Eur Spine J 2008;17:289–99.
53. MacMillan DW, McNally DS, Garbutt G, et al. Stress distribution inside intervertebral discs: the validity of experimental 'stress profilometry'. Proc Inst Mech Eng H 1996;210:81–7.
54. Moneta GB, Videman T, Kaivanto K, et al. Reported pain during lumbar discography as a function of anular ruptures and disc degeneration. A re-analysis of 833 discograms. Spine 1994;17:1968–74.
55. Smith BM, Hurwitz EL, Solsberg D, et al. Interobserver reliability of detecting lumbar intervertebral disc high-intensity zone on magnetic resonance imaging and association of high intensity zone with pain and anular disruption. Spine 1998;23:2074–80.
56. Lim CH, Jee WH, Sou BC, et al. Discogenic lumbar pain: association with MR imaging and CT discography. Eur J Radiol 2005;54:431–7.
57. Kokkonen SM, Kurunlahti M, Tervonen O, et al. Endplate degeneration observed on magnetic resonance imaging of the lumbar spine. Correlation with pain provocation and disc changes observed on computed tomography discography. Spine 2002;27:2274–8.
58. McNally DS, Shackleford IM, Goodship AE, et al. In vivo stress measurement can predict pain on discography. Spine 1996;21:2500–87.
59. Thomson KJ, Dagher M, Eckel TS, et al. Modic changes on MR images as studied with provocative diskography: clinical relevance–a retrospective study of 2457 disks. Radiology 2009;250:849–55.
60. Braithwaite I, White J, Saifuddin A, et al. Vertebral endplate (Modic) changes on lumbar spine MRI: correlation with pain reproduction at lumbar discography. Eur Spine J 1998;7:363–8.
61. Ito M, Incorvaia KM, Yu SF, et al. Predictive signs of discogenic lumbar pain on magnetic resonance imaging with discography correlation. Spine 1998; 23:1252–60.
62. Sandhu HS, Sanchez-Caso LP, Parvataneni HK, et al. Association between findings of provocative discography and vertebral endplate changes as seen on MRI. J Spinal Disord 2000;13:438–43.
63. Kang CH, Kim YH, Lee SH, et al. Can magnetic resonance imaging accurately predict concordant pain provocation during provocative disc injection? Skeletal Radiol 2009;38:877–85.
64. Peng B, Hou S, Wu W, et al. The pathogenesis and clinical significance of a high-intensity zone (HIZ) of lumbar intervertebral disc on MR imaging in the patient with discogenic low back pain. Eur Spine J 2006;15:583–7.
65. Chen J, Ding Y, Lv R, et al. Correlation between MR imaging and discography with provocative concordant pain in patients with low back pain. Clin J Pain 2011;27:125–30.
66. Saifuddin A, Braithwaite I, White J, et al. The value of lumbar spine magnetic resonance imaging in the demonstration of anular tears. Spine 1998;23:453–7.
67. Lam KS, Carlin D, Mulhollad RC. Lumbar disc high-intensity zone: the value and significance of provocative discography in the determination of the discogenic pain source. Eur Spine J 2000;9:36–41.
68. Carragee EJ, Paragoudakis SJ, Khurana S. Lumbar high-intensity zone and discography in subjects without low back problems. Spine 2000; 25:2987–92.

69. Weishaupt D, Zanetti M, Hodler J, et al. Painful lumbar disk derangement: relevance of endplate abnormalities at MR imaging. Radiology 2001;218:420–7.
70. Ricketson R, Simmons JW, Hauser BO. The prolapsed intervertebral disc. The high-intensity zone with discography correlation. Spine 1996;21:2758–62.
71. Coppes MH, Marani E, Thomeer RT, et al. Innervation of 'painful' lumbar discs. Spine (Phila Pa 1976) 1997;22:2342–50.
72. Freemont AJ, Peacock TE, Goupille P, et al. Nerve ingrowth into diseased intervertebral disc in chronic back pain. Lancet 1997;350:178–81.
73. Johnson WE, Evans H, Menage J, et al. Immunohistochemical detection of Schwann cells in innervated and vascularised human intervertebral discs. Spine 2001;26:2550–7.
74. Ozawa T, Ohtori S, Inoue G, et al. The degenerated lumbar intervertebral disc is innervated primarily by peptide-containing sensory nerve fibers in humans. Spine 2006;31:2418–22.
75. Peng B, Wu W, Hou S, et al. The pathogenesis of discogenic low back pain. J Bone Joint Surg Br 2005; 87:62–7.
76. Peng B, Hao J, Hou S, et al. Possible pathogenesis of painful intervertebral disc degeneration. Spine 2006;31:560–6.
77. Schwarzer AC, Aprill CN, Derby R, et al. The relative contributions of the disc and zygapophyseal joint in chronic low back pain. Spine 1994;19:801–6.
78. Manchikanti L, Singh V, Pampati V, et al. Evaluation of the relative contributions of various structures in chronic low back pain. Pain Physician 2001;4:308–16.
79. De Palma MJ, Ketchum JM, Saullo T. What is the source of chronic low back pain and does age play a role? Pain Med 2011;12:224–33.

Imaging the Intervertebral Disk
Age-Related Changes, Herniations, and Radicular Pain

Filippo Del Grande, MD, MBA, MHEM[a,*],
Timothy P. Maus, MD[b], John A. Carrino, MD, MPH[c]

KEYWORDS

• Intervertebral disk • Disk herniation • Degeneration • End plate

KEY POINTS

- Radicular pain requires both compression of neural tissue and an inflammatory response.
- Standard imaging can only detect nerve root displacement or compression; this is in part the basis of the specificity fault: many disk herniations are asymptomatic.
- The natural history of disk herniations is resolution; larger herniations, extrusions, and sequestrations are more likely to resolve.
- There is no relationship between the size, type, or change in disk herniations over time and patient outcomes.

INTRODUCTION

The articulations of the spinal motion segment, consisting of the intervertebral disk in the anterior column and the zygapophyseal joints in the posterior column, inevitably undergo age-related changes in response to a variety of insults, as described by Bogduk elsewhere in this issue. This article focuses on the intervertebral disk, specifically when fissures sufficiently weaken the posterior annulus so as to allow herniation of nuclear material into the outer annular lamellae as a contained protrusion or breach the annulus and pass into the epidural space as an extrusion. Such displaced nuclear material may directly impinge on neural tissue as well as initiate an inflammatory response in the epidural space, producing radicular pain and neural dysfunction. This article examines the imaging of age-related changes in the disc and the sequelae of internal disk disruption, disk herniation: appropriate nomenclature, the reliability and relative merits of imaging modalities, the imaging natural history of disk herniations, and most importantly, its clinical significance. The imaging professional cannot lose sight of the ultimate goal of imaging disk herniations: to improve the outcomes of patients with radicular pain syndromes and radiculopathy. The lumbar segment of the spine will receive primary attention.

The evaluation of disk herniations by imaging most frequently occurs in the setting of radicular pain or radiculopathy. Radiculopathy implies the presence of objective signs of neural dysfunction including motor weakness, sensory loss/paresthesias, or diminished deep tendon reflexes; it is typically accompanied by radiating limb pain which is described as intermittent, lancinating, electric, or burning. This pain differs from the referred pain from somatic sources, such as facet or sacroiliac (SI) joint

[a] Section of Musculoskeletal Radiology, The Johns Hopkins Medical Institutions, Russell H. Morgan Department of Radiology and Radiological Science, 601 North Caroline Street, JHOC 5165, Baltimore, MD 21287, USA; [b] Department of Radiology, Mayo Clinic, 200 First Street SW, Rochester, MN 55905, USA; [c] Musculoskeletal Radiology, The Russell H. Morgan Department of Radiology and Radiological Science, Johns Hopkins University School of Medicine, 601 North Caroline Street, JHOC 5165, Baltimore, MD 21287, USA
* Corresponding author.
E-mail address: fdelgra1@jhmi.edu

Radiol Clin N Am 50 (2012) 629–649
doi:10.1016/j.rcl.2012.04.014
0033-8389/12/$ – see front matter

radiologic.theclinics.com

inflammatory synovitis, which is characterized as constant, deep, dull, and aching. Radicular pain frequently extends into the distal limb, whereas somatic referred pain is seldom experienced below the knee or elbow. Lumbar somatic referred pain from facet or SI joints is often maximal after a period of immobility, arising from bed, prolonged standing or sitting, which eases with continued motion. Lumbar radicular pain may exist in isolation without objective evidence of radiculopathy; it is typically worse with axial load and upright posture and relieved by recumbency. Lumbar radicular pain may be accompanied by allodynia, pain provoked by light touch, but in general is not manifest in cutaneous innervation; it is best described as having a radicular, not dermatomal, distribution.

PATHOGENESIS OF RADICULAR PAIN DUE TO DISK HERNIATION

Mixter and Barr[1] initially described the disk herniation as the cause of sciatica in 1934; this observation, and the ability to relieve pain and neurologic dysfunction by surgical extirpation of the offending herniation, provided the basis for the first 70 years of spine imaging. Myelography, computed tomography (CT), CT/myelography, and magnetic resonance (MR) imaging were deemed useful in patients with radicular pain or radiculopathy because of their ability to first indirectly, and later directly, visualize the disk herniation and neural compression. Over the past few decades, however, the pathogenesis of radicular pain/radiculopathy has been shown to be more complex. Mulleman and colleagues[2,3] reviewed the evidence supporting an inflammatory component as essential in the cause for radicular pain. Clinical observations supporting the role of inflammation in radicular pain include[2,3]

1. Surgical relief of neural compression is not uniformly clinically successful; pain may persist despite adequate decompression
2. Large disk herniations may be asymptomatic
3. The severity of symptoms has no relationship with herniation size or shape
4. Imaging features of herniation have little prognostic value
5. Conservative therapy is often effective

There is also experimental data to refute the exclusive role of mechanical compression and include an inflammatory factor in the generation of radicular pain.

1. The imaging natural history of disk herniation is resorption.[4] Resorption is mediated by macrophage-produced metalloproteases and neovascularization.[5,6]
2. The disk nucleus pulposis (NP) has been shown to be immunogenic (it is sequestered from the vascular space), and its presence can induce an inflammatory response mediated by phospholipase A2; Interleukins (IL) 1α, 1β, and 6; tumor necrosis factor α (TNFα); and nitric oxide.[2]
3. In a pig model, introduction of NP into the epidural space, without nerve compression, induced nerve dysfunction and histologic evidence of nerve fiber degeneration.[7]
4. NP alone induces nerve dysfunction, but concomitant compression is necessary to cause pain.[2]

There is also evidence, in animal and human models, that nerve compression alone is insufficient to cause radicular pain, hence there must be an associated inflammatory (chemical) reaction. Kulisch and colleagues[8] performed disk resections on volunteers under local anesthesia; traction on a nerve not having contact with disk produced modest discomfort only, similar traction on a nerve contacting herniated disk reproduced radicular pain.[8] Several investigators, in a series of animal experiments, demonstrated the following: NP applied to a spinal nerve induces nerve dysfunction; this dysfunction is reduced by anti-inflammatory agents; the dysfunction is due to substances secreted by NP cell membranes; TNFα is the most likely agent although IL-1, interferon-Υ, and nitric oxide synthetase may contribute.[2] A subsequent randomized controlled trial of the transforaminal epidural administration of etanercept (a TNFα antagonist) in patients with lumbar radiculopathy yielded positive results.[9] Hence radiculopathy and radicular pain are the product not only of nerve compression but also an inflammatory response, likely mediated at least in part by TNFα. Structural imaging studies can only view a necessary, but insufficient, component of the lesion generating radicular pain.

ANATOMY AND NOMENCLATURE OF AGE-RELATED CHANGES AT THE DISCOVERTEBRAL COMPLEX OF THE LUMBAR SPINE

The discovertebral complex is formed by the intervertebral disk and the adjacent cartilaginous vertebral end plate (**Fig. 1**). These components comprise a cartilaginous joint called an amphiartrosis.[10] The central nucleus pulposis is composed of 70% to 90% water; this is bound within proteoglycans.[10,11] The proteoglycans constitute about 65% of the dry weight of the nucleus; collagen comprises 15% to 20%. The

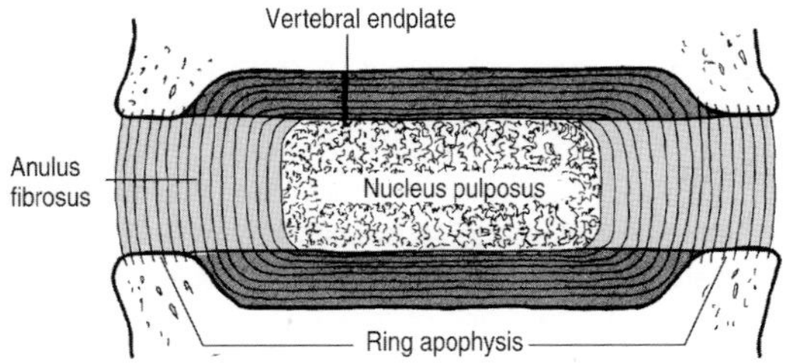

Fig. 1. Detailed structure of the vertebral end plate. The collagen fibers of the inner two-thirds of the anulus fibrosus sweep around into the vertebral end plate forming its fibrocartilaginous component. The peripheral fibers of the anulus are anchored into the bone of the ring apophysis. (*From* Bogduk N. Clinical anatomy of the lumbar spine and sacrum. Philadelphia: Elsevier; 2005. p. 14; with permission.)

proteoglycan units, including their bound water, together with the collagen, constitute the nuclear matrix.[11] Chondrocytes are sparsely dispersed in the nucleus, primarily near the cartilaginous end plates and are responsible for proteoglycan and collagen synthesis. In infancy and childhood, the nuclear compartment makes up the vast majority of the volume of the disk; the annulus is small and discrete from it. As the disk ages, the boundary zone between nucleus and annulus becomes indistinct with progressive incorporation of nuclear volume into the annulus.

The healthy nucleus acts as a fluid, and applied axial load is dispersed radially, constrained by the fibrous annulus. The annulus also comprises 60% to 70% water along with collagen and proteoglycans; collagen is dominant in the annulus.[11] The annulus is organized as 10 to 20 concentric sheets (lamellae) of collagen fibers; each lamella has its fibers oriented at 65 to 70° from the longitudinal axis of the body. The orientation shifts its direction of angulation in alternating layers. Lamellae are often not complete circular layers but end with fusion to an adjacent lamellae, which is most common in the posterolateral quadrant of the disk.[11] The vertical ends of the lamellae in the outer annulus tightly bind it to the ring apophysis of the vertebrae. The collagen fibers of the inner annular lamellae are contiguous with the collagen of the cartilaginous end plate. The annulus serves to constrain the fluidlike nucleus, bulging slightly as it accepts radial load dispersed by the nucleus in response to axial-applied load. Axial load is transmitted to the subjacent end plate with slight temporal delay and attenuation of energy.

The cartilaginous end plate is 0.6 to 1.0 m thick, composed of hyaline and fibrocartilage; as the disk ages, the fibrocartilage dominates. The collagen fibers in this fibrocartilage are contiguous with those of the annulus, now oriented horizontally, enclosing the nuclear compartment in a complete capsule of collagen.[11] The end plate is tightly bound to the disk, less firmly fixed to the underlying subchondral bone. The intimate contact of end plate with marrow is critical to nutrient diffusion into the cartilaginous end plate and nuclear matrix.

With aging, the number of viable chondrocytes in the nucleus diminishes; the synthesis rate and concentration of proteoglycans decreases and the proportion of collagen in the nucleus increases.[11] The water binding capacity of the nucleus decreases; it becomes more fibrous and stiffer. The nucleus is less able to bear and disburse load, transferring load to the posterior annulus. If the annulus remains intact, the joint expresses this added load by increasing its surface area, and osteophytes develop. If the annulus fails, fissures develop across annular lamellae; these may ultimately reach the disk periphery. This process of internal disk disruption may cause axial pain, as described by Bogduk elsewhere in this issue. It also sets the stage for the expression of degraded nuclear material through these fissures as a disk herniation.

The manifestations of age-related changes of the disk on MR imaging, most commonly referred to as degenerative change, consist primarily of diminished T2 signal within the nuclear compartment. The boundary between nucleus and annulus becomes indistinct, and the normal band of T2 hypointensity at the equator of the disk, the intranuclear cleft, may no longer be apparent. Pfirrmann and colleagues[12] analyzed 300 lumbar MR images in 60 patients with a mean age of 40 years, and proposed a 5-part grading system for lumbar disk degeneration using midsagittal T2-weighted imaging. Parameters were T2 signal in the nuclear compartment and disk space height; there was good to excellent interobserver and intraobserver agreement (**Box 1**, **Fig. 2**).[12]

The nomenclature of age-related changes of the disk, pathologic degeneration, and disk herniation has historically been chaotic because varied conceptual constructs of disk change over time coexist in the literature, and varied specialties have adopted different terminology. Multiple spine imaging and surgical societies proposed a lexicon of nomenclature in 2001; it represents the best effort to date to provide a uniform basis for communication.[13]

In this terminology, spondylosis deformans (**Fig. 3**) is used to encompass normal changes of aging, including loss to T2 signal and anterior and lateral osteophytes. As the annulus bears more

Box 1
Grading of lumbar disk changes based on Pfirrmann classification[12]

Grade I: Homogenous bright white disk structure and normal disk height.

Grade II: Inhomogeneous disk structure with or without horizontal bands.

Grade III: Inhomogeneous disk structure. The distinction between nucleus pulposus and annulus fibrosus is unclear and the disk height is normal or slightly decreases.

Grade IV: Low signal disk with indistinct interface between annulus fibrous and nucleus pulposus. Disk height is normal or moderately decreased.

Grade V: Disk is collapsed.

load due to nuclear matrix degradation, there are reactive changes, primarily osteophyte formation. Nathan[14] described the presence of anterior and lateral osteophytes in all cadavers at the age of 40, whereas posterior osteophytes were present only in a minority of cadavers at the age of 80. These age-related changes are typically relatively uniform across the spine. Loss of disk space height, posterior osteophytes, radial annular fissures, and large amounts of nitrogen gas in the nuclear compartment are not features of normal aging, in this description.[13]

Intervertebral osteochondrosis is the term applied to pathologic, although not necessarily symptomatic, disk changes.[13] This includes posterior osteophyte formation, large amounts of nuclear gas, loss of disk space height, profound loss of normal T2 nuclear signal, end-plate erosive changes, and reactive marrow changes as initially described by Modic and colleagues in 1988.[15]

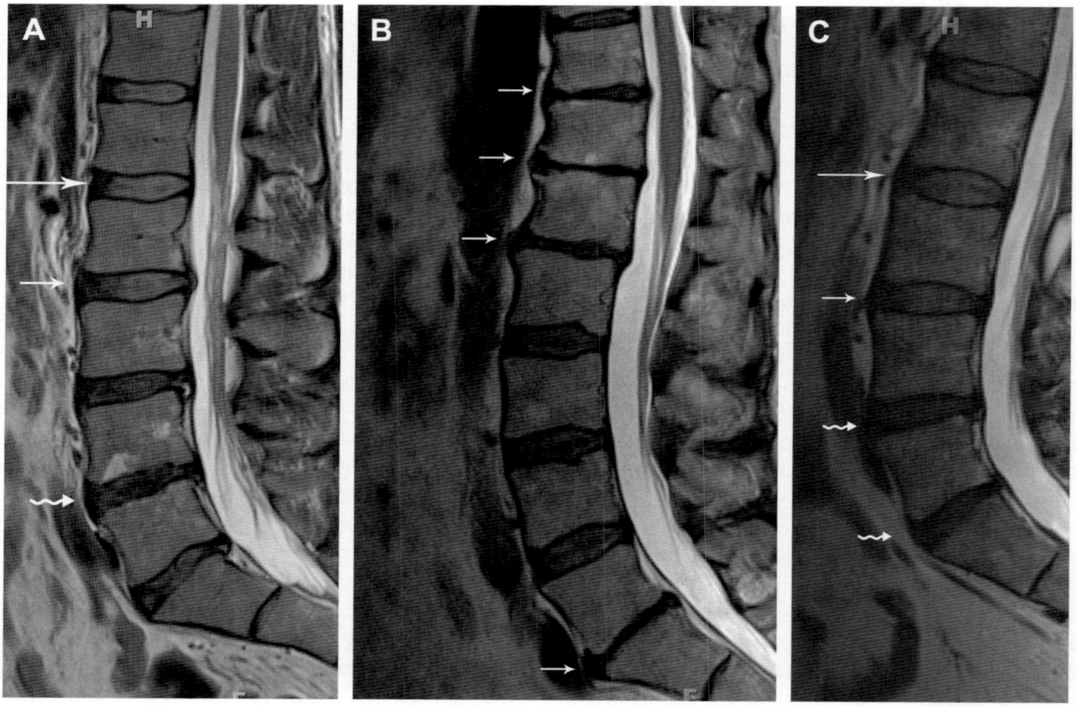

Fig. 2. (*A–C*) Spectrum of disk degeneration using the Pfirrmann classification. (*A*) demonstrates a slightly inhomogeneous disk with normal height corresponding to grade II change (*long white arrow*) at level L1-L2; and the L2-L3 disk shows intermediate signal intensity with slightly decreased height corresponding to grade III degeneration (*short white arrow*). The L4-L5 disk is inhomogeneous with loss of distinction between nucleus pulpous and annulus fibrous and moderately decreased height (*squiggly arrow*), corresponding to grade IV change. (*B*) Homogenous black, collapsed disks corresponding to degeneration grade V are present at T11-T12, T12-L1, L1-L2, and L5-S1 (*arrows*). (*C*) The L2-L3 level has a normal disk, grade I (*long white arrow*), the L3-L4 level shows a slightly inhomogeneous disk corresponding to disk degeneration of grade II (*short white arrow*), and the L4-L5 and L5-S1 levels show gray to black disks with moderate decrease in height corresponding degeneration grade IV (*squiggly arrows*).

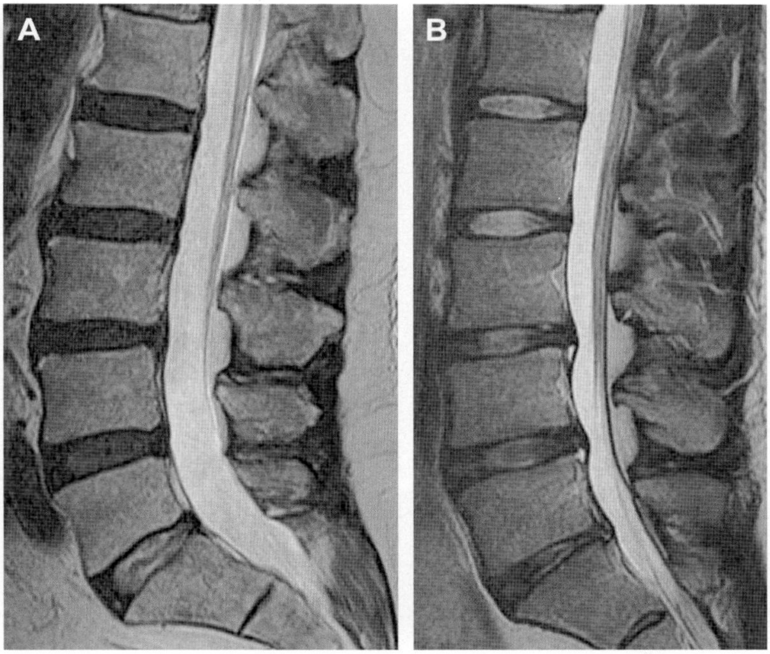

Fig. 3. Normal aging (spondylosis deformans) versus pathologic degeneration (osteochondrosis). (*A*) Spondylosis deformans: midsagittal T2-weighted MR image of a 62-year-old man with modest back pain. Loss of T2 signal in multiple disks is apparent, but there is preservation of the height of the disk space, no disk contour abnormality, and a widely patent central canal. (*B*) Osteochondrosis: midsagittal T2-weighted MR image of a 32-year-old man with disabling back pain. Note the loss of T2 signal and disk height at L3-L5 with small disk herniations and high-intensity zones at L3 and L4. Early central canal narrowing. (*From* Maus T. Imaging the back pain patient. Phys Med Rehabil Clin N Am 2010;21(4):725–66; with permission.)

This process, and its imaging findings, typically involves one or more individual disks and is not uniform throughout the lumbar spine.

MODIC END-PLATE CHANGES

Modic changes provides an insight into the physiologic and histologic changes occurring in the disk-end-plate complex in response to insults and altered load bearing as the nuclear matrix degrades. Modic type I changes are characterized by decreased signal intensity on T1-weighted sequences and increased signal intensity on T2-weighted sequences. Histologically, the subchondral marrow is infiltrated by fibrovascular tissue. Modic II changes are characterized by increased signal intensity on T1- and T2-weighted sequences; the histologic correlate is yellow or fatty marrow replacement. Type III changes are characterized by decreased signal intensity on T1- and T2-weighted images and histologically correspond to sclerosis **Fig. 4.**[15]

Several publications[16–19] evaluated the prevalence, distribution, and natural history of changes in the end plate . The reported prevalence of Modic changes is variable, but type II changes are generally more common than Type I. Kuisma and associates[16] identified a distribution of 30% of type I changes, 66% of type II changes, and 4% of type III changes among 228 middle-aged working men. Eighty percent of all Modic changes occurred at the L4-L5 or L5-S1 levels. The investigators suggested that Modic changes occurring at the L5-S1 level, Modic type I changes, and extensive expression of Modic changes are more closely associated with pain.[16] Karchevsky and colleagues[18] studied the morphology and the epidemiology of the reactive end-plate bone marrow changes. Of the 100 patients studied, 40.5% had type I changes, 57.3% had type II changes, and 2.1% had type III changes. The most affected segment was the anterior end plate of the L4-L5 level; there was a positive correlation with weight and male gender.[18]

In an additional study, Kuisma and colleagues[17] followed 60 conservatively treated patients with sciatica between the ages of 23 and 76 to assess the dynamics of changes in the end plate. At baseline, the prevalence for all Modic changes was 23%; 10% showed mixed Modic type I and type II changes, whereas 90% showed Modic type II change. During the observational period of 3 years the investigators found that 14% of the 70 disks with Modic changes converted to another type, and the lesions that did not convert extended. The investigators found that 80% of the conversions occurred from type II to mixed type I/II or to type I changes. These investigators suggested that Modic type II changes are probably less stable than previously thought.[17,20,21] Hutton and

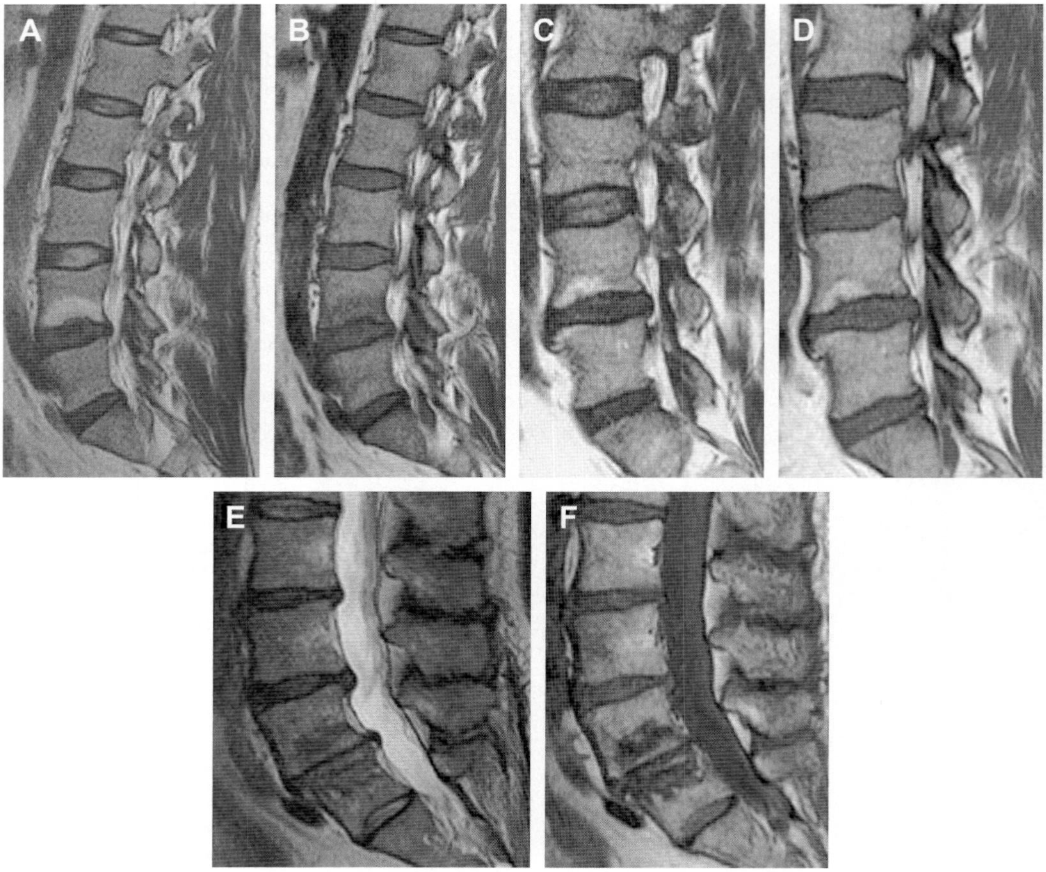

Fig. 4. End-plate (Modic) changes. (*A*) Sagittal T2-weighted MR image shows hyperintense signal in marrow adjacent to L4 inferior end plate in a 44-year-old man with axial pain. Note the loss of T2 signal in L4 and L5 disks. (*B*) Matched sagittal T1-weighted MR image in same patient shows hypointense T1 signal adjacent to L4 inferior end plate; this is type I marrow change, vascularized granulation tissue. (*C*) Sagittal T2-weighted MR image in a 46-year-old man with radicular pain. Note the increased T2 signal about anterior aspect of L4 disk; there is also T2 signal loss at the L4 and L5 levels. (*D*) Matched sagittal T1-weighted MR image in the same patient demonstrates increased T1 signal about L4 disk; this is type II marrow change, fatty infiltration. (*E*) Sagittal T2-weighted MR image in a patient exhibiting type III marrow change at the L4 interspace. Note the marked loss of disk space height and low T2 signal. (*F*) Matched T1 sagittal image in the same patient as (*E*) demonstrates the low T1 signal about the L4 disk in type III end plate change. (*From* Maus T. Imaging the back pain patient. Phys Med Rehabil Clin N Am 2010;21(4):725–66; with permission.)

colleagues[19] assessed the dynamics of Modic changes by reviewing 2 MR images of 490 end plates in 49 subjects with an average time interval of 695 days. Of the end plates with Modic type I changes, 36% progressed to Modic type II, 8% to Modic type III, and 6% to Modic type 0 (normal). Of the 22 Modic type II changes on the baseline MR image, 4 converted to Modic I whereas the others remain unchanged.[19]

The data in literature are thus rather disparate. Modic type II change is most common and Modic type III change is quite rare. Earlier literature had suggested a typical progression from the more active inflammatory state of Modic type I to a more quiescent Modic type II state; this has been challenged more recently. The correlation of Modic change with axial back pain of disk origin (discogenic pain) is discussed by Aprill and Maus later in this issue.

HIGH-INTENSITY ZONE (ANNULAR FISSURE)

The high-intensity zone was described by Aprill and Bogduk[21] as an imaging finding marking the presence of internal disk disruption and correlating strongly both with the presence of a grade 4 annular fissure on post-diskography CT and concordant pain reproduction at provocation diskography. The inflammatory nature of this finding is manifest in its T2 hyperintensity (similar to CSF) and gadolinium enhancement (**Fig. 5**). The literature support for its correlation with discogenic pain will be discussed in detail by Aprill and Maus elsewhere in this issue.

DISK HERNIATION NOMENCLATURE

When radial annular fissures accompany nuclear matrix degradation, the stage is set for disk herniation; mechanical compression of neural elements and an inflammatory response induced by TNFα and other mediators combine to produce radicular pain or radiculopathy. Imaging to date has primarily been directed toward detecting the displaced disk material and its relationship to neural elements. A combined task force of the North American Spine Society, the American Society of Spine Radiology, and the American Society of Neuroradiology established the consensus terminology describing disk herniation.[13] Disk herniation is the over-arching term, defined as "a localized displacement of disc material beyond the limit of the intervertebral disc space. The disc material may be nucleus, cartilage, fragmented apophyseal bone, annular tissue, or any combination thereof."[13]

The classification divides the surface of the disk into 4 quadrants (**Figs. 6–8**, **Table 1**). A localized herniation is arbitrarily defined as involving less than 50% of the disk circumference; generalized disk displacement of more than 50% of the circumference is a bulging disk. A localized displacement of the disk of less than 25% of its circumference is a focal herniation; disk displacement between 25% and 50% is a broad-based herniation. The distinction between protrusion and extrusion (see **Fig. 6**; **Fig. 9**) is one of shape. In a protrusion the width

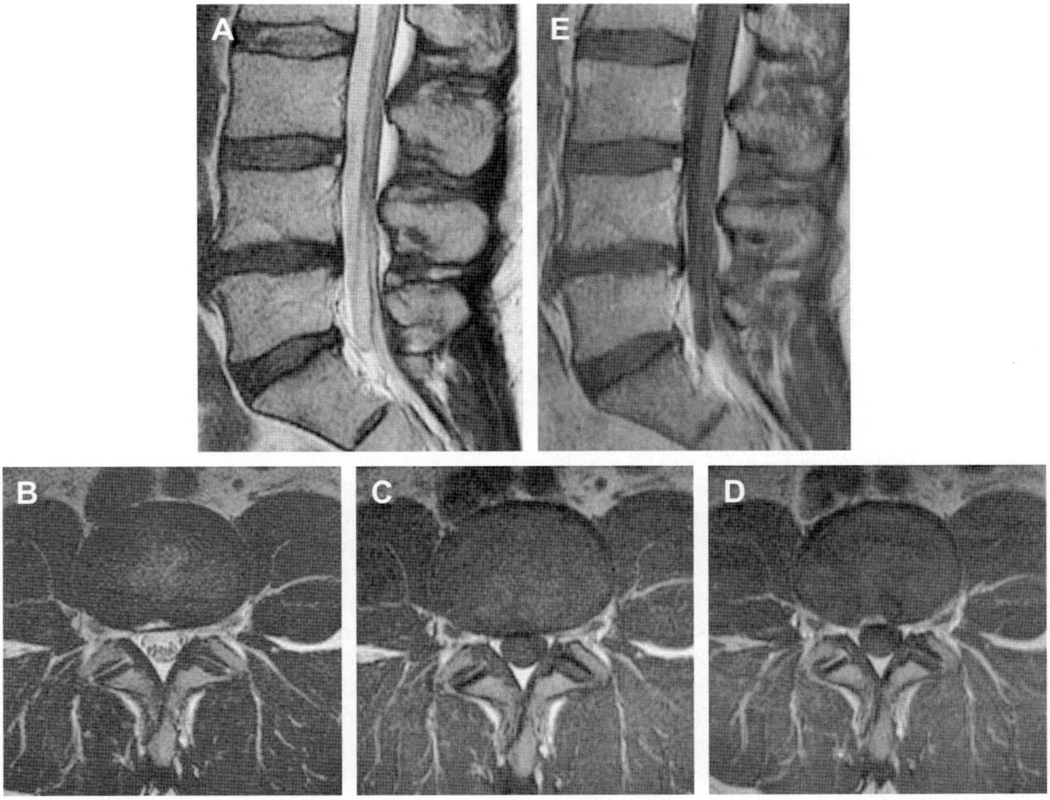

Fig. 5. High-intensity zone (HIZ). (*A*) Sagittal T2-weighted image in a 44-year-old man with axial pain shows HIZ within posterior annulus of L3 disk. Note also disk degeneration at L4 and L5. (*B*) Axial T2-weighted image at L3 demonstrates the HIZ within the bulging L3 posterior annulus. (*C*) Axial T1-weighted image at L3 shows only the mild contour abnormality (bulge). (*D*) Post-gadolinium axial T1-weighted image reveals enhancement with in the HIZ consistent with vascularized granulation tissue. (*E*) Sagittal post-gadolinium T1 image also demonstrates the enhancement in the posterior annulus of L3. (*From* Maus T. Imaging the back pain patient. Phys Med Rehabil Clin N Am 2010;21(4):725–66; with permission.)

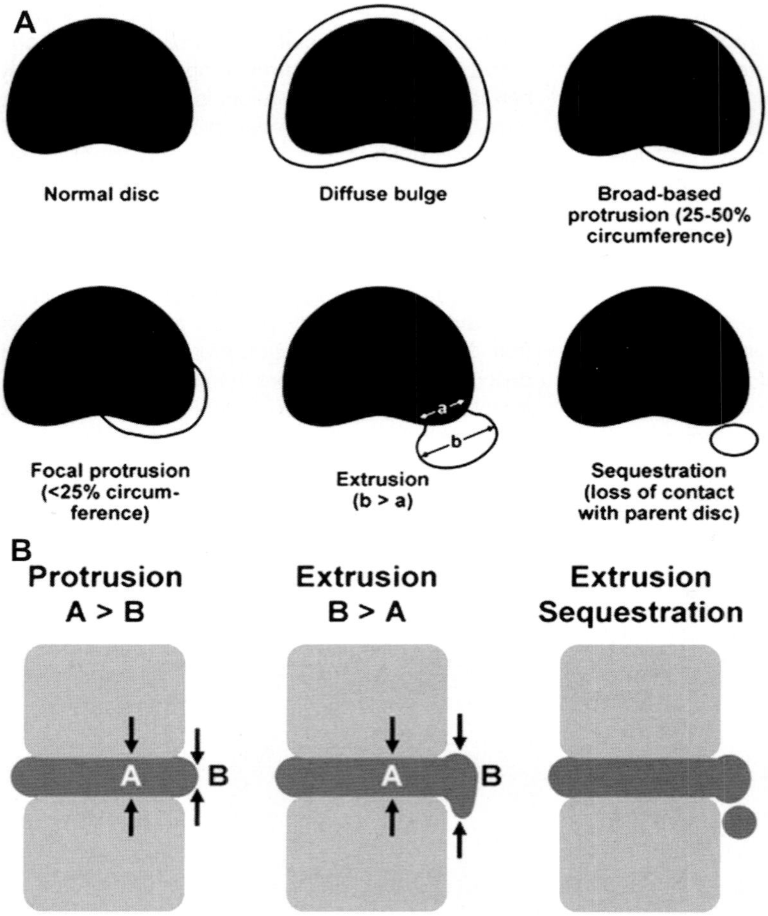

Fig. 6. Disk herniations. (*A*) Disk herniation configurations in the axial plane. (*B*) Disk herniation configurations in the sagittal plane. (*From* Maus T. Imaging the back pain patient. Phys Med Rehabil Clin N Am 2010;21(4):725–66; with permission.)

of the displaced disk material, in any plane, does not exceed the width of its base or the aperture through which the disk material had left its normal position. In an extrusion, the width of the displaced disk material exceeds its base or aperture in any plane. The presence of an extrusion shape suggests that there has been complete disruption of the outer annulus, and disk material has entered the epidural space. Sequestration is the term for loss of continuity of a disk fragment with the parent disk from which it arose. Displacement of disk material away from the parent disk is termed migration. Migration can occur caudally or cranially. A herniated disk can further be considerate contained or uncontained. A contained disk herniation is one in which the outer annulus fibrosis is intact, an uncontained herniation is when the annulus in completely disrupted. The shape definitions of protrusion and extrusion apply to this, but only by implication not direct observation. CT or MR imaging can only rarely directly establish containment, only post-CT diskography can make this distinction.

Description of displaced disk material (see **Fig. 7**) in the axial plane is defined by zones: the central zone, defined by the medial margins of the facets; the subarticular zone, extending from the medial facet margin to the medial pedicle margin; the foraminal zone, extending from the medial to lateral margins of the pedicle; and the extraforaminal zone, peripheral to the lateral pedicle margin. A right-sided focal disk herniation may therefore be described as right central, right subarticular, right foraminal, or right extraforaminal. Similarly, location in the sagittal plane (superior–inferior) is defined by levels in relationship to the vertebral end-plate and pedicle margins. Extending from superior to inferior, the designations include the disk level, suprapedicular level, pedicle level, infrapedicular level, and the subsequent disk level. Although an element of subjectivity remains inherent in any usable system of terminology, careful adherence to the above

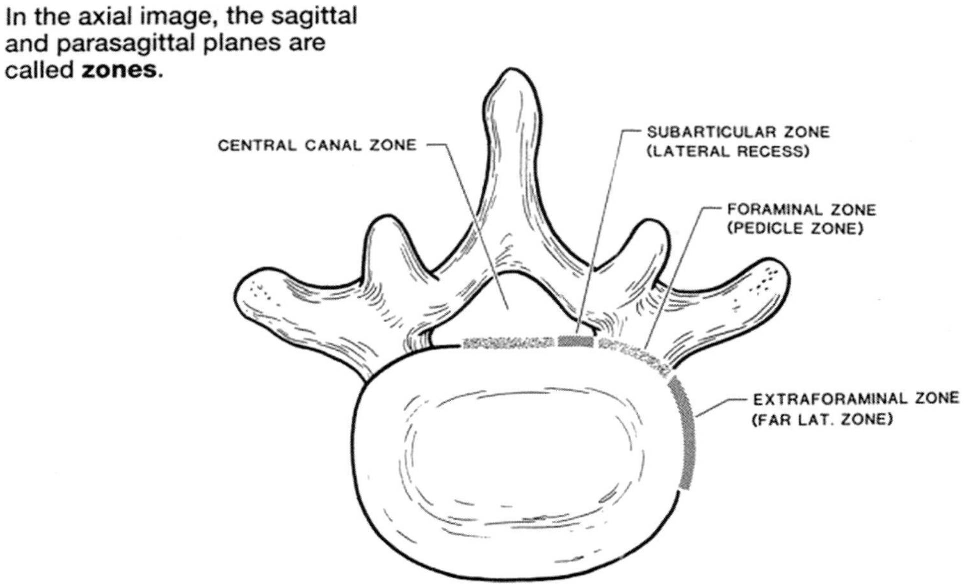

Fig. 7. Schematic representation of the anatomic "zones" identified on axial images. The anterior zone (not illustrated) is delineated from the extraforaminal zone by an imaginary coronal line in the center of the vertebral body. (*From* Wiltse LL, Berger PE, McCulloch JA. A system for reporting the size and location of lesions of the spine. Spine 1997;22:1534–7; with permission.)

descriptors should allow a more coherent discussion of disk pathology.

IMAGING MODALITIES

As noted by Chou and colleagues earlier in this issue, imaging is not indicated in the initial presentation of a patient with radicular pain or radiculopathy. The American College of Radiology considers spine imaging appropriate only when there are red flag features that suggest the presence of an underlying systemic disease, in the face of progressive neurologic deficits, or cauda equina syndrome.[22] The American Pain Society and American College of Physicians further emphasize that imaging should be recommended only when the patient with radiculopathy is a candidate for a therapeutic intervention, such as epidural steroid injection of surgery.[23] There is no benefit from imaging in planning conservative therapy.

If the patient has failed clinically directed conservative therapy, it is reasonable to consider imaging. This should occur in the context of a risk-benefit assessment, with appropriate consideration of potential harms of imaging, as discussed by Chou and colleagues elsewhere in this issue. When imaging is performed on a patient with radiculopathy or radicular pain, the first step is to obtain radiographs in an upright physiologic position. The advantages of physiologic imaging are discussed earlier in this issue. Oblique or flexion-extension radiographs have no role in the initial evaluation of the patient.[24] Radiographs serve to establish spine enumeration, coronal and sagittal balance, and

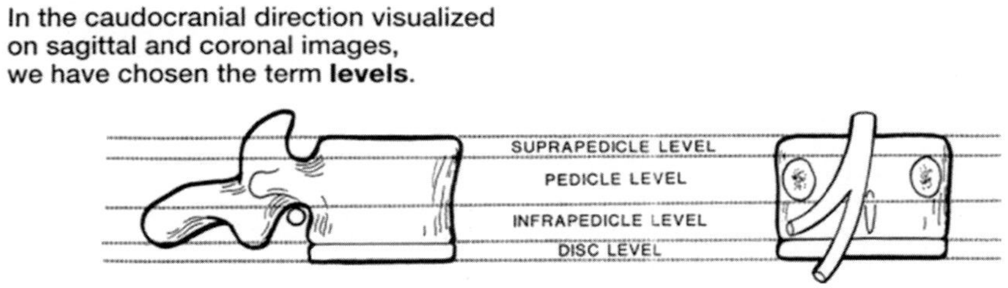

Fig. 8. Schematic representation of the anatomic "levels" identified on cranio-caudal images. (*From* Wiltse LL, Berger PE, McCulloch JA. A system for reporting the size and location of lesions of the spine. Spine 1997;22:1534–7; with permission.)

Table 1
Classification of disk herniation

Area of the Disk	Shape of the Disk	Axial Location	Sagittal Location
<25%	Extrusion	Central	Discal
	Focal protrusion	R/L central[1]	Pedicular
25%–50%	Broad-based protrusion	R/L subarticular	Infrapedicular
		R/L foraminal	Suprapedicular
		R/L extraforaminal	

Abbreviations: L, left; R, right.

a low sensitivity screen for undiagnosed sinister conditions. The common age-related changes seen on radiographs are seldom clinically useful. Advanced imaging in the form of CT, CT myelography, or MR imaging may provide more useful information in patients with radiculopathy.

CT has undergone a revolution in the last decade with the advancement of multidetector technology. A dataset for the lumbar or cervical spine can be obtained in a few seconds, eliminating motion artifact and dramatically improving patient tolerance. This dataset can then be reconstructed in any plane without the loss of spatial resolution or additional radiation exposure. CT provides superior imaging of cortical and trabecular bone compared with MR imaging. CT also

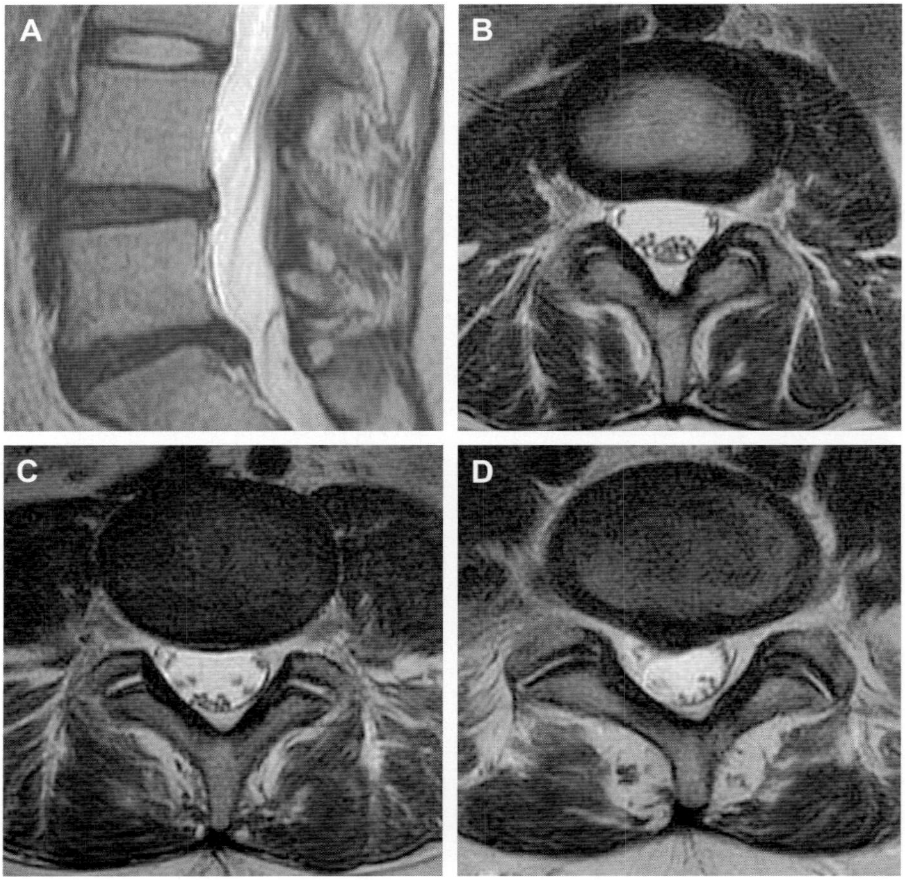

Fig. 9. Disk protrusion and extrusion. Sagittal T2 (*A*), and axial T2 images at L3 (*B*), L4 (*C*) and L5 (*D*). Normal disk at L3, broad central protrusion at L4 and right central extrusion with caudal migration at L5. This suggests, but does not directly demonstrate, that there has been complete disruption of the L5 annulus.

provides reasonable contrast resolution and can identify root compressive lesions such as disk herniations in the vast majority of cases. Radiation dose must always be considered when using CT, particularly in younger patients, and in serial examinations. In the cervical spine, CT or CT myelography may add value in their ability to distinguish bony osteophyte from soft disk, which may alter the surgical approach. One by-product of the rapid recent technological advance of CT is that the literature contains no comparative studies between MR imaging and the current generation of multidetector CT scanners in the detection and characterization of disk herniations.

Thornbury and colleagues,[25] in 1993, demonstrated little difference in the accuracy of MR imaging, CT Myelography, or CT alone in the assessment of herniated disk-related root compressive disease. In a review article by Jarvik and Deyo,[26] the sensitivity of CT in the detection of lumbar disk herniation ranged from 62% to 90%; for MR imaging the sensitivity ranged from 60% to 100%. The specificity of CT ranged from 70% to 87% and for MR imaging from 47% to 97%. According to Janssen and colleagues,[27] sensitivity and specificity are higher in MR imaging than in CT and CT-myelography. The investigators studied 60 patients who underwent surgery on 102 disk levels. The correlation between preoperative finding and surgical finding was much higher with MR imaging (96%) than CT (57%) and higher than CT-myelography (84%).[27] A more recent study by van Rijn and colleagues[28] found no evidence that CT was inferior to MR imaging in the detection of disk herniation. There was, however, more interobserver variability in detecting root compressive lesions with CT than MR imaging. This study used 2-slice CT scanners. There are no studies comparing current generation 64- to 256-slice CT with MR imaging.

CT-myelography is a minimally invasive modality that plays a problem-solving role in the lumbar region, and it is recommended for patients with contraindications to MR imaging, or in the postoperative spine in which metal artifacts may obscure critical anatomy on MR imaging. Intrathecal contrast media allows for accurate detection of root impingement and central lateral recess and foraminal stenosis.

MR imaging has long been considered the best single diagnostic test for imaging the cervical, thoracic, and lumbar spine for disk herniation in patients with radicular pain syndromes, despite the modest evidence basis. The superior contrast resolution of MR imaging allows direct visualization of herniated disk material and its relationship to neural tissue, including intrathecal contents. With the use of gadolinium, there is an opportunity to display the inflammatory reaction critical to the pathophysiology of radicular pain or radiculopathy. There are no studies to assess the potential degree of specificity this may add. In the postoperative spine, enhanced imaging allows discrimination of scar from recurrent disk, which is discussed elsewhere in this issue.

MR IMAGING: RELIABILITY

Lurie and colleagues[29] analyzed MR images of randomly selected patients with intervertebral disk herniations from the Spine Patient Outcome Research Trial (SPORT). They noted high ($\kappa = 0.81$) interobserver agreement for disk morphology when classified as normal/bulge, protrusion and extrusion/sequestration. There was only moderate interobserver agreement for thecal sac ($\kappa = 0.54$) and nerve root compression ($\kappa = 0.47$).[29] Pfirrmann and colleagues[30] proposed a grading system for nerve root compression. The investigators divided the relationship of the herniated disk and the nerve root into 4 categories: no compromise, contact with the nerve root, deviation of the nerve root, and compression of the nerve root. The interobserver reliability ($\kappa = 0.62$–0.67) and intraobserver reliability ($\kappa = 0.72$–0.77) were good. The correlation for higher grade of nerve root involvement (compression) was greater than for lower grade nerve root involvement.

Carrino and colleagues[31] reviewed 111 MR imaging studies of patients between the ages of 18 and 87 to assess intraobserver and interobserver agreement for non-disk contour degenerative findings. They reported good interobserver agreement in rating disk degeneration ($\kappa = 0.66$) and moderate interobserver agreement in rating spondylolisthesis, Modic changes, facet arthrosis, and high-intensity zones (κ ranging from 0.44 to 0.59). Intraobserver agreement was overall good for the same changes, with κ values ranging from 0.66 to 0.74.

DISK HERNIATION: SPECIFICITY

The specificity challenges associated with imaging of the disk and disk herniations have been well known for decades. Age-related changes in the disk occur progressively throughout adult life without any relation to symptoms. Recent studies have addressed the prevalence of age-related disk findings (primarily T2 signal loss) in younger populations, primarily in Scandinavian countries; these are population-based studies of MR imaging regardless of symptoms. Kjaer and colleagues,[32] studying children aged 13 years, found a 21% prevalence of disk "degeneration". In a study of adolescents, Salminen and colleagues[33] found a 31% prevalence of disk "degeneration" in 15-year-olds, which increased to 42% in 18-year-olds. Takatalo and colleagues[34] evaluated 558 young adults aged 20 to 22 years. Using the 5-point Pfirrmann classification of disk degeneration, they noted disk changes of grade III or higher in 47% of these young adults. There was a higher prevalence in men (54%) than in women (42%). Multilevel changes were identified in 17%. In a much earlier study of asymptomatic workers, Hult[35] noted radiographic evidence of narrowing of disk space, osteophytes, and vacuum phenomena in 56% of those aged between 40 and 44 years, which increased to 95% in subjects aged between 50 and 59 years. These studies clearly identify these common findings in the disk as normal changes of aging or maturation.

The literature reveals similar results when the prevalence of disk herniations in normal subjects is examined. Hitselberger and Witten[36] studied plain myelography of asymptomatic volunteers and noted that 31% of patients demonstrated disk herniations. A study of lumbar spine CT in asymptomatic volunteers by Wiesel and colleagues[37] showed that in subjects older than 40 years, 20% had disk herniations. Similarly, Boden and colleagues[38] evaluated MR images of the lumbar spine in asymptomatic volunteers; in patients older than 60 years, 36% had disk herniations, 79% exhibited annular bulges and 93% had disk "degeneration" or age-related change. Jarvik and colleagues[39] noted that only extrusions, moderate to severe central canal stenosis, and direct visualization of neural compression were likely to be significant and would separate patients with pain from asymptomatic volunteers.

One of the consequences of this specificity challenge in the evaluation of disk herniations is that there will always be a background of asymptomatic disease on which may be superimposed changes causal of a current radiculopathy or radicular pain syndrome. Only a close concordance, a key in lock fit, of an imaging finding and an individual patient's pain syndrome can suggest causation, which further implies that the imager must know the nature of a radicular pain syndrome if he/she is to suggest a causal lesion. Close communication between clinician and imager via the medical record, an intake document at the imaging site detailing the pain syndrome, or direct patient interview by the imager is necessary.

SENSITIVITY

The major sensitivity fault of spine imaging is discussed elsewhere in this issue. Both anterior and posterior column structures may change under axial load and physiologic positioning, especially extension. Disk herniations that do not appear to contact neural tissue in recumbent imaging studies may result in significant compression in the physiologic state. Zamani and colleagues[40] noted an increase in disk bulging in 40% of disks showing age-related changes when imaged in an erect extended position. Weishaupt and colleagues[41] observed that more instances of disk-neural contact were seen in images obtained in the seated position than those obtained in the supine position; there were also small increases in the frequency of neural deviation or compression, particularly in images generated in the seated extension position. Neural foraminal narrowing in the seated position was significantly associated with increased pain.[41] Willen and Danielson[42] demonstrated that in 14% of patients with sciatica significant additional information was demonstrated on images obtained under extension and axial load, including accentuation of disk herniation, lateral recess or foraminal stenosis, distension of a synovial cyst, or reduction in dural sac cross-sectional area to stenotic dimensions.[42]

IMAGING OBSERVATIONS IN DISK HERNIATIONS

MR imaging can beautifully demonstrate disk herniations and their effect on the thecal sac and nerve roots, particularly on T2-weighted images. Disk extrusions and sequestered fragments on T2-weighted images often show greater signal intensity than the parent disk; this may be a reflection of inflammation. Within the lateral recess or neural foramen, such T2 hyperintense fragments can be difficult to detect against the high-signal fat on fast-spin echo T2 images. Careful scrutiny of matched T1 images reveals the lesion, now hypointense against the bright intraforaminal fat. The greater spatial resolution of CT myelography may identify subtle lateral recess or foraminal lesions less well seen on MR imaging.

Ninety percent of lumbar disk herniations occur at the L4 or L5 interspace levels.[43] The vector of disk displacement in most herniations is posterolateral, an interesting correlate with the higher proportion of incomplete annular lamellae in this quadrant. In the lumbar spine, the exiting nerve passes immediately inferior to the vertebral pedicle and exits the foramen above the interspace level. Therefore, most disk herniations do not affect the exiting nerve, but rather impinge on the traversing nerve, which exits under the next lower vertebral pedicle. For example, a posterolateral L4-L5 disk herniation results in an L5 radicular pain syndrome or radiculopathy. For a lumbar disk herniation to affect the like-numbered nerve, it must be an extrusion with cephalad migration of disk material into the neural foramen. The imager must know the pain syndrome to assess the nerve root in question (**Fig. 10**).

ROLE OF CONTRAST MEDIUM IN DISK HERNIATION

Gadolinium enhancement is not usually used or required in examination of the unoperated spine. Unenhanced imaging can only detect the mechanical compression of a nerve, not the inflammatory response which is also necessary to provoke radicular pain. T2 hyperintensity on short tau

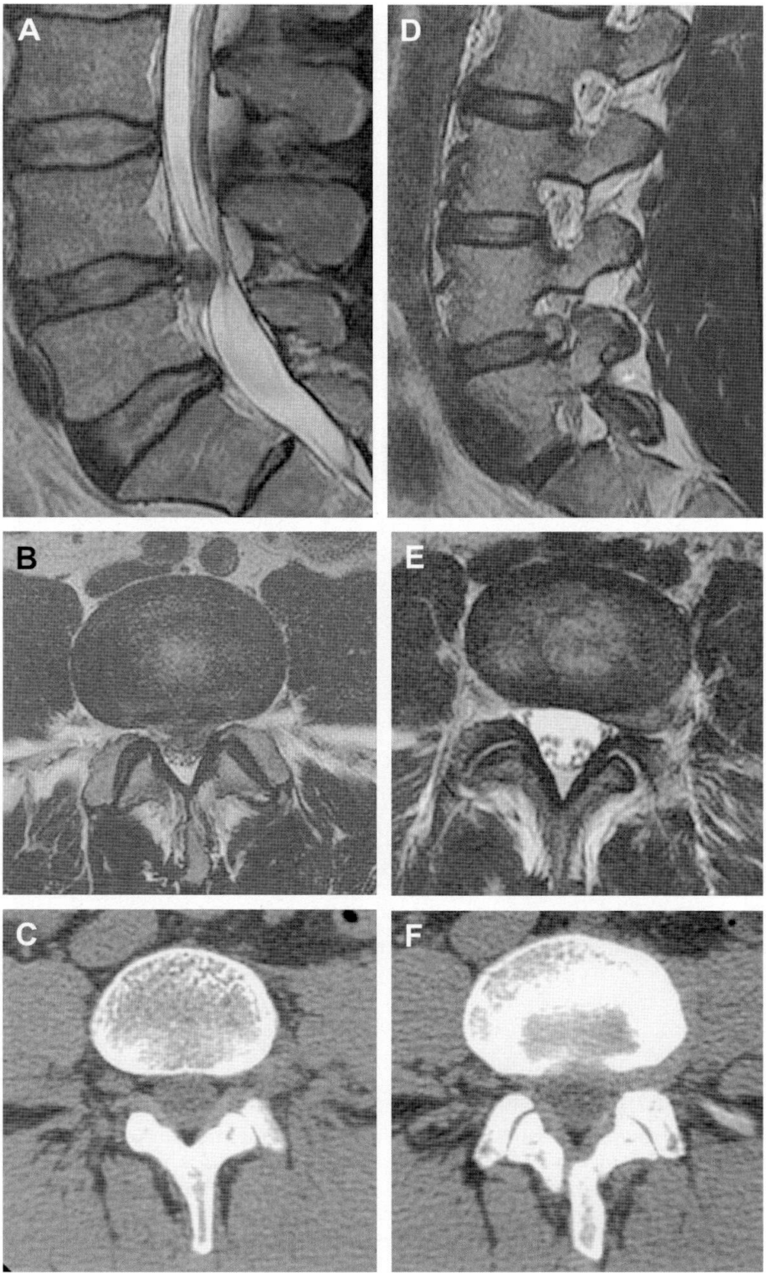

Fig. 10. Disk herniations. (*A*) Sagittal T2-weighted image in a patient with left L5 radicular pain reveals a large extrusion with cranial and caudal migration of disk material. The extrusion severely narrows the thecal sac, but the patient had no signs of cauda equina syndrome only unilateral pain. (*B*) Axial T2-weighted image in the same patient at the L4 level. Note the compression of the thecal sac. (*F*) Axial CT image at the L4 interspace in a patient with acute left L4 radicular pain who is unable to tolerate MR imaging. Note the broad-based left-sided herniation. (*C*) CT image of the same patient cephalad to the disk reveals extruded disk material in left L4 foramen. Compare with normal fat surrounding right-sided nerve. (*D*) Sagittal T2-weighted MR image in another patient with left L4 radicular pain. L4 disk extrusion with migration of extruded material into foramen displaces the nerve superiorly. (*E*) Axial T2-weighted MR image at L4 disk level well demonstrates the foraminal extrusion. (*From* Maus T. Imaging the back pain patient. Phys Med Rehabil Clin N Am 2010;21(4):725–66; with permission.)

inversion recovery or fat-saturated images may identify this reaction. If gadolinium is given, it will often be observed that the soft tissue seen on unenhanced images, thought to be herniated disk material, is largely enhancing inflammatory/granulation tissue about a small disk fragment (**Fig. 11**). When confronted by a patient with clinically evident radicular pain or radiculopathy and no evidence of a neural compressive lesion on standard imaging, it may be reasonable to consider an enhanced examination, which may reveal an inflammatory process associated with a disk whose annulus is incompetent,[44] which is sometimes referred to as a chemical radiculitis, first described by Marshall and colleagues.[45] The neural compressive component of the lesion may only be present on imaging with axial load and physiologic positioning.

The use of gadolinium in the postoperative spine is discussed elsewhere in this issue.

NATURAL HISTORY OF LUMBAR DISK HERNIATIONS

The natural history of disk herniation is spontaneous regression (**Fig. 12**).[4,46–53] Moreover, there is a general agreement that extruded disks, large herniations, and sequestrations have a greater tendency to resolution when compared with small herniations and disk bulges.[48,49,51] Maigne and colleagues[48] followed up 48 patients with up to 48 months' follow-up CT scans and observed that

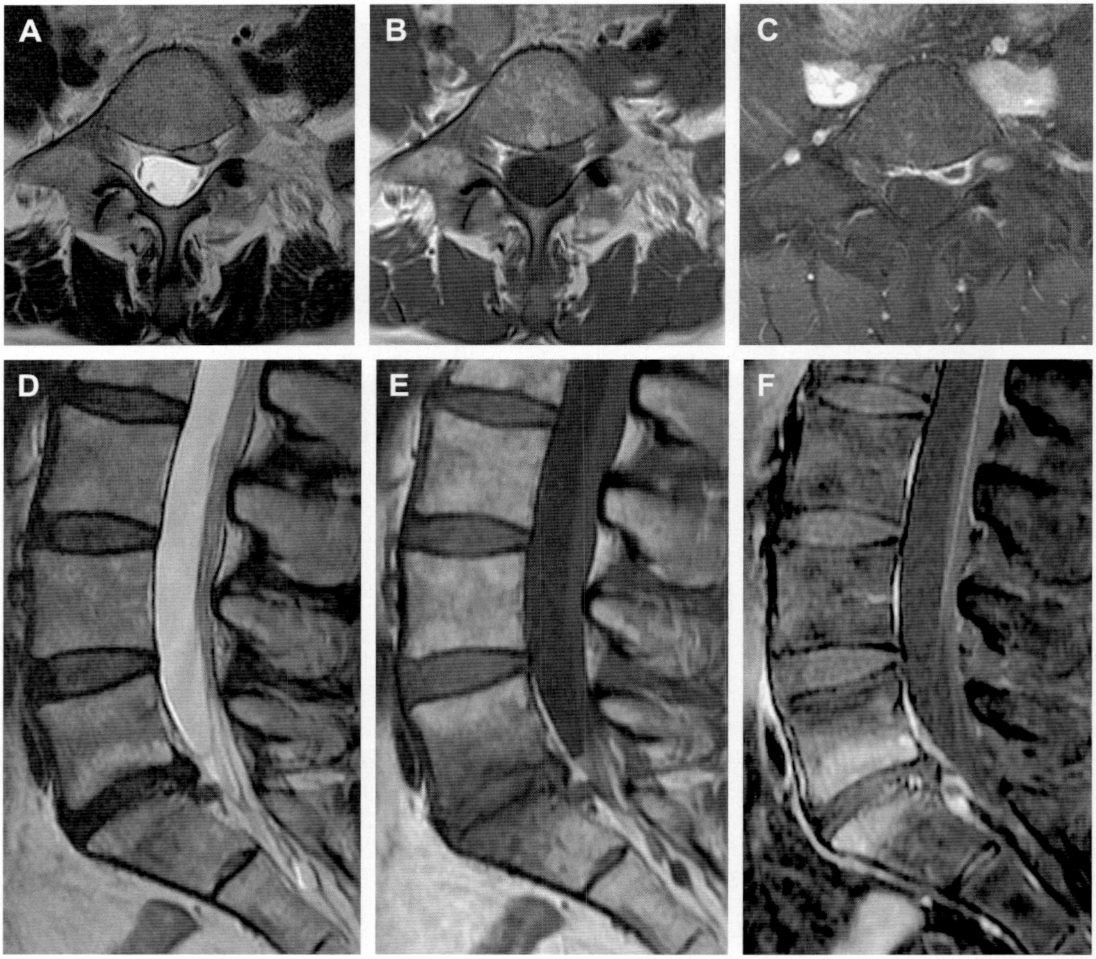

Fig. 11. Enhancing inflammatory reaction surrounding sequestration. This patient presented with left leg pain. Axial T2 (*A*) and T1 (*B*) images at the level of the L5 pedicle demonstrate a sequestered disk fragment having migrated cephalad from the L5 disk. Fat-saturated enhanced T1 image (C) at the same level shows that the sequestered fragment is small, but surrounded by enhancing inflammatory tissue. Sagittal T2 (*D*), T1 (*E*) and fat-saturated enhanced T1 (*F*) images in another patient similarly show inflammatory enhancement about a caudally migrated L5 sequestration. Note also the enhancing Modic I change.

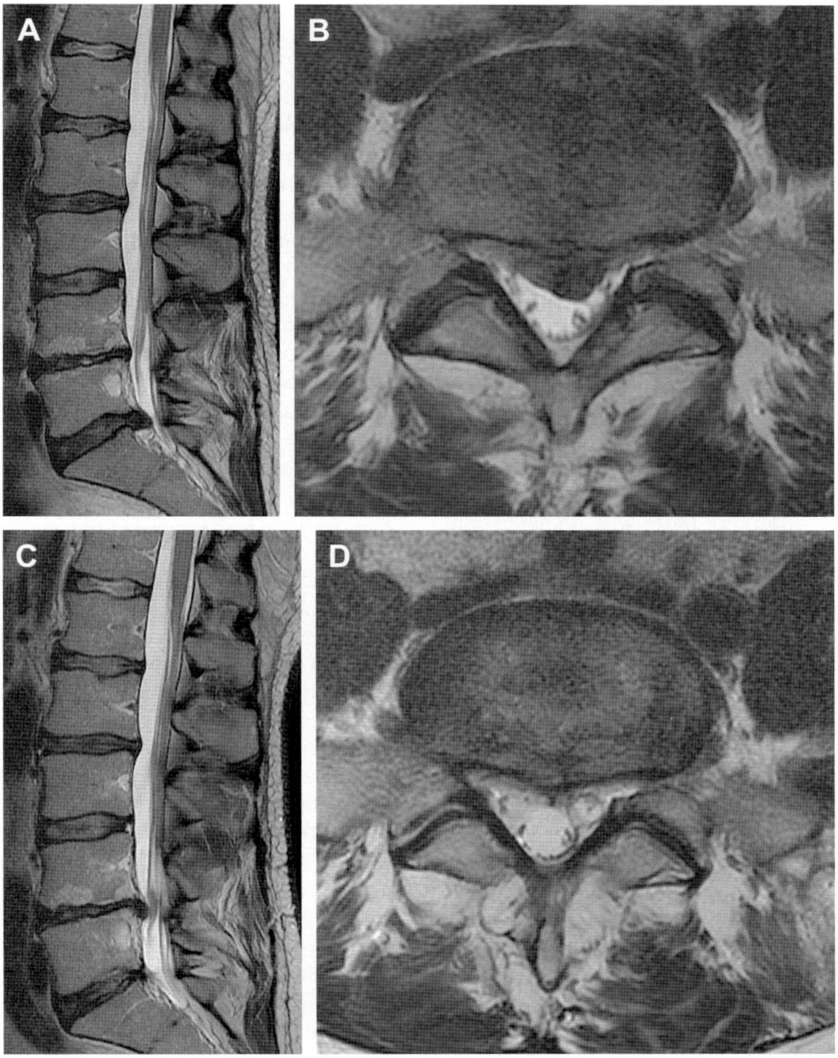

Fig. 12. Disk herniation resolution. This patient presented in 2006 with left S1 radicular pain because of a moderately large left central L5 disk extrusion. Sagittal T2 image (*A*) and axial T2 image at L5 (*B*). He was treated with a left S1 transforaminal epidural steroid injection with clinical resolution of pain. He presented 4 years later with new left L5 distribution pain. 2010 MR images (sagittal T2 image [*C*], and axial T2 image at L5 [*D*]) show that the L5 extrusion has completely resolved; a new L4 extrusion has developed.

the largest herniations had the greatest tendency to decrease in size. Bush and colleagues confirmed these results in 165 patients with a 1-year follow-up CT. In this study, 76% of disk herniation and 26% of disk bulges showed partial or complete resolution.[49] The large extrusion or sequestration has entered the highly vascular epidural space, initiating a significant inflammatory response as described previously. This inflammatory response is integral to the profound pain these patients feel but will ultimately resorb the extruded disk material. This is the basis of transforaminal epidural steroid administration in patients who have failed conservative therapy. If the inflammatory response can be attenuated and the patient is allowed to remain functional, natural history will bear out with resolution of the herniated disk material and the radicular pain syndrome over time. Annular bulges or contained protrusions have not breached the annulus to initiate a similar degree of inflammatory response; these herniations tend to be stable over time.

CORRELATION OF DISK HERNIATION IMAGING WITH CLINICAL STATE

The spine imaging correlates with axial discogenic pain are discussed in detail by Aprill and Maus elsewhere in this issue. The correlation of disk herniation imaging with the clinical presentation of radicular pain or radiculopathy has been well studied. The basic specificity fault is described previously. As noted in a systematic review by Chou and colleagues,[54] there is no value in imaging patients at the initial presentation of back or limb pain. In another study not included in that review, Modic and colleagues[55] examined 246 patients who presented with acute back pain or radiculopathy; all underwent MR imaging, but were randomized to either providing the imaging results to the patient and clinician or withholding them. A safety board did not intervene because there were no imaging findings requiring acute intervention in any patient. Patients were followed for 2 years and had a 6-week follow-up MR imaging. Sixty percent of patients had disk herniations at presentation, but there was no significant difference in the prevalence of herniations between back pain or radiculopathy patients. There was no relationship between herniation type, size, or change over time and patient outcome. Disk herniations characterized as extrusions showed a trend toward greater resolution. The presence of a herniation was a positive prognostic sign, as might be expected given its natural history. The investigators concluded that MR imaging does not have value in planning conservative care. They emphasized that a surgical decision should be based on clinical parameters, not imaging.[55]

This is reinforced by the study of Cribb and colleagues,[56] who followed 15 patients with massive disk herniations who were not surgical candidates or declined surgery. All the herniations were extrusions or sequestrations occupying more than 66% of the spinal canal cross-sectional area. Fourteen of the 15 herniations diminished in size by more than 80% (area) in the 2-year follow-up period. One patient underwent discectomy for persistent pain despite significant decrease in size of the herniation. The one patient whose herniation did not decrease in size had complete symptom resolution; no patient developed cauda equina syndrome.[56] In another study by Masui and colleagues, disk herniations were treated conservatively and followed for 7 years; 71% of herniations had diminished in size at 2 years, 95% at 7 years.[57] Clinical outcomes were unrelated to the size of the herniation or age-related changes in the disk. A prospective observational study by Carragee and colleagues[58] performed lumbar MR images on 200 asymptomatic subjects; over the next 5 years, a subset of these subjects presented for medical care because of significant back or leg pain, at which time another MR imaging was performed. Eighty-four percent of the subjects presenting with pain had either no change or regression of baseline changes. The only positive correlates were new root compressive lesions in 2 patients with radicular pain. There were no imaging predictors of functional disability; as has been well documented, psychosocial factors are the principle determinates of disability, not imaging. Providing value in imaging the patient with radicular pain demands knowledge of the clinical state to appropriately filter out the plethora of insignificant imaging findings; direct observation of nerve displacement or compression concordant with the pain pattern may help to plan subsequent intervention. The decision to undertake interventions should be clinical, not based on imaging features.

CERVICAL DISK HERNIATIONS

This article, and the issue as a whole, concentrates on the lumbar spine. It would remiss, however, not to illustrate similarities and contrasts in the imaging of patients with cervical or thoracic radicular pain.

The cervical intervertebral disks differ structurally from the lumbar disks. The cervical disks are thicker anteriorly than posteriorly and have a less well-defined nuclear/annular structure. There is no discrete annulus at the posterior disk margin. The cervical disks function less to disburse axial load. As in the lumbar region, age-related changes in the cervical spine are common, asymptomatic, and increase in prevalence with age. Matsumoto and colleagues[59] studied nearly 500 asymptomatic patients using MR imaging and noted loss of T2 signal within cervical disks in 12% to 17% of patients in their 20s but in 86% to 89% of patients older than 60 years. Asymptomatic cervical cord compression was seen in 7.6% of patients, largely older than the age of 50. Similarly, Boden and colleagues[38] studied 63 asymptomatic subjects using MR imaging and noted cervical disk "degeneration" in 25% of those younger than 40 years, and in excess of 60% of patients older than 40 years. Asymptomatic subjects older than 40 years had a 5% rate of disk herniations and a 20% rate of foraminal stenosis. Teresi and colleagues[60] studied 100 asymptomatic subjects using MR imaging and noted asymptomatic cervical cord compression in 7% and either disk protrusion or annular bulge in 57% of subjects older than 64 years.

The natural history of cervical disk herniations parallels the lumbar region. Cervical disk herniations may undergo spontaneous regression, a finding that correlates with improvement in a patient's symptoms.[61] Similar to the lumbar region, extrusions, migrated disk material, and laterally situated disk herniations are more likely to undergo spontaneous regression.[62] As most lesions causing cervical radicular pain are not purely soft disk, but at least in part bony, overall regression of the root compressive lesion is less likely than in the lumbar region.

Cervical radiculopathy is a common clinical problem but less so than lumbar radicular pain or

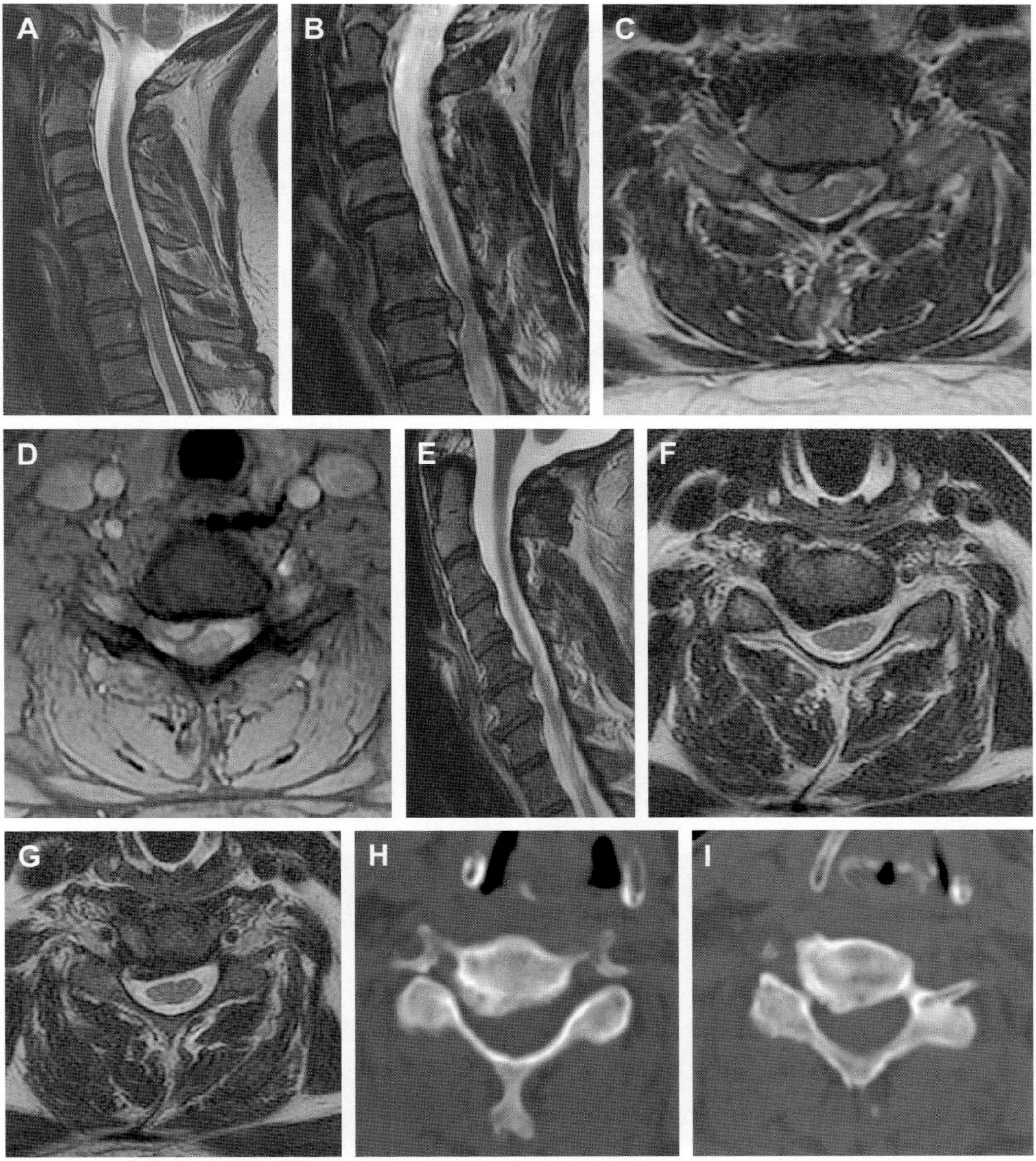

Fig. 13. Cervical disk herniation and foraminal compromise. Patient with prior C5-C6 fusion presents with right C7 radiculopathy. Sagittal T2 images (*A, B*) demonstrate C6 disk extrusion; note the extruded material is of higher T2 signal than disk of origin, a common observation. This is confirmed on axial fast-spin echo T2 (*C*) and gradient recalled echo T2 (*D*) images. In another patient with a right C6 radiculopathy, sagittal T2 image (*E*), and axial FSE T2 images (*F, G*) at the C5-C6 interspace suggest a disk–osteophyte complex and uncovertebral joint osteophytes compromise the C5-C6 foramen. The primary bony nature of the process in confirmed on CT images. (*H, I*) In the cervical spine, compressive lesions are more likely to be osseous than soft disk alone.

radiculopathy. In population-based data from Rochester, Minnesota, cervical radiculopathy had an annual incidence of 107.3 per 100,000 for men and 63.5 per 100,000 for women.[63] The most common cause of cervical radiculopathy is a foraminal constriction of multifactorial origin including uncovertebral joint hypertrophy, facet arthropathy, and loss of disk space height. Only 22% of cervical radiculopathies in this study were the result of herniated disk (**Fig. 13**).[63] When herniations were present, the spinal nerves most commonly involved were C6 and C7.[63] Generally the herniated disk is located posterolaterally, compromising the nerve root at the entrance to the neural foramen; occasionally the herniated disk is centrally located and causes myelopathy. Cervical nerves exit in the inferior aspect of the foramen; hence the exiting, not the traversing, nerve is most likely to be impacted by a disk herniation or a disk–osteophyte complex. The cervical nerves exit above the like-numbered pedicle; a C5 disk herniation compromising the C5-C6 neural foramen will impinge on the exiting C6 nerve.

The 2010 North American Spine Society evidence-based guidelines on cervical radiculopathy extensively reviewed the literature on imaging; the guideline recommendation is that MR imaging be performed as the initial imaging test, with CT myelography used in MR imaging-incompatible patients or when MR imaging is discordant from the clinical presentation.[64] MR imaging approaches the diagnostic accuracy of CT myelography without invasion or ionizing radiation. CT myelography may be crucial when the nature of the compressive lesion, bone versus soft disk, may change an operative approach. The higher spatial resolution of CT myelography may reveal subtle lateral recess and foraminal lesions that are less conspicuous on MR imaging.

THORACIC DISK HERNIATIONS

Symptomatic thoracic disk herniations are uncommon; operation for symptomatic thoracic disk disease constitutes less than 1% to 2% of all disk surgeries.[65] As in other segments, there is a high

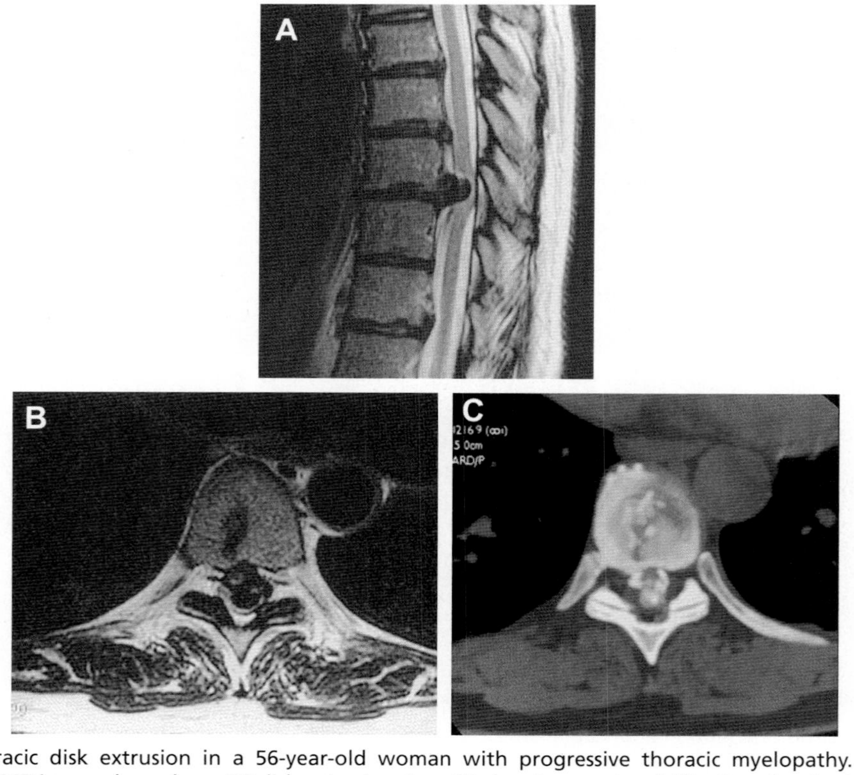

Fig. 14. Thoracic disk extrusion in a 56-year-old woman with progressive thoracic myelopathy. (*A*) Sagittal T2-weighted MR image shows large T8 disk extrusion. Low T2 signal suggests calcification. Smaller T7 disk extrusion. (*B*) Only a thin rim of cord is seen dorsal to the extrusion on T2-weighted axial MR. Axial CT image (*C*) demonstrates coarse calcification in the disk extrusion. Note the linear sclerosis in the end plate, a finding often accompanying disk herniations. At surgery, the T8 disk perforated the dura; it was resected successfully. (*From* Maus TP. Imaging of the spine and nerve roots. Phys Med Rehabil Clin N Am 2002;13:487–544; with permission.)

rate of asymptomatic degenerative disk disease in the thoracic region. Wood and colleagues[66] studied 90 asymptomatic patients using MR imaging. In this population, 73% of the patients had positive thoracic imaging findings, 37% had disk herniations, 53% demonstrated disk bulges, and 29% had asymptomatic cord deformity. In a follow-up study, the investigators reexamined a subgroup of their asymptomatic patients[67] and showed that there was little demonstrable change over time in the size of asymptomatic disk herniations. There was a nonstatistically significant trend for small herniations to increase in size and for large herniations to diminish. New asymptomatic herniations appeared within the follow-up interval; no herniations became symptomatic.

The majority of symptomatic thoracic disk herniations occur in the mid thoracic and lower thoracic spine. In the surgical series of Levi and colleagues,[65] T6 and T7 were the most common levels of operation. In the larger series of Stillerman and colleagues[68] (82 patients), the T8 through T11 levels most commonly required intervention. In this series, 76% of patients presented with pain, 61% with either motor or sensory dysfunction, and 24% with bladder dysfunction. Nearly two-thirds of the disk herniations showed evidence of calcification on CT imaging. At surgery, 7% showed intradural extension. Thoracic disk herniations at the level of the conus or high cauda equina can mimic lumbar radicular disease.[69] Hence, the conus must be included in lumbar MR imaging.

Imaging of thoracic disk herniations is done using MR imaging or CT myelography (**Fig. 14**). As the central canal and vertebral bodies diminish in size in the thoracic region, spatial and contrast resolution become more critical. CT myelography has the greatest spatial resolution and may better demonstrate the presence of calcification within thoracic disks. MR imaging is noninvasive and can detect signal abnormality within the cord, which may serve as a marker of cord edema or venous hypertension, verifying the physiologic significance of a disk herniation. All imaging evaluation for thoracic disk disease must include careful enumeration of the segmental level involved. If a lesion that may require surgical or percutaneous intervention is detected, the imaging study should be extended to include sagittal images from the sacrum to the skull base. Communication between radiologist and surgeon or spine interventionalist is critical to avoid wrong segment interventions.

SUMMARY

Age-related changes in the disk are ubiquitous and unrelated to symptoms. Disk herniations may occur when there is degradation of the nuclear matrix and failure of the annulus. Radicular pain requires both an element of mechanical compression of neural tissue and an inflammatory response, likely mediated by TNFα. Imaging of disk herniations suffers from the specificity fault seen in all spine imaging; disk herniations are frequently asymptomatic. The imager must know the nature of the pain syndrome to suggest a causal relationship with an imaging finding. The natural history of disk herniation is resolution. There is no relationship between the size, type, or change in disk herniations over time and patient outcomes. Patient disability due to disk herniation is primarily related to psychosocial factors not imaging. Selection of patients with radiculopathy or radicular pain for interventions, including surgery, must occur on clinical grounds, not based on imaging appearance.

REFERENCES

1. Mixter WJ, Barr JS. Rupture of the intervertebral disc with involvement of the spinal canal. N Engl J Med 1934;211:210–5.
2. Mulleman D, Mammou S, Griffoul I, et al. Pathophysiology of disk-related sciatica. I.–Evidence supporting a chemical component. Joint Bone Spine 2006; 73(2):151–8.
3. Mulleman D, Mammou S, Griffoul I, et al. Pathophysiology of disk-related low back pain and sciatica. II. Evidence supporting treatment with TNF-alpha antagonists. Joint Bone Spine 2006; 73(3):270–7.
4. Saal JA, Saal JS, Herzog RJ. The natural history of lumbar intervertebral disc extrusions treated nonoperatively. Spine 1990;15:683–6.
5. Haro H, Crawford HC, Fingleton B, et al. Matrix metalloproteinase-7-dependent release of a tumor necrosis factor-a in a model of herniated disc resorption. J Clin Invest 2000;105:143–50.
6. Haro H, Kato T, Komori H, et al. Sequential dynamics of inflammatory cytokines, angiogenesis inducing factor and matrix degrading enzymes during spontaneous resorption of the herniated disc. J Orthop Res 2004;22:895–900.
7. Olmarker K, Rydevik B, Nordborg C. Autologous nucleus pulposus induces neurophysiologic and histologic changes in porcine cauda equina nerve roots. Spine 1993;18:1425–32.
8. Kulisch SD, Ulstrom CL, Michael CJ. The tissue origin of low-back pain and sciatica: a report of pain response to tissue stimulation during operations on the lumbar spine using local anesthesia. Orthop Clin North Am 1991;22:181–7.
9. Cohen SP, Bogduk N, Dragovich A, et al. Randomized, double-blind, placebo-controlled, dose-response,

and preclinical safety study of transforaminal epidural etanercept for the treatment of sciatica. Anesthesiology 2009;110(5):1116–26.
10. Modic MT, Ross JS. Lumbar degenerative disk disease. Radiology 2007;245(1):43–61.
11. Bogduk N. Clinical anatomy of the lumbar spine and sacrum. New York: Elsevier; 1987.
12. Pfirrmann CW, Metzdorf A, Zanetti M, et al. Magnetic resonance classification of lumbar intervertebral disc degeneration. Spine (Phila Pa 1976) 2001;26(17): 1873–8.
13. Fardon DF, Milette PC, Combined Task Forces of the North American Spine Society, American Society of Spine Radiology, and American Society of Neuroradiology. Nomenclature and classification of lumbar disc pathology. Recommendations of the Combined task Forces of the North American Spine Society, American Society of Spine Radiology, and American Society of Neuroradiology. Spine (Phila Pa 1976) 2001;26(5):E93–113.
14. Nathan H. Osteophytes of the vertebral column. An anatomical study of their development according to age, race, and sex, with consideration as to their etiology and significance. J Bone Joint Surg Am 1962;44:243–68.
15. Modic MT, Steinberg PM, Ross JS, et al. Degenerative disk disease: assessment of changes in vertebral body marrow with MR imaging. Radiology 1988;166(1 Pt 1):193–9.
16. Kuisma M, Karppinen J, Niinimaki J, et al. Modic changes in endplates of lumbar vertebral bodies: prevalence and association with low back and sciatic pain among middle-aged male workers. Spine (Phila Pa 1976) 2007;32(10):1116–22.
17. Kuisma M, Karppinen J, Niinimaki J, et al. A three-year follow-up of lumbar spine endplate (Modic) changes. Spine (Phila Pa 1976) 2006;31(15):1714–8.
18. Karchevsky M, Schweitzer ME, Carrino JA, et al. Reactive endplate marrow changes: a systematic morphologic and epidemiologic evaluation. Skeletal Radiol 2005;34(3):125–9.
19. Hutton MJ, Bayer JH, Powell J, et al. Modic vertebral body changes: the natural history as assessed by consecutive magnetic resonance imaging. Spine (Phila Pa 1976) 2011;36(26):2304–7.
20. Rahme R, Moussa R. The modic vertebral endplate and marrow changes: pathologic significance and relation to low back pain and segmental instability of the lumbar spine. AJNR Am J Neuroradiol 2008; 29(5):838–42.
21. Aprill C, Bogduk N. High-intensity zone: a diagnostic sign of painful lumbar disc on magnetic resonance imaging. Br J Radiol 1992;65(773):361–9.
22. Bradley W. Low back pain. AJNR Am J Neuroradiol 2007;28(5):990–2.
23. Chou R, Qaseem A, Snow B, et al. Diagnosis and treatment of low back pain: a joint clinical practice guideline from the American College of Physicians and the American Pain Society. Ann Intern Med 2007;147:478–91.
24. Hall FM. Back pain and the radiologist. Radiology 1980;137(3):861–3.
25. Thornbury JR, Fryback DC, Turski PA, et al. Disk-cased nerve compression in patients with acute low-back pain: diagnosis with MR, CT myelography, and plain CT. Radiology 1993;186:731–8.
26. Jarvik JG, Deyo RA. Diagnostic evaluation of low back pain with emphasis on imaging. Ann Intern Med 2002;137(7):586–97.
27. Janssen ME, Bertrand SL, Joe C, et al. Lumbar herniated disk disease: comparison of MRI, myelography, and post-myelographic CT scan with surgical findings. Orthopedics 1994;17(2):121–7.
28. van Rijn JC, Klemetso N, Reitsma JB, et al. Observer variation in the evaluation of lumbar herniated discs and root compression: spiral CT compared with MRI. Br J Radiol 2006;79:372–7.
29. Lurie JD, Tosteson AN, Tosteson TD, et al. Reliability of magnetic resonance imaging readings for lumbar disc herniation in the Spine Patient Outcomes Research Trial (SPORT). Spine (Phila Pa 1976) 2008;33(9):991–8.
30. Pfirrmann CW, Dora C, Schmid MR, et al. MR image-based grading of lumbar nerve root compromise due to disk herniation: reliability study with surgical correlation. Radiology 2004;230(2):583–8.
31. Carrino JA, Lurie JD, Tosteson AN, et al. Lumbar spine: reliability of MR imaging findings. Radiology 2009;250(1):161–70.
32. Kjaer P, Leboeuf-Yde C, Sorensen JS, et al. An epidemiologic study of MRI and low back pain in 13-year-old children. Spine 2005;30:798–806.
33. Salminen JJ, Erkintalo MO, Pentti J, et al. Recurrent low back pain and early disc degeneration in the young. Spine 1999;24:1316–21.
34. Takatalo J, Karppinen J, Niinimaki J, et al. Prevalence of degenerative imaging findings in lumbar magnetic resonance imaging among young adults. Spine 2009;34:1716–21.
35. Hult L. Cervical, dorsal and lumbar spinal syndromes. Acta Orthop Scand Suppl 1954;17:1–102.
36. Hitselberger WE, Witten RM. Abnormal myelograms in asymptomatic patients. J Neurosurg 1968;28: 204–6.
37. Wiesel SW, Tsourmas N, Feffer HL, et al. A study of computer-assisted tomography. I. The incidence of positive CAT scans in an asymptomatic group of patients. Spine 1984;9:549–51.
38. Boden SD, McCowin PR, Davis DO, et al. Abnormal magnetic-resonance scans of the cervical spine in asymptomatic subjects. A prospective investigation. J Bone Joint Surg Am 1990;72(8):1178–84.
39. Jarvik JJ, Hollingworth W, Heagerty P, et al. The Longitudinal Assessment of Imaging and Disability

of the Back (LAID Back) study. Spine (Phila Pa 1976) 2001;26(10):1158–66.
40. Zamani AA, Moriarty T, Hsu L, et al. Functional MRI of the lumbar spine in erect position in a superconducting open-configuration MR system: preliminary results. J Magn Reson Imaging 1998;8:1329–33.
41. Weishaupt D, Schmid MR, Zanetti M, et al. Positional MR imaging of the lumbar spine: does it demonstrate nerve root compromise not visible at conventional MR imaging? Radiology 2000;215:247–53.
42. Willen J, Danielson B. The diagnostic effect from axial loading of the lumbar spine during computed tomography and magnetic resonance imaging in patients with degenerative disorders. Spine 2001; 26:2607–14.
43. Ross JS, Brant-Zawadzki M, Moore KR, et al. Diagnostic imaging spine. Salt Lake City (UT): Amirys; 2007.
44. Peng B, Wu W, Li Z, et al. Chemical radiculitis. Pain 2007;127(1–2):11–6.
45. Marshall LL, Trethewie ER, Curtain CC. Chemical radiculitis. A clinical, physiological and immunological study. Clin Orthop Relat Res 1977;(129):61–7.
46. Teplick JG, Haskin ME. Spontaneous regression of herniated nucleus pulposus. AJR Am J Roentgenol 1985;145(2):371–5.
47. Fagerlund MK, Thelander U, Friberg S. Size of lumbar disc hernias measured using computed tomography and related to sciatic symptoms. Acta Radiol 1990;31(6):555–8.
48. Maigne JY, Rime B, Deligne B. Computed tomographic follow-up study of forty-eight cases of nonoperatively treated lumbar intervertebral disc herniation. Spine (Phila Pa 1976) 1992;17(9):1071–4.
49. Bush K, Cowan N, Katz DE, et al. The natural history of sciatica associated with disc pathology. A prospective study with clinical and independent radiologic follow-up. Spine (Phila Pa 1976) 1992; 17(10):1205–12.
50. Bozzao A, Gallucci M, Masciocchi C, et al. Lumbar disk herniation: MR imaging assessment of natural history in patients treated without surgery. Radiology 1992;185(1):135–41.
51. Jensen TS, Albert HB, Soerensen JS, et al. Natural course of disc morphology in patients with sciatica: an MRI study using a standardized qualitative classification system. Spine (Phila Pa 1976) 2006;31(14): 1605–12 [discussion: 1613].
52. Autio RA, Karppinen J, Niinimaki J, et al. Determinants of spontaneous resorption of intervertebral disc herniations. Spine (Phila Pa 1976) 2006; 31(11):1247–52.
53. Monument MJ, Salo PT. Spontaneous regression of a lumbar disk herniation. CMAJ 2011;183(7):823.
54. Chou R, Fu R, Carrino JA, et al. Imaging strategies for low-back pain: systematic review and meta-analysis. Lancet 2009;373(9662):463–72.
55. Modic MT, Obuchowski NA, Ross JS, et al. Acute low back pain and radiculopathy: MR imaging findings and their prognostic role and effect on outcome. Radiology 2005;237(2):597–604.
56. Cribb GL, Jaffray DC, Cassar-Pullicino VN. Observations on the natural history of massive lumbar disc herniation. J Bone Joint Surg Br 2007;89(6): 782–4.
57. Masui T, Yukawa Y, Nakamura S, et al. Natural history of patients with lumbar disc herniation observed by magnetic resonance imaging for minimum 7 years. J Spinal Disord Tech 2005;18(2):121–6.
58. Carragee E, Alamin T, Cheng I, et al. Are first-time episodes of serious LBP associated with new MRI findings? Spine J 2006;6(6):624–35.
59. Matsumoto M, Fujimura Y, Suzuki N, et al. MRI of cervical intervertebral discs in asymptomatic subjects. J Bone Joint Surg Br 1998;80:19–24.
60. Teresi LM, Lufin RB, Reicher MA, et al. Asymptomatic degenerative disc disease and spondylolysis of the cervical spine: MR imaging. Radiology 1987; 164:82–8.
61. Bush K, Chaudhuri R, Hillier S, et al. The pathomorphologic changes that accompany the resolution of cervical radiculopathy: a prospective study with repeat magnetic resonance imaging. Spine 1997; 22:183–6.
62. Mochida K, Komori H, Okawa A, et al. Regression of cervical disc herniation observed on magnetic resonance images. Spine 1998;23:990–7.
63. Radhakrishnan K, Litchy WJ, O'Fallon WM, et al. Epidemiology of cervical radiculopathy. A population-based study from Rochester, Minnesota, 1976 through 1990. Brain 1994;117(Pt 2):325–35.
64. North American Spine Society. Evidence-based guidelines for multidisciplinary spine care, diagnosis and treatment of cervical radiculopathy from degenerative disorders. Burr Ridge (IL): North American Spine Society; 2010.
65. Levi N, Gjerris F, Dons K. Thoracic disc herniation: unilateral transpedicular approach in 35 consecutive patients. J Neurosurg Sci 1999;43:37–42.
66. Wood KB, Garvey TA, Gundrey C, et al. Magnetic resonance imaging of the thoracic spine: evaluation of asymptomatic individuals. J Bone Joint Surg Am 1995;77:1631–8.
67. Wood KB, Blair JM, Aepple DM, et al. The natural history of asymptomatic thoracic disc herniations. Spine 1997;22:525–9.
68. Stillerman CB, Chen TC, Douldwell WE, et al. Experience in the surgical management of 82 symptomatic herniated thoracic discs and review of the literature. J Neurosurg 1998;88:623–33.
69. Lyu RK, Chang HS, Tang LM, et al. Thoracic disc herniation mimicking acute lumbar disc disease. Spine 1999;24:416–8.

Imaging of Spinal Stenosis
Neurogenic Intermittent Claudication and Cervical Spondylotic Myelopathy

Timothy P. Maus, MD

KEYWORDS

• Spinal stenosis • Claudication • Myelopathy cervical spondylotic myelopathy (CSM) • Neurogenic intermittent claudication (NIC) • Diffusion tensor imaging (DTI) • Foraminal stenosis

KEY POINTS

- Lumbar spinal stenosis is an anatomic observation; it may cause the clinical syndrome of neurogenic intermittent claudication (NIC).
- The pathophysiology of NIC remains controversial; the best evidence suggests venous congestion from multiple sites of compression initiates an inflammatory reaction causing neural dysfunction and irritability.
- The imager must identify all sites of neural compression in the central canal, subarticular recess, and foramen.
- The clinical syndrome of cervical spondylotic myelopathy (CSM) occurs in the setting of cervical central canal compromise, frequently with underlying congenital narrowing.
- Intramedullary signal change, enhancement, and diffusion characteristics can aid in selecting CSM patients for decompressive surgery.

SPINAL STENOSIS

Although spinal stenosis is one of the most common reasons for spinal imaging, and most radiologists likely perceive they "know it when they see it," it remains a more elusive phenomenon when one carefully examines the literature. It is first important to distinguish between the anatomic observation of central canal narrowing and the clinical syndromes that it may provoke: neurogenic intermittent claudication (NIC) and/or radiculopathy in the lumbar spine, or myelopathy in the cervical or thoracic spine. Anatomic central canal narrowing is a frequent observation in an asymptomatic population, and increases in prevalence as an asymptomatic finding with age.[1] Compromise of the central canal, with or without associated subarticular recess (lateral recess) or foraminal compromise, provides the necessary but insufficient anatomic substrate for the clinical syndromes of NIC, radiculopathy, or myelopathy.

This article initially examines the literature describing the pathophysiology and imaging of NIC caused by lumbar central canal, lateral, and foraminal stenosis, followed by consideration of thoracic central canal compromise, and finally the pathophysiology and imaging literature of cervical spondylotic myelopathy (CSM). It is assumed that the reader can make the observations regarding compromise of the various spinal compartments; the emphasis is on the clinical significance of these observations as they affect the patient's clinical care and ultimate outcome.

NEUROGENIC INTERMITTENT CLAUDICATION

NIC caused by central and/or lateral and foraminal stenosis in the lumbar spine is a clinical syndrome of significant frequency and debility in the elderly population. The North American Spine Society (NASS) 2011 evidence-based guidelines on the diagnosis and treatment of spinal stenosis define

Department of Radiology, Mayo Clinic, 200 First Street SW, Rochester, MN 55905, USA
E-mail address: timpmaus@gmail.com

Radiol Clin N Am 50 (2012) 651–679
doi:10.1016/j.rcl.2012.04.007

it in this fashion: "degenerative lumbar spinal stenosis describes a condition in which there is diminished space available for the neural and vascular elements in the lumbar spine secondary to degenerative changes in the spinal canal. When symptomatic, this causes a variable clinical syndrome of gluteal and lower extremity pain and/or fatigue, which may occur with or without back pain. Symptomatic lumbar spinal stenosis has certain characteristic provocative and palliative features. Provocative features include upright exercise such as walking or positionally induced neurogenic claudication. Palliative features commonly include symptomatic relief with forward flexion, sitting and /or recumbency."[2(p8)] The most common symptoms in patients with lumbar spinal stenosis are back pain (prevalence of 95%), claudication (91%), leg pain (71%), weakness (33%), and voiding disturbances (12%).[3] There may be a paucity of physical findings, even in the presence of symptoms. NIC as a result of lumbar spinal stenosis is the most common cause of spine surgery in patients older than 65 years.[4] Critical points regarding NIC are summarized in **Box 1**.

> **Box 1**
> **Lumbar spinal stenosis**
>
> Decompression procedures for lumbar spinal stenosis are the most common spine surgery in the elderly.
>
> Neurogenic intermittent claudication (NIC) is a clinical syndrome; spinal stenosis is an anatomic observation.
>
> The pathophysiology of NIC remains controversial; the best evidence suggests venous congestion from multiple sites of compression initiates an inflammatory reaction and Wallerian degeneration with blood–nerve barrier disruption and intraradicular edema.
>
> The imager must identify all sites of neural compression: central canal, subarticular zone (lateral recess), and neural foramen.
>
> The reliability of imaging identification of compromise of the central canal, subarticular zone, and foramen is dependent on precise, well-defined criteria, not gestalt.
>
> Beware the specificity fault: the correlation between quantitative measures of central canal or dural sac size and patient symptoms or function is poor.
>
> Beware the sensitivity fault: dynamic lesions, present only with extension and axial load, may make recumbent imaging insensitive.
>
> Although magnetic resonance imaging is widely accepted as the primary imaging modality in assessment of NIC, there is no literature establishing its superiority over computed tomography (CT) or CT/myelography.

Prevalence, Natural History

Despite the significance of lumbar spinal stenosis and NIC, there is relatively little epidemiologic literature. A study from Denmark suggested an annual incidence of symptomatic disease of 272 per million inhabitants.[5] This is a fourfold higher incidence than symptomatic cervical central canal compromise. In the United States, Kalichman and colleagues[6] used data from the Framingham study to establish the prevalence of congenital and acquired lumbar central canal stenosis in a community population. Using the anterior-posterior dimension of the central canal derived from computed tomography (CT) studies (12 mm = relative stenosis, 10 mm = absolute stenosis), they noted congenital central canal narrowing of relative degree in 4.7% of the population and absolute stenosis in 2.6%. Acquired stenosis was identified in 22.5% (relative) and 7.3% (absolute) of individuals. Their review of the literature noted a range of prevalence of acquired lumbar stenosis from 1.7% to 13.1%. As would be expected, the congenital central canal stenosis did not change with age, but the prevalence of acquired stenosis (absolute) increased from 4% in patients younger than 40 years to 14.3% in patients older than 60. The presence of absolute central canal stenosis was significantly associated with low back pain in this study population; it was not significantly associated with leg pain. The correlation between imaging findings and symptomatology is discussed in detail below.

There is even less high-quality literature describing the natural history of lumbar spinal stenosis in the absence of medical or surgical therapy. The NASS systematic review suggests that, in the absence of reliable evidence, it is likely that the natural history of patients with clinically mild to moderately symptomatic degenerative stenosis is favorable in one-third to one-half of patients.[2] In patients with mild to moderately symptomatic stenosis, rapid or catastrophic neurologic decline is a rare phenomenon. There is no reliable evidence to define the natural history of clinically or radiographically severe stenosis, as all studies have excluded patients with severe neurologic compromise; they were considered immediate surgical candidates.

Pathophysiology

The pathogenesis of NIC in lumbar spinal stenosis has been a subject of investigation for half a century. Verbiest[7] initially described mechanical compression of the nerve roots of the cauda equina as a cause of NIC in 1954. Subsequent investigators have postulated that arterial or venous ischemia, perhaps exacerbated by restriction of cerebrospinal fluid (CSF) flow (which participates in nerve root nutrition), are major contributors to the clinical syndrome. The current preponderance of evidence would favor venous congestion secondary to mechanical compression. This hypothesis emphasizes the importance of multiple levels of compression, and the physiologic effects of lumbar extension. Both of these observations have significant relevance to imaging.

Takahashi and colleagues[8] demonstrated in a porcine model that blood flow within the cauda equina was reduced by 64% in the segment between 2 zones of modest (10 mm Hg) compression, providing early evidence that there are profound microcirculatory changes even in an uncompressed segment of nerve between 2 zones of compression. Olmarker and Rydevik[9] postulated that venous stasis between 2 zones of modest compression may cause proinflammatory compounds to leak from capillaries, stimulating a local inflammatory response. Also in a porcine model, they demonstrated reduced amplitude of action potentials in nerves subjected to 2 zones of modest compression. Furthermore, when 2 vertebral segments rather than 1 separated the zones of compression, there was a significant further reduction in the amplitude of action potentials. Thus, venous congestion can precipitate neural dysfunction.

Kobayashi and colleagues,[10] in a canine model, examined cauda equina histology after the application of a modest stenosis (30% of cross-sectional area) to the dural tube. The cauda equina demonstrated congestion and dilatation of intraradicular veins and an inflammatory cellular infiltrate. There was disruption of the blood–nerve barrier, both at the site of the compression and also in more distant sites of Wallerian degeneration. The necrotic debris created by Wallerian degeneration stimulates macrophage activity; macrophages are known to generate inflammatory molecules, such as interleukin-1 and tumor necrosis factor α. Macrophages may also stimulate cytotoxic activity by the release of nitric oxide and proteases. They are considered the chief effector cells causing an inflammatory neuritis that results in aberrant ectopic neural discharge and conduction disturbance leading to the pain and neural dysfunction of NIC.[10] In this canine model, the histologically demonstrated disruption of the blood–nerve barrier correlated with strong gadolinium enhancement on magnetic resonance imaging (MRI). It should be emphasized, paralleling the evidence presented earlier on the genesis of radicular pain caused by disc herniations, that an inflammatory reaction is intimately involved in the generation of pain.

There are thus experimental data to suggest that multilevel central canal compromise may provoke clinical symptoms even at modest levels of compression owing to venous congestion and a secondary inflammatory response. There are clinical studies supporting this contention. Sato and Kikuchi[11] stratified 81 patients with lumbar central canal stenosis caused by spondylosis and degenerative spondylolisthesis into those with a single-level stenosis at the L4-L5 level and a second group with 2-level stenosis at L3-L4 and L4-L5. The patients with 2-level stenosis were significantly more likely to have neurogenic claudication symptoms than those with single-level stenosis. It was also observed that in 2-level stenosis, the symptomatic expression most closely matched the radicular distribution of the more caudal of the 2 stenotic levels; in those patients with compromise at the L3 and L4 disc levels, the pain pattern matched that of the traversing L5 roots.

The study of Porter and Ward[12] noted that the sites of compression may be either in the central canal or the neural foramina. In their cohort of 49 patients with symptomatic NIC, 94% had either a multilevel central canal stenosis or central canal plus neural foraminal stenosis. They defined neural foraminal stenosis as a foraminal diameter smaller than 4 mm (the plane of the dimension was not specified). Symptomatic single-level stenosis was rare. Drawing on the earlier work of Takahashi and colleagues[9] and Olmarker and Rydevik,[9] they postulated that modest compression at 2 distant sites will cause venous congestion over a long segment and this will be exacerbated by the dynamic effects of walking (ie, vasodilatation of the arterioles and capillaries will worsen the venous hypertension and capillary stasis rendering a long segment of nerve ischemic and irritable, ultimately producing pain). This hypothesis can explain bilateral and unilateral claudication with a varied combination of central and lateral lesions, which may be near normal venous pressure in the static state but then exceed venous pressure under the stress of walking. It also emphasizes the importance of imaging detection of all stenotic zones, both within the central canal, the subarticular recess, and the neural foramina. Failure to address all zones of stenosis during a decompression procedure may result in an undesirable clinical result.

The work of Morishita and colleagues[13] emphasized the importance of the neural foramen as a potential zone of compression, particularly with dynamic changes in posture. In 2006, they studied 41 patients with central canal stenosis or disk herniations; intraoperatively, micro catheters with pressure transducers were placed in the neural foramina of L5. Action potentials were measured in the anterior tibial musculature. Intraforaminal pressures significantly increased when the patient posture was passively moved from lumbar flexion to extension. The amplitude of the action potentials diminished in concert with the rise in intraforaminal pressure. These patients did not have foraminal stenosis by imaging. The findings suggest that the neural foramen may be a site of venous constriction with the spine in extension even in the absence of stenosis detectable by imaging. This stenosis may act in concert with central or subarticular recess compromise to produce symptoms in positions of lumbar extension, such as walking. In a second study, Morishita and colleagues[14] again measured intraoperative L5 intraforaminal pressures during passive positional changes of the lumbar spine in a cohort of patients with spinal stenosis. These patients were stratified into single or 2 levels of central canal compromise, as well as into greater or lesser disability. The group with greater disability had significantly greater rises in intraforaminal pressures in the movement from flexion to extension. The patients who had 2-level central canal compromise had greater disability even though the rises in intraforaminal pressure were more modest. The study suggests that there is a cumulative effect of multiple sites of central canal compromise that conspire with the rise in intraforaminal pressures during lumbar extension to produce neural ischemia, presumably via venous congestion. One can postulate that static foraminal stenosis would further exacerbate this process. All levels of neural compromise, central, subarticular, and foraminal, are potentially significant and must be detected by imaging.

Imaging

Congenital spinal stenosis

It is widely accepted, although poorly documented, that in a portion (10%–15%) of patients who present with NIC, the spinal canal is congenitally or developmentally narrow, and only modest spondylotic changes are necessary to produce clinical symptoms (**Figs. 1** and **2**). Szpalski and Gunzburg,[15] in a recent review article on lumbar spinal stenosis, contended that there is a Gaussian distribution of both canal size and dural sac size; when a canal size is too small for the dural sac it contains, stenosis occurs. In this construct, disregarding the true achondroplasia syndromes, so-called congenitally narrow canals are merely the extreme of Gaussian distribution of healthy subjects. In contrast, Singh and colleagues[16] studied the morphologic characteristics of a cohort of surgically treated patients carrying the clinical diagnosis of congenital lumbar stenosis. They noted that these patients had a significantly shorter pedicle length and, as a result, smaller cross-sectional spinal canal area when compared with controls matched for age and sex. The patients with a congenitally narrowed lumbar central canal typically exhibit these morphologic characteristics over several vertebral segments, maximal at the L3 level. This contrasts with purely "degenerative" stenosis, which is often more focal, particularly at the L4 disc level.[16] Patients with congenital central canal stenosis tend to present at a younger age (40–50) and with less spondylotic change than typical. In this cohort of patients, congenital narrowing could be recognized on lateral radiographs by identifying a pedicle length to vertebral body ratio of less than 0.43 at the L3 vertebral level.

The common terminology of "congenital" spinal stenosis may in fact be flawed; "developmental" may be a more accurate designation. These morphologic changes may not simply represent genetic variation, but rather reflect a developmental insult. Papp and colleagues[17] studied patients with "congenital" spinal canal stenosis and noted significant correlations with prenatal factors. The spinal canal at the L3 level (>L4>L5) was found to be the most sensitive to the influence of prenatal events. In a multiple regression analysis, external factors accounted for 43% of the variance of the spinal canal cross-sectional area at L3; gestational age was by far the most significant factor. Shorter gestational age resulted in a smaller adult spinal canal. Significant factors of less importance included low placental weight, greater maternal age, primiparity, low socioeconomic class, and low birth weight. The L3 and L4 vertebral bodies are fully developed by age 1; L5, in contrast, is not fully mature until age 6. There is little opportunity for catch-up growth at L3 or L4 following a prenatal insult.[17] The trunk and limbs can recover from a prenatal disturbance, as they continue to grow until adulthood, resulting in normal external patient morphology concealing a mid-lumbar developmental stenosis.

Acquired spinal stenosis

The great majority of patients presenting with NIC have acquired "degenerative" spondylotic change as their primary cause of central canal, subarticular recess, and/or foraminal compromise. As noted by Dr Bogduk earlier in this issue, the term "degenerative" is unduly pejorative and may contribute to negative patient perceptions regarding their prognosis. Maturational or age change is preferred.

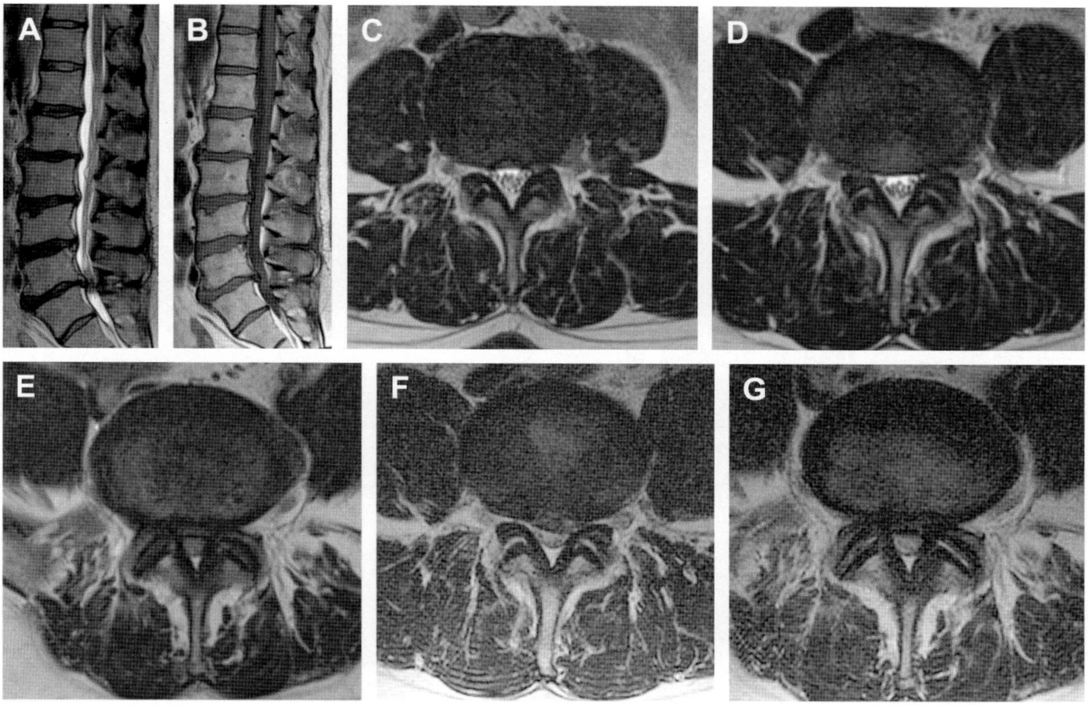

Fig. 1. MRI of developmental stenosis. Sagittal T2-weighted (*A*) and T1-weighted (*B*) images from 2010, with axial T2-weighted images at L3 (*C*), L4 (*D*), and L5 (*E*) discs. MRI axial T2-weighted images from 2003 at L4 (*F*) and L5 (*G*). There is developmental narrowing of the lower lumbar spinal canal with a reduced anterior-posterior diameter. Note the presence of a transitional segment, considered S1. This renders the L5 disc more vulnerable to age-related change. This 57-year-old man developed significant NIC in 2003, at which time he had a left-sided disc herniation at L4, and concentric severe stenosis at L5. Multilevel central canal compromise is more likely to be symptomatic. He refused surgery. In 2010 the L4 herniation had resorbed. He has persistent but much improved symptoms.

The changes that result in compromise of the central canal are rooted in the 3-joint structure of the spine motion segment: the disc and the paired facet joints. In the anterior column, degradation of the nuclear compartment of the disc places excessive load on the posterior annulus, resulting in endplate hypertrophs, or with annular failure, disc herniation. These changes encroach on the ventral aspect of the central canal or LRs. Loss of disc space height obligates narrowing of the neural foramina, and contributes to increased facet load and ultimately arthrosis; facet capsular hypertrophy and superior articular process (SAP) osteophytes compromise the subarticular recesses. Synovial cysts, particularly at the L4 level, may contribute to central canal, subarticular recess, or foraminal compromise. The reduced height of the segment, and loss of elasticity of the ligamentum flavum, result in its buckling centrally as a dominant cause of loss of cross-sectional area of the central canal. The ligamentum flavum may also thicken, although it is unclear if this represents true hypertrophy.[18] It is known to undergo fibrotic chondrometaplastic change, diminishing its elasticity, and to calcify more commonly in patients presenting with NIC.[15] Thickening of the ligamentum flavum has also been associated with arthropathy in the adjacent facet joints, suggesting there may be an inflammatory component to this process, independent of simple mechanical buckling of ligament into the central canal as a result of loss of disc height.[19] These several anterior and posterior column phenomena conspire to narrow the central canal most commonly at the L4-5 disc level, followed by L3-L4, L5-S1, and L1-L2.[20]

This cascade of age changes compromise the central canal, subarticular recesses, and/or neural foramina; there are a number of measurable parameters that could quantify the degree of stenosis depicted by radiography, myelography, CT, or MRI. Verbiest,[7] in his early descriptions of the entity of spinal stenosis, suggested that a 10-mm to 12-mm anterior-posterior (AP) diameter of the dural sac on conventional myelography constituted relative stenosis, with a measurement of less than 10 mm denoting absolute stenosis. Steurer

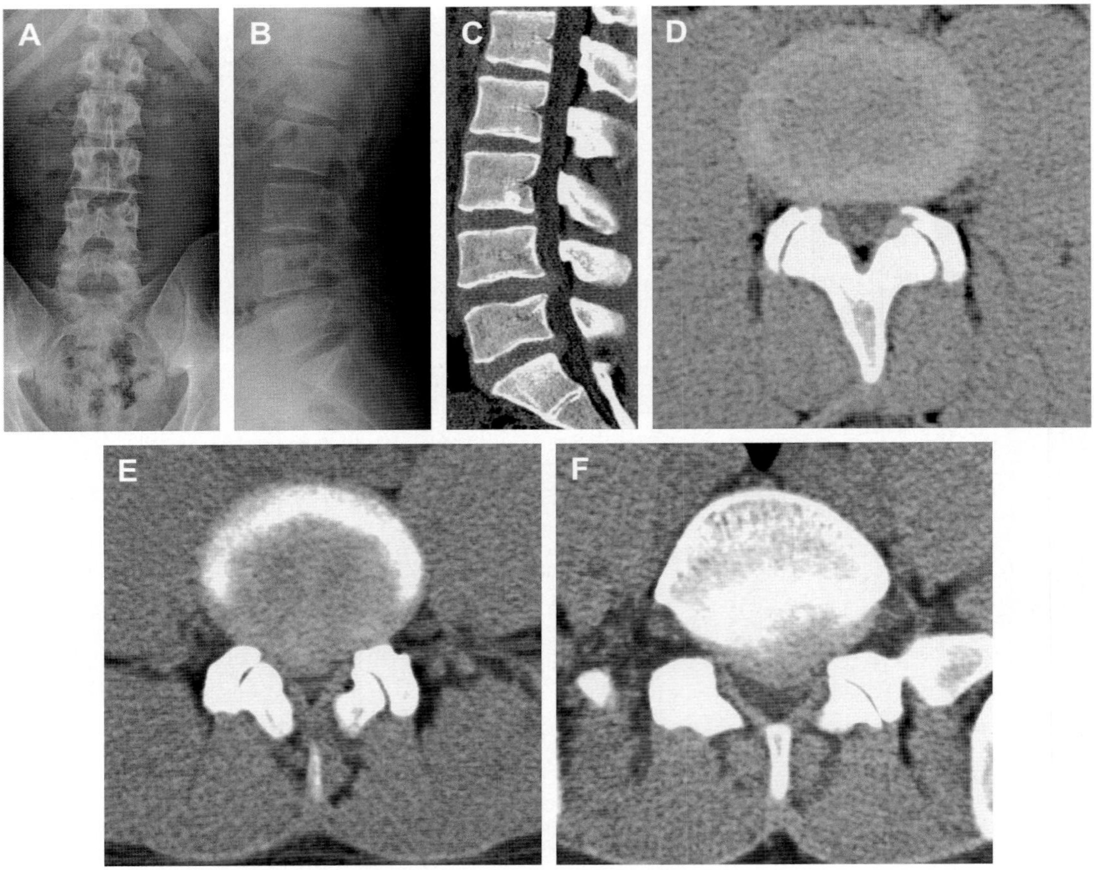

Fig. 2. CT of developmental stenosis. This 24-year-old man presented with incapacitating leg pain with walking and voiding disturbance. His standing radiographs (*A, B*) show only short pedicles at L4 and L5. He was not MRI compatible. Sagittal CT reconstruction (*C*) demonstrates disc herniations at L4 and L5 that severely constrict the thecal sac. Axial CT images at L3 (*D*), L4 (*E*), and L5 (*F*) confirm severe central canal stenosis at both L4 and L5 owing to the disc herniations and a small canal. This case is unusual in that congenital central canal narrowing is usually maximal at L3. It does demonstrate the ability of CT to provide all the needed information for surgical planning.

and colleagues,[21] in a 2011 review, surveyed the numerous measurements applied by various investigators in the intervening decades in 25 unique studies and 4 systematic reviews. These parameters are detailed in **Tables 1** and **2**.

The most common descriptors of central stenosis include the AP dimension of the osseous canal or the dural sac and the cross-sectional area of the dural sac. Dural sac AP dimension of less than 10 mm or dural sac cross-sectional area of less than 100 mm^2 constitutes stenosis. Descriptors of lateral recess or subarticular stenosis include the height and depth of the recess and the subarticular recess angle. Height is defined as the shortest distance between the most anterior point of the SAP and the posterior vertebral body, depth as the distance from the SAP to the junction of the pedicle and the vertebral body, and recess angle as the angle formed by the posterior vertebral body and the pars interarticularis. Although defined differently by different investigators, there is little real distinction between height and depth. Subarticular recess stenosis is typically defined as height less than 2 mm, depth less than 3 mm, or angle smaller than 30°. Descriptors of foraminal stenosis most commonly used suggest a diameter of 2 to 3 mm or smaller as indicative of stenosis. Steurer and colleagues[21] correctly observed that the lack of a uniform quantitative description of anatomic central canal, subarticular recess, or foraminal stenosis confounds the evaluation of the role of imaging in the diagnosis of the clinical entity of NIC. This criticism was echoed by Genevay and associates,[22] who lamented the high degree of variability in the eligibility criteria for studies examining neurogenic claudication caused by lumbar spinal

Table 1
Sites of measurement, measurement points, and radiologic definitions for central lumbar spinal stenosis

Imaging Method	Author	Site of Measurement	Level, Where Measured (Measurement Points)	Definition of Stenosis (Cut-Off Values)
Magnetic resonance imaging				
		Antero-posterior diameter of spinal canal		
	Fukusaki[102]		Not reported	<15 mm
	Koc[103]		Not reported	<12 mm
		Midsagittal diameter of thecal sac		
	Herzog[104]		Midbody of each vertebra	Compression of thecal sac area in % of normal midsagittal diameter: Grade 1: anterior <15%, posterior <10%; Grade 2: anterior 15%–30%, posterior 10%–20%; Grade 3: anterior >30%, posterior >20%
		Cross-sectional area of dural tube or sac		
	Hamanishi[30]		Intervertebral levels: L2/3, L3/4, L4/5	<100 mm^2, at more than 2 of 3 intervertebral levels
	Mariconda[105]		Not reported	<130 mm^2
	Laurencin[106]		Motion segment: intervertebral disc level coincident with flexible joint; stable segment: level coincident with the midpedicle unaffected by stenosis	Stenosis ratio: Cross-sectional area of dural sac of motion segment divided by stable segment cross-sectional dural sac area: Level: L3–L4 <0.66 L4–L5 <0.62 L5–S1 <0.73
		Ligamentous interfacet distance		
	Herzog[104]		Distance between the inner surface of flaval ligaments on a line connecting the joint space of facet joints at the level of the intervertebral disc	<10 mm (L2–L3) <10 mm (L3–L4) <12 mm (L4–L5) <13 mm (L5–S1)
		Transverse diameter of spinal canal		
	Koc[103]		Not reported	<15 mm

(*continued on next page*)

Table 1
(continued)

Imaging Method	Author	Site of Measurement	Level, Where Measured (Measurement Points)	Definition of Stenosis (Cut-Off Values)
	Ullrich[107]		4 zones of measurement: upper, middle, lower zone of vertebral body and disc space	<16 mm
Computed tomography				
		Antero -posterior diameter of spinal canal		
	Bolender[111]		5-mm intervals from L2 to L5	<13 mm
	Haig[33]		Not reported	≤11.95 mm
	Lee[108]		Not reported	<15 mm (suggesting narrowing) <10 mm (usually diagnostic)
	Ullrich[107]		Four zones of measurement: upper, middle, lower zone of vertebral body and disc space	<11.5 mm
	Verbiest[109]		Not reported	<12 mm (relative) <10 mm (absolute)
		Antero-posterior diameter of dural sac		
	Kalichman[6]		Midvertebral body level	10–12 mm (relative) <10 mm (absolute)
	Herzog[104]		Midbody of each vertebra	Compression of thecal sac area in % of normal midsagittal diameter: Grade 1: anterior < 15%, posterior < 10%; Grade 2: anterior 15%–30%, posterior 10%–20%; Grade 3: anterior >30%, posterior >20%
	Jönsson[110]		Disc level	≤10 mm
		Cross-sectional area of dural sac		
	Bolender[111]		5-mm intervals from L2 to L5	100–130 mm^2 (early stenosis) <100 mm^2 (present stenosis)

(*continued on next page*)

Table 1
(continued)

Imaging Method	Author	Site of Measurement	Level, Where Measured (Measurement Points)	Definition of Stenosis (Cut-Off Values)
	Laurencin[106]		Motion segment: intervertebral disc level coincident with flexible joint; stable segment: level coincident with the midpedicle unaffected by stenosis	Stenosis ratio: Area of motion segment divided by stable segment area Level: L3–L4 <0.66 L4–L5 <0.62 L5–S1 <0.73
	Schönström[111]		On each CT scan slice	<100 mm^2
	Schönström[112]		Not reported	75–100 mm^2 (moderate) <75 mm^2 (severe)
	Ullrich[107]		4 zones of measurement: upper, middle, lower zone of vertebral body and disc space	<145 mm^2
			Ligamentous interfacet distance	
	Herzog[104]		Intervertebral disc level	<10 mm (L2–L3) <10 mm (L3–L4) <12 mm (L4–L5) <13 mm (L5–S1)
	Wilmink[113]		Pedicular, infrapedicular and/or disc level	<11 mm (L4–L5)
Myelography conventional		Anteroposterior diameter of contrast column		
	Airaksinen[114]		Narrowest point	>12 mm 10–12 mm <10 mm Subtotal block Total block
	Bolender[111]		Intervertebral level	<13 mm
	Herno[115]		Not reported	<12 mm
	Jönsson[110]		Disc level	≤10 mm
	Sortland[116]		Disc level	<10.5 mm (lower limit) <5.5–7.0 mm (considerable)
	Verbiest[117]		Superior and inferior boarders of the laminae	10–12 mm (relative) <10 mm (absolute)
Myelography-computed tomography	Mariconda[105]		Not reported	<130 mm^2

Available at: http://www.biomedcentral.com/1471-2474/12/175. Accessed November 19, 2011.
From Steurer J, Roner S, Gnannt R, et al. Quantitative radiologic criteria for the diagnosis of lumbar spinal stenosis: a symptomatic literature review. BMC Musculoskelet Disord 2011;12:175; with permission.

Table 2
Sites of measurement, measurement points, and radiologic definitions for lateral lumbar spinal stenosis (subarticular recess)

Imaging Method	Author	Site of Measurement	Level, Where Measured	Definition Of Stenosis (Cut-Off Values)
Computed tomography		Lateral recess height		
	Ciric[118]	Not reported		5 mm (normal) ≤3 mm (highly indicative) ≤2 mm (diagnostic)
	Strojnik[119]		Between the most medial point of the superior articular facet and the posterior point of the vertebral body	≤3.6 mm
		Depth of lateral recess		
	Dincer[120]		Between superior articular facet and the top part of the pedicle.	>5 mm (normal) 4–5 mm (Group 3) 3–4 mm (Group 2) 2–3 mm (Group 1)
	Mikhael[121]		Between the posterior surface of the vertebral body and the anteromedial portion of the superior articular facet at the level of the superior border of the corresponding level	>5 mm (normal) 3–5 mm (suggestive) ≤3 mm (definitive)
		Lateral recess angle		
	Strojnik[119]		Between the bottom and the roof of the triangular space (= lateral recess)	<30°

Available at: http://www.biomedcentral.com/1471-2474/12/175.

From Steurer J, Roner S, Gnannt R, et al. Quantitative radiologic criteria for the diagnosis of lumbar spinal stenosis: a symptomatic literature review. BMC Musculoskelet Disord 2011;12:175; with permission.

stenosis, both radiological and clinical. The lack of a validated classification criterion impairs the quality of knowledge of this condition.

The multiplicity of quantitative parameters suggests that no single measurement has proven satisfactory. Indeed, the very notion of a readily quantifiable measure of stenosis may be flawed. There is wide individual variation in the size of the central canal and dural tube; the relative mismatch of these structures, exacerbated by spondylotic change, produces the increased pressure that results in venous congestion and Wallerian degeneration. Thus, any imaging criteria must address not just size of the dural tube or central canal, but imaging manifestations of crowding or compression of the neural elements. This was well described by Speciale and colleagues[23]; in examining the reliability of rating of central canal stenosis they noted a very poor correlation between the cross-sectional area of the spinal canal and the degree of crowding of neural elements. Some patients in whom the central canal was stenotic by cross-sectional area criteria showed little crowding of neural elements, whereas other patients exhibited adequate cross-sectional area but significant crowding of the cauda equina. A qualitative assessment of crowding is indeed what most radiologists examine, and is the basis of the simplistic criteria put forth by the joint study commission of radiological and surgical societies in 2001.[24] This lexicon of spine "degenerative " conditions defines central canal stenosis as mild if there is compromise of one-third or less of the expected canal area, moderate if the compromise is one-third to two-thirds, and severe if the compromise exceeds two-thirds. This more subjective standard better addresses the crowding of neural elements, but has reliability challenges, described later.

The observation of nerve root redundancy as a qualitative marker of central canal compromise dates from the original description of the entity of spinal stenosis by Verbiest.[7] This is presumed to originate from mechanical entrapment of the root at the site of compression, with subsequent elongation of the nerve above this site under the tensile stress of physiologic flexion and extension motion. Although frequently observed, this sign has been subjected to little study. Redundant nerve roots are present in 34% to 42% of surgical candidates with clinical NIC.[25] In a 2007 study by Min and colleagues,[25] redundant nerve roots were more commonly seen in older patients, but there was no significant association with duration of symptoms, diameter of the spinal canal, preoperative symptom intensity, or surgical outcomes. There was a nonsignificant trend toward poorer surgical outcomes in patients with redundant roots.

Degenerative spondylolisthesis

Degenerative spondylolisthesis was initially described by McNab as "spondylolisthesis with an intact neural arch."[26] It is highly associated with disk failure at this level, as well as significant facet arthrosis; it frequently results in single-level central canal compromise. Degenerative anterolisthesis is present in 4% to 14% of elderly patients.[27] It is most frequent at the L4 level, followed by the L5 and L3 levels. It is significantly more common in women than men.[27]

As degenerative spondylolisthesis is usually present at a single segmental level, it most commonly causes radiculopathy or radicular pain rather than NIC.[15] Associated foraminal stenosis or modest central canal or LR compromise at other levels can provoke NIC (**Fig. 3**).

Reliability of imaging parameters

Speciale and associates[23] studied the reliability of a normal, mild, moderate, severe classification of central canal stenosis. They observed only fair interobserver reliability ($\kappa = 0.26$). Stratified by specialties, reliability was higher among radiologists ($\kappa = 0.40$), followed by neurosurgeons ($\kappa = 0.21$) and orthopedic surgeons ($\kappa = 0.15$). Intraobserver reliability was poor at $\kappa = 0.11$. Linear regression models showed that the classification was highly correlated with central canal area; that is, although the grade of stenosis at a given spinal level showed wide variability among observers, smaller canals were invariably diagnosed as more severely stenotic than larger canals. In this study, the observers were not given criteria or examples defining the mild, moderate, or severe classification.

In contrast, Lurie and associates[28] studied the reliability of subjective grading of stenosis of the central canal, subarticular recesses, and neural foramina and measurement of central canal and dural sac area aided by specific definitions and imaging examples of the criteria. Stenosis was subjectively rated as none, mild, moderate, or severe using the Fardon and Millette definitions; nerve root compromise in the foramen was categorized as none, touching, displacing, or compressing. Inter-reader reliability in assessing the central canal was substantial, with $\kappa = 0.73$. There was moderate to substantial reliability for foraminal stenosis and nerve root impingement ($\kappa = 0.58$ and 0.51, respectively). Reliability for subarticular stenosis was only moderate at $\kappa = 0.49$. Intrareader reliability was greater than inter-reader reliability for all features. These results emphasize the importance of clear definition of criteria for reliable grading of stenosis by subjective scales.

Specificity: correlation of imaging findings with clinical state

The ultimate challenge in establishing the utility of diagnostic imaging in the diagnosis of NIC is the lack of a gold standard against which to measure imaging parameters. Surgical findings may be subjective. Clinical outcomes are highly dependent on the technical success of the instituted surgical therapy, and the outcome instruments used in any such measurement. Comparison against the best available cross-sectional imaging results in a circular argument.

The specificity fault in imaging of central canal stenosis can be seen in studies of asymptomatic volunteers. Boden and associates[1] noted significant central canal stenosis on MRI in 21% of asymptomatic subjects older than 60. Jarvik and colleagues[29] demonstrated that asymptomatic stenosis on MRI increases in prevalence with age: moderate to severe central canal stenosis was seen in 7% of subjects younger than 45, 6% of subjects age 45 to 55, 11% of subjects age 55 to 65, and in 21% of subjects older than 65.

Several studies involving patients with NIC suggested quantitative imaging correlates, which may aid in the diagnosis. The study of Hamanishi and colleagues[30] showed that a decrease in the dural

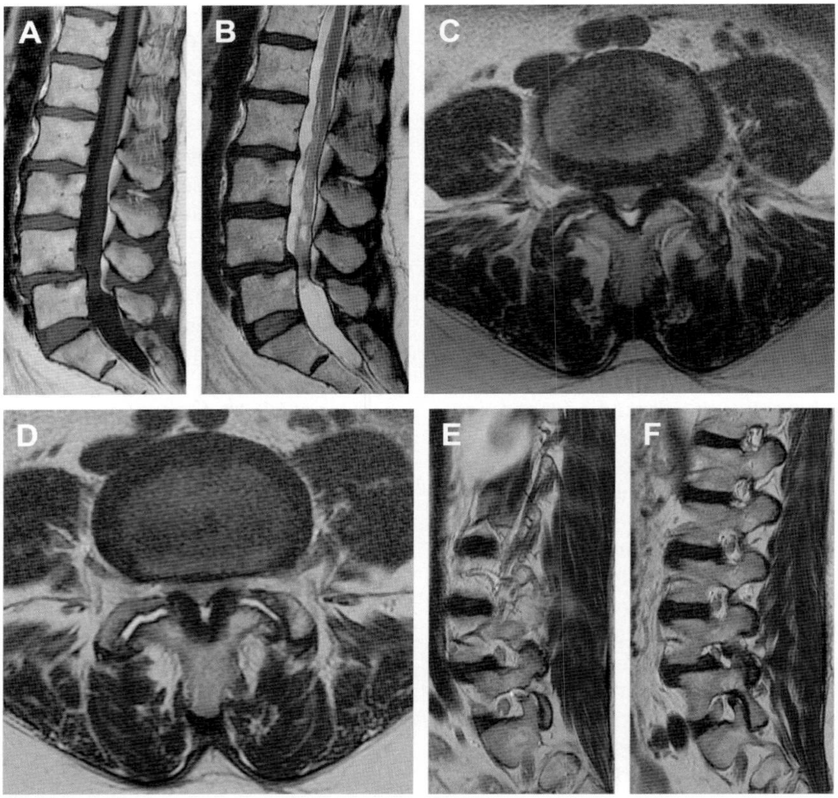

Fig. 3. Degenerative spondylolisthesis. Sagittal T1-weighted (*A*) and T2-weighted (*B*) images demonstrate grade 1 anterolisthesis of L4 on L5 with central canal compromise. Axial T2-weighted images through the L4 disc space (*C, D*) confirm severe central canal stenosis. Paramedian T2 sagittal images through the left and right foramina (*E, F*) show only modest foraminal narrowing on the right. This patient presented with a radicular pain syndrome (bilateral L5) rather than NIC, likely owing to the single-level compressive disease.

cross-sectional area (DCSA) to less than 100 mm^2 at more than 2 of 3 lumbar levels (L2–3, L3–4, L4–5) was highly associated with the presence of clinical NIC. Similarly, Bolender and colleagues[31] suggested that a DCSA of 100 mm^2 or less on CT was unequivocal evidence of central canal compromise. Schönström and Hansson,[32] in a cadaver study, demonstrated that a DCSA of 75 mm^2 or less corresponded to the initial increase in pressure in the cauda equina and represented a more physiologic marker of central canal stenosis.

On the contrary, numerous studies examining patients with NIC have shown a poor correlation between imaging parameters of stenosis and clinical state. Haig and colleagues[33] studied 126 patients stratified into 3 groups: those with no back pain, those with mechanical back pain, and those with NIC by clinical diagnosis. MRI measurements did not differentiate between patients with clinical NIC and controls by better than chance. Sirvanci and colleagues[34] examined 63 patients undergoing decompressive surgery for NIC. Morphologic stenosis was assessed by dural cross-sectional area (normal was greater than 100 mm^2; 76 to 100 mm^2 was moderately stenotic; less than 76 mm^2 was severely stenotic) and a 4-point grading of subarticular and foraminal stenosis. There was no correlation between any of the measured parameters in any spine compartment and patient disability as measured by the Oswestry Disability Index (ODI). This applied to both patients with multilevel central stenosis and a subset with degenerative spondylolisthesis.

Yasar and colleagues[35] performed a prospective analysis of 125 patients with a clinical diagnosis of NIC and anatomic central canal stenosis (DCSA <100 mm^2) who underwent surgical decompression. Preoperative evaluation included time to first claudicatory symptoms (FST) on treadmill testing, maximum walking distance (MWD), and ODI. There was no correlation between DCSA and the FST, MWD, or ODI preoperatively or at a 3-month postoperative evaluation. Results emphasize that the decision to operate and assessment at follow-up are better done with functional than anatomic parameters.

Geisser and colleagues,[36] in a 2007 study of 50 patients with clinical NIC, showed no correlation between the AP dimension of the spinal canal (using 10-mm or 13-mm criteria for stenosis) and functional assessments of patient disability. Zeifang and colleagues,[37] in a 2008 evaluation of 63 patients, found no correlation between MWD and DCSA. Although the NASS guidelines[2] conclude that there is insufficient evidence to recommend for or against a correlation between clinical symptoms or function and the presence of anatomic narrowing of the spinal canal on cross-sectional imaging, the preponderance of evidence argues against such a correlation in this author's judgment.

Sensitivity: dynamic lesions

There is also a basic sensitivity flaw in advanced imaging. NIC is by definition intermittent; most patients with NIC report exacerbation of symptoms with extension and weight bearing. The cross-sectional area of the central spinal canal, subarticular zone or lateral recess, and neural foramina are maximized with flexion positioning; the dimensions of these structures diminish with extension and axial load. Intradiscal pressures are significantly lower in a recumbent position than when sitting or standing. Schmid and associates[38] noted a 40 mm^2 reduction in cross-sectional area of the dural sac at the L3-4 level in moving from flexion to extension. Danielson and Willen[39] studied asymptomatic volunteers and noted a significant decrease in the DCSA with axial loading in 56% of the subjects, most commonly at L4-5. This finding was more common with increasing age. Decrease in DCSA with loading was less frequent in healthy volunteers than in a population of patients with NIC. In Willen and Danielson's study,[40] 80% of symptomatic patients crossed a threshold of relative (100 mm^2) or absolute (75 mm^2) in DCSA when axial load was applied using a loading device on a standard MRI scanner. Willen and colleagues[41] reported on the follow-up of 25 patients who underwent lumbar decompression based on central canal compromise detected solely on images obtained under axial load; 96% of the patients were improved or much improved regarding their clinical NIC after decompression. The proportion of patients with a walking capacity of 500 m increased from 4% preoperatively to 87% postoperatively. The NASS guidelines suggest that MRI or CT with axial loading is a useful adjunct to standard imaging in patients who have clinical signs or symptoms of NIC, a DCSA of less than 110 mm^2 at 1 or more levels, and suspected but not verified central or lateral stenosis on unloaded MRI or CT.[2]

A 2009 study by Hansson and associates[42] identified the ligamentum flavum as the greatest dynamic contributor to central canal compromise with axial load and extension. The average cross-sectional area of the central canal diminished by 23 mm^2 at the L3 disk level and 14 mm^2 at the L4 level under load. The ligamentum flavum was responsible for 50% of the reduction at the L3 level and 85% of the reduction at the L4 level. Madsen and associates[43] attempted to distinguish between the effects of axial load and extension; their work suggested that lumbar spine extension is the dominant cause of reduction in DCSA in the standing patient. Axial load was less significant. The study of Feng and colleagues[44] similarly identified a direct correlation between the degree of lumbar angular motion and the observed reduction in central canal diameter in the movement from flexion to extension. These studies would suggest that recumbent imaging in lumbar extension, with standard MRI scanners, may improve the sensitivity to the detection of dynamic lesions without the cost and diminished signal-to-noise ratio of dedicated upright scanners. This remains to be demonstrated in direct comparative studies.

Imaging modalities: CT, CT/myelography, MRI

There are no comparative effectiveness studies addressing the use of CT versus CT/myelography versus MRI in the documentation of central canal, subarticular recess, or foraminal stenosis using current technologies. The NASS systematic review of this question revealed that there is little strong evidence preferring MRI over CT or CT/myelography.[2] The studies of Kent and colleagues,[45] Bischoff and colleagues,[46] Modic and colleagues,[47] and Schnebel and colleagues[48] show good agreement between the modalities and no substantive evidence for the superiority of any modality. Based primarily on its noninvasive character, and lack of radiation exposure, NASS suggests MRI as the most appropriate initial study in patients with clinically suspected NIC; CT/myelography or CT alone are appropriate examinations in the non–MRI-compatible patient (**Figs. 4** and **5**).[2]

Gadolinium

MRI studies in patients with clinical evidence of NIC are typically performed without the administration of intravenous gadolinium, with the exception of the postoperative setting. Given the specificity challenges of purely anatomic imaging, the more physiologic parameter of gadolinium enhancement may have a role. This is not a new observation; Jinkins[49] in 1993 observed abnormal

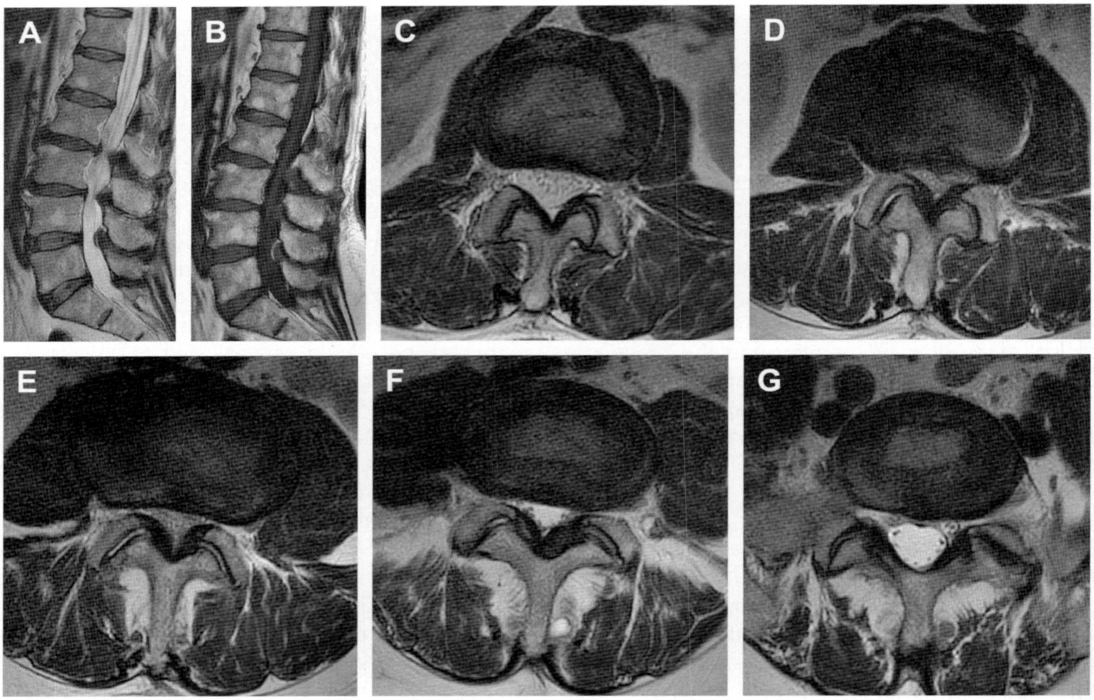

Fig. 4. Multilevel central canal stenosis, NIC. This 62-year-old exhibits classic symptoms of NIC, with bilateral buttock and lower extremity pain with walking; his tolerance is less than 1 block. Sagittal T2-weighted (*A*) and T1-weighted (*B*) images demonstrate mild loss of disc space height and annular bulges at L2 and L3; the dominant element constricting the spinal canal is the ligamentum flavum. Axial T2 images at L1 to L5 (*C–G* respectively) confirm the severe central canal compromise at L2 and L3 primarily because of ligamentum flavum.

intrathecal nerve root enhancement at the site of stenosis on enhanced MRI in patients with NIC. He postulated that this represented breakdown of the blood–nerve barrier at sites of nerve root injury with subsequent Wallerian degeneration. This has been elegantly confirmed in a canine model by the recent work of Kobayashi and colleagues.[10] Histologic examination demonstrated congestion and dilatation of intraradicular veins and an inflammatory cellular infiltrate at sites of gadolinium enhancement. Gadolinium enhancement may provide added specificity in the correlation of imaging and the clinical symptomatology of NIC; this remains to be proven in clinical studies **Fig. 6**.

Recent Observations

A 2010 study by Barz and colleagues[50] described the "nerve root sedimentation sign" as a marker of symptomatic NIC. In patients without central canal compromise, the roots of cauda equina lie in the dorsal aspect of the dural sac on supine MRI. A positive sedimentation sign was defined as the absence of nerve root sedimentation to the dorsal dural sac on at least 1 image of axial MRI at a level above or below the zone of compression; the 2 nerve roots leaving the dural sac at the next most caudal segment are exceptions. This retrospective study used a total of 200 patients: 100 patients with low back pain but without clinical NIC, and a DCSA greater than 120 mm^2, and a cohort of 100 patients with clinical NIC, a maximum walking distance of less than 200 m, and a DCSA of less than 80 mm^2 on at least 1 level. There was no correlation between the smallest DCSA and patient disability as measured by the ODI. The sedimentation sign, however, was identified in 94 of the patients in the NIC cohort but in none of the low back pain group. It remains to be demonstrated that this sign provides additional specificity over quantitative measurement of the DCSA.

THORACIC SPINAL STENOSIS

Symptomatic central canal stenosis in the thoracic segment of the spine owing to age-related change is far less common than in the cervical and lumbar regions, likely because of the added mechanical stability imparted by the rib cage. Systemic disease

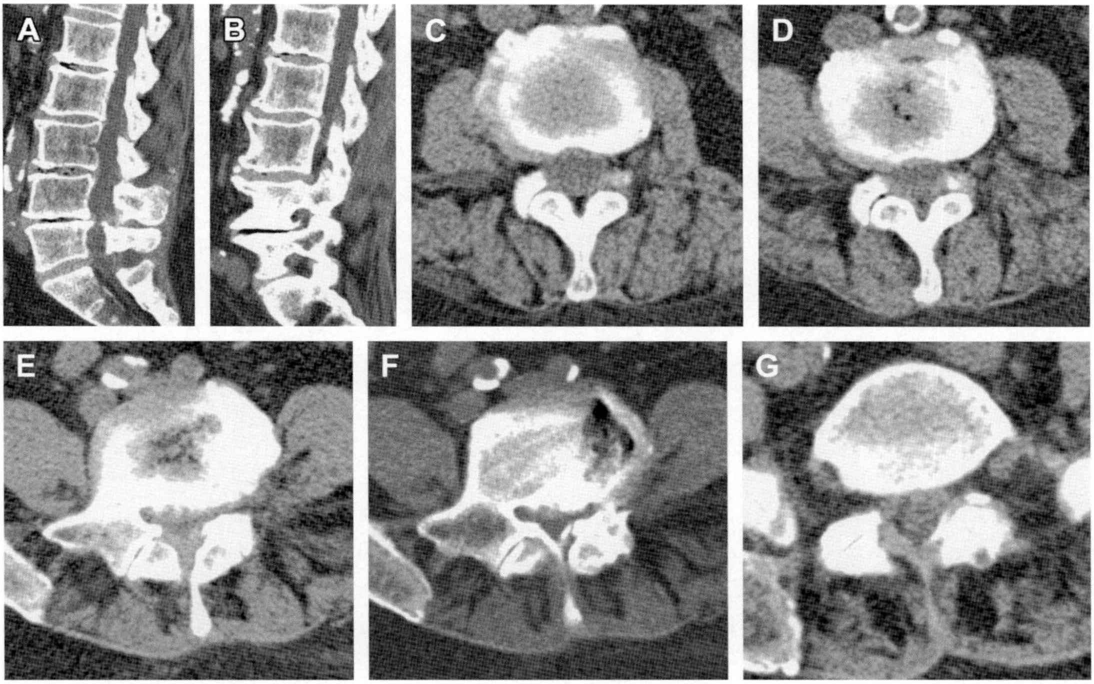

Fig. 5. CT of central canal, lateral recess, and foraminal stenosis. This 90-year-old woman complains of left leg pain reproducibly brought on by walking 20 to 30 m. She was MRI incompatible. Midsagittal CT reconstruction (*A*) shows severe central canal stenosis at the L4 interspace level. Left paramedian sagittal image reveals left L4 foraminal stenosis (*B*). Axial CT images at L2 (*C*), L3 (*D*), L4 (*E, F*), and L5 (*G*) illustrate that CT can well demonstrate the severe central canal stenosis at L4, and also demonstrate the left subarticular recess and foraminal stenosis at that level. All sites of possible neural (and venous) compression must be identified.

accounts for a correspondingly greater proportion of cases. Systemic processes leading to thoracic central canal compromise include achondroplasia, osteochondrodystrophy, Scheuermannn disease, diffuse idiopathic skeletal hyperostosis (DISH), and Paget disease. Age-related causes and select unique entities are addressed in the following paragraphs.

Compromise of the thoracic spinal canal may be manifest clinically as myelopathy, radiculopathy, or a mixed presentation. In a surgical series reported by Palumbo and colleagues,[51] all patients reported pain at presentation; half exhibited a clinical myelopathy. In another surgical series of Chang and associates,[52] a myelopathy picture dominated in 86% (spastic paraparesis, hyperreflexia, sensory level), whereas 14% exhibited a mixed pattern (paraparesis, radicular pain, and normal deep tendon reflexes). In this series, back pain was less frequent.

The segmental level of canal compromise is most commonly reported to be in the lower thoracic region. In the Palumbo and colleagues' series[51] the stenotic zone was always in the lower half of the thoracic spine; two-thirds bridged the thoracolumbar junction, and most were multilevel. The larger series by Chang and colleagues[52] had 54% of cases with lesions in the T9 to T12 region, with 25% from T5 to T8, and the remainder in the upper thoracic region. Earlier surgical series also demonstrated stenotic segments exclusively in the lower thoracic spine. Thoracic spine mobility, particularly flexion-extension motion, is greatest near the thoracolumbar junction, likely the biomechanical underpinning to this distribution of age-related pathology.

Posterior element age-related changes play a greater role in the genesis of thoracic central canal compromise. This takes the form primarily of unilateral or bilateral facet joint hypertrophy. Thoracic disc herniations or disc-osteophyte complexes may also contribute. Both the ventral and dorsal contributions to thoracic central canal compromise are well seen on CT, CT/myelography, and MRI.

Ossification of the thoracic ligamentum flavum (OTLF), although rare in a white population, is a well-recognized cause of myelopathy or mixed myelo-radiculopathy in an Asian population. The prevalence of OTLF in an Asian population is

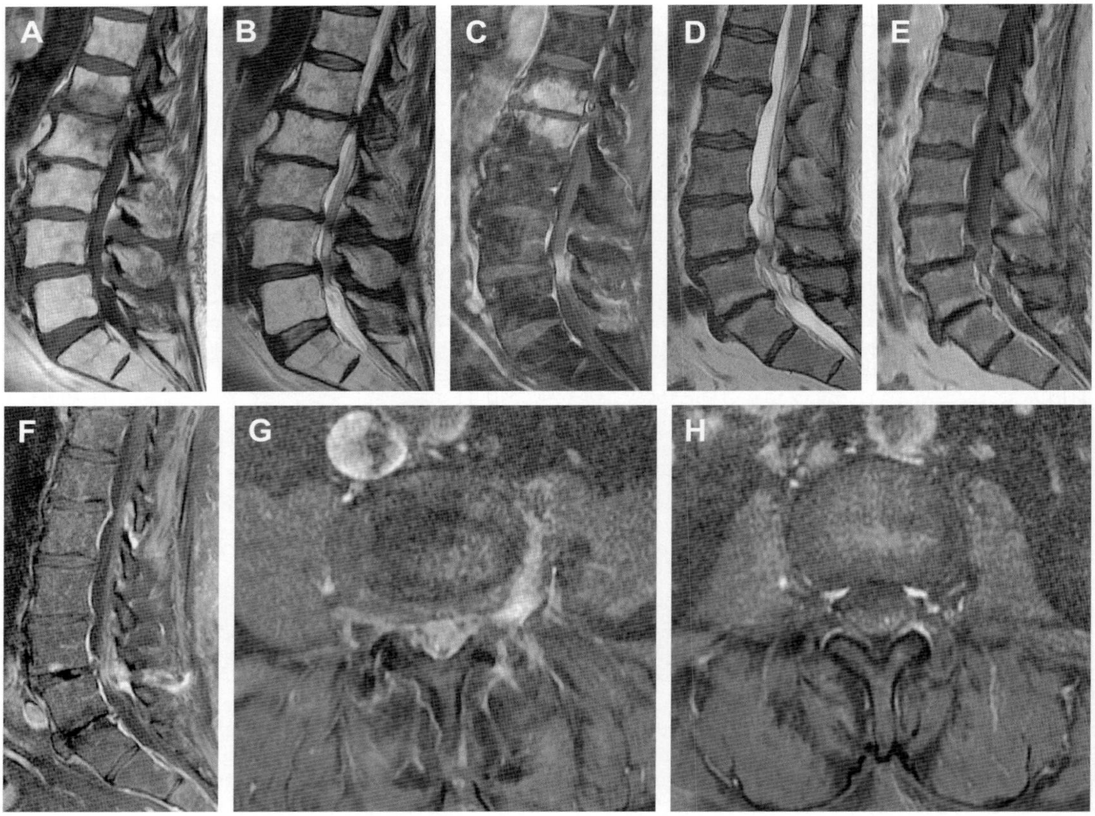

Fig. 6. Cauda equina enhancement. This 68-year-old man has severe NIC, with a walking tolerance of only 10 to 20 m. Sagittal T1-weighted (*A*) and T2-weighted (*B*) images demonstrate a congenitally narrow spinal canal in AP dimension. There is Modic 1 change about the L1 interspace with significant central canal compromise; slight anterolisthesis of L4 on L5 with severe central canal compromise. Sagittal T1 fat-saturated post gadolinium image (*C*) shows enhancement in the cauda equina at the L4 level, implying breakdown of the blood–nerve barrier. In another case of an elderly man with NIC , sagittal T2 image (*D*) shows central canal compromise maximal at L5; note that L5 is transitional in character. Redundant nerve roots are evident. Post gadolinium T1-weighted image (*E*) suggests intrathecal enhancement, which is much more conspicuous on fat-saturated, enhanced T1 image (*F*). Note also enhancement in the interspinous ligament (Baastrup disease). Axial T1 fat-saturated images demonstrate the cauda equina enhancement at L3 (*G*). Axial image at L1 level (*H*) for comparison shows no intrathecal enhancement. (*Courtesy of* Dr Felix Diehn.)

estimated as 6.2% of men and 4.8% of women.[53] The ossified, thickened ligamentum flavum is readily demonstrated by either CT or MRI, and is typically seen in the lower third of the thoracic region. Its pathogenesis is poorly understood. It may be associated with ossification of the posterior longitudinal ligament (OPLL), which is discussed later in this article.

Epidural lipomatosis is a rare cause of central canal compromise in the thoracic or lumbar spine; it may be idiopathic or secondary to endogenous or exogenous steroid excess. Obesity is a common factor in both groups. Excess epidural fat acts as a mass compressing the dural sac, most commonly from a dorsal vector in the thoracic region; it is more likely to be circumferential in the lumbar region. A recent literature review by Al- Khawaja and associates[54] noted that thoracic involvement was more frequent in secondary versus idiopathic cases; lumbar involvement dominated in idiopathic cases. Conservative therapy with weight reduction (and removal of any endocrine stimulus) was beneficial when no neurologic compromise was evident; in the face of neurologic deficit, surgery was indicated. Surgical intervention was moderately successful (50%–60% full recovery) with the exception of secondary thoracic involvement, where surgical outcomes were much poorer (**Fig. 7**).

CERVICAL STENOSIS

Cervical spondylotic myelopathy (CSM) is the most common cause of spinal cord dysfunction

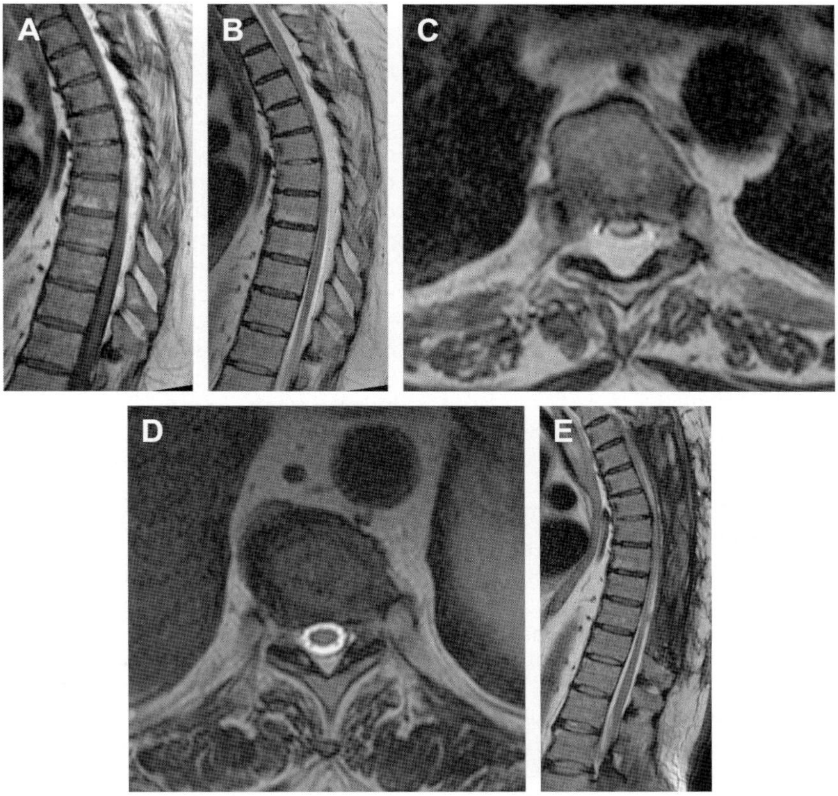

Fig. 7. Thoracic epidural lipomatosis. This 73-year-old morbidly obese man developed progressive myelopathy over several months. T1-weighted (*A*) and T2-weighted (*B*) sagittal MRI images of the thoracic spine demonstrate severe epidural lipomatosis situated dorsally. Axial T2-weighted images at (*C*) and below (*D*) the zone of maximal stenosis show cord deformity and intramedullary T2 hyperintensity at the apex of the thoracic kyphosis. Surgical decompression was performed without benefit (*E*).

in patients older than 55 years.[55] This section examines the pathophysiology of CSM, the role of imaging in the detection and characterization of the underlying anatomic abnormality, and the use of imaging in the selection of patients for therapeutic interventions, particularly surgical decompression. It is insufficient to simply describe morphologic alterations in cervical spondylosis; the imager must be familiar with the literature identifying the clinical significance of imaging findings, guide the use of advanced imaging, and inform its use in patient selection for decompression. The prognostic significance of MRI findings in CSM are discussed in depth. The critical points are summarized in **Box 2**.

Stookey[56] originally described CSM in 1928. Although its pathophysiology remains incompletely understood, it is widely acknowledged to involve static factors causing stenosis of the cervical canal and dynamic factors causing repetitive cord injury.[55] These mechanical factors both directly injure neural tissue and initiate secondary ischemia, inflammation, and apoptosis. The histologic characteristics of CSM include cystic cavitation and gliosis of the central gray matter and demyelination of the medial portions of the white matter long tracks. There is Wallerian degeneration in the posterior columns and posterolateral tracts cephalad to the site of compression. Loss of anterior horn cells and corticospinal tract degeneration are seen at and caudal to the site of compression.[55] Imaging correlates are discussed later in this section.

Pathogenesis: Static Factors

The developmentally narrow spinal canal is a more universal substrate for CSM than is the case with NIC in the lumbar region. The sagittal diameter of the adult spinal cord is nearly constant, measuring about 8 mm from C3 to C7; the cervical cord enlargement occurs primarily in the transverse plane.[57] The normal cervical spinal canal sagittal diameter (posterior vertebral body to spinolaminar

Box 2
Cervical spinal stenosis

The clinical syndrome of cervical spondylotic myelopathy (CSM) very frequently occurs in the setting of a congenitally narrowed spinal canal.

Fixed stenosis, dynamic injury with motion, and a secondary cascade of ischemia, inflammation, and cell death cause the clinical syndrome of CSM.

The specificity fault common to all spine imaging persists in the cervical region: patients meeting objective criteria of central canal stenosis may be asymptomatic.

Intramedullary T2 hyperintensity may reflect a spectrum of pathology, from reversible edema to demyelination and cystic necrosis; more intense and well-defined T2 hyperintensity suggests irreversible injury.

Intramedullary T1 hypointensity implies irreversible necrotic change.

Intramedullary gadolinium enhancement is a negative prognostic finding in patients with CSM.

Diffusion tensor imaging is more sensitive than T2 hyperintensity in the detection of early cord injury; decreased fractional anisotropy values at the site of compression are the most reliable parameter.

line) is 17 to 18 mm (C3–C7) in a white population; such subjects will rarely develop sufficient age-related change to provoke CSM. Edwards and LaRocca[58] observed that patients with developmentally narrowed midcervical sagittal diameters smaller than 10 mm were often myelopathic, patients with canals of 10 to 13 mm were at risk for CSM, canals of 13 to 17 mm were seen in patients with symptomatic spondylosis but rarely myelopathy, and subjects with canals larger than 17 mm were not prone to develop spondylosis.

Morishita and colleagues[57] recently examined the kinematics of subjects with congenitally narrow cervical canals, and noted significant differences when compared with normal canals. In congenitally narrowed canals, there is more segmental mobility in the lower cervical segments, C4-5 to C6-7, and significantly greater disc age-related change in the lower cervical spine. Hence, the individual with a congenitally narrowed canal is at risk both because of the limited space available for the cord, and a greater propensity to age-related spondylotic change (**Fig. 8**).

Acquired cervical central canal stenosis encompasses age-related spondylotic change (most common), OPLL, and ossification of the ligamentum flavum (OLF). As in the lumbar region, age-related degradation of the matrix of the disc nucleus transfers load to the annulus, resulting in disc-osteophyte complexes or protrusions encroaching on the ventral canal. Increased loading of the uncovertebral joints provokes hypertrophic change, compromising the lateral recesses and proximal neural foramina. These anterior column changes excessively load the facet joints, with resultant hypertrophy. The ligamentum flavum loses elasticity and buckles centrally. This cascade of events circumferentially narrows the canal and may directly compress the cord, exiting spinal nerves, and the anterior spinal artery. In Morio and colleagues' surgical series,[59] the most common levels of compromise were C3-4 (27%), C4-5 (37%), and C5-6 (29%). This series included patients with spondylosis only and patients with OPLL.

OPLL is a multifactorial disease, whose genetic basis is a defect in the nucleotide pyrophosphatase (NPPS) gene.[55] The prevalence is 1.9% to 4.3% of the Japanese population, and approximately 3.0% in Korea and Taiwan. It is implicated in up to 25% of the North American and Japanese cases of CSM.[59] It has a significant association (up to 50%) with DISH, and is considered by some a subtype of DISH.[60] It is progressive with age. OPLL imaging characteristics are discussed later in this section.

OLF is more common in the thoracic spine, where it was previously described. It may also extend into the cervical spine; its prevalence in the Japanese population older than 65 years is up to 20%.[55]

Pathogenesis: Dynamic Factors

In addition to static compression, dynamic forces contribute to repetitive cord injury. Chen and colleagues[60] measured dynamic flexion-extension changes in cadavers; the flexion to extension motion increased disc bulging by 10.8% of the canal diameter, and ligamentum flavum bucking by 24.3% of the canal diameter. Zhang and colleagues[61] performed flexion and extension MRI studies on patients with CSM. The cross-sectional area of the central canal was greater in the neutral position than in either flexion or extension; it was greater in flexion than extension. There was functional cord impingement in 12% of patients in flexion, 34% in the neutral position, and 74% in extension. Muhle and colleagues[62] noted an increase in central canal stenosis in 48% of patients moving from the neutral to an extension position, with 20% exhibiting cord

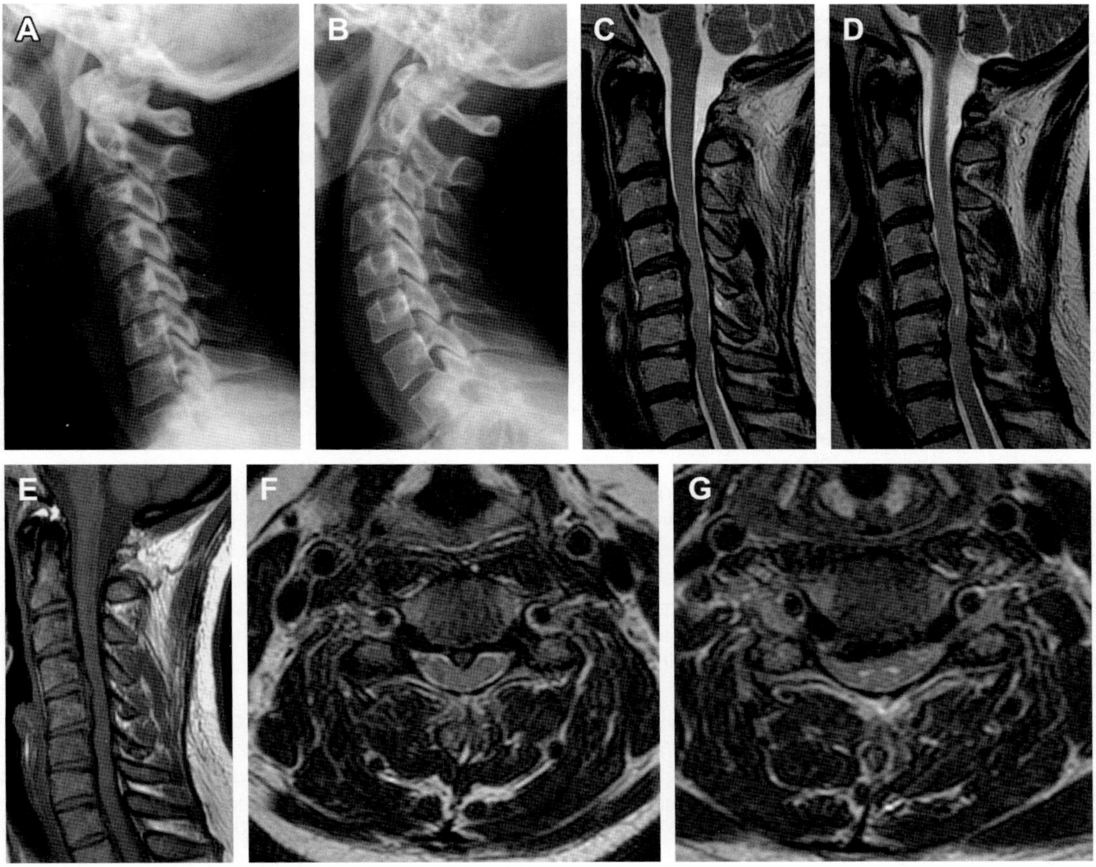

Fig. 8. Developmental cervical stenosis. This 36-year-old woman presented with very subtle bilateral hand incoordination, neck pain, and left arm symptoms. Her lateral radiograph (*A*) shows no lamina posterior to the articular pillar. Compare with a normal lateral radiograph (*B*). Sagittal T2-weighted (*C, D*) and T1-weighted (*E*) images show cord deformity from the C4 through C6 interspaces. T2 hyperintensity in the cord caudal to C5 interspace. Axial fast spin-echo (FSE) T2 image at the C4 to C5 interspace (*F*) reveals central disc herniation compressing the cord. Axial FSE T2 image at the C5 to C6 interspace (*G*) shows disc-osteophyte complex eccentric to the right deforming the cord. Focal intramedullary T2 hyperintensity may reflect irreversible injury.

compromise; the movement from neutral into flexion increased central canal stenosis in 24% and cord compromise in 11%. Cervical neural foramina diminish in cross-sectional area in extension, and increase slightly in flexion.[62]

In addition to the mechanical trauma to the cord imparted by static compression or dynamic compression and tension, secondary biochemical processes, especially ischemia, contribute to the development of CSM.[55] Ventral compression of the cord compromises flow through the arterioles arising from the anterior spinal artery in the ventral sulcus; dorsal compression reduces perfusion to the central gray matter. Oligodendrocytes are extremely sensitive to ischemic injury; resultant apoptotic cell death may cause the demyelination characteristically seen in CSM. Recent animal evidence further supports the role of an inflammatory cascade and Fas-mediated apoptosis in CSM.[63] In an animal model, an antibody directed against the Fas-ligand diminished the inflammatory response and increased neurologic recovery from compressive injury.[63] Such medical management may become a useful adjuvant to surgical decompression.

Imaging

Imaging of patients with CSM may include radiographs, CT, CT/myelography, and MRI. Imaging parameters, reliability, specificity challenges, correlation with clinical CSM, and imaging predictors of response to surgical decompression are discussed.

Historically, radiographic assessment of cervical anatomic stenosis relied on the AP dimension of the central canal as measured from the posterior vertebral body to the spinolaminar line. As noted previously, the normal sagittal diameter from C3 through C7 is considered to be 17 to 18 mm. Edwards and LaRocca[58] noted that a cervical canal with a sagittal diameter smaller than 13 mm was at risk for myelopathy; absolute stenosis was defined as being smaller than 10 mm. To compensate for magnification variables, Pavlov and Torg (Pavlov and colleagues[64]) promulgated the ratio of the sagittal diameter of the spinal canal to the sagittal diameter of the mid-vertebral body; a value greater than 1 was regarded as normal, and a value less than 0.82 was considered absolute stenosis. More recent studies have shown a poor correlation between the Pavlov/Torg ratio and the space available for the cord, suggesting its usefulness is limited.[65]

The advent of cross-sectional imaging has allowed us to directly measure the diameters and cross-sectional areas of the cervical spinal canal and the cervical cord. MRI has also given us the ability to evaluate physiologic parameters: T2 hyperintensity, T1 hypointensity, gadolinium enhancement, and, with diffusion tensor imaging (DTI), fractional anisotropy (FA) and apparent diffusion coefficient (ADC).

Reliability

A 2010 study by Naganawa and associates[66] demonstrated good intraobserver and interobserver reliability in evaluation of the cross sections of the cervical canal and spinal cord with both CT/myelography and MRI. They noted that dural sac diameter and cross-sectional area measurements were slightly but significantly larger with CT/myelography than fast spin-echo T2-weighted MRI; conversely, the diameters and cross-sectional areas of the spinal cord were slightly but significantly larger with MRI. These findings may reflect halation by the myelographic contrast material, overestimating the CSF space. They also evaluated a semiquantitative 4-point rating scale of the degree of stenosis; the interobserver kappa values were 0.69 for CT/myelography and 0.68 for MRI. MRI graded the stenosis as slightly, but significantly, more severe than CT/myelography, likely because of the halation effect. This study examined fast spin-echo T2-weighted images; it could be anticipated that T2* (gradient echo) imaging would have further accentuated this effect. Note that the very good reliability figures in this study may reflect the use of defined criteria and representative images in training observers. A similar 2009 study by Song and associates[67] found no significant difference in interobserver or intraobserver reliability between CT/myelography and MRI. With its superior spatial resolution, CT/myelography was somewhat better in assessment of foraminal stenosis, and much better in discriminating bony versus soft tissue lesions. MRI was more reliable in identifying direct nerve root compression. An earlier (1999) study by Shafaie and colleagues[68] showed a poorer agreement between MRI and CT/myelography; given the interval evolution in technology, this is of questionable relevance.

Imaging specificity: correlation with pathophysiology, clinical state

As in the lumbar region, there is a basic specificity fault in all cervical imaging: subjective and quantitative evidence of central canal compromise may be seen in asymptomatic subjects. The prevalence of asymptomatic findings increases with age. Teresi and colleagues[69] studied asymptomatic volunteers 65 and older with MRI; 57% exhibited cervical disc protrusions and 7% had frank cord compression. Hayashi and colleagues[70] noted 10% of subjects older than 60 to demonstrate significant stenosis in canal diameter (<13 mm) without signs or symptoms. Matsumoto and colleages,[71] in a large study of 500 asymptomatic subjects, observed direct cervical cord compression in 8%.

When a population of patients with a clinical diagnosis of CSM is studied, the correlations appear more favorable. The transverse area of the spinal cord as measured by MRI correlates well with the severity of myelopathy and the pathologic changes seen in the cord in CSM.[72,73]

The physiologic parameters of T2 hyperintensity or T1 hypointensity have provided further insight into the evolution of CSM. Takahashi and colleagues[74] initially suggested that T2 hyperintensity within the cord represents the myelomalacia or gliosis seen pathologically in patients with CSM. Ramanauskas and colleagues[75] considered that early in the process of myelomalacia evolution, T2 hyperintensity may reflect edema; this may progress to cystic necrosis of the central gray matter, which will ultimately manifest itself as T1 hypointensity and T2 hyperintensity. Al-Mefty and associates[76] considered T2 hyperintensity to represent myelomalacia, with T2 hyperintensity accompanied by T1 hypointensity to reflect cystic necrosis or syrinx formation. Direct correlation with histology in a canine model by Al-Mefty and associates[76] showed motor neuron loss, necrosis, and cavitation in areas of cord signal abnormality. Correlation with human autopsy findings led Ohshiro and colleagues[77] to conclude that T2 hyperintensity alone represents edema, gliosis, and minimal gray matter cell loss, whereas T1 hypointensity heralds necrosis, myelomalacia, and spongiform change. The observation that T2 hyperintensity may resolve led Taneichi and colleagues[78] to ascribe it to reversible edema, whereas stable T2 hyperintensity reflects gliosis (**Fig. 9**).

From these studies, and additional outcomes studies detailed in the following paragraphs, we can conclude that

1. Intramedullary T2 hyperintensity represents a range of reversible (edema) and irreversible (demyelination, gliosis, cystic necrosis) pathology
2. Faint and indistinct T2 hyperintensity is more likely to reflect reversible edema
3. Very intense and well-defined T2 hyperintensity more likely represents fixed gliosis or cystic necrotic change
4. Intramedullary T1 hypointensity represents irreversible necrosis and myelomalacia.

A 2010 study by Ozawa and colleagues[79] and a 2011 study by Cho and colleagues[80] compared patients with CSM who exhibited gadolinium enhancement with a nonenhancing control group. The zone of enhancement was always within and smaller than a zone of T2 hyperintensity at the site of maximal compression, with extension caudally; it was typically seen in the posterior or posterolateral cord. There was no correlation of enhancement with preoperative clinical symptoms. Enhancement disappeared in most patients within 1 year of surgical decompression; patients who exhibited preoperative enhancement had a poorer postoperative prognosis than those who did not (**Fig. 10**).

Floeth and colleagues[81] studied 20 patients with CSM using 18F-fluorodeoxyglucose (18F-FDG) positron emission tomography (PET) in the setting of a single-level stenosis at C3-4 or C4-5. All the patients with CSM showed a significant decrease in 18F-FDG uptake in the lower cord below the stenosis, relative to healthy controls. A cohort of these patients also exhibited increased uptake at the level of the stenosis. The patients with increased 18F-FDG uptake at the stenosis had a significantly shorter duration of symptoms, a more precipitous decline in function

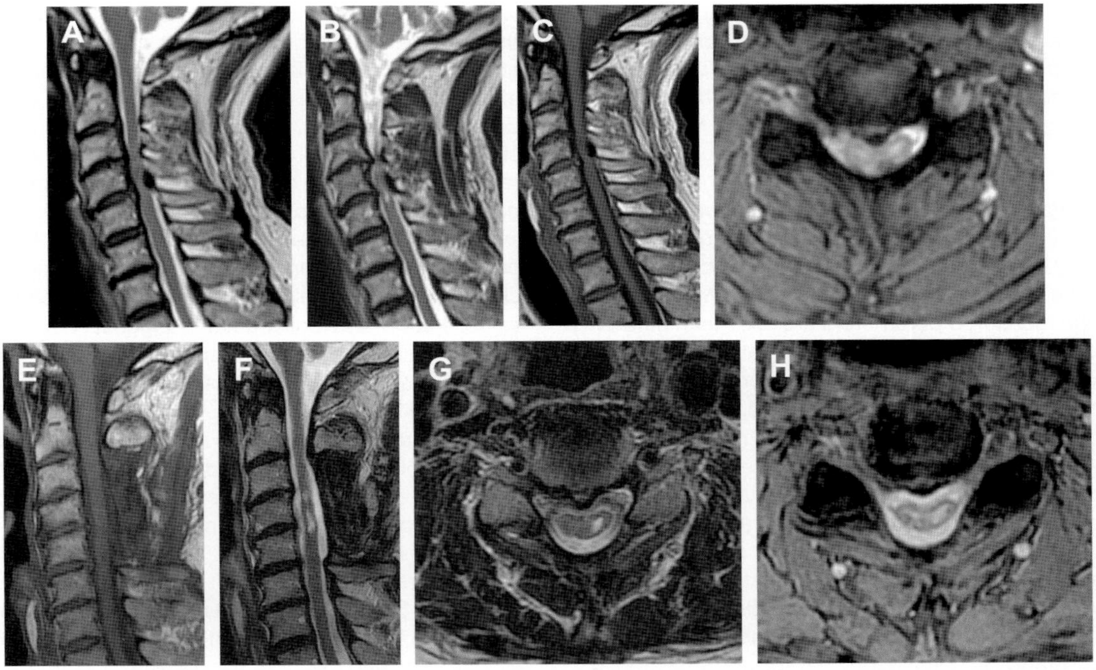

Fig. 9. Cervical spondylotic myelopathy. This patient had a moderate myelopathy preoperatively. Sagittal T2 (*A, B*) and T1 (*C*) images show severe central canal stenosis at the C4 level with impingement from both ventral and dorsal vectors. Discrete, well-marginated T2 hyperintensity is seen off the midline (*B*). Axial gradient echo T2-weighted image (*D*) confirms the cord deformity, central disc protrusion, and left >right T2 hyperintensity. Post decompression sagittal T1 and T2 images (*E, F* respectively) show that the central canal is well decompressed, with some reexpansion of the cord. The zone of T2 hyperintensity, however, has expanded, also demonstrated on axial FSE (*G*) and gradient echo (*H*) images. The patient had a fixed deficit without clinical improvement. The well-marginated intramedullary T2 hyperintensity preoperatively was a negative prognostic sign, as was the postoperative expansion of the T2 hyperintensity.

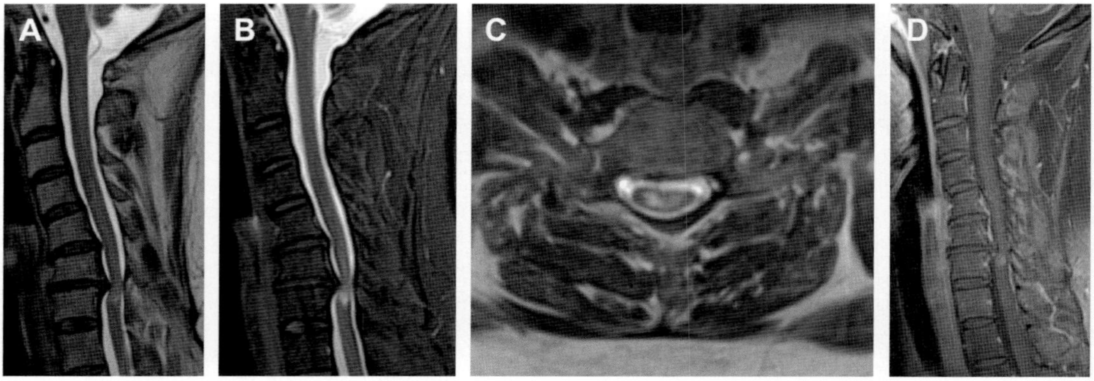

Fig. 10. Intramedullary enhancement. This 48-year-old woman had intractable upper extremity pain and dysesthesia involving the right lateral forearm. There were also long tract signs. T2 FSE (*A*) and T2 FSE with fat saturation (*B*) demonstrate significant cord deformity at the C6 to C7 interspace level, with focal T2 hyperintensity in the right side of the cord, as seen on the axial FSE image (*C*). Post gadolinium sagittal T1-weighted image with fat saturation (*D*) shows enhancement at the site of T2 hyperintensity, a negative prognostic sign. Patient has static dysesthesias after decompression.

in the 3 months before decompression, and ultimately exhibited significant improvement after decompression. Patients without increased uptake at the stenotic zone did not recover neurologic function after decompression. Animal experiments have shown increased immunoreactivity (postulated to cause increased metabolic activity) in neurons and glial cells in the early stages of cord compression; chronic compression leads to cell loss, atrophy, and diminished metabolic activity.[81]

Imaging correlates: diffusion tensor imaging

Early reports suggest DTI may offer greater accuracy in identification of symptomatic cord compromise than T2 hyperintensity or T1 hypointensity. The measured parameters are FA, mean diffusivity (MD), or ADC. The ADC or MD values reflect overall diffusivity in the tissue irrespective of directional dependence. Anisotropy (directional dependence) of diffusion in white matter tracts results from linearly oriented membrane structures (ie, axons and myelin). Diminished FA values may reflect loss of directionally oriented membrane structures, increased extracellular edema, or both. Animal studies have demonstrated that diminished FA values are seen in mechanical disruption, tearing of fibers and myelin sheaths, Wallerian degeneration, and demyelination.[82] Kara and colleagues[83] speculate that decreased FA values in the spinal cord devoid of T2 signal abnormality represent early demyelination owing to oligodendrocyte ischemia and subsequent apoptosis. Direct histologic confirmation of this attractive hypothesis is not yet available.

Several recent studies have addressed DTI in patients with CSM. Kara and colleagues[83] examined 16 patients with a clinical diagnosis of CSM but no T2 hyperintensity within the cord. All of the patients showed a statistically significant reduction in FA values and an increase in ADC values at the site of maximum stenosis, prompting the hypothesis that low FA reflects early demyelination. Facon and colleagues[82] studied DTI parameters in 15 patients with cervical or thoracic cord compressive lesions, both spondylotic and metastatic. FA values in the compressed cord were reduced compared with healthy controls in 10 patients; ADC values were significantly increased in only 2 patients. Seven patients showed T2 hyperintensity in the cord. One patient with an acute clinical onset of myelopathy had an increased FA value. Facon and colleagues[82] suggest this may be because of acutely restricted diffusivity; all other compressive processes have shown decreased FA.

Budzik and colleagues[84] studied 20 patients with symptomatic CSM and 15 volunteers. FA values were significantly lower at the compressed levels in patients than at comparable uncompressed levels in volunteers. There was a significant correlation between clinical state as measured by validated functional scores and the FA values. There was no such correlation between clinical state and the T2 hyperintensity; T2 hyperintensity did not correlate with FA or MD values. Patients who exhibited T1 hypointensity in the cord showed very low FA values.

Finally, Kerkovsky and colleagues[85] studied 52 patients with CSM and 13 volunteers using DTI. They demonstrated good interobserver reproducibility in DTI values. The patients all exhibited cord compression, but were stratified into those exhibiting signs and symptoms of CSM and those with nonspecific neck pain. The morphologic parameters of AP dimension of the central canal or cross-sectional area of the spinal canal did not discriminate between symptomatic and asymptomatic patients. The FA values were significantly reduced and ADC values elevated at the site of maximal compression in the symptomatic patients with CSM compared with the patients with cord compression but no symptoms. The FA and ADC values also discriminated between the 2 patient subgroups versus healthy controls.

DTI holds significant promise in identifying patients early in the course of CSM who are at risk for progression. Currently available evidence suggests diminished FA is more sensitive in the detection of cord injury than T2 hyperintensity and is better correlated with symptoms. This may assist in selection of patients for surgical decompression, although additional work remains to be done.

Imaging: prognosis, selection of patients for decompression

The ultimate goal of imaging must be to improve the clinical outcomes of patients. In the CSM population, this currently implies timely and appropriate selection of patents for therapeutic interventions, primarily surgical decompression. There is a large body of literature that has examined the role of imaging in predicting clinical response to surgical decompression; this literature is reviewed, hopefully adding clarity to a sometimes confusing mass of work. The imaging parameters under consideration include the cross- sectional area of the cord, intramedullary T2 hyperintensity, including its degree of intensity and multifocality, intramedullary T1 hypointensity, change or stability of intramedullary signal after decompression, recovery of cord cross-sectional area after decompression, and intramedullary gadolinium enhancement. The correlates are summarized in **Box 3**.

There is a consensus that there is a negative correlation in surgical prognosis with cross-sectional area of the cord at the site of compression; patients with greater degrees of cord compression do less well.[72,86,87]

There is reasonable consensus that symptomatic patients with CSM who have no intramedullary signal change have a better prognosis for surgical decompression than those who exhibit T2 hyperintensity.[74,75,80,86,88,89] There are contradictory studies in which focal T2 hyperintensity did not greatly affect prognosis.[87,90,91] The studies of Shin and colleagues,[92] Zhang and colleagues,[61] Yasutsugu and colleagues,[93] and Mastronardi and colleagues[86] all semiquantitatively scored the intensity of T2 signal elevation on 3-point or 4-point scales; patients with intense T2 signal abnormality had the longest duration of disease and the poorest objective recovery rates. More intense and well-defined intramedullary T2 signal likely reflects fixed cavitary disease as opposed to reversible edema. The study of Avadhani and colleagues[94] also used a 3-point evaluation of T2 intensity, but did not see a difference in recovery rates. The systematic review of patient selection by Mummaneni and colleagues [95] noted there is also evidence that multilevel intramedullary T2 hyperintensity predicts a poorer outcome from surgical decompression than single-level T2 hyperintensity.

There is a strong consensus that intramedullary T1 hypointensity is a very poor prognostic sign for recovery following cervical decompression.[59,76,86,90,91,94–96] The diminished T1 signal represents cavitary change or necrotic tissue. Patients exhibiting intramedullary T1 hypointensity recovered less well than patients with T2 hyperintensity alone, and much less well than patients without intramedullary signal abnormality. As noted previously, intramedullary gadolinium enhancement is a negative prognostic sign for postoperative recovery.[79,80]

Box 3
CSM prognostic factors for surgical decompression

1. Intramedullary T2 hyperintensity diminishes prognosis relative to normal signal.
   a. Intense, focal T2 hyperintensity is a more negative prognostic sign than ill-defined hyperintensity.
   b. Multilevel T2 hyperintensity is a more negative prognostic sign than single-level change.
   c. Resolution of T2 hyperintensity postoperatively improves prognosis.
   d. Expansion of T2 hyperintensity postoperatively diminishes prognosis.
2. Intramedullary T1 hypointensity greatly diminishes prognosis.
   a. Evolution of T1 hypointensity postoperatively diminishes prognosis.
3. Intramedullary gadolinium enhancement greatly diminishes prognosis.
4. Increased metabolic activity at the site of compression on 18F-FDG PET improves prognosis over no increased activity.
5. Postoperative residual compression and failure of reexpansion of the cord cross section are negative prognostic signs.

The regression of intramedullary T2 hyperintensity following surgical decompression has also been studied. The consensus of multiple studies is that patients who undergo regression of T2 hyperintensity on postoperative MRI examinations recover better than those in whom T2 hyperintensity is stable.[59,74,86,89,90] Mastronardi and colleagues[86] reported several patients who exhibited regression of T2 hyperintensity on intraoperative imaging obtained immediately after decompression, emphasizing that T2 hyperintensity may reflect rapidly reversible edema. Patients with preoperative T1 hypointensity never exhibited improvement in this signal abnormality postoperatively in any study.

Avadhani and colleagues[94] described patients who developed T1 hypointensity postoperatively; as would be anticipated, they did very poorly.[94] Yagi and colleagues[97] described a cohort of patients who developed expansion of a zone of T2 hyperintensity postoperatively. The recovery rates were significantly reduced in these patients; the development of increasing T2 hyperintensity was significantly related to development of instability (defined as >3 mm subluxation) postoperatively, as well as residual cord compression.

Postoperative cord morphology may also affect prognosis; it is not surprising that patients with no residual cord compression did better.[59,90] Evidence of cord reexpansion in the postoperative period is also a positive prognostic sign.[59,86]

Ossification of the Posterior Longitudinal Ligament

As is noted previously, OPLL is implicated in up to 25% of patients with cervical myelopathy, and it is

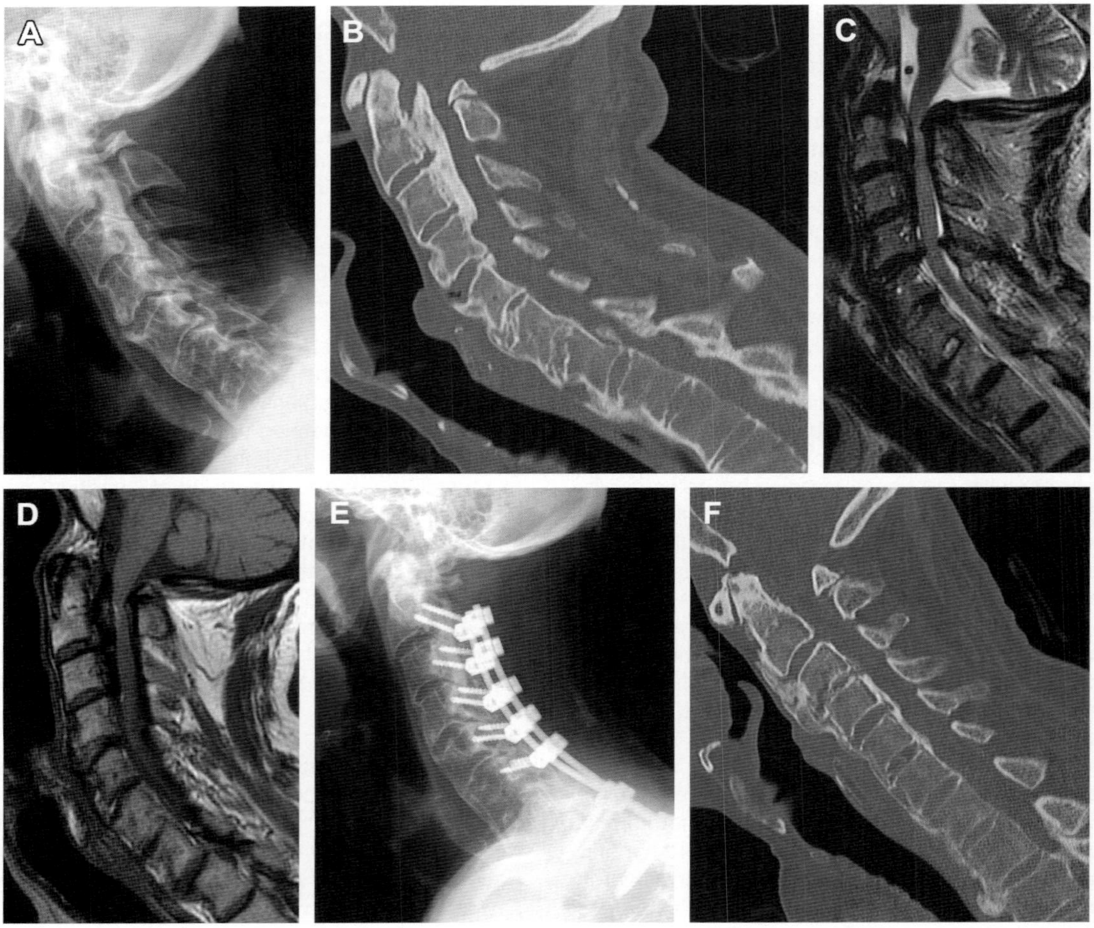

Fig. 11. OPLL. This 77-year-old white man had slowly progressive myelopathy on clinical examination. Lateral radiograph (*A*) demonstrates OPLL in the upper cervical spine; note the coexistent manifestations of DISH. CT sagittal reconstruction (*B*) and sagittal T2-weighted (*C*) and T1-weighted (*D*) images better depict the severe cord deformity at C2. The patient underwent C2 to T2 instrumented fusion, and C1 to C5 decompression (*E*). He is neurologically intact. Another patient (*F*) demonstrates coexistence of DISH and OPLL.

typically grouped with age-related changes into the CSM population. Most of the previously referenced studies describing the pathophysiologic correlates of imaging and prognostic signs for decompression include large proportions of patients with OPLL. Like age-related causes of structural central canal narrowing, it is often asymptomatic. The ossification is most common in the cervical region, where it causes static narrowing of the canal; repeated impact of the ventral cord on the bony mass also contributes to myelopathic injury. Patients may present in their 40s and 50s with pain, chronic myelopathy, or acute neurologic injury after modest trauma. The natural history of the ossification is progression.[96] From this flows the recommendation for surveillance imaging and close clinical follow-up (**Fig. 11**).

The ligamentous ossification may be identified on radiographs, CT, and MRI. On lateral radiographs, reduction of the sagittal canal diameter available for the cord by more than 60% correlates strongly with myelopathy.[98] The ossification is located from C2 to C4 in 70% of cases, T1 to T4 in 15%, and L1 to L3 in 15%.[98] On CT, the ossification may be classified as segmental (posterior to individual vertebrae: 39%), continuous (bridging across vertebrae: 27%), mixed type (29%), and other (ossification posterior to discs, variable sagittal extension: 5%).[98] It may also be classified as central or laterally deviated. Matsunaga and colleagues[99] noted that clinical myelopathy was more frequent in the laterally deviated type. They also observed that myelopathy was more frequent when the range of flexion-extension motion was greater, emphasizing the importance of dynamic trauma to the cord.

CT imaging is also critical to identify characteristics that suggest penetration of the dura. CSF leaks are a significant risk in anterior decompression surgery, particularly when the dura is ossified/inseparable from the bony ligamentous mass. Hida and colleagues[100] described the single-layer and double-layer signs. A double-layer sign describes ossification continuous with the dorsal vertebral body, an intervening layer of hypodense hypertrophied PLL, and another central ossified layer. The single-layer sign implies a single homogeneous ossified mass. The double-layer sign is strongly associated with no identifiable dural plane at surgery and significant risk of postoperative CSF leak. Epstein[101] noted that a large laterally deviated single-layer mass that hooked in a "C" configuration was also seen in association with local dural penetration.

On MRI, mature ligamentous ossification is of diminished signal intensity on all sequences; early OPLL may have inhomogeneous signal and exhibit slight enhancement.[98] When mature, there is no enhancement, allowing differentiation from epidural fibrosis. The secondary signal alterations in the cord are described previously.

SUMMARY

This article has reviewed pertinent pathophysiology, imaging findings, and the predictive value of imaging when evaluating patients with the clinical syndromes of NIC and CSM. Key points are summarized in the boxed comments. It should be apparent that several of the themes of this volume are carried through: (1) imaging has significant specificity and sensitivity faults; (2) the imager must understand the clinical state to provide useful information to the referring physician; and (3) imaging parameters that are based in physiology will be more valuable than a purely morphologic evaluation of spinal structures.

REFERENCES

1. Boden SD, Davis DO, Dina TS, et al. Abnormal magnetic-resonance scans of the lumbar spine in asymptomatic subjects. A prospective investigation. J Bone Joint Surg Am 1990;72(3):403–8.
2. North American Spine Society. Evidence-based clinical guidelines for multidisciplinary spine care, diagnosis and treatment of degenerative lumbar spinal stenosis. Burr Ridge (IL): North American Spine Society; 2011.
3. Amundsen T, Weber H, Lilleås F, et al. Lumbar spinal stenosis. Clinical and radiologic features. Spine 1995;20(10):1178–86.
4. Deyo RA. Treatment of lumbar spinal stenosis: a balancing act. Spine J 2010;19(7):625–7.
5. Johnsson KE, Sass M. Cauda equina syndrome in lumbar spinal stenosis: case report and incidence in Jutland, Denmark. J Spinal Disord Tech 2004; 17:334–5.
6. Kalichman L, Cole R, Kim D, et al. Spinal stenosis prevalence and association with symptoms: the Framingham Study. Spine J 2009;9(7):545–50.
7. Verbiest H. A radicular symptom from developmental narrowing of the lumbar vertebral canal. J Bone Joint Surg Br 1954;36:230–7.
8. Takahashi K, Olmarker K, Porter RW, et al. Double level cauda equina compression: an experimental study with continuous monitoring of intraneural blood flow in the porcine cauda equina. J Orthop Res 1993;11:104–9.
9. Olmarker K, Rydevik B. Single-level versus double-level nerve root compression: an experimental study on the porcine cauda equina with analysis of nerve impulse conduction properties. Clin Orthop 1992;(279):35–9.

10. Kobayashi S, Uchida K, Takeno K, et al. Imaging of cauda equina edema in lumbar canal stenosis by using gadolinium-enhanced MR imaging experimental constriction injury. AJNR Am J Neuroradiol 2006;27:346–53.
11. Sato K, Kikuchi S. Clinical analysis of two-level compression of the cauda equina and the nerve roots in lumbar spinal canal stenosis. Spine 1997; 16:1898–904.
12. Porter RW, Ward D. Cauda equina dysfunction: the significance of two-level pathology. Spine 1992;17: 9–15.
13. Morishita Y, Hida S, Naito ME, et al. Measurement of the local pressure of intervertebral foramen and the electrophysiological values of the spinal nerve roots in the vertebral foramen. Spine 2006; 31:3076–80.
14. Morishita Y, Hida S, Naito M, et al. Neurogenic intermittent claudication in lumbar spinal canal stenosis. The clinical relationships between the local pressure of the intervertebral foramen and the clinical findings in lumbar spinal canal stenosis. J Spinal Disord Tech 2009;22:130–4.
15. Szpalski M, Gunzburg R. Lumbar spinal stenosis in the elderly: an overview. Eur Spine J 2003;12(2): S170–5.
16. Singh K, Samartzis D, Vaccaro AR, et al. Congenital lumbar spinal stenosis: a prospective control-matched, cohort radiographic analysis. Spine J 2005;5:615–22.
17. Papp T, Porter R, Craig C, et al. Significant antenatal factors in the development of lumbar spinal stenosis. Spine 1997;22(16):1805–10.
18. Schonstron NR, Hansson GH. Thickness of the lumbar ligamentum flavum as a function of load: an in vitro experimental study. Clin Biomech 1991; 6:19–24.
19. Chokshi FH, Quencer RM, Smoker WR. The "thickened" ligamentum flavum: is it buckling or enlargement? AJNR Am J Neuroradiol 2010;31(10):1813–6.
20. Siebert E, Prüss H, Klingebiel R, et al. Lumbar spinal stenosis: syndrome, diagnostics and treatments. Nat Rev Neurol 2009;5:392–403.
21. Steurer J, Roner S, Gnannt R, et al. Quantitative radiologic criteria for the diagnosis of lumbar spinal stenosis: a symptomatic literature review. BMC Musculoskelet Disord 2011;12:175.
22. Genevay S, Atlas SJ, Katz JN. Variation in eligibility criteria from studies of radiculopathy due to a herniated disc and of neurogenic claudication due to lumbar spinal stenosis: a structured literature review. Spine (Phila PA 1976) 2010;35(7):803–11.
23. Speciale AC, Pietrobon R, Urban CT, et al. Observer variability in assessing lumbar spinal stenosis severity on magnetic resonance imaging and its relation to cross-sectional spinal canal area. Spine 2002;27(10):1082–6.
24. Fardon DF, Milette PC. Nomenclature and classifications of lumbar disc pathology. Recommendations of the Combined Task Forces of the North American Spine Society, American Society of Spine Radiology, and American Society of Neuroradiology. Spine (Phila Pa 1976) 2001;26(5):E93–113.
25. Min JH, Jang JS, Lee SH. Clinical significance of redundant nerve roots of the cauda equina in lumbar spinal stenosis. Clin Neurol Neurosurg 2008;110(1):14–8.
26. McNab I. Spondylolisthesis with an intact neural arch: the so-called pseudo-spondylolisthesis. J Bone Joint Surg Br 1950;32:325–33.
27. Kauppila LI, Eustace S, Kiel D, et al. Degenerative displacement of lumbar vertebrae: a 25-year follow-up study in Framingham. Spine 1998;23:1868–73.
28. Lurie JD, Tosteson AN, Tosteson TD, et al. Reliability of readings of magnetic resonance imaging features of lumbar spinal stenosis. Spine (Phila Pa 1976) 2008;33(14):1605–10.
29. Jarvik JJ, Hollingworth W, Heagerty P, et al. The longitudinal assessment of imaging and disability of the back (LAIDBack) study: baseline data. Spine (Phila PA 1976) 2001;26(10):1158–66.
30. Hamanishi C, Matukura N, Fujita M, et al. Cross-sectional area of the stenotic lumbar dural tube measured from the transverse views of magnetic resonance imaging. J Spinal Disord 1994;7(5): 388–93.
31. Bolender NF, Schonstrom NG, Spengler DM. Role of computed tomography and myelography in the diagnosis of central spinal stenosis. J Bone Joint Surg Am 1985;67(2):240–6.
32. Schönström N, Hansson T. Pressure changes following constriction of the cauda equina. An experimental study in site. Spine (Phila Pa 1976) 1988;13(4):385–8.
33. Haig AJ, Geisser ME, Tong HC, et al. Electromyographic and magnetic resonance imaging to predict lumbar spinal stenosis, low back pain, and no back symptoms. J Bone Joint Surg 2007; 89:358–66.
34. Sirvanci M, Bhatia M, Ganiyusufoglu KA, et al. Degenerative lumbar spinal stenosis: correlation with Oswestry disability index and MR imaging. Eur Spine J 2008;17(5):679–85.
35. Yasar B, Simşek S, Er U, et al. Functional and clinical evaluation for the surgical treatment of degenerative stenosis of the lumbar spinal canal. J Neurosurg Spine 2009;11(3):347–52.
36. Geisser ME, Haig AJ, Tong HC, et al. Spinal canal size and clinical symptoms among persons diagnosed with lumbar spinal stenosis. Clin J Pain 2007;23:780–5.
37. Zeifang F, Schiltenwolf M, Abel R, et al. Gait analysis does not correlate with clinical and MR imaging parameters in patients with symptomatic

lumbar spinal stenosis. BMC Musculoskelet Disord 2008;9:89.
38. Schmid MR, Stucki G, Duewell S, et al. Changes in cross-sectional measurements of the spinal canal and intervertebral foramina as a function of body position: in vivo studies on an open-configuration MR system. AJR Am J Roentgenol 1999;172(4):1095–102.
39. Danielson B, Willen J. Axially loaded magnetic resonance image of the lumbar spine in asymptomatic individuals. Spine (Phila Pa 1976) 2001;26(23):2601–6.
40. Willen J, Danielson B. The diagnostic effect from axial loading of the lumbar spine during computed tomography and magnetic resonance imaging in patients with degenerative disorders. Spine 2001;26(23):2607–14.
41. Willen J, Wessberg PJ, Danielson B. Surgical results in hidden lumbar spinal stenosis detected by axial loaded computed tomography and magnetic resonance imaging: an outcome study. Spine 2008;33(4):E109–15.
42. Hansson T, Suzuki N, Hebelka H. The narrowing of the lumbar spinal canal during loaded MRI: the effects of the disc and ligamentum flavum. Eur Spine J 2009;18:679–86.
43. Madsen R, Jensen TS, Pope M, et al. The effect of body position and axial load on spinal canal morphology: an MRI study of central spinal stenosis. Spine (Phila Pa 1976) 2008;33(1):617.
44. Feng W, Wang J, Zou J, et al. Effect of lumbar angular motion on central canal diameter: positional MRI study in 491 cases. Chin Med J 2010;123(11):1422–5.
45. Kent DL, Haynor DR, Larson EB, et al. Diagnosis of lumbar spinal stenosis in adults: a metaanalysis of the accuracy of CT, MR, and myelography. AJR Am J Roentgenol 1992;158(5):1135–44.
46. Bischoff RJ, Rodriquez RP, Gupta K, et al. A comparison of computed tomography-myelography, magnetic resonance imaging, and myelography in the diagnosis of herniated nucleus pulposus and spinal stenosis. J Spinal Disord 1993;6(44):289–95.
47. Modic MT, Masaryk T, Boumphrey F, et al. Lumbar herniated disk disease and canal stenosis: prospective evaluation by surface coil MR, CT, and myelography. AJR Am J Roentgenol 1986;147(4):757–65.
48. Schnebel B, Kingston S, Watkins R, et al. Comparison of MRI to contrast CT in the diagnosis of spinal stenosis. Spine 1989;14(3):332–7.
49. Jinkins R. Gd-DTPA enhanced MR of the lumbar spinal canal in patients with claudication. J Comput Assist Tomogr 1993;17:555–62.
50. Barz T, Melloh M, Staub LP, et al. Nerve root sedimentation sign: evaluation of a new radiological sign in lumbar spinal stenosis. Spine (Phila Pa 1976) 2010;35(8):892–7.
51. Palumbo MA, Hilibrand AS, Hart RA, et al. Surgical treatment of thoracic spinal stenosis: a 2 to 9 year follow-up. Spine (Phila Pa 1976) 2001;26(5):558–66.
52. Chang UK, Choe WJ, Chung CK, et al. Surgical treatment for thoracic spinal stenosis. Spinal Cord 2001;39(7):362–9.
53. Xiong L, Zeng QY, Jinkins JR. CT and MRI characteristics of ossification of the ligament flava in the thoracic spine. Eur Radiol 2001;11:1798–802.
54. Al-Khawaja D, Seex K, Eslick GD. Spinal epidural lipomatosis—a brief review. J Clin Neurosci 2008;15(12):1323–6.
55. Baptiste DC, Fehlings MG. Pathophysiology of cervical myelography. Spine J 2006;6(Suppl 6):190S–7S.
56. Stookey B. Compression of the spinal cord due to ventral extradural cervical chondromas. Arch Neurol Psychiatry 1928;20:275–91.
57. Morishita Y, Naito M, Hymanson H, et al. The relationship between the cervical spinal canal diameter and the pathological changes in the cervical spine. Eur Spine J 2009;18(6):877–83.
58. Edwards WC, LaRocca H. The developmental segmental sagittal diameter of the cervical spinal patients with cervical spondylosis. Spine (Phila Pa 1976) 1983;8(1):20–7.
59. Morio Y, Teshima R, Nagashima H, et al. Correlation between operative outcomes of cervical compression myelography and MRI of the spinal cord. Spine 2001;26(11):123.
60. Chen IH, Vasavada A, Panjabi M. Kinematics of the cervical spine canal: changes with sagittal plane loads. J Spinal Disord 1994;7(2):93–101.
61. Zhang L, Zeitoun D, Rangel A, et al. Preoperative evaluation of the cervical spondylotic myelopathy with flexion-extension magnetic resonance imaging: about a prospective study of fifty patients. Spine (Phila Pa 1976) 2011;36(17):E1134–9.
62. Muhle C, Weinert D, Falliner A, et al. Dynamic changes of the spinal canal in patients with cervical spondylosis at flexion and extension using magnetic resonance imaging. Invest Radiol 1998;33(8):444–9.
63. Yu WR, Liu T, Kiehl TG, et al. Human neuropathological and animal model evidence supporting a role for Fas-mediated apoptosis and inflammation in cervical spondylotic myelopathy. Brain 2011;134(Pt 5):1277–92.
64. Pavlov H, Torg JS, Robie B, et al. Cervical spinal stenosis: determination with vertebral body ratio method. Radiology 1987;164(3):771–5.
65. Prasad SS, O'Malley M, Caplan M, et al. MRI measurements of the cervical spine and their correlation to Pavlov's ratio. Spine (Phila Pa 1976) 2003;28(12):1263–8.
66. Naganawa T, Miyamoto K, Ogura H, et al. Comparison of magnetic resonance imaging and computed tomogram-myelography for evaluation

of cross sections of cervical spine morphology. Spine (Phila Pa 1976) 2011;36(1):50–6.
67. Song KJ, Choi BW, Kim GH, et al. Clinical usefulness of CT-myelogram comparing with the MRI in degenerative cervical spinal disorders: is CTM still useful for primary diagnostic tool? J Spinal Disord Tech 2009;22:353–7.
68. Shafaie FF, Wippold FJ, Gado M, et al. Comparison of computed tomography myelography and magnetic resonance imaging in the evaluation of cervical spondylotic myelopathy and radiculopathy. Spine 1999;24:1781–5.
69. Teresi LM, Lufkin RB, Reicher MA, et al. Asymptomatic degenerative disk disease and spondylosis of the cervical spine: MR imaging. Radiology 1987; 164(1):83–8.
70. Hayashi H, Okada K, Hamada M, et al. Etiologic factors of myelopathy. A radiographic evaluation of the aging changes in the cervical spine. Clin Orthop Relat Res 1987;(214):200–9.
71. Matsumoto M, Fujimura Y, Suzuki N, et al. MRI of cervical intervertebral discs in asymptomatic subjects. J Bone Joint Surg Br 1998;80(1):19–24.
72. Okada Y, Ikata T, Katoh S, et al. Morphologic analysis of the cervical spinal cord, dural tube, and spinal canal by magnetic resonance imaging in normal adults and patients with cervical spondylotic myelopathy. Spine (Phila Pa 1976) 1994; 19(20):2331–5.
73. Fujiwara K, Fujimoto M, Owaki H, et al. Cervical lesions related to the systemic progression in rheumatoid arthritis. Spine 1998;23:2052–6.
74. Takahashi M, Yamashita Y, Sakamoto, et al. Chronic cervical cord compression: clinical significance of increased signal intensity on MR imaging. Radiology 1989;173:219–24.
75. Ramanauskas WL, Wilner HI, Metes JJ, et al. MR imaging of compressive myelomalacia. J Comput Assist Tomogr 1989;13:399–404.
76. Al-Mefty O, Harkey LH, Middleton TH, et al. Myelopathic cervical spondylotic lesions demonstrated by magnetic resonance imaging. J Neurosurg 1988;68:217–22.
77. Ohshiro I, Hatayama A, Kaneda K, et al. Correlation between histopathologic features and magnetic resonance images of spinal cord lesions. Spine 1993;18:1140–9.
78. Taneichi H, Abumi K, Kaneda K, et al. Monitoring the evaluation of intra medullary lesions in cervical spinal cord injury. Qualitative and quantitative analysis with sequential MR imaging. Paraplegia 1994;32:9–18.
79. Ozawa H, Sato T, Hyodo H, et al. Clinical significance of intramedullary Gd-DTPA enhancement in cervical myelopathy. Spinal Cord 2010;48(5): 415–22.
80. Cho YE, Shin JJ, Kim K, et al. The relevance of intramedullary high signal intensity and gadolinium (Gd-DTPA) enhancement to the clinical outcome in cervical compressive myelography. Eur Spine J 2011;20(12):2267–74.
81. Floeth FW, Stoffels G, Herdmann J, et al. Prognostic value of 18F-FDG PET in monosegmental stenosis and myelopathy of the cervical spinal cord. J Nucl Med 2011;52(9):1385–91.
82. Facon D, Ozanne A, Fillard P, et al. MR diffusion tensor imaging and fiber tracking in spinal cord compression. AJNR Am J Neuroradiol 2005;26(6): 1587–94.
83. Kara B, Celik A, Karadereler S, et al. The role of DTI in early detection of cervical spondylotic myelopathy: a preliminary study with 3-T MRI. Neuroradiology 2011;53(8):609–16.
84. Budzik JF, Balbi V, Le Thuc V, et al. Diffusion tensor imaging and fibre tracking in cervical spondylotic myelopathy. Eur Radiol 2011;21(2):426–33.
85. Keřkovský M, Bednařík J, Dušek L, et al. Magnetic resonance diffusion tensor imaging in patients with cervical spondylotic spinal cord compression: correlations between clinical and electrophysiological findings. Spine (Phila Pa 1976) 2012;37(1):48–56.
86. Mastronardi L, Elsawaf A, Roperto R, et al. Prognostic relevance of the post operative evolution of intramedullary spinal cord changes in signal intensity on magnetic resonance imaging after anterior decompression for cervical spondylotic myelopathy. J Neurosurg Spine 2007;7(6):615–22.
87. Wada E, Ohmura M, Yonenobu K. Intramedullary changes of the spinal cord in cervical spondylotic myelopathy. Spine 1995;20:2226–32.
88. Matsuda Y, Miyazaki K, Tada K, et al. Increased MR signal intensity due to cervical myelopathy. Analysis of 29 surgical cases. J Neurosurg 1991;74: 887–92.
89. Mehalic TF, Pezzuti RT, Applebaum BI. Magnetic resonance imaging and cervical spondylotic myelopathy. Neurosurgery 1990;26(2):217–26 [discussion: 226–7].
90. Suri A, Chabbra RP, Mehta VS, et al. Effect of intramedullary signal changes on the surgical outcome of patients with cervical spondylotic myelopathy. Spine J 2003;3(1):33–45.
91. Fernandez de Rota JJ, Meschian S, Fernandez de Rota A, et al. Cervical spondylotic myelopathy due to chronic compression: the role of signal intensity changes in magnetic resonance images. J Neurosurg Spine 2007;6:17–22.
92. Shin JJ, Jin BH, Kim KS, et al. Intramedullary high signal intensity and neurological status as prognostic factors in cervical spondylotic myelopathy. Acta Neurochir (Wien) 2010;152(10):1687–94.
93. Yasutsugu Y, Fumihiko K, Hisatake Y, et al. MR T2 image classification in cervical compression myelopathy predictor of surgical outcomes. Spine (Phila Pa 1976) 2007;32:167–8.

94. Avadhani A, Rajasekaran S, Shetty AP. Comparison of prognostic value of different MRI classifications of signal intensity change in cervical spondylotic myelopathy. Spine J 2010;10(6):475–85.
95. Mummaneni PV, Kaiser MG, Matz PG, et al. Preoperative patient selection with magnetic resonance imaging, computed tomography, and electroencephalography: does the test predict outcome after cervical surgery? J Neurosurg Spine 2009; 11(2):119–29.
96. Smith ZA, Buchanon CC, Raphael D, et al. Ossification of the posterior longitudinal ligament: pathogenesis, management, and current surgical approaches. A review. Neurosurg Focus 2011;30(3):E10.
97. Yagi M, Ninomiya K, Kihara M, et al. Long-term surgical outcome and risk factors in patients with cervical myelopathy and a change in signal intensity of intramedullary spinal cord on magnetic resonance imaging. J Neurosurg Spine 2010;12(1):59–65.
98. Epstein N. Ossification of the cervical posterior longitudinal ligament: a review. Neurosurg Focus 2002;13(2):ECP1.
99. Matsunaga S, Nakamura K, Seichi A, et al. Radiographic predictors for the development of myelopathy in patients with ossification of the posterior longitudinal ligament: a multicenter cohort study. Spine (Phila Pa 1976) 2008;33(24):2648–50.
100. Hida K, Iwasaki Y, Koyanagi I, et al. Bone window computed tomography for detection of dural defect association with cervical ossified posterior longitudinal ligament. Neurol Med Chir (Tokyo) 1997; 37(2):173–5 [discussion: 175–6].
101. Epstein NE. Identification of ossification of the posterior longitudinal ligament extending through the dura on preoperative computed tomographic examinations of the cervical spine. Spine (Phila Pa 1976) 2001;26(2):182–6.
102. Fukusaki M, Kobayashi I, Hara T, et al. Symptoms of spinal stenosis do not improve after epidural steroid injection. Clin J Pain 1998;14(2):148–51.
103. Koc Z, Ozcakir S, Sivrioglu K, et al. Effectiveness of physical therapy and epidural steroid injections in lumbar spinal stenosis. Spine (Phila Pa 1976) 2009;34(10):985–9.
104. Herzog RJ, Kaiser JA, Saal JA, et al. The importance of posterior epidural fat pad in lumbar central canal stenosis. Spine (Phila Pa 1976) 1991;16(6 Suppl): S227–33.
105. Mariconda M, Fava R, Gatto A, et al. Unilateral laminectomy for bilateral decompression of lumbar spinal stenosis: a prospective comparative study with conservatively treated patients. J Spinal Disord Tech 2002;15(1):39–46.
106. Laurencin C, Lipson S, Senatus P, et al. The stenosis ratio: a new tool for the diagnosis of degenerative spinal stenosis. Int J Surg Investig 1999;1(2):127–31.
107. Ullrich C, Binet E, Sanecki M, et al. Quantitative assessment of the lumbar spinal canal by computed tomography. Radiology 1980;134(1):137–43.
108. Lee B, Kazam E, Newman A. Computed tomography of the spine and spinal cord. Radiology 1978;128(1):95–102.
109. Verbiest H. The significance and principles of computerized axial tomography in idiopathic developmental stenosis of the bony lumbar vertebral canal. Spine (Phila Pa 1976) 1979;4(4):369–78.
110. Jönsson B, Annertz M, Sjöberg C, et al. A prospective and consecutive study of surgically treated lumbar spinal stenosis. Part I: Clinical features related to radiographic findings. Spine (Phila Pa 1976) 1997;22(24):2932–7.
111. Schonstrom N, Bolender N, Spengler D. The pathomorphology of spinal stenosis as seen on CT scans of the lumbar spine. Spine (Phila Pa 1976) 1985;10(9):806–11.
112. Schonstrom N, Willen J. Imaging lumbar spinal stenosis. Radiol Clin North Am 2001;39(1):31–53.
113. Wilmink J, Korte J, Penning L. Dimensions of the spinal canal in individuals symptomatic and nonsymptomatic for sciatica: a CT study. Neuroradiology 1988;30(6):547–50.
114. Airaksinen O, Herno A, Turunen V, et al. Surgical outcome of 438 patients treated surgically for lumbar spinal stenosis. Spine (Phila Pa 1976) 1997;22(19):2278–82.
115. Herno A, Airaksinen O, Saari T. Computed tomography after laminectomy for lumbar spinal stenosis. Patients' pain patterns, walking capacity, and subjective disability had no correlation with computed tomography findings. Spine (Phila Pa 1976) 1994;19(17):1975–8.
116. Sortland O, Magnaes B, Hauge T. Functional myelography with metrizamide in the diagnosis of lumbar spinal stenosis. Acta Radiol Suppl 1977; 355:42–54.
117. Verbiest H. Neurogenic intermittent claudication in cases with absolute and relative stenosis of the lumbar vertebral canal (ASLC and RSLC), in cases with narrow lumbar intervertebral foramina, and in cases with both entities. Clin Neurosurg 1973;20:204–14.
118. Ciric I, Mikhael MA, Tarkington JA, et al. The lateral recess syndrome. A variant of spinal stenosis. J Neurosurg 1980;53(4):433–43.
119. Strojnik T. Measurement of the lateral recess angle as a possible alternative for evaluation of the lateral recess stenosis on a CT scan. Wien Klin Wochenschr 2001;113(Suppl 3):53–8.
120. Dincer F, Erzen C, Basgöze O, et al. Lateral recess syndrome and computed tomography. Turkish Neurosurgery 1991;2:30–5.
121. Mikhael M, Ciric I, Tarkington J, et al. Neuroradiological evaluation of lateral recess syndrome. Radiology 1981;140(1):97–107.

Lumbar Diskogenic Pain, Provocation Diskography, and Imaging Correlates

Timothy P. Maus, MD[a,*], Charles N. Aprill, MD[b,c]

KEYWORDS

• Diskography • Provocation diskography • Diskogenic pain • Annular fissure
• High intensity zone (HIZ) • Modic end plate change

KEY POINTS

- Diskogenic pain is the most common cause of axial back pain.
- Provocation diskography is the reference standard for the diagnosis of diskogenic pain.
- There is ultimately no pathoanatomic gold standard for diskogenic pain against which to measure the accuracy of provocation diskography or imaging.
- Provocation diskography requires reproduction of concordant pain with disk pressurization as well as grade 3 or 4 annular disruption.
- Careful analysis of MR imaging features can provide a reasonable prediction of the likelihood of diskogenic pain.
- There is no well-validated minimally invasive or surgical therapy for diskogenic pain.

Diskogenic pain refers to pain mediated by the intrinsic innervation of the intervertebral disk. It is experienced as pain centered at the symptomatic spine segment (axial pain) without radicular features or radiculopathy. There is no pathoanatomic gold standard for diskogenic pain; histologic examination cannot identify a painful disk. The current reference standard test for diskogenic pain is disk stimulation or provocation diskography. Provocation diskography remains controversial, invasive, and potentially harmful to the disk. There is an understandable desire for an imaging diagnostic standard for diskogenic pain. This article reviews the history of provocation diskography and its current use in the diagnosis of lumbar diskogenic pain. Provocation diskography technique is beyond the scope of this imaging issue. Rather, the extensive literature on imaging correlates of diskogenic pain is examined.

DISKOGENIC (AXIAL) BACK PAIN

Historical and clinical perspectives are important for imaging professionals to understand the essence of diskogenic pain. Mixter and Barr[1] described the prolapsed disk as a cause of low back and leg pain in 1934. Although the historical impact of that work was immense, many misinterpreted the study and believed disk prolapse to be the primary cause of back pain. In the following decades, many patients with disk prolapse (protrusion) and predominantly axial back pain were treated with surgical decompression (laminectomy and partial discectomy). The poor outcomes propelled the search for a more accurate diagnosis.[2]

Internal disk disruption (IDD) was first described by Crock in 1970.[3] IDD is the pathoanatomic process underpinning back pain arising from an intervertebral disk. As described by Bogduk

[a] Department of Radiology, Mayo Medical School, 200 First Street SW, Rochester, MN 55905, USA; [b] Departments of Radiology and Physical Medicine and Rehabilitation, Louisiana State University Health Science Center New Orleans, LA, USA; [c] Interventional Spine Specialists, 1919 Veterens Memorial Blvd, Suite 101, Kenner, LA 70062, USA
* Corresponding author.
E-mail address: timpmaus@gmail.com

Radiol Clin N Am 50 (2012) 681–704
doi:10.1016/j.rcl.2012.04.013

elsewhere in this issue, IDD is an entity distinct from normal age changes in the disk, even though imaging manifestations may overlap. The condition usually follows a memorable event, such as a sudden axial load while lifting or shear and torsion forces transmitted to the spine during rapid acceleration incidents. The affected disks are rendered painful by pathologic changes of the internal disk structure, regardless of disk contour.

The clinical features are protean. Patients affected with severe IDD present with a variety of symptoms, but back pain is primary.[4] The dominant pain is midline and immediate paraspinous in the lumbar region. Pain spreading to the lower flanks and buttocks is a common complaint and may be unilateral or bilateral. The discomfort is generally characterized as deep and aching and is typically aggravated by axial loading, whether sitting or standing. Sitting intolerance is a major feature of the syndrome. Patients often extend both arms while sitting on an examination table, seemingly unloading their low back. There may be episodic sharp pain associated with trunk movements, which are usually guarded and often limited, especially in flexion. Many patients have difficulty recovering from standing flexion. They often assist recovery by placing their hands on their thighs and slowly climbing up to full upright position.

Although diskogenic pain is predominantly axial, somatic referred pain to the lower extremities is common. Lower extremity pain is usually unilateral but occasionally bilateral. Lower extremity pain associated with IDD is widespread, ill defined, and described as an intolerable ache deep in the limb. This is different from the radicular pain associated with disk herniation. Primary radicular pain is sharp, lancinating, electric in character, and usually well defined in a band-like distribution. Physical examination features of dural tension are usually absent in diskogenic pain. Abnormal neurologic findings are uncommon. There are often complaints of altered sensation, such as nondermatomal paresthesias, vague weakness, and descriptions, such as "my leg just gives out," but objective motor or reflex changes are rare.

IDD is associated with psychological distress. Crock and Bedbrook[4] described psychological responses to the condition, including acute psychotic reactions and reactions to prolonged disease. Superimposed chronic illness behavior has been studied more recently and a patient's psychological status is relevant in establishing an accurate diagnosis.[5]

DISKOGRAPHY

Iophendylate (Myodil or Pantopaque), an oil-based contrast agent, became available in the 1940s and was the preferred agent for myelography in Great Britain and the United States for the successive 3 decades. This allowed visualization of the thecal sac and its contents; the imager remained blind to the epidural space and internal disk structure. In cadaveric studies, Knut Lindblom,[6] a radiologist, injected "red lead", a radiopaque material, into disks and recognized radial disk ruptures on radiographs. Seeking to develop a technique for direct study of the disk in patients with clinical signs of neural compression but normal lumbar myelograms, diskography was introduced by Lindblom in 1948.[7]

The first report of diskography in the United States was in 1951.[8] Cloward and Buzaid[9] subsequently described a technique and indications for lumbar diskography. In his classic 1960 monograph, Fernstrom[10] noted that back and leg pain could occur whether or not there is nerve compression, introducing the concept of radicular (mechanical or compressive) and diskogenic (biochemical or irritative) pain sources. This prefigures biochemical studies to be discussed later. Diskography in these early descriptions was a purely morphologic test, and it ultimately fell prey to the specificity fault seen in all spine imaging based on structure alone. Structural alterations are common, are generally asymptomatic, and increase with age.

PROVOCATION DISKOGRAPHY

Although the disk at this time was thought devoid of intrinsic innervation, diskographers began to report associations between morphologic abnormality and pain production during injection of contrast into the disk; morphologically normal disks were seldom painful, whereas disks with contour abnormalities or leaks into the epidural space were frequently painful.[11,12] Massie and Stevens[13] reported on diskography in 52 normal subjects and 570 patients; they noted that structurally abnormal disks were more common with advancing age but also occurred more commonly in patients than asymptomatic subjects. Structurally abnormal disks in control subjects were seldom painful during contrast injection, whereas in back pain patients a painful disk was frequently encountered. This introduced the concept of pain provocation as critical to the diagnosis of the painful disk.

Provocation diskography was dealt a significant setback by the methodologically flawed 1968 study of Holt,[14] which reported a false-positive rate of 37% in diskography performed on a cohort of asymptomatic prisoners. This was subsequently refuted in the more rigorous study of Walsh and colleagues.[15] In this study of patients and normal subjects, with careful blinding, only structurally abnormal disks in back pain patients were painful on injection; normal disks in asymptomatic subjects were not painful. Coincident with the interlude between Holt's and Walsh and colleagues' studies, important anatomic observations were made. The validity of provocation diskography had been questioned based on the contention that the intervertebral disk was an insensate tissue without intrinsic nociception. This was corrected with the histologic description of intrinsic nerve endings in the outer third of the annulus fibrosis, accompanied by peptides characteristic of nociception, such as calcitonin gene-related peptide, vasoactive intestinal peptide, and substance P.[16–18]

The addition of postdiskography CT allowed further characterization of the anatomic basis of IDD. The distribution of contrast within radially directed annular fissures was classified by the Dallas diskogram scale.[19] Annular disruption was graded on a 4-point scale with 0 being normal and grades 1, 2, and 3 representing penetration to the inner, mid, and outer annulus respectively. Grade 4 denotes a complex fissure extending over 30° of arc within the lamellae of the outer annulus (see article by Bogduk elsewhere in this issue). Vanharanta and colleagues[20] then demonstrated that pain provocation correlated with the extent of annular disruption; 77% of disks provoking exact reproduction of patients' typical pain with injection exhibited grade 3 disruption. Reciprocally, grade 3 disks were painful in 75% of cases; grade 0 or 1 disks were seldom painful to injection. Moneta and coworkers[21] demonstrated that annular fissures were distinct from other age-related "degenerative" change; pain provocation was associated with grades 3 and 4 fissures, not other age-related features. Derby added further refinement with the observation that pain provocation at low pressures of injection was better predictive of positive surgical outcomes than provocation at higher levels of pressure.[22]

CLINICAL DIAGNOSIS OF DISKOGENIC PAIN BY PROVOCATION DISKOGRAPHY

Lumbar diskogenic pain is mediated by the intrinsic innervation of the intervertebral disk (**Fig. 1**). The normal adult disk is avascular; its central nuclear compartment is aneural. The outer third of the annulus fibrosis contains nociceptive nerve endings of several types; the innervation is most dense in the posterior and posterolateral disk. Afferent signaling at the posterolateral disk occurs via somatic branches from the ventral ramus and the sinuvertbral nerve (recurrent meningeal nerve), which also passes into the ventral neural foramen to provide innervation to the posterior disk annulus, the ventral epidural space, the ventral dura, and the posterior longitudinal ligament.[23] The lateral margins of the disk receive innervation by the gray rami communicans, which continues to the anterolateral disk where it synapses with the ganglia of the sympathetic trunk.

In addition to its native innervation, the disk afflicted with IDD may also acquire innervation. Fissures that reach the outer annulus stimulate a granulomatous reparative response, with penetration of neovascularity and unmyelinated nerve endings along fissures deep into the annulus, the outer nuclear compartment, and the cartilaginous end plate.[24] These deeply seated nerves and the normal outer annular innervation may be sensitized by inflammatory cytokines; disks with characteristics of IDD have been shown to be immunoreactive to substance P and calcitonin gene-related peptide and demonstrate increased levels of nitric oxide; prostaglandin E2; interleukins 2, 6, and 8; phospholipase A_2; and tumor necrosis factor α (TNF-α).[25]

Diskography can be postulated to stimulate the intrinsic and acquired innervation of the disk by annular distension or end plate deflection. When there are extensive inflammatory mediators present, as during an acute flair of back pain, the sensitization of nociception results in pain with minimal elevation of intradiscal pressure. This is described as a "chemically sensitized" disk, one in which typical pain is provoked at modest pressures, in the range of 15 PSI over opening pressure (the pressure at which contrast first enters the disk). Clinical pain may be omnipresent. In a more quiescent situation, pain during diskographic distension may only be produced at higher pressure (15–50 PSI); this is labeled a "mechanically sensitized" disk. Clinical expression may be sitting and standing intolerance.[25]

Significant caveats apply. If there is a breach in the annulus, the disk may decompress freely into the epidural space. It may not be possible to pressurize the disk to nociceptive levels and there is the potential of a false-negative investigation. Because the endpoint of diskography is a subjective one, account must be taken for variation in pain perception; in this instance, an internal control must be sought. For a pain response on disk stimulation to be valid, it must be observed in the setting of pressurization of a morphologically normal disk that does not produce pain. The work of Derby and colleagues[21] suggests an upper limit to pressurization of the disk; pressurization significantly above 50 PSI may provoke false-positive pain responses.[22] To be considered positive, a pain response must be concordant, matching in location and character the index pain.

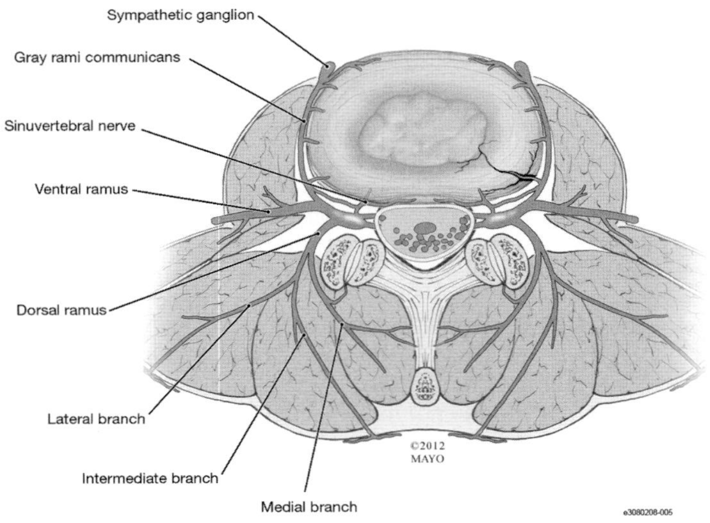

Fig. 1. Innervation of the lumbar intervertebral disk. Somatic branches of the ventral ramus and the sinuvertebral nerve innervate the posterolateral disk, the quadrant most vulnerable to IDD and subsequently herniations. Branches of the gray rami communicans supply the more lateral disk. The disk may also acquire innervation penetrating deep in the annulus along radial fissures. (*Courtesy of* Mayo Clinic, Rochester, Minnesota; with permission.)

The most rigorous criteria for provocation diskography are those published in the practice guidelines of the International Spine Intervention Society (ISIS).[26] A positive diskogram must demonstrate:

1. Provocation (by injection into the disk nuclear compartment) of the patient's typical pain (concordant pain)
2. Concordant pain reproduced at an intensity level of 7/10
3. Pain must be reproduced at low to intermediate pressure of injection (<50 PSI above opening pressure)
4. Stimulation of adjacent disks must not reproduce pain
5. Postdiskography CT demonstrating a grade 3 or 4 disruption.

A point system provides added account for disks painful at low pressures and other possible variations of clinical scenarios encountered during diskography. Greater certainty of diagnosis is attached to pain provocation at less than 15 PSI.

Provocation diskography is considered the reference standard for the diagnosis of diskogenic pain (**Fig. 2**). Diskogenic pain (IDD) is now broadly acknowledged as the most common cause of axial, nonradicular lumbar pain. There is a historical contention that the majority of low back pain does not have a discoverable, anatomically specific cause. Systematic application of diagnostic anesthetic and provocation procedures has refuted this concept. Depalma reported on 170 cases of axial low back pain in which a systematic clinical and diagnostic procedural algorithm identified a pain source.[27] No cases remained undiagnosed. The intervertebral disk was the most common pain generator, accounting for 42% of cases (**Table 1**). Patients with diskogenic pain (IDD) were significantly younger than patients with facet or sacroiliac joint pain. As age increased, the probability of IDD as a pain source decreased and the probability of facet or sacroiliac pain increased, up to approximately age 70.[27] A later multivariable analysis also showed a gender relationship, with IDD more prevalent in young men.[28] The high prevalence of IDD as a cause of axial pain is also supported by multiple earlier studies (**Table 2**).

VALIDITY

Although now accepted as the reference standard for the diagnosis of diskogenic pain by several scientific societies, diskography remains controversial. Carragee and colleagues[5,35–38] produced a series of reports of provocation diskography performed on populations asymptomatic of low back pain; these suggest false-positive rates in specific settings of bone graft donor site pain (50%); no low back pain and no other chronic pain (10%); chronic cervical pain (40%); postdiskectomy patients (35%); patients with established somatization disorders (75%). In patients with modest low back pain not requiring treatment, they reported a false-positive rate of 36%. These data and all other studies in asymptomatic patients have been subsequently reviewed by Wolfer and colleagues.[39] With rigorous application of ISIS criteria, the false-positive rate in all the pooled studies was 9.3% per patient and 6% per disk. In patients without confounding factors, such as

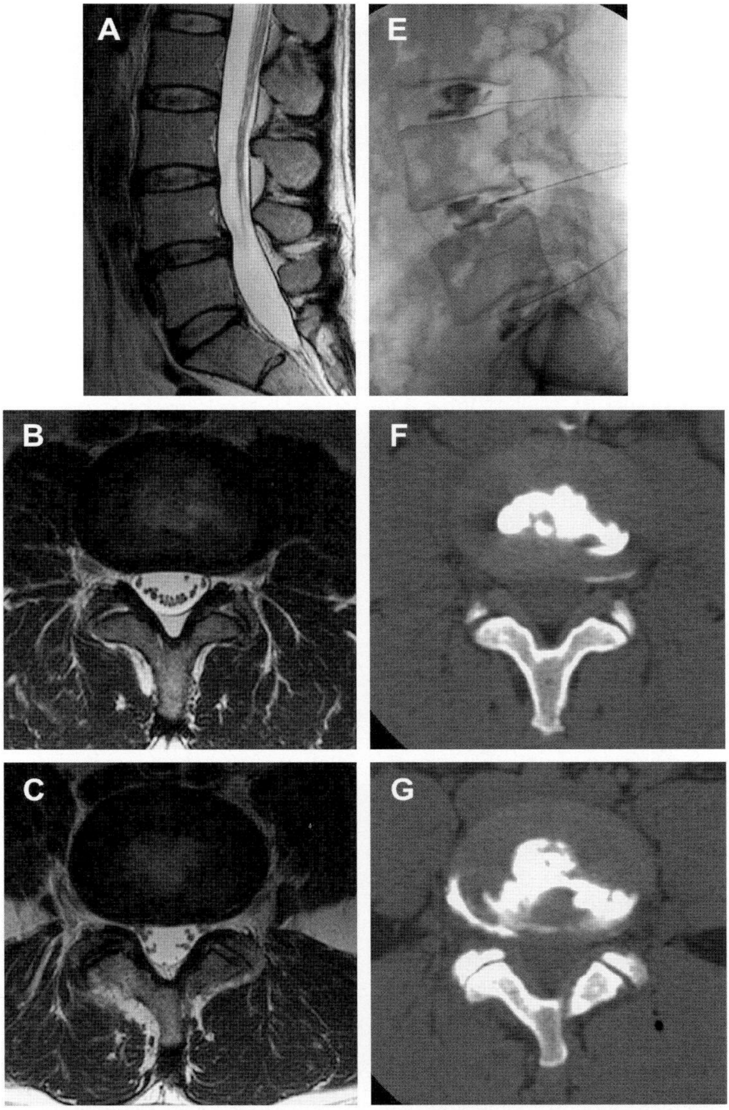

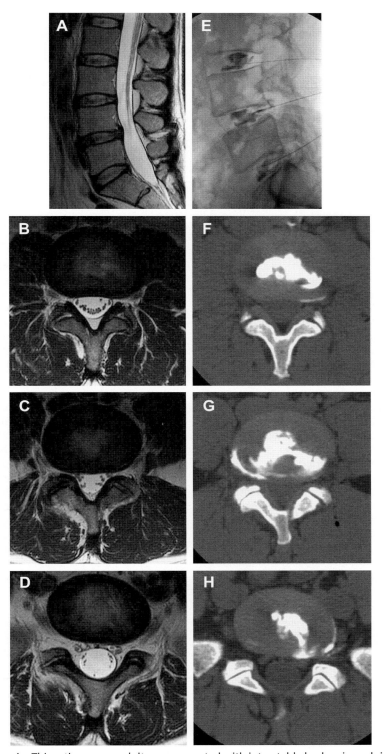

Fig. 2. Diskogenic pain. This active young adult man presented with intractable back pain and sitting intolerance. Sagittal T2-weighted MR imaging (*A*) and axial T2-weighted images at the L3 (*B*), L4 (*C*), and L5 (*D*) disks show modest T2 signal loss in all disks and a broad-based central protrusion at L4. Lateral fluoroscopic image (*E*) from provocation diskography and axial CT images postdiskography at L3 (*F*), L4 (*G*), and L5 (*H*) reveal grade 4 fissures at L4 and L5 with extension to the outer annulus and circumferential spread within annular lamellae. Diskography is more sensitive than MR imaging to the structural changes of IDD. Pressurization of the L4 disk reproduced his typical pain. The L3 and L5 disks were nonpainful.

Table 1
Prevalence of sources of axial low back pain and age correlation

Pain Source	Prevalence (%)	Mean Age (SD)
IDD	41.8	43.7 (10.3)
Facet joint	30.6	59.6 (13.1)
Sacroiliac joint	18.2	61.4 (17.7)
Vertebral insufficiency fracture	2.9	79.0 (11.8)
Pelvic insufficiency fracture	1.8	71.3 (11.7)
Baastrup disease	1.8	75.3 (4.7)
Fusion hardware	2.9	59.6 (19.4)

Data from DePalma MJ, Ketchum JM, Saullo T. What is the source of chronic low back pain and does age play a role? Pain Med 2011;12(2):224–33.

prior surgery or chronic pain states, the false-positive rates were 3.0% per patient and 2.1% per disk. Carragee and colleagues' studies properly noted the difficulty in diagnosis of diskogenic pain in the setting of chronic pain states or somatization disorders. They also highlighted the challenge of central hyperalgesia, in which a structure not intrinsically painful may seem painful when stimulated in the presence of an actual pain source innervated by the same or adjacent cord segments.[26] The nervous system lacks sufficient granularity to distinguish between the pain sources; this explains the iliac crest donor site pain observation. It may, therefore, be necessary to exclude other pain generators at the same segmental level as a painful disk via physical examination, imaging, or anesthetic procedures.

Lumbar diskography, as a part of a diagnostic algorithm, including clinical examination, imaging, and systematically applied anesthetic or provocation procedures, represents the current best means of establishing or excluding a diagnosis of diskogenic pain (**Box 1**). There is inherent value in achieving a specific diagnosis of diskogenic pain, because it should preclude further costly or invasive diagnostic work-up or the application of invasive therapies applied nonspecifically or directed at a different pain generator. A diagnosis of diskogenic pain unfortunately does not reveal well-validated therapies. Over the past decades, many destructive, device-based intradiscal therapies using various means of delivering energy (lasers, radiofrequency, thermal heating, and plasma field generation) or chemicals (corticosteroids, methylene blue, and ozone) have been introduced as treatments for diskogenic pain. Only intradiscal electrothermotherapy has shown benefit above placebo effect in a randomized controlled trial, but the therapeutic effect was sufficiently small that it is no longer widely used. Surgical fusion has been used for many years in the treatment of intractable diskogenic pain. This occurs despite the lack of convincing evidence of the clinical benefit of fusion. A recent meta-analysis of randomized controlled trials of fusion for axial back pain showed only a marginal, nonsignificant functional

Table 2
Prevalence of sources of axial low back pain

Pain Source	Author, Year	Age (Mean, Y)	Prevalence (%)
IDD	Schwarzer et al,[29] 1995	36.7	39
	Manichkanti et al,[30] 2001	~47	26
	DePalma et al,[27] 2011	43.7	42
Facet	Schwarzer et al,[31] 1994	38.4	15
	Schwarzer et al,[32] 1995	59	32
	Manichkanti et al,[30] 2001	~47	27
	DePalma et al,[27] 2011	59.6	30.6
Sacroiliac joint	Maigne et al,[33] 1996	45.3	18.5
	Schwarzer et al,[34] 1995	32.8	13–30
	DePalma et al,[27] 2011	61.4	18.2

Box 1
Diskogenic pain

1. Diskogenic pain is the most common cause of axial back pain.
2. Diskogenic pain is more common in younger subjects, especially men.
3. Facet and sacroiliac joint increase in prevalence as the cause of axial pain with advancing age.
4. Diskogenic pain is characterized as deep and aching, often associated with sitting or standing intolerance.
5. There is no pathoanatomic gold standard for diskogenic pain.
6. Provocation diskography is the reference standard for the diagnosis of diskogenic pain.
7. Diskography was originally developed as a morphologic test; morphology alone is not useful.
8. Provocation diskography requires reproduction of concordant pain at low pressures of injection, grade 3 or 4 annular disruption on postdiskography CT, and a nonpainful control disk.
9. With meticulous technique, provocation diskography should have a false-positive rate of less than 3% in uncomplicated patients.
10. False-positive rates of diskography are higher in patients with chronic pain syndromes.

improvement in surgical patients; there was also a 16% pooled complication rate in surgical patients.[40] A 2009 systematic review for the American Pain Society practice guidelines concluded that fusion is no more effective than intensive rehabilitation.[41] There is conflicting evidence regarding the ability of diskography to improve outcomes in surgical fusion.[25] Diskography has been use in planning fusion procedures as a means of identifying a painful disk and confirming that adjacent disks are nonpainful. This is not well supported by evidence. Diskography may function as a harm-sparing procedure when it identifies diskogenic pain at multiple levels, disqualifying a patient from a futile surgical procedure.

Unique intradiscal procedures have been developed to attempt to achieve greater specificity compared with that of provocation diskography.[42] Analgesic diskography refers to the injection of local anesthetics into the disk under study in hopes of rendering it and the patient pain-free for the duration of the pharmacologic effect of the agent. This is conceptually attractive but could be confounded by failure of the anesthetic to distribute to all disk nociception or to leak from the disk and anesthetize the epidural space. Functional analgesic diskography describes a proprietary device system in which a balloon-tipped catheter is anchored in the disk. This allows administration of anesthetic agents before provocative maneuvers that typically induce a patient's pain. The clinical utility of analgesic diskography and its variants remains unclear.

IMAGING CORRELATES OF DISKOGENIC PAIN

Although provocation diskography is the reference standard for the diagnosis of diskogenic pain, it is reasonable to consider if the diagnosis can be made by imaging alone. Earlier articles have pointed out the specificity fault inherent in spine imaging: manifestations of disk "degeneration" are ubiquitous, usually asymptomatic, and primarily represent normal age change. In a population of symptomatic patients with suspected diskogenic pain, however, are there imaging findings that correlate with positive provocation diskography? As evidence begins to emerge suggesting that diskography may harm the disk, a non-invasive imaging diagnosis takes on greater significance.

Diskography has until recently been considered a minimally invasive and nondestructive test. There is now in vitro and in vivo evidence suggesting that disk puncture or diskography may contribute to disk dysfunction and degeneration. Korecki and colleagues[43] noted that in a bovine disk model, single punctures with a 25-gauge needle resulted in biomechanical degradation of disk function with cyclic loading. Carragee and coworkers[44] demonstrated on 10-year follow-up MR imaging that asymptomatic subjects who had undergone investigational diskography showed more degenerative phenomena than matched control subjects. Although the clinical significance of these reports remains uncertain, noninvasive diagnosis would be desirable.

The evaluation of imaging findings that predict diskogenic pain is complicated by its nonspecific clinical nature and the lack of a pathologic or surgical gold standard. Although there is extensive literature examining imaging findings purporting to identify diskogenic pain, comparing and collating numerous studies is confounded by shifting definitions and fixed preconceptions among investigators. This literature must be read critically, because in many instances the unstated motivation in validating imaging findings of diskogenic pain is the performance of therapeutic interventions. Existing data have lent themselves to diametrically opposed interpretations by different physician groups and societies, illustrating the importance of perspective and motivation.

In regard to diskogenic pain, imaging is primarily limited to static morphology. It is largely unknown whether there may be dynamic structural processes that only become evident with extension and axial load, which may serve as markers for painful disks. Looking at imaging more broadly, the ability to quantitatively or qualitatively detect inflammatory cytokines or other biochemical mediators of the pain generation process and map them to specific spatial locations may be what is ultimately necessary to truly localize diskogenic pain.

The changes seen in the intervertebral disk with aging in asymptomatic subjects and in low back pain patients are of multifactorial origin. There are mechanical, traumatic, nutritional, and genetic factors involved, as described by Bogduk. The consensus terminology agreed on by multiple spine imaging, medical, and surgical societies uses the term, *spondylosis deformans*, originally introduced by Schmorl and Junghanns, to describe normal aging phenomenon; this primarily reflects changes in the annulus fibrosis and adjacent vertebral apophyses resulting in anterior and lateral end plate osteophytes.[45] Such osteophytes are present in 100% of skeletons of individuals over 40 years of age.[46] *Intervertebral osteochondrosis* is the term used to describe pathologic (although not necessarily symptomatic) change; it involves failure of the nucleus pulposis to effectively disperse axial load with concurrent changes in the vertebral end plates and fissuring in the annulus fibrosis.[45] Pathologic changes in this process include posterior vertebral osteophytes, end plate erosions, extensive annular fissuring, and reactive bone marrow changes. When the disk–end plate complex undergoes IDD with annular failure, herniation may occur. The currently accepted lexicon of herniation is described by Del Grande and colleagues elsewhere in this issue.

As noted by Bogduk, the pathoanatomic correlate of the painful disk (diskogenic pain) is best described as IDD, a diagnosis that can only be made at provocation diskography. Imaging findings that are potentially predictive of diskogenic pain may include those observable with x-ray–based studies (radiographs or CT), such as vertebral osteophytes, end plate sclerosis, loss of disk space height, and vacuum phenomenon (nitrogen gas) within the disk. There are also soft tissue findings, which are only observable with MR imaging, including alterations in disk contour (bulges, protrusions, and extrusions), T2 signal loss within the disk nucleus, focal T2 hyperintensity in annular fissures (the high intensity zone [HIZ]), and changes in the end plate and sub–end plate marrow (Modic changes).

The existing literature that seeks to identify imaging findings predictive of diskogenic pain deals primarily with MR imaging findings, which are the focus of this discussion. The findings evaluated include (1) loss of disk space height, (2) alterations of disk contour, (3) generalized alterations in T2 signal within the disk, (4) end plate marrow changes, and (5) the presence of HIZs or fissures within the posterior disk annulus. These imaging features are examined initially as independent variables with subsequent discussion of the more limited literature in which they are combined in a multivariate analysis. A significant portion of the presented data was drawn from a systematic review of imaging and clinical markers of axial pain generators in the lumbar spine performed by Hancock and colleagues.[47] Additional studies not included in that report or published subsequent to it have been added. A common set of measures was compiled from the many studies: sensitivity, specificity, positive predictive value (PPV), negative predictive value (NPV), and likelihood ratios (LRs). When imaging features were quantified (T2 signal loss in the disk was reported as normal, moderate, or severe), a threshold was used. Original data were combined and recalculated to reflect setting a detection threshold as moderate (including moderate and severe cases) or severe only. Because the diagnosis of diskogenic pain may provoke therapeutic interventions (most of which carry risk and have unproved efficacy), emphasis was placed on those measurements that inform about false-positive results: specificity (true negatives/true negatives + false positives) and PPV (true positives/true positives + false positives). These measures can be conflicting when class sizes vary and are dependent on the prevalence of the condition studied.[48] LRs are prevalence independent, given by sensitivity/(1 − specificity). The higher the positive LR (+LR), the more likely it is that a patient with a positive test does have the disease, here diskogenic pain; +LR greater than 2 is considered useful, where the confidence interval (CI) does not cross 1.0. The lower a negative LR (−LR), the more likely a patient with a negative test does not have the disease; −LR less than 0.5 is considered informative when the CI does not include 1.0.

Before proceeding with examination of individual imaging findings, the gold standard dilemma must be considered. There is no surgical or pathologic marker of a painful vertebral disk. The most restrictive current standard for a painful disk is a concordant response to manometrically controlled provocation diskography, with nonpainful control levels, as defined by the practice guidelines of ISIS.[26] Examination of the same body of evidence regarding the validity of diskography has resulted in diametrically opposed recommendations regarding its use by different physician societies. The ISIS,[26] the North American Spine Society,[49] and the International Association for the Study of Pain[50] accept diskography as a useful diagnostic tool in back pain patients and recommend its use. The American Pain Society rejects diskography as a diagnostically useful test.[51] A comprehensive review of diskography in the journal of the American Society of Regional Anesthesia and Pain Medicine notes that whereas CT diskography is the gold standard for the assessment of structural disk alteration, there is no convincing evidence that the use of diskography as a selection tool improves surgical outcomes.[25] Any analysis of imaging findings in diskogenic pain patients thus remains based on a reference standard (provocation diskography) that is ultimately unproved against a pathoanatomic gold standard. This is further confounded by evolution of the criteria for a positive diskogram within the past 2 decades. The literature correlating imaging findings with diskography outcomes often uses varying or unstated criteria for a positive diskogram and must be read critically. For the purposes of this discussion, only concordant pain responses were considered to represent a positive diskogram. A significant concordant pain response without specification of pain intensity or use of manometry is defined as Walsh criteria[15] for the remainder of this article. Inclusion of the requirement for a normal control disk elevates the criteria to that of IASP.[50] None of the studies meaningfully used manometric control or met the ISIS criteria for positive diskography.[26]

LOSS OF DISK HEIGHT

The reports of Ito and colleagues,[52] Lim and colleagues,[53] and O'Neill and colleagues[54] studied loss of disk space height as an imaging finding that may correlate with positive provocation diskography; data are summarized in **Table 3**. The studies of Ito and colleagues and O'Neill and colleagues both suggest that in a population of symptomatic patients with axial pain considered diskogenic in nature, severe disk space narrowing, although an uncommon imaging finding (approximately 10% of disk), is strongly predictive of a painful disk. Specificity of this finding was at least 97% in these studies with PPVs of 78% and 90%, respectively. The study of Lim and colleagues was less supportive. **Fig. 3** illustrates the disk height and T2 signal loss correlation.

Alterations of Disk Contour

The studies of O'Neill and colleagues[54] and Kang and colleagues[55] included data correlating disk contour abnormalities and diskography; data are summarized in **Table 4**. Both studies showed a statistically significant correlation of disk contour abnormality with positive provocation diskography. In O'Neill and colleagues' study, a disk bulge was the most useful contour abnormality parameter, with a +LR of 5.3. Multivariate analyses of these data are discussed later. **Fig. 4** illustrates the disk herniation correlation with diskography.

Disk Degeneration (T2 Signal Loss)

Studies addressing the correlation between MR imaging evidence of disk "degeneration" and diskogenic pain identified by diskography reach back approximately 20 years.[52–59] The definition of disk degeneration is variable; most classifications rely primarily on loss of T2 nuclear signal, in association with loss of the boundary between nucleus and annulus, as well as loss of disk space height. The difficulty in drawing conclusions from the existing literature in regard to the usefulness of imaging parameters in predicting diskogenic pain at provocation diskography is illustrated by these several studies, summarized in **Table 5**. Although the definitions of disk degeneration on MR imaging are inconsistent, the authors have recalculated the original data into threshold values in an attempt to provide a more uniform basis for comparison. Diskographic criteria for diskogenic pain have evolved significantly over the 18-year span bridged by these studies; the varying criteria are noted in the table.

Acknowledging these shortcomings, some general conclusions can be advanced from the data. The NPV of disks of normal nuclear signal is uniformly high and –LRs are highly informative; disks of normal nuclear signal are rarely painful. Severe disk degeneration, manifest as uniformly dark T2 signal, with or without loss of disk space height, is a finding of high specificity (88%–96% in studies using a 3-part classification system) and strongly informative +LR. Disks with severe T2 signal loss are rarely nonpainful. The utility of this finding is reduced by its low prevalence (it is found in 13%–25% of disks undergoing diskography in patients with diskogenic pain) and low sensitivity (23%, 24%, 37%, and 70% in the studies with 3-part classification system). Disks with intermediate signal loss may be painful but with less certainty.

Table 3
Loss of disk height

Author, Year	Diskogram Criteria	Height Loss Criteria	Prevalence	Sensitivity	Specificity	PPV	NPV	+LR	−LR
Ito et al,[52] 1998	Walsh	Moderate + severe	44%	87%	69%	46%	95%	2.8 (2.0–4.1)	0.2 (0.1–0.6)
		Severe	9%	30%	97%	78%	83%	11.9 (2.7–53.3)	0.7 (0.5–0.9)
Lim et al,[53] 2005	Walsh	Reduced?	22%	30%	82%	48%	68%	1.7 (0.8–3.5)	0.9 (0.7–1.1)
O'Neill et al,[54] 2008	IASP	Moderate + severe	47%	73%	81%	81%	74%	3.9 (3.0–5.2)	0.3 (0.3–0.4)
		Severe	10%	18%	98%	90%	52%	8.0 (3.2–19.7)	0.8 (0.8–0.9)

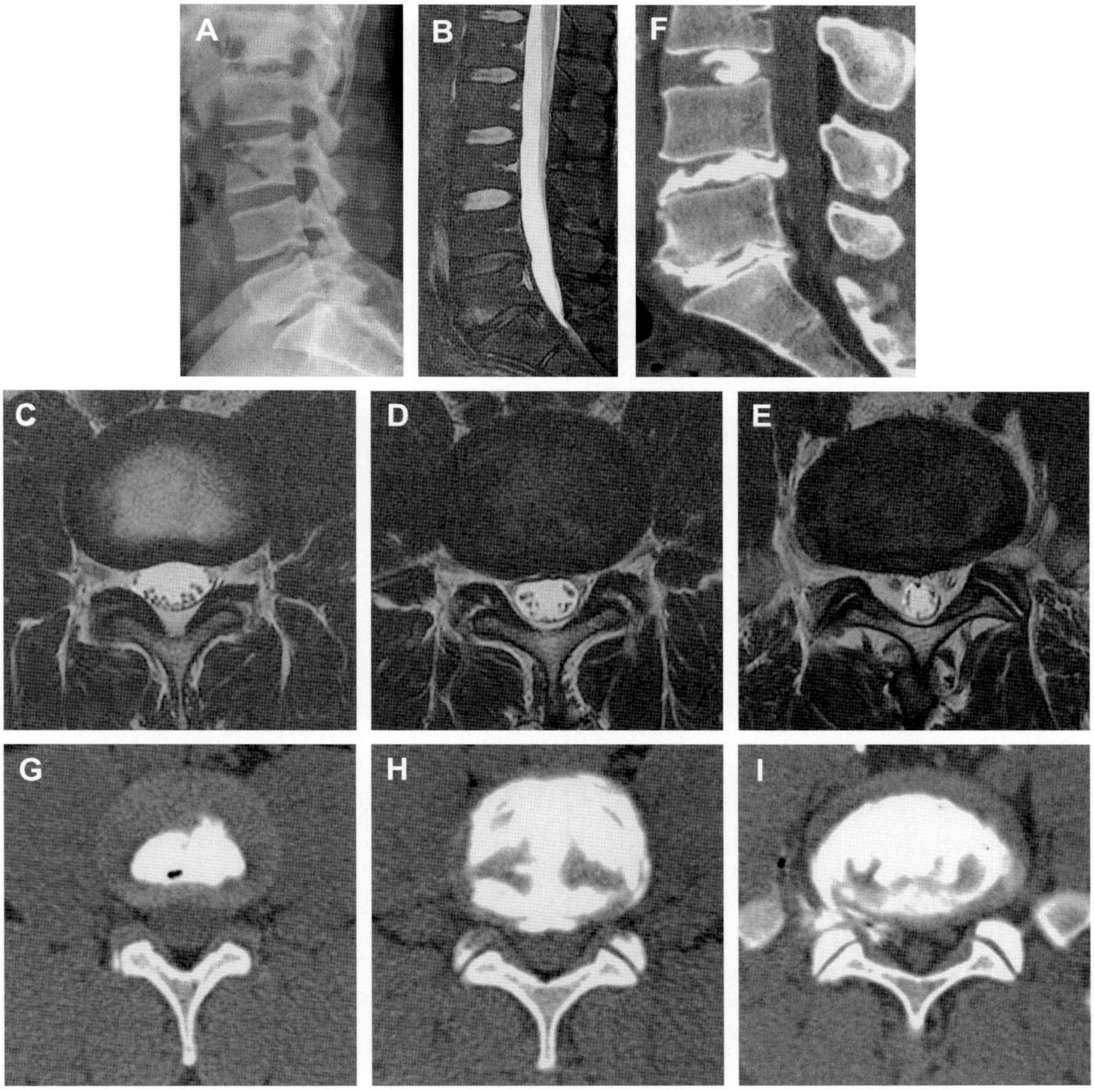

Fig. 3. Disk height and signal loss. (*A*) Lateral radiograph of a 50-year-old man with intractable axial pain. Note loss of height of lumbosacral disk, which contains gas. There is slight retrolisthesis of L4 on L5 and L5 on S1. Sagittal fat-saturated T2-weighted MR imaging (*B*) shows loss of T2 signal in L4 and L5 disk; normal upper lumbar disks. Axial T2-weighted images at L3 (*C*), L4 (*D*), and L5 (*E*) demonstrate normal L3 disk, loss of T2 signal in L4 with a small central herniation, and a broad bulge at L5. Sagittal CT diskogram (*F*) and axial images at L3 (*G*), L4 (*H*), and L5 (*I*) show normal L3 disk, extensive annular disruption at L4 and L5 with leak of contrast from the right posterolateral annulus at L5. Patient had concordant axial pain at L4 and L5 with a normal control disk at L3.

End Plate and Subchondral Marrow (Modic) Changes

The functional unity of the disk and the cartilaginous end plate is manifest in signal changes within the end plate and adjacent subchondral marrow, which accompany nuclear matrix degradation. End plate marrow changes were originally classified by Modic in 1988 (**Fig. 5**).[60] Type I change represents ingrowth of vascularized granulation tissue into sub–end plate marrow; it exhibits hypointense T1 and hyperintense T2 signal on MR imaging and may enhance with gadolinium. Type II change exhibits elevated T1 and T2 signal and reflects fatty infiltration of sub–end plate marrow. Type III change is hypointense on T1 and T2; it

Table 4
Disk contour abnormality

Author, Year	Diskogram Criteria	Disk Contour	Prevalence	Sensitivity	Specificity	PPV	NPV	+LR (CI)	−LR (CI)
O'Neill et al,[54] 2008	IASP	Bulge	23%	38%	93%	85%	58%	5.3 (3.2–8.7)	0.7 (0.6–0.7)
O'Neil	IASP	Protrusion	18%	29%	93%	93%	54%	4.3 (2.5–7.2)	0.8 (0.7–0.8)
O'Neil	IASP	Extrusion	5%	7%	98%	76%	49%	3.0 (1.1–7.9)	0.9 (0.9–0.0)
Kang et al,[55] 2009	IASP	Focal + broad-based protrusion	32%	68%	81%	54%	89%	3.51 (2.4–5.2)	0.4 (0.3–0.6)

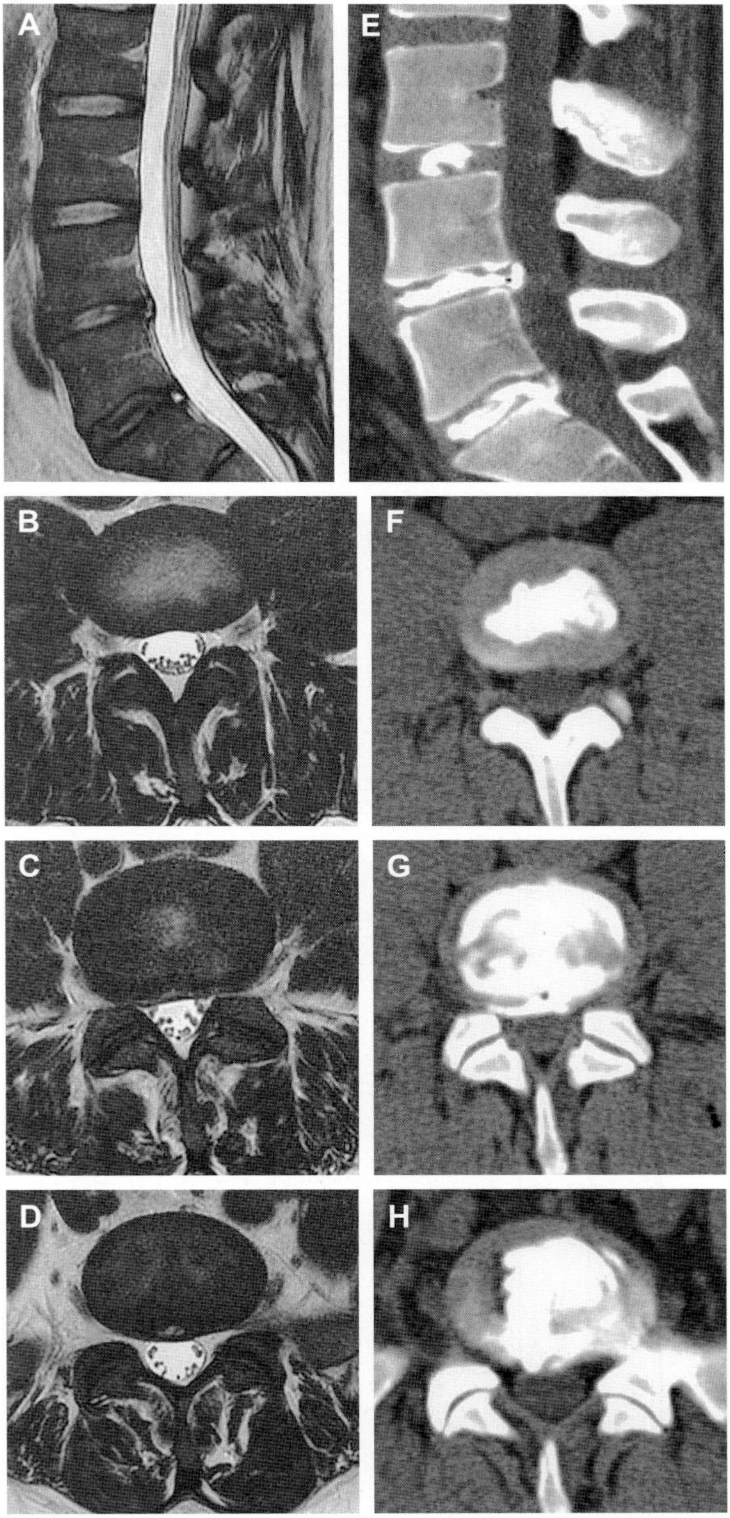

Fig. 4. Disk herniation and HIZ. (*A*) Patient with axial back pain; sagittal T2-weighted MR imaging shows T2 signal loss and herniations at L4 and L5 with HIZ at L5. Axial T2 images show a normal L3 disk (*B*), broad-based protrusion at L4 (*C*), and small central extrusion at L5 with caudal migration of disk material (*D*). Sagittal CT diskogram (*E*) and axial images at L3 (*F*), L4 (*G*), and L5 (*H*) show a normal L3 disk; diffuse, complex fissure with protrusion at L4; and more focal radial fissure leading to a small extrusion at L5. There was concordant pain at L4 and L5 at low pressures of injection (<20 PSI above opening pressure); L3 was a normal control disk.

Table 5
T2 signal loss

Author, Year	Diskogram Criteria	T2 Signal Criteria	Prevalence	Sensitivity	Specificity	PPV	NPV	+LR (CI)	−LR (CI)
Osti and Fraser,[56] 1992	Walsh	Moderate + severe	47%	70%	64%	50%	80%	1.9 (1.3–2.7)	0.49 (0.3–0.8)
		Severe only	13%	23%	92%	60%	70%	2.8 (1.1–7.0)	0.83 (0.7–1.0)
Horton and Daftari,[57] 1992	Walsh	Moderate + severe	69%	95%	43%	44%	94%	1.6 (1.2–2.2)	0.18 (0.04–0.9)
		Severe only	20%	37%	88%	58%	74%	2.8 (1.1–7.3)	0.72 (0.5–1.0)
Ito et al,[52] 1998	Walsh	Moderate + severe	63%	96%	46%	34%	97%	1.7 (1.4–2.2)	0.14 (0.03–0.6)
		Severe only	25%	70%	89%	64%	91%	5.7 (3.0–11.0)	0.36 (0.2–0.7)
Weishaupt et al,[58] 2001	IASP	3–5 of 5 Grade Pearce[41]	65%	98%	59%	64%	98%	2.3 (1.8–3.1)	0.05 (0.01–0.3)
Lim et al,[53] 2005	Walsh	4 and 5 of 5 Grade Pearce	62%	88%	52%	50%	89%	1.8 (1.4–2.4)	0.25 (0.1–0.6)
Lei et al,[59] 2008	IASP	3 and 4 of 4 Point Woodward	57%	94%	77%	78%	94%	4.0 (2.5–6.4)	0.07 (0.02–0.2)
O'Neill et al,[54] 2008	IASP	Moderate + severe	62%	90%	67%	75%	86%	2.7 (2.2–3.3)	0.16 (0.1–0.2)
		Severe only	15%	24%	96%	87%	54%	6.0 (3.0–11.7)	0.79 (0.7–0.9)
Kang et al,[55] 2009	IASP	3, 4, and 5 on Pfirrmann[42] 5-point scale	70%	95%	39%	34%	96%	1.6 (1.3–1.8)	0.12 (0.03–0.5)

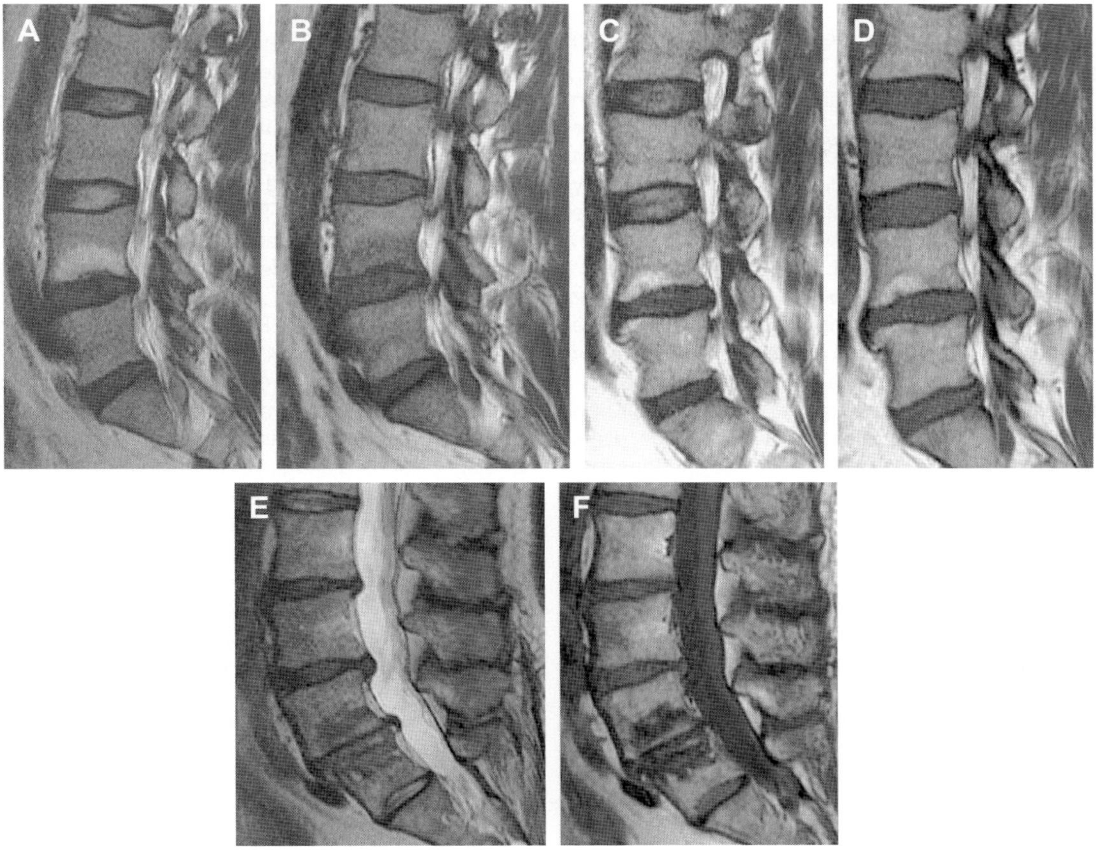

Fig. 5. End plate (Modic) change. (*A*, *B*) T2-weighted and T1-weighted MR images, respectively, show high T2 and low T1 signal at L4 inferior end plate consistent with the vascularized granulation tissue of type I end plate change. (*C*, *D*) T2-weighted and T1-weighted MR images in another patient demonstrate elevated T1 and T2 signal about the L4 interspace, reflecting the fatty infiltration of type II end plate change. (*E*, *F*) T2-weighted and T1-weighted MR images show low T2 and T1 signal about the L4 interspace, indicative of type III end plate change.

correlates with bony sclerosis. Type I change is thought to represent an active inflammatory state, with type II more quiescent and type III postinflammatory. Ohtori and colleagues[61] noted elevated levels of protein gene product 9.5–immunoreactive nerve fibers and TNF-α immunoreactive cells in the cartilaginous end plates of patients with Modic changes. The immunoreactive nerve ingrowth was seen exclusively in patients with the diskogenic low back pain. TNF-α immunoreactive cells were more common in type I end plate changes.

Modic end plate changes do carry an association with low back pain, in particular type I change. Toyone and colleagues[62] found that 73% of patients with type I change had low back pain as opposed to 11% of type II patients. Likewise, Albert and Maniche[63] reported low back pain in 60% of patients with Modic changes but in only 20% of those without Modic changes. Type I change was more strongly associated with low back pain than type II change. Modic type I change may also be associated with segmental instability; in the study of Toyone and colleagues,[62] 70% of patients with type I change were found to have segmental hypermobility (>3 mm translation on flexion-extension films). Hypermobility was seen in only 16% of those with type II change. Similarly, in post-fusion patients, the studies of Butterman and colleagues[64] and Lang and colleagues[65] showed persistent type I change in patients ultimately shown to have pseudarthroses. Patients with solid fusions tend to have type II change or resolution of all Modic changes. The studies of Chataigner and colleagues[66] and Esposito and colleagues[67] evaluated Modic change as a predictor of fusion outcome; patients with type I change at the operative level on preprocedure imaging tended to have much better outcomes than patients operated on with isolated disk "degeneration" or disk "degeneration" plus type II end plate change.

Again, there are disparate data, presented in **Table 6**,[52–55,58,59,68,69] when considering the value of Modic-type end plate changes as predictors of diskogenic pain. The studies discussed previously suggested that type I Modic change would be more strongly correlated with positive provocation diskography than type II; that conclusion is not borne out by the data, which suggest that either type I or type II Modic change correlate with positive diskography, although not uniformly. The studies of Braithwaite and colleagues,[68] Weishaupt and colleauges,[58] Lei and colleagues,[59] and O'Neill and colleagues[54] had few false-positive results (ie, disks with adjacent type I or type II end plate changes that were nonpainful). The specificity, PPV, and +LRs in these studies were high. The usefulness of the MR imaging finding is only hampered by its infrequency. The studies of Kokkonen and colleagues,[69] Lim and colleagues,[53] and Kang and colleagues,[55] however, showed no association between end plate change and diskogenic pain, with significant numbers of false-positive results. The Kokkonen and colleagues[69] and Lim and colleagues[53] articles provide scant description of the diskography technique, which raises concerns about their validity. Kang and colleagues'[55] article, however, describes appropriate technique in detail. The compelling results presented by Weishaupt and colleagues[58] suggest a threshold for marrow change is significant; with a threshold at 25% of vertebral body height, there were no false-positive results in his series. A reasonable conclusion is that Modic type I or II marrow change of this severity (25% vertebral height) is an infrequent but highly specific finding, with a high PPV for diskogenic pain.

High Intensity Zone

In 1992, Aprill and Bogduk described the HIZ as an imaging marker of a painful disk at provocation diskography.[70] Their definition of the HIZ is "high-intensity signal (bright white) located in the substance of the posterior annulus fibrosis, clearly dissociated from the signal of the nucleus pulposis in that it is surrounded superiorly, inferiorly, posteriorly and anteriorly by the low intensity (black) signal of the annulus fibrosis and is appreciably brighter than that of the nucleus pulposis." This finding was identified on a midsagittal T2-weighted image; it may occur centrally in an otherwise normal annulus or in a bulging annulus or be located superiorly or inferiorly behind the edge of the vertebral body in a severely bulging annulus. The prevalence of this finding was assessed in the MR imaging examinations of 500 consecutive patients. The per-patient prevalence was 29%; the per-disk prevalence of an HIZ was 6%. There was excellent reliability in identification of this finding, with independent observers in agreement on the presence or absence of an HIZ in 411 of 412 disks. The finding was best demonstrated on spin-echo T2-weighted images and not well demonstrated on gradient-echo images. The vast majority of HIZs were present at the L4 and L5 disk levels, confirmed on later studies. **Fig. 6** demonstrates an HIZ to diskography correlation.

The relationship of the HIZ to pain production was evaluated in a subset of 41 patients, selected for the presence of an HIZ on prediskography MR imaging. Diskography was performed using IASP criteria with the requirement of a nonpainful control disk for a diagnosis of diskogenic pain. Pain responses were tabulated both as "exact" reproduction of pain as well as "similar" pain. Correlations of pain provocation and diskography with the HIZ are seen in **Table 7**. In the 41 patients, 118 disks were tested; the per-disk prevalence of the HIZ was 34% reflecting the selection bias in this nonconsecutive series. In detecting exact pain, the HIZ had a sensitivity of 82% and specificity of 89%, a 70% PPV, and a +LR of 7.3. When the diskographic criteria was relaxed to exact or similar pain, the specificity rose to 97% with a PPV of 95%; there were only 2 false-positive cases where a disk bearing an HIZ was nonpainful. The investigators postulated that the HIZ represents a complex grade 4 fissure where the nuclear material has been trapped within the lamellae of the annulus fibrosis and become inflamed, accounting for the T2 signal intensity, which is brighter than that of the parent nucleus. They advanced the HIZ finding as pathognomonic of a symptomatic disk. The publication of these findings elicited considerable interest and many subsequent studies[52,54,55,58,59,70–76] attempting to verify or refute its conclusions. The several studies are presented in **Table 7**; a few are highlighted.

In 2000, Carragee and colleagues[75] evaluated the presence and significance of the HIZ in both symptomatic and asymptomatic subjects. The definition of HIZ was expanded to include bright signal in the posterolateral quadrants of the annulus rather than only those seen on the midsagittal images, as originally described. Quantitated signal intensity was required to be within 10% of that exhibited by cerebrospinal fluid to be considered an HIZ; areas of elevated but less intense signal were tracked as medium intensity zones. Diskography was performed with Walsh criteria, requiring 3/5 intensity concordant pain. The methods section states that pressure measurements occurred but no statement is made

Table 6
End plate (Modic) changes

Author, Year	Diskogram Criteria	Modic Type	Prevalence Per Disk	Sensitivity	Specificity	PPV	NPV	+LR	−LR
Braithwaite et al,[68] 1998	Walsh	I + II	25% Imaged 15% Tested	24%	96%	91%	47%	6.0 (1.7–21.2)	0.80 (0.7–0.9)
		I	4% Tested	5%	100%	100%	42%	7.4 (0.4–131)	0.95 (0.9–1.0)
		II	12% Tested	18%	96%	89%	48%	4.4 (1.2–16.1)	0.86 (0.8–0.9)
Ito et al,[52] 1998	Walsh	I + II + III?	9%	23%	94%	56%	80%	4.0 (1.3–12.8)	0.82 (0.7–1.0)
Weishaupt et al,[58] 2001	IASP	I	14%	29%	97%	88%	66%	9.9 (2.4–41.6)	0.73 (0.6–0.9)
		II	9%	19%	99%	90%	63%	12.75 (1.7–97.3)	0.83 (0.7–0.9)
		I + II	22%	48%	96%	88%	72%	10.86 (3.5–34.1)	0.55 (0.4–0.7)
		I + II Moderate + severe	16%	38%	100%	100%	69%	52.1 (3.2–844)	0.63 (0.5–0.8)
Kokkonen et al,[69] 2002	Walsh	I	17%	19%	85%	41%	65%	1.25 (0.5–3.0)	0.96 (0.8–1.20)
		II	19%	19%	80%	35%	64%	0.96 (0.4–2.2)	1.0 (0.8–1.2)
		I + II	36%	38%	65%	38%	65%	1.1 (0.6–1.8)	0.95 (0.7–1.3)
Lim et al,[53] 2005	Walsh	I + II	14%	9%	83%	21%	62%	0.6 (0.2–1.7)	1.1 (0.9–1.3)
Lei et al,[59] 2008	IASP	I + II?	14%	32%	98%	94%	62%	19.25 (2.7–140)	0.69 (0.6–0.8)
O'Neill et al,[54] 2008	IASP	I	4%	6%	99%	88%	49%	6.94 (1.6–29.9)	0.95 (0.9–1.0)
		II	4%	7%	99%	90%	50%	8.32 (1.9–35.5)	0.93 (0.9–1.0)
		I + II	8%	14%	98%	89%	51%	7.63 (2.8–21.2)	0.88 (0.8–0.9)
Kang et al,[55] 2009	IASP	I + II	13%	14%	87%	26%	76%	1.08 (0.5–2.6)	0.99 (0.9–1.1)

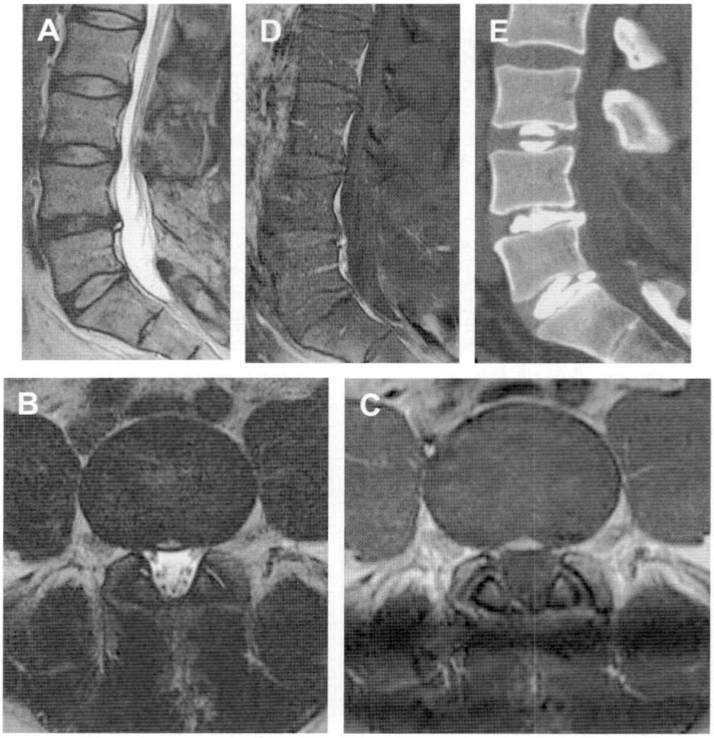

Fig. 6. HIZ. (*A*) Sagittal T2-weighted MR imaging shows loss of T2 signal in the L4 disk with an HIZ in the posterior annulus. There has been previous decompression, but no disk resection. (*B*) Axial T2-weighted MR imaging at L4 interspace demonstrates the HIZ in the posterior annulus. (*C*) Axial enhanced T1-weighted MR image showing enhancement in the HIZ also demonstrated in the sagittal fat-saturated T1 image (*D*). (*E*) Sagittal postdiskogram CT demonstrates annular fissure at L4 leading to HIZ.

regarding how this altered diagnostic criteria nor are any data presented. Forty-two symptomatic patients (109 disks) and 54 asymptomatic subjects (143 disks) were studied. In the symptomatic group, 59% of patients had HIZ disks whereas in the asymptomatic group only 24% had HIZ disks (significant, $P = .001$). In symptomatic patients, 30% of disks had an HIZ; only 9% of disks in asymptomatic subjects contained in HIZ (significant, $P<.0001$). The statistics for the symptomatic group are presented in **Table 7**; an HIZ disk has an 84% specificity, a 73% PPV, and a +LR of 2.8 for diskogenic pain. These data are supportive of the HIZ as a useful marker for the painful disk. The investigators, however, point out that the presence of an HIZ disk was strongly predictive of a positive pain response at diskography in both the symptomatic (73%) and asymptomatic (69%) groups. The asymptomatic group had also been stratified by psychometric evaluation; in participants with either chronic pain or abnormal psychometric studies, all HIZ disks produced pain with pressurization. The investigators contend that the similar painful response rate of HIZ disks in symptomatic and asymptomatic subjects devalues the HIZ as a useful finding, because the total weight of diagnosis depends on the concordance versus nonconcordance of the pain response. The medium intensity zone did not predict diskogenic pain, suggesting a threshold effect for the significance of the HIZ, as noted in the original description.

O'Neill and colleagues' study[54] of 2008 modified the Aprill and Bogduk criteria to include HIZ lesions connected to the nuclear compartment by a thin line of high T2 signal or consisted only of a thin horizontal line of high T2 signal within the annulus. They also included posterior, posterolateral, and lateral lesions. HIZ lesions were further segregated by intensity of T2 signal on a 3-part scale (mild, moderate, and markedly hyperintense). Contingency tables were constructed from the published data and the **Table 7** statistics calculated for 3 thresholds of HIZ detection—markedly intense cases, markedly and moderately intense cases, and combining all 3. As the threshold tightened, the specificity and +LR rose; the PPV remained high for all 3 threshold levels. For only markedly hyperintense HIZs, the specificity was 98%, the PPV 86%, and the +LR 6.8, supporting Bogduk's

Table 7
High intensity zone

Author, Year	Diskogram Criteria	HIZ Criteria	Prevalence Per Disk	Sensitivity	Specificity	PPV	NPV	+LR (CI)	−LR (CI)
Aprill and Bogduk,[70] 1992	IASP Exact pain	Aprill	34%[a]	82%	89%	78%	91%	7.3 (3.9–13.7)	0.21 (0.1–0.4)
	Exact or similar pain	Aprill	—	63%	97%	95%	72%	18.4 (4.6–72.7)	0.38 (0.3–0.5)
Schellhas et al,[71] 1996	IASP	Schellhas[b]	60%[a]	97%	83%	87%	97%	5.7 (3.5–9.3)	0.03 (0.01–0.11)
Ricketson et al,[72] 1996	Walsh	Aprill	9%	12%	92%	57%	54%	1.5 (0.4–5.6)	0.96 (0.8–1.1)
Saifuddin et al,[73] 1998	Walsh	Aprill	18%	27%	94%	89%	47%	4.8 (1.7–14.2)	0.77 (0.7–0.9)
Ito et al,[52] 1998	Walsh	Aprill	20%	52%	89%	60%	87%	4.8 (2.3–10.2)	0.54 (0.4–0.8)
Smith et al,[74] 1998	Walsh	Aprill	13%	27%	90%	40%	80%	2.6 (1.2–5.6)	0.82 (0.7–1.0)
Carragee et al,[75] 2000	Walsh	Carragee[c]	30%	45%	84%	73%	62%	2.8 (1.5–5.5)	0.7 (0.5–0.9)
Weishaupt et al,[58] 2001	IASP	Aprill	20%	27%	85%	56%	62%	1.8 (0.8–3.7)	0.86 (0.7–1.0)
Peng et al,[76] 2006	Walsh	Aprill	12%	NC	NC	100%	NC	NC	NC
Lei et al,[59] 2008	Walsh	Aprill	19%	25%	87%	62%	57%	1.8 (0.8–4.1)	0.87 (0.7–1.1)
O'Neill et al,[54] 2008	IASP	O'Neill[d] 1 + 2 + 3 intensity grades	28%	44%	89%	82%	60%	4.1 (2.7–6.1)	0.62 (0.5–0.7)
		2 + 3	16%	26%	95%	86%	54%	5.7 (3.0–10.9)	0.78 (0.7–0.8)
		3	9%	15%	98%	86%	52%	6.8 (2.7–17.1)	0.87 (0.8–0.9)
Kang et al,[55] 2009	IASP	Aprill	26%	57%	84%	53%	86%	3.46 (2.2–5.5)	0.52 (0.4–0.7)

[a] Nonconsecutive series, with presence of an HIZ as an inclusion criteria. Sensitivity and prevalence values are not meaningful due to this selection bias.
[b] Includes lesions with thin line of T2 hyperintensity within annulus or connecting nucleus to HIZ.
[c] Includes posterolateral lesions, HIZ signal intensity within 10% of cerebrospinal fluid T2 signal.
[d] Schellhas criteria plus posterolateral and lateral lesions.

comment that "low intensity zones may well occur in asymptomatic volunteers, but that when 'activated' (ostensibly inflamed), these fissures become painful and assume a higher signal intensity."[48]

Again, general conclusions are confounded by alterations in the definition of the parameter under study (HIZ) by various investigators, and significant variability of the reference standard test, provocation diskography. The Aprill and Bogduk,[70] Schellhas and colleauges,[71] Weishaupt and colleauges,[58] O'Neill and colleauges,[54] and Kang and colleauges[55] studies used IASP criteria, with a negative control disk; the remaining studies did not. No studies used ISIS criteria with mamometry. Schelhas and colleagues,[71] Carragee and colleagues[75] and O'Neill and colleagues[54] expanded the definition of the HIZ. The data of O'Neill and colleagues[54] suggest a threshold effect, with higher levels of T2 signal having greater specificity and PPV for pain production. It is reasonable to conclude from the several studies that the HIZ is a finding of modest frequency in patients investigated for diskogenic pain, with a per-patient prevalence approaching 30%. When present, the preponderance of data suggests that an HIZ predicts a painful disk with high specificity, PPV, and +LR. There is likely a threshold effect for signal intensity.

Multivariate Analysis

The studies of Kang and colleagues[55] and O'Neill and colleagues[54] included multivariate analyses. O'Neill and colleagues showed that the disk structural findings—loss of disk height, loss of nuclear signal, and disk contour abnormalities correlated strongly with each other; the inflammatory findings, HIZ and end plate change did not, with the exception of HIZ and disk contour abnormality. The rank correlations of the MR imaging findings with a positive diskogram were signal abnormality greater than disk height greater than disk contour greater than HIZ greater than end plate change. Disk signal change alone was as accurate as other individual parameters or combinations thereof. This was most evident at the 2 extremes of the ROC curve: when disk signal is normal, it is highly unlikely the disk is painful regardless of other findings; and when there is severe signal loss, the disk is highly likely to be painful. Other parameters become useful when disk signal is intermediate. The investigators noted that disk bulge was most helpful when signal loss was intermediate, resulting in a sensitivity of 80% and a specificity of 79%. In the presence of intermediate signal loss, the findings of moderate loss of disk space height or presence of an HIZ boosted the specificity further, at the cost of sensitivity.

Kang and colleagues[55] introduced a new MR imaging classification system combining the findings previously addressed as independent variables: class 1, normal or bulging disk without an HIZ; class 2, normal or bulging disk with an HIZ; class 3, disk protrusion without HIZ; and class 4, disk protrusion with HIZ. Disk extrusions and sequestrations were excluded from the analysis. Logistic regression analysis showed that class 4, disk protrusion with HIZ had the strongest correlation with concordant pain at diskography. This combination had a specificity of 87% and a PPV of 98%. This finding had a prevalence of 13% and a sensitivity of 45%.

SUMMARY: IMAGING CORRELATES OF LUMBAR DISKOGENIC PAIN

Noninvasive imaging identification of diskogenic pain is challenging: (1) There is no pathologic or surgical gold standard. (2) The existing reference standard, provocation diskography, is subjective in its interpretation, and has evolved over time in its criteria for a positive test. None of the studies reviewed in this article used the most current and restrictive criteria, those of ISIS. (3) The imaging findings likely have threshold effects, where only a significant expression of the finding (intensity of an HIZ or extent of marrow change) is a useful predictor of diskogenic pain. Most studies do not account for this. (4) Imaging findings are likely technique dependent to an unknown degree, and imaging techniques are evolving. An HIZ may be seen with greater conspicuity on thinner slices than thicker ones; it was originally described with spin-echo T2-weighted sequences, whereas most current T2-weighted imaging uses fast spin-echo (FSE) or turbo spin-echo (TSE) sequences. Is a bright signal in the posterior annulus on a short tau inversion recovery (STIR) or fat-saturated FSE equivalent to the original description? Will marrow edema be better seen on a T1 fluid-attenuated inversion recovery (FLAIR) sequence or a conventional spin-echo sequence? These questions are unanswered.

From the morass of data, useful information can emerge. This is what can be reasonably concluded from existing research, in reference to a population of symptomatic patients suspected of diskogenic pain:

1. The disk structural markers—loss of disk space height, loss of nuclear T2 signal, and disk herniation—correlate strongly with one another; loss of nuclear signal is most significant.
2. Severe T2 nuclear signal loss or severe loss of disk space height strongly predicts a painful disk.

3. Normal T2 nuclear signal virtually excludes a painful disk.
4. When nuclear signal is intermediate, the inflammatory markers of the HIZ and end plate marrow change come into play.
5. A truly HIZ is infrequent but strongly predicts a painful disk.
6. When an HIZ is seen in combination with a disk protrusion, it strongly predicts a painful disk.
7. Marrow end plate changes of type I or type II involving greater than 25% of the vertebral body are uncommon but strongly predict a painful disk.

These imaging predictors of diskogenic pain, when applied to a select population of patients with axial back pain, in whom other pain generators have been excluded, could perhaps be used to initiate a proven therapy possessing a good safety profile. No such therapy exists. Diskography remains the reference standard for the diagnosis of diskogenic pain.

On the horizon are advanced MR imaging techniques, which may allow better characterization of disk nuclear matrix degradation and perhaps identification of a painful disk. Watanabe and colleagues[77] used 3-T MR imaging to generate axial T2 maps of the intervertebral disk, which may allow earlier detection of disk nuclear matrix degradation. Johannessen and associates[78] used a novel pulse sequence, T1ρ relaxation, to study disks in human cadavers; this was performed on a standard 1.5-T imager. Their work showed a strong correlation between T1ρ signal and sulfated-glycosaminoglycan content in the nucleus.[78] Sodium (as opposed to proton) MR imaging has also been reported as a means of quantification of the proteoglycan content in the nuclear compartment of the disk.[79] These studies demonstrate that to be valuable in the diagnosis of diskogenic pain, imaging must move beyond macroscopic descriptions of morphology to the realm of biochemical imaging, quantifying the change in nuclear constituents over time. In addition to biochemical degradation, imaging also needs to more precisely identify inflammatory mediators in the disk and adjacent cartilaginous end plate. Perhaps then noninvasive diagnosis of diskogenic pain will be possible.

EPILOGUE: CERVICAL DISKOGRAPHY AND DISKOGENIC PAIN

This discussion has purposely focused on the lumbar spine. The lumbar spine segment is most commonly afflicted with diskogenic pain, and the literature regarding its pathogenesis and evaluation with imaging and provocation diskography, although challenging, is of greatest depth. As noted by Bogduk, the cervical intervertebral disk is structurally distinct from the lumbar disk. There is no posterior annulus, and the small nuclear compartment disappears early in life; the residual fibrocartilaginous plate normally develops fissures as mere age-related change.[26] Thus, there are no morphologic features at diskography that contribute to a diagnosis of diskogenic pain. Diagnosis is reliant entirely on the provocation of concordant pain, with the requirement of nonpainful control disks.

As in the lumbar segment, structural age changes (loss of T2 signal, loss of disk space height, and contour abnormality) are ubiquitous on cervical MR imaging studies. Matsumoto and colleagues[80] studied 2480 cervical disks in 497 asymptomatic subjects with MR imaging and noted loss of T2 signal in 17% of men and 12% of women between ages 20 and 30, and 89% of men and 86% of women over 60 years of age. In another study by Okada and colleagues,[81] 89% of asymptomatic subjects (mean age 49) exhibited structural age changes on MR imaging; another group of patients (mean age 46) with symptomatic lumbar disk herniations but asymptomatic of neck pain showed cervical disk age-related change in 98%. There is a paucity of literature addressing the correlation of imaging findings with cervical diskography. An early study by Parfenchuck and colleagues[82] in 1994 showed only a modest ability of MR imaging findings of T2 signal loss or disk contour abnormality to predict a positive cervical diskogram (sensitivity 73% and specificity 67%). Schellhas and colleagues' 1996 study[83] suggested MR imaging cannot reliably predict a positive cervical diskogram. A more recent study by Zheng and colleagues[84] again demonstrated only a modest predictive value of MR imaging using parameters of T2 signal loss and disk contour abnormality (sensitivity 73% and specificity 49%). The inflammatory disk parameters, which proved to have such high specificity in the lumbar region, are either unusual and little studied (Modic change) or have no anatomic existence (HIZ) in the cervical region. Occasionally, foci of elevated T2 signal are observed in the posterior cervical disk, but in the absence of a posterior annulus, the anatomic correlate is unclear. Imaging identification of diskogenic pain in the cervical spine remains elusive. Cervical diskography remains the reference standard.

REFERENCES

1. Mixter WJ, Barr JS. Rupture of the intervertebral disc with involvement of the spinal canal. N Engl J Med 1934;211:210–5.

2. Morgan FP, King T. Primary instability of lumbar vertebrae as a common cause of low back pain. J Bone Joint Surg Br 1957;39(1):6–22.
3. Crock HV. A reappraisal of intervertebral disc lesions. Med J Aust 1970;1(20):983–9.
4. Crock HV, Bedbrook GM. Practice of spinal surgery. Internal Disc Disruption. New York: Springer-Verlag, Wein; 1983. P. 35–56.
5. Carragee EJ, Tanner CM, Khurana S, et al. The rate of false-positive lumbar discography in selected patients without low back symptoms. Spine 2000; 25(11):1373–80 [discussion: 1381].
6. Lindblom K. Protrusions of the disks and nerve compression in the lumbar region. Acta Radiol 1944;25:195–212.
7. Lindblom K. Diagnostic puncture of intervertebral disks in sciatica. Acta Orthop Scand 1948;17(3–4):231–9.
8. Wise RE, Weiford EC. X-ray visualization of the intervertebral disc; report of a case. Cleve Clin Q 1951; 18(2):127–30.
9. Cloward RB, Buzaid LL. Discography; technique, indications and evaluation of the normal and abnormal intervertebral discs. Am J Roentgenol Radium Ther Nucl Med 1952;68(4):552–64.
10. Fernstrom U. A discographical study of ruptured lumbar intervertebral discs. Acta Chir Scand Suppl 1960;258:1–60.
11. Feinberg SB. The place of diskography in radiology as based on 2,320 cases. Am J Roentgenol Radium Ther Nucl Med 1964;92:1275–81.
12. Friedman J, Goldner MZ. Discography in evaluation of lumbar disk lesions. Radiology 1955;65(5):653–62.
13. Massie WK, Stevens DB. A critical evaluation of discography. J Bone Joint Surg Am 1967;49:1243–4.
14. Holt EP. The question of lumbar discography. J Bone Joint Surg Am 1968;50(4):720–6.
15. Walsh TR, Weinstein JN, Spratt KF, et al. Lumbar discography in normal subjects. A controlled, prospective study. J Bone Joint Surg Am 1990;72(7):1081–8.
16. Bogduk N. The innervation of the lumbar spine. Spine (Phila Pa 1976) 1983;8(3):286–93.
17. Yoshizawa H, O'Brien JP, Thomas-Smith W, et al. The neuropathology of intervertebral discs removed for low-back pain. J Pathol 1980;132:95–104.
18. Weinstein J, Claverie W, Gibson S. The pain of discography. Spine (Phila Pa 1976) 1988;13(12):1344–8.
19. Sachs BL, Vanharanta H, Spivey MA, et al. Dallas discogram description. A new classification of CT/discography in low-back disorders. Spine (Phila Pa 1976) 1987;12(3):287–94.
20. Vanharanta H, Sachs BL, Spivey MA, et al. The relationship of pain provocation to lumbar disc deterioration as seen by CT/discography. Spine (Phila Pa 1976) 1987;12(3):295–8.
21. Moneta GB, Videman T, Kaivanto K, et al. Reported pain during lumbar discography as a function of anular ruptures and disc degeneration. A re-analysis of 833 discograms. Spine (Phila Pa 1976) 1994; 19(17):1968–74.
22. Derby R, Howard MW, Grant JM, et al. The ability of pressure-controlled discography to predict surgical and nonsurgical outcomes. Spine (Phila Pa 1976) 1999;24(4):364–71 [discussion: 371–2].
23. Bogduk N. Clinical anatomy of the lumbar spine and sacrum. 3rd edition. New York: Churchill Livingston; 1997.
24. Peng B, Wu W, Hou S, et al. The pathogenesis of discogenic low back pain. J Bone Joint Surg Br 2005; 87(1):62–7.
25. Cohen SP, Larkin TM, Barna SA, et al. Lumbar discography: a comprehensive review of outcome studies, diagnostic accuracy, and principles. Reg Anesth Pain Med 2005;30(2):163–83.
26. Bogduk N, editor. Practice guidelines for spinal diagnostic procedures. San Francisco (CA): International Spine Intervention Society; 2004.
27. DePalma MJ, Ketchum JM, Saullo T. What is the source of chronic low back pain and does age play a role? Pain Med 2011;12(2):224–33.
28. Depalma MJ, Ketchum JM, Saullo TR. Multivariable analyses of the relationships between age, gender, and body mass index and the source of chronic low back pain. Pain Med 2012;13(4):498–506.
29. Schwarzer AC, Aprill CN, Derby R, et al. The prevalence and clinical features of internal disc disruption in patients with chronic low back pain. Spine 1995;20(17):1878–81.
30. Manchikanti L, Singh V, Pampati V, et al. Evaluation of the relative contributions of various structures in chronic low back pain. Pain Physician 2001;4(4):308–16.
31. Schwarzer AC, Aprill CN, Derby R, et al. Clinical features of patients with pain stemming from the lumbar zygapophysial joints. Is the lumbar facet syndrome a clinical entity? Spine (Phila Pa 1976) 1994;19(10):1132–7.
32. Schwarzer A, Wang SC, Bogduk N, et al. Prevalence and clinical features of lumbar z joint pain: a study in an Australian population w/chronic low back pain. Ann Rheum Dis 1995;54:100–6.
33. Maigne JY, Aivaliklis A, Fabrice P. Results of sacroiliac joint double block and value of sacroiliac pain provocation tests in 54 patients with low back pain. Spine 1996;21(16):1889–92.
34. Schwarzer AC, Aprill CN, Bogduk N. The sacroiliac joint in chronic low back pain. Spine 1995; 20:31–7.
35. Carragee EJ, Tanner CM, Yang B, et al. False-positive findings on lumbar discography. Reliability of sub- jective concordance assessment during provocative disc injection. Spine 1999;24:2542–7.
36. Carragee EJ, Chen Y, Tanner CM, et al. Provocative discography in patients after limited lumbar discectomy: a controlled, randomized study of pain response in symptomatic and asymptomatic subjects. Spine 2000;25:3065–71.

37. Carragee EJ, Alamin TF, Miller J, et al. Provocative discography in volunteer subjects with mild persistent low back pain. Spine J 2002;2:25–34.
38. Carragee EJ, Alamin TF, Carragee JM. Low-pressure positive discography in subjects asymptomatic of signifi- cant low back pain illness. Spine 2006;31: 505–9.
39. Wolfer LR, Derby R, Lee JE, et al. Systematic review of lumbar provocation discography in asymptomatic subjects with a meta-analysis of false-positive rates. Pain Physician 2008;11(4):513–38.
40. Ibrahim T, Tleyjeh IM, Gabbar O. Surgical versus non-surgical treatment of chronic low back pain: a meta-analysis of randomised trials. Int Orthop 2008;32(1):107–13.
41. Chou R, Baisden J, Carragee EJ, et al. Surgery for low back pain: a review of the evidence for an American Pain Society Clinical Practice Guideline. Spine (Phila Pa 1976) 2009;34(10):1094–109.
42. Derby R, Baker R, Wolfer L. Analgesic discography in diagnosis. In: Deer T, editor. Management and treatment of discogenic pain. Philadelphia: Elsevier; 2012.
43. Korecki C, Costi J, Iatridis J. Needle puncture injury affects intervertebral disc mechanics and biology in an organ culture model. Spine 2008;33(3):235–41.
44. Carragee E, Don A, Hurwitz E, et al. Does discography cause accelerated progression of degenerative changes in the lumbar disc: a ten-year matched cohort study. Spine 2009;34(21):2338–45.
45. Fardon DF, Milette PC. Nomenclature and classification of the lumbar disc pathology: recommendations of the combined task forces of the North American Spine Society, American Society of Spine Radiology, and American Society of Neuroradiology. Spine 2001;26:E93–113.
46. Nathan H. Osteophytes of the vertebral column: an anatomic study of their development according to age, race, and sex with consideration as to their etiology and significance. J Bone Joint Surg 1962; 44:243–68.
47. Hancock M, Maher C, Latimer, et al. Systematic review of tests to identify the disc. SIJ, or facet joint as the source of low back pain. Eur Spine J 2007;16: 1539–50.
48. Bogduk N. Point of view: predictive signs of discogenic lumbar pain on magnetic resonance imaging with discography correlation. Spine 1998;23(11):1259–60.
49. Guyer R, Ohhnmeiss D. Lumbar discography. Spine J 2003;3(Suppl 3):11S–27S.
50. Manchikanti L, Glaser S, Wolfer L, et al. Systematic review of lumbar discography as a diagnostic test for chronic low back pain. Pain Physician 2009; 12(3):541–59.
51. Chou R, Loeser J, Owens D, et al. Interventional therapies, surgery, and interdisciplinary rehabilitation for low back pain: evidence based clinical practice guidelines from the American Pain Society. Spine 2009;34(10):1066–77.
52. Ito M, Incorvaia K, Yu S, et al. Predictive signs of discogenic lumbar pain on magnetic resonance imaging with discography correlation. Spine 1998; 23:1252–8.
53. Lim C, Jee W, Son B, et al. Discogenic lumbar pain: association with MRI imaging and CT discography. Eur J Radiol 2005;54(3):431–7.
54. O'Neill C, Kurganshy M, Kaiser J, et al. Accuracy of MRI for diagnosis of discogenic pain. Pain Physician 2008;11:311–26.
55. Kang C, Kim Y, Lee S, et al. Can magnetic resonance imaging accurately predict concordant pain provocation during provocative disc injection? Skeletal Radiol 2009;38:877–85.
56. Osti O, Fraser R. MRI and discography of annular tears and intervertebral disc degeneration. J Bone Joint Surg Br 1992;74(3):431–5.
57. Horton C, Daftari T. Which disc visualized by magnetic resonance imaging is actually a source of pain? Spine 1992;17(Suppl 6):S164–71.
58. Weishaupt D, Zanetti M, Hodler J, et al. Painful lumbar disk derangement: relevance of endplate abnormalities at MR imaging. Radiology 2001;218: 420–7.
59. Lei D, Rege A, Koti M, et al. Painful disc lesion: can modern biplanar magnetic resonance imaging replace discography. J Spinal Disord Tech 2008;21:430–5.
60. Modic M, Steinberg P, Ross J, et al. Degenerative disk disease: assessment of changes in vertebral body marrow with MR imaging. Radiology 1988; 166(1 pt 1):193–9.
61. Ohtori S, Inoue G, Ito K, et al. Tumor necrosis factor-immunoreactive cells and PGP 9.5-immunoreactive nerve fibers in vertebral endplates of patients with discogenic low back pain and Modic type 1 or type 2 changes on MRI. Spine 2006;31(9):1026–31.
62. Toyone T, Takahashi K, Kitahara H, et al. Vertebral bone-marrow changes in degenerative lumbar disc disease: an MRI study of 74 patients with low back pain. J Bone Joint Surg Br 1994;76:757–64.
63. Albert HB, Manniche C. Modic changes following lumbar disc herniation. Eur Spine J 2007;16(7): 977–82.
64. Buttermann GR, Heithoff KB, Ogilvie JW, et al. Vertebral body MRI related to lumbar fusion results. Eur Spine J 1997;6:115–20.
65. Lang P, Chafetz N, Genant HK, et al. Lumbar spinal fusion: assessment of functional stability with magnetic resonance imaging. Spine 1990;15:581–8.
66. Chataigner H, Onimus M, Polette A. Surgery for degenerative lumbar disc disease: should the black disc be grafted? Rev Chir Orthop Reparatrice Appar Mot 1998;84:583–9 [in French].
67. Esposito P, Pinheiro-Franco JL, Froelich S, et al. Predictive value of MRI vertebral end-plate signal changes

(Modic) on outcome of surgically treated degenerative disc disease: results of a cohort study including 60 patients. Neurochirurgie 2006;52:315–22.
68. Braithwaite IJ, White J, Saifuddin A, et al. Vertebral end-plate (Modic) changes on lumbar spine MRI: correlation with pain reproduction at lumbar discography. Eur Spine J 1998;7:363–8.
69. Kokkonen S, Kurunlahti M, Tervonen O, et al. Endplate degeneration observed on magnetic resonance imaging of the lumbar spine. Spine 2002; 27(20):2274–8.
70. Aprill C, Bogduk N. High-intensity zone: a diagnostic sign of painful lumbar disc on magnetic resonance imaging. Br J Radiol 1992;65(773):361–9.
71. Schellhas K, Pollei S, Gundry C, et al. Lumbar disc high-intensity zone. correlation of magnetic resonance imaging and discography. Spine 1996;21(1): 79–86.
72. Ricketson R, Simmons J, Hauser W. The prolapsed intervertebral disc: the high intensity zone with discography correlation. Spine 1996; 21(23):2758–62.
73. Saifuddin A, Braithwaite I, White J, et al. The value of magnetic resonance imaging in the demonstration of annular tears. Spine 1998;23(4):453–7.
74. Smith B, Hurwitz E, Solsberg D, et al. Interobserver reliability of detecting lumbar intervertebral disc high-intensity zone on magnetic resonance imaging and association of high–intensity zone with pain and annular disruption. Spine 1998;23(19):2074–80.
75. Carragee E, Paragioudakis S, Khurana S. Lumbar high-intensity zone and discography in subjects without low back problems. Spine 2000;25(23): 2987–92.
76. Peng B, Hou S, Wu W. The pathogenesis and clinical significance of a high-intensity zone (HIZ) of lumbar intervertebral disc on MRI imaging in the patient with discogenic low back pain. Eur Spine J 2006;15(5): 583–7.
77. Watanabe A, Benneker L, Boesch C, et al. Classification of intervertebral disk degeneration with axial T2 mapping. AJR Am J Roentgenol 2007;189: 936–42.
78. Johannessen W, Auerbach J, Wheaton A, et al. Assessment of human disc degeneration and proteoglycan content using T1ρ-weighted magnetic resonance imaging. Spine 2006;31(11):1253–7.
79. Wang C, McArdle E, Fenty M, et al. Validation of sodium magnetic resonance imaging of intervertebral disc. Spine 2010;35(5):505–10.
80. Matsumoto M, Fujimura Y, Suzuki N, et al. MRI of cervical intervertebral discs in asymptomatic subjects. J Bone Joint Surg Br 1998;80:19–24.
81. Okada E, Matsumoto M, Fujiwara H, et al. Disc degeneration of cervical spine on MRI in patients with lumbar disc herniation: comparison study with asymptomatic volunteers. Eur Spine J 2011;20(4): 585–91.
82. Parfenchuck TA, Janssen ME. A correlation of cervical magnetic resonance imaging and discography/computed tomographic discograms. Spine (Phila Pa 1976) 1994;19(24):2819–25.
83. Schellhas KP, Smith MD, Gundry CR, et al. Cervical discogenic pain. Prospective correlation of magnetic resonance imaging and discography in asymptomatic subjects and pain sufferers. Spine (Phila Pa 1976) 1996;21(3):300–11.
84. Zheng Y, Liew SM, Simmons ED. Value of magnetic resonance imaging and discography in determining the level of cervical discectomy and fusion. Spine (Phila Pa 1976) 2004;29(19):2140–5 [discussion: 2146].

Imaging of Posterior Element Axial Pain Generators

Facet Joints, Pedicles, Spinous Processes, Sacroiliac Joints, and Transitional Segments

Amy L. Kotsenas, MD

KEYWORDS

• Baastrup disease • Bertolotti syndrome • Facet synovitis • Fat-suppressed MR imaging • ^{18}F-FDG PET/CT • Interspinous bursitis • Posterior elements • SPECT

KEY POINTS

- The role of the posterior elements in generating axial back and neck pain is well established.
- Morphologic imaging findings are nonspecific and are frequently present in asymptomatic patients.
- Edema, inflammation, and hypervascularity are more specific for sites of pain generation.
- Physiologic imaging techniques such as fat-suppressed magnetic resonance imaging, single-photon emission computed tomography (CT), or ^{18}F-fluorodeoxyglucose positron emission tomography combined with CT are more sensitive for edema, inflammation, and hypervascularity than morphologic imaging alone.

INTRODUCTION

Radiologists and referring clinicians evaluating patients with low back pain (LBP) or radicular symptoms tend to focus on the anterior spinal column, specifically on disc pathology, often overlooking the role of the posterior elements in pain generation. Facet joints, pedicles, spinal ligaments, spinous processes, transitional lumbosacral segments, and sacroiliac (SI) joints have all been implicated as sources of axial back and neck pain, and may be causal of radicular symptoms. Imaging of the posterior elements in LBP remains controversial, primarily because of the specificity fault seen in all spine imaging. Morphologic changes on radiography, computed tomography (CT), and magnetic resonance (MR) imaging are common in asymptomatic individuals. Conversely, posterior element causes of LBP and neck pain may remain underrecognized secondary to use of MR imaging techniques which fail to demonstrate the bone marrow edema, soft-tissue inflammation, and hypervascularity often associated with posterior element pain generators. Inclusion of fat-suppressed T2-weighted or fat-suppressed contrast-enhanced (CE) T1-weighted images into a standard spinal MR imaging protocol increases the conspicuity of these findings. Nuclear medicine bone scanning with single-photon emission computed tomography (SPECT), SPECT/CT, and/or ^{18}F-fluorodeoxyglucose positron emission tomography combined with CT (FDG-PET/CT) are additional physiologic imaging techniques that may identify sites of posterior element pain. This article focuses on the use of appropriate imaging techniques to diagnose posterior element–associated spine pain and discusses imaging findings associated with posterior element pain generators (**Box 1**).

The author has nothing to disclose.
Division of Neuroradiology, Department of Radiology, Mayo Clinic, 200 1st Street Southwest, Rochester, MN 55905, USA
E-mail address: kotsenas.amy@mayo.edu

Radiol Clin N Am 50 (2012) 705–730
doi:10.1016/j.rcl.2012.04.008

Box 1
Posterior element pain generators

- Facet joints
- Ligamentum flavum
- Pedicles and pars interarticularis
- Spinous processes and interspinous ligaments
- Transitional lumbosacral segments and pseudoarticulations
- Sacroiliac joints

ANATOMY OF THE POSTERIOR SPINAL COLUMN

The 3-column spine model was originally described by Denis in 1983 to explain injury and instability patterns, and remains useful today.[1] It consists of anterior (anterior half of the vertebral body, intervertebral disc and annulus fibrosus, and anterior longitudinal ligament), middle (posterior half of the vertebral body, intervertebral disc and annulus fibrosus, and posterior longitudinal ligament), and posterior columns (pedicles, facet joints, laminae, spinous processes, ligamentum flavum, and interspinous ligaments). This article focuses on the elements of the posterior column.

The functional unit of the spine consists of the 2 adjacent vertebral bodies, the intervening intervertebral disc, and the bilateral paired facet joints.[2] The superior articular process of the lumbar facet joint has a concave surface and faces dorsomedially to meet the inferior articular process of the level above. The inferior articular process has a convex surface and faces anterolaterally, typically resulting in a parasagittal oblique orientation to the lumbar facet joint articulation. The obliquity of the facet joints varies greatly from patient to patient, but is generally greatest at the L4-L5 and L5-S1 levels, accounting in part for greater susceptibility of these 2 levels to disc protrusions and degenerative spondylolisthesis.[3,4] The superior and inferior articular processes are joined by the pars interarticularis (**Fig. 1**).

The paired facet joints at each level are true synovial joints lined by hyaline cartilage surfaces, surrounded by a synovial membrane and fibrous capsule. The cervical and lumbar facet joints are primarily innervated by medial branches of the primary dorsal rami that arise from the spinal nerve just peripheral to the dorsal root ganglion.[5,6] These nerves carry both sensory and motor information. Each dorsal ramus supplies two adjacent facet joints, one at the level of its emergence from the spinal canal and the other one vertebral segment inferiorly. Therefore, each facet joint is supplied by branches from 2 adjacent spinal segments (**Fig. 2**).[2] The medial branch also supplies the periosteum of the lamina and continues along the

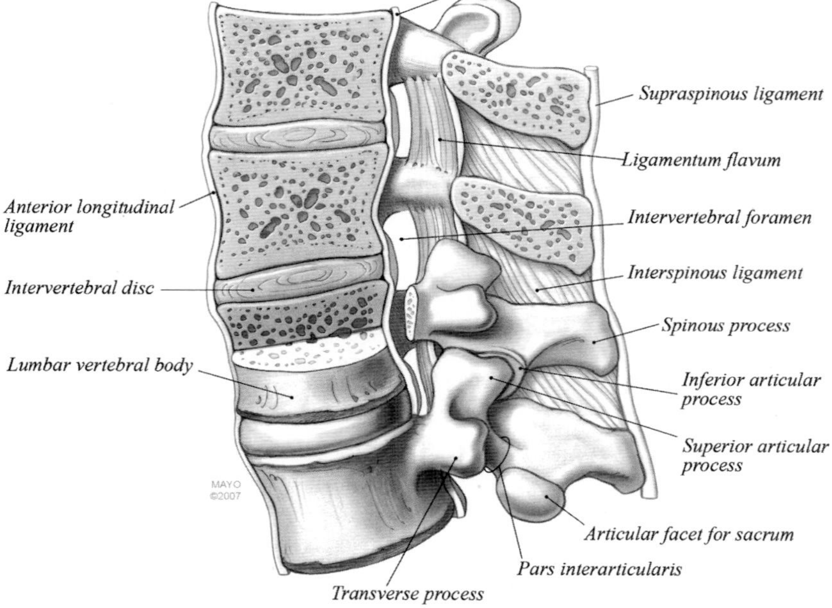

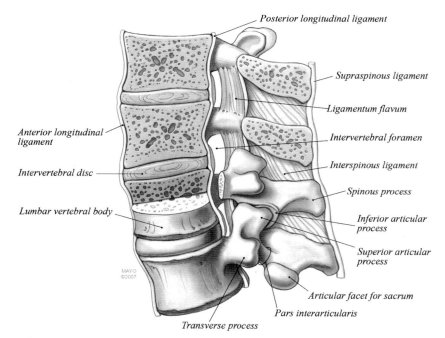

Fig. 1. Bony and ligamentous anatomy of the posterior spinal elements. (*Courtesy of* Mayo Clinic, Rochester, MN; with permission.)

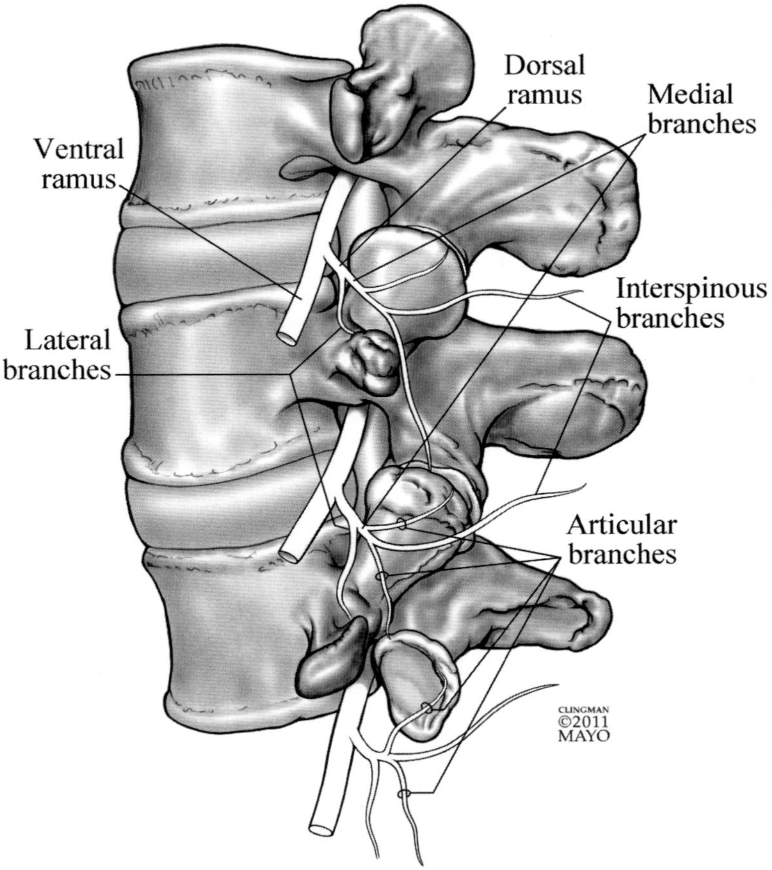

Fig. 2. Innervation of the posterior elements. The posterior elements are primarily innervated by the medial branches of the primary dorsal ramus. Each facet joint is innervated by branches from 2 adjacent spinal levels. (*Courtesy of* Mayo Clinic, Rochester, MN; with permission.)

inferior border of the spinous process to innervate the interspinous soft tissues; it also supplies motor innervation to the multifidus muscle.[6]

The posterior ligamentous complex consists of the paired ligamentum flavum, the interspinous ligaments, the supraspinous ligament, and the facet joint capsules. These ligaments normally provide stability. The paired ligamenta flava connect adjacent laminae at each level from C2 to the lumbosacral junction. The ligamenta flava are loosely attached to the facet joint capsule at their lateral margin and extend medially to the base of the spinous process in the midline, at which point they may be discontinuous. These ligaments are thin and broad in the cervical region and become thicker in the lumbar region. The interspinous ligaments connect adjacent spinous processes, extending from the ligamentum flavum anteriorly to the supraspinous ligament posteriorly. The supraspinous ligament merges with the ligamentum nuchae at its cranial end at C7, then extends inferiorly along the tips of the spinous processes, becoming progressively thicker, to the lumbosacral junction. The supraspinous ligament is fused with the posterior margin of the interspinous ligaments at each level.[7] Alteration in biomechanics (excessive lordosis, loss of disc-space height, vertebral articulations) can result in ligamentous degeneration: calcification, ossification, bone proliferation at sites of attachment, granulomatous reaction, and perivascular cellular infiltration.

A retrodural and retroligamentous potential space providing communication between bilateral cervical facet joints at a single level was first described by Okada in 1981.[8] Subsequent reports have described similar communication between facet joints and the interlaminar region, interspinous region, contralateral facet joints, and pars interarticularis defects in both the cervical and lumbar regions via a retrodural space lying posterior to the ligamentum flavum.[9] This potential space can serve as a conduit of inflammatory reaction and, rarely, infection, between posterior element structures usually considered distinct entities.

The SI joints are large, C-shaped, true diarthrodial synovial joints demonstrating great variability in size and shape. The SI joints are lined by a synovial membrane surrounded by a fibrous articular capsule, and contain a small synovial fluid-filled space in their anterior and inferior portion. Anteriorly, the articular capsule is a well-defined fibrous capsule with thin ligamentous connections between the sacrum and ileum. Posteriorly there is an extensive network of ligamentous connections between the sacrum and ileum with ligamentous fusion to a less well-defined posterior joint capsule. Unlike most synovial joints, the SI joints are not lined by hyaline cartilage on both articulating surfaces. Only the sacral surface is lined with hyaline cartilage. The ileal surface is lined by a thin layer of fibrocartilage, which may account for greater susceptibility of the iliac side of the joint to degenerative change.[10] Innervation of the SI joints has been a source of controversy; current consensus suggests the dominant innervation arises from the dorsal rami of L5 through S4.[11,12]

Transitional spinal segments can occur in as many as 30% of patients, typically involving the last lumbar or first sacral segment.[13] The transitional segment demonstrates anatomic features of both lumbar-type and sacral-type vertebral bodies with frequent asymmetry from left to right side, particularly in the configuration of the facet joints. Sacralization of the lowest lumbar segment can range from an enlarged transverse process articulating with the ileum to complete incorporation of the lowest segment into the sacrum. Lumbarization of the sacrum results in elevation of S1 above the sacral fusion mass and assumption of a lumbar anatomic configuration. Lumbarization and sacralization, therefore, can have a very similar imaging appearance, and accurate counting of spinal segments from C2 inferiorly is required to precisely define anatomy.[7]

PHYSIOLOGIC AND FUNCTIONAL IMAGING TECHNIQUES

It is often difficult to identify the source of a patient's LBP or neck pain because history and physical examination findings are nonspecific; degenerative or age-related changes in the spine are highly prevalent even in asymptomatic patients, and pain patterns may overlap secondary to rich anastomoses of pain-sensing neural structures.[14] Both conventional CT and MR imaging techniques can demonstrate the structural and anatomic changes of spondylosis such as sclerosis, joint-space narrowing, and osteophytosis. However, these findings are common in both asymptomatic and symptomatic patients and often fail to correspond to the site of the patient's pain. Physiologic imaging with fat-suppressed T2-weighted and/or CE T1-weighted MR imaging, radionuclide bone scanning, or FDG-PET/CT and functional imaging with weight bearing or axial loading may demonstrate findings more specific to the subset of degenerative age-related changes that are actually responsible for the patient's pain (**Box 2**).

Fat-Suppressed MR Imaging Techniques

MR imaging and CT are very sensitive to morphologic degenerative changes that may cause LBP. However, these findings are very common, and marked degenerative changes may be identified even in asymptomatic patients. Inflammatory changes and hyperemia may be more specific findings for the source of a patient's back pain, but these changes are difficult to detect on the standard T1-weighted and fast spin-echo (FSE) T2-weighted sequences most commonly used for spine imaging, because of the relatively increased signal intensity of both marrow fat and edema or enhancement on these sequences.[15] Bone marrow edema and soft-tissue inflammation are much more conspicuous on fat-suppressed T2-weighted images; the hypervascularity associated with soft tissue inflammation can best be seen on fat-suppressed CE T1-weighted images. Fat-suppressed T2-weighted and CE T1-weighted sequences therefore enable the clear visualization of facet joint effusions, subchondral bone marrow edema, and paraspinal soft-tissue inflammation that may be overlooked with conventional non–fat-suppressed MR imaging techniques (**Fig. 3**).[15–17]

To increase the conspicuity of edema and inflammation on MR imaging, several distinct

Box 2
Physiologic imaging techniques

- Fat-suppressed MR imaging techniques
  - Short T1 inversion recovery (STIR)
  - Fat-saturation fast spin-echo (FSE) T2-weighted or contrast-enhanced (CE) T1-weighted
  - Water-excitation FSE T2-weighted or CE T1-weighted
  - 3-point Dixon water-fat separation (IDEAL)
- Nuclear medicine bone scintigraphy
- ^{18}F-fluorodeoxyglucose positron emission tomography combined with CT (FDG-PET/CT)
- Weight-bearing/axial-loading imaging

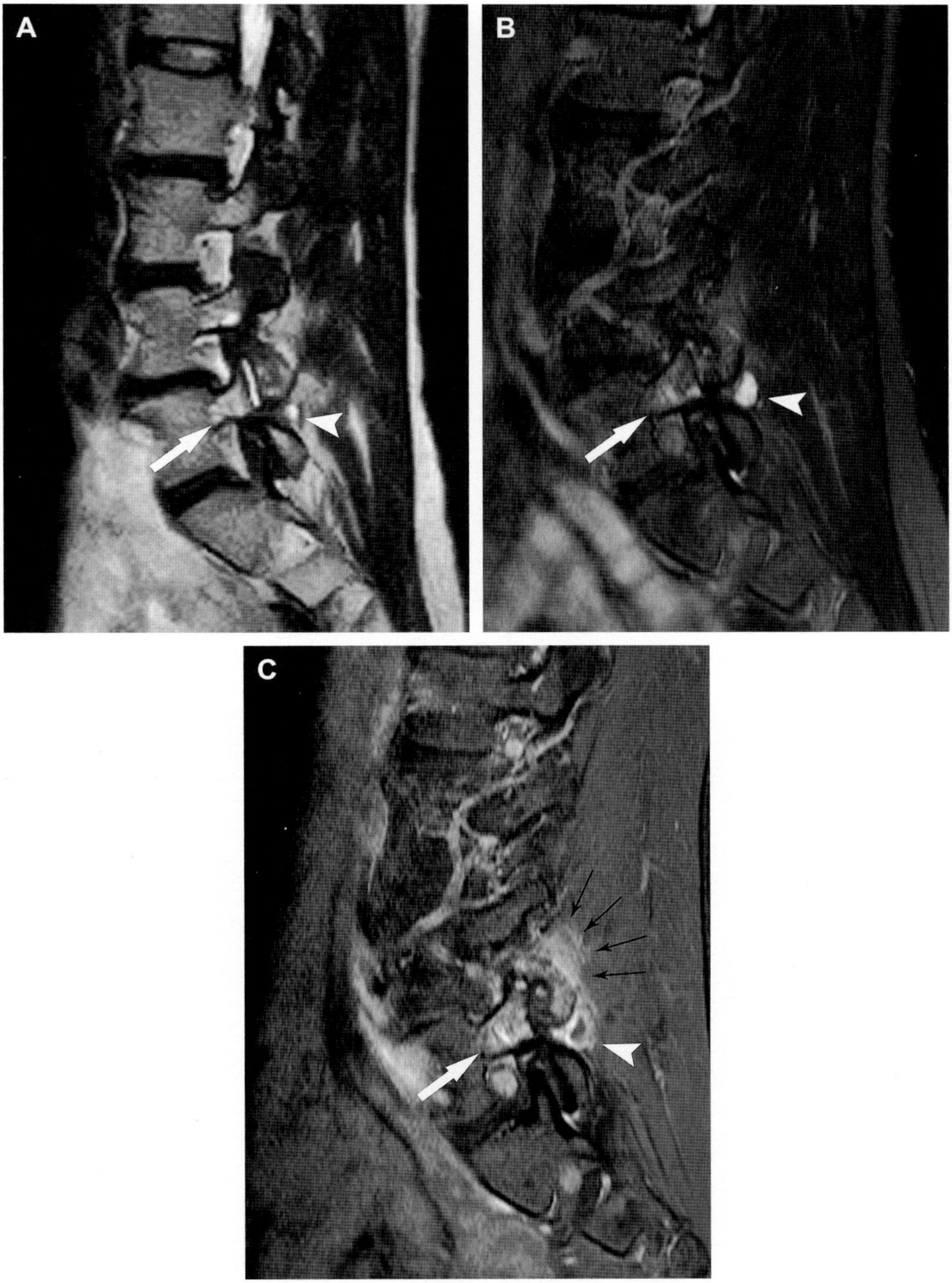

Fig. 3. Fat-suppression MR techniques. A 45-year-old woman presents with LBP worse with sitting. L5 pedicle edema (*white arrow*) and posterior L4-L5 facet synovial cyst (*white arrowhead*) are poorly visualized on standard fast spin-echo (FSE) T2-weighted sagittal sequence (*A*), and are much better demonstrated on fat-saturated FSE T2-weighted (*B*) and fat-saturated contrast-enhanced (CE) T1-weighted sagittal images (*C*). The fat-saturated CE T1-weighted sagittal sequence (*C*) best demonstrates facet edema and extensive periarticular soft tissue inflammation (*black arrows*).

fat-suppression techniques can be used: the short T1 inversion recovery (STIR) sequence,[18,19] fat-saturated[20] or water-excitation[21] T2-weighted or CE T1-weighted sequences, or Dixon-based fat separation methods.[22,23] Each of these techniques relies on either the difference between fat and water in relaxation time (T1 or T2) or in the resonant frequency (chemical shift).

Fat has a very short T1 relaxation rate, and therefore has a high signal on most T1-weighted sequences as well as on FSE T2-weighted techniques. The difference in T1 relaxation between water and lipid can be used to selectively suppress or null the signal from short T1 tissues, such as fat, using the STIR sequence. A short inversion time is chosen close to the T1 value of fat, approximately 100 milliseconds, so that the signal intensity of fat is close to zero when the 90° inversion pulse is applied.[19] STIR sequences with long spin-echo times resemble fat-saturated T2-weighted images. However, unless the inversion time chosen exactly matches the T1 of fat tissue, some fat signal will remain and the T1 signal from other non–fat-containing short T1 tissues may also be suppressed; this results in a lower signal-to-noise ratio with this technique than with other fat-suppression techniques. The advantages of STIR are that it is relatively insensitive to magnetic field inhomogeneity such as with the presence of implanted metallic hardware, and can also be used at lower scanner field strengths.[24] However, because the T1 signal is suppressed, STIR cannot be used for CE imaging.

The chemical shift, or small difference in resonance frequency between fat and water related to differences in the local magnetic environment around their respective protons, allows for fat saturation or water excitation.[20,21] Both use a frequency-selective spectral pulse before the spin-echo pulse sequence to either saturate signal from fat or excite signal from water. These techniques are reliable in areas with large amounts of fat such as bone marrow or paraspinal soft tissue, do not affect signal from non–fat-containing tissues, and can be applied to either T1-weighted or FSE T2-weighted sequences. However, in the presence of local magnetic field inhomogeneities, such as with shorter bore scanners and in patients with implanted metallic hardware, incomplete or nonuniform fat saturation can result (**Fig. 4**A). The chemical shift decreases with the strength of the magnetic field, so fat saturation is also of lower quality at lower field strengths.[24]

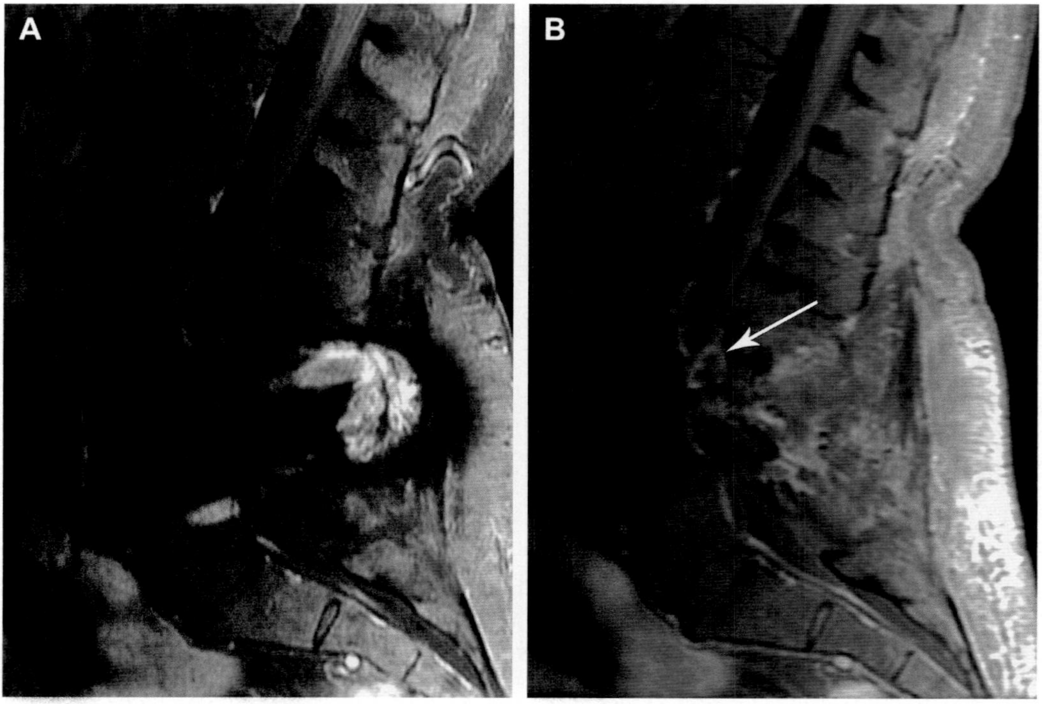

Fig. 4. Fat-suppression MR techniques. A 61-year-old woman, status post laminectomy and instrumented fusion, presents with LBP. Conventional fat-saturated CE T1-weighted sequence (*A*) is limited by the presence of susceptibility artifact related to the presence of metallic hardware. Fat suppression is incomplete and inhomogeneous, and signal from intraspinal structures is lost. CE T1-weighted IDEAL sequence (*B*) clearly demonstrates a peripherally enhancing synovial cyst above the L4 pedicle screw (*white arrow*).

Dixon techniques were originally developed for fat and water separation by using information from both the phase and frequency of water and fat obtained from 2 separate acquisitions and then applying a subtraction technique. Three-point Dixon techniques use phase and frequency information from 3 acquisitions to estimate field inhomogeneity and to separate fat and water.[23] The iterative decomposition of water and fat with echo asymmetry and least-squares estimation (IDEAL) technique is a recently introduced 3-point Dixon technique that is less susceptible to artifact from implanted metallic hardware.[22,23] This sequence can be used for both FSE T2-weighted and CE T1-weighted images (**Fig. 4**B).

Nuclear Medicine Bone Scintigraphy and FDG-PET/CT

Nuclear medicine bone scintigraphy with ^{99m}Tc–methylene diphosphonate (^{99m}Tc-MDP) has long been used to identify occult destructive neoplastic and infectious processes in patients with LBP, but is increasingly recognized for its ability to also identify benign pathology associated with LBP.[25] Nuclear medicine bone scintigraphy provides a whole-body anatomic survey while also allowing for evaluation of tissue function. Uptake of ^{99m}Tc-MDP is primarily related to osteoblastic activity, but is also related to the degree of blood flow, so this radiotracer will accumulate in areas of hypervascularity.[26] Anatomic localization is imprecise with routine bone-scan technique secondary to poor spatial resolution. SPECT is a tomographic technique that increases sensitivity for spine pathology and improves spatial resolution, allowing more precise localization of abnormal uptake to specific posterior element structures in the spine.[26,27] A recent study suggests that combining nuclear medicine SPECT with standard CT will further improve diagnostic accuracy and anatomic localization.[28] Foci of increased radiotracer uptake may be seen in the posterior elements associated with facet arthrosis/synovitis, acute or subacute pars interarticularis defects/fractures, and Baastrup phenomenon of the spinous processes. It can identify facet arthropathy with active findings related to inflammation and hypervascularity, which therefore is more likely to benefit from treatment (**Fig. 5**).[29]

FDG-PET combined with CT provides both metabolic and anatomic information. The improved specificity for benign versus malignant disease over that of nuclear medicine bone scintigraphy with MDP may be in part related to better localization with the CT component. Increased uptake associated with degenerative change in the spine was found in 22% of 150 patients in one study of whole-body FDG-PET/CT.[30] This finding is likely secondary to the inflammatory component that accompanies these degenerative changes. Increased uptake is most severe in patients with milder changes on CT and decreases in intensity as the CT changes progress, suggesting that CT changes represent the end-stage result of the inflammatory process.

Functional Imaging

Many patients with LBP complain of pain only in the upright position or with standing and/or walking. With CT or MR imaging performed in a recumbent position, abnormalities are frequently absent or minimal in this patient population. Imaging such patients in the upright position, or with axial loading that mimics an upright position, is known to show increased abnormality of disc and posterior element.[31,32] This basic sensitivity fault of spine imaging is discussed more fully in an article elsewhere in this issue by Nassr. Recently 3-dimensional rotational myelography using flat-panel detectors has been described.[33] Rotational time is increased compared with CT, which may introduce motion artifacts. However, this technique allows reconstruction in any plane and can also be performed with the patient in the upright position.[34] This technique may have potential to demonstrate increased spinal stenosis with the patient in the upright position (Kent Thielen, Rochester, MN, unpublished data, November 2011).

FACET JOINTS

Facet, or zygapophyseal, joints are true synovium-lined diarthrodial joints. Facet degeneration, or age-related changes, are common, beginning in the first 2 decades of life, with increasing prevalence with age, and becoming nearly universal in patients older than 60 years.[35] There is no gender predilection.[36] Clinical examination findings such as morning stiffness and mechanical pain exacerbated with bending, rotation, or extension, and relieved with gentle flexion, and pain with palpation over the suspected joint can suggest facet-mediated pain, but ultimately are nonspecific.[37] Schwarzer and colleagues[38] reported a 45% false-positive diagnostic rate for facetogenic pain when physical examination findings alone were correlated with diagnostic medial branch blocks.

Further complicating diagnosis is the fact that facet degeneration is often an asymptomatic finding at imaging. It could be argued that in a more select population of patients with LBP, structural evidence of facet degeneration might predict a painful joint.

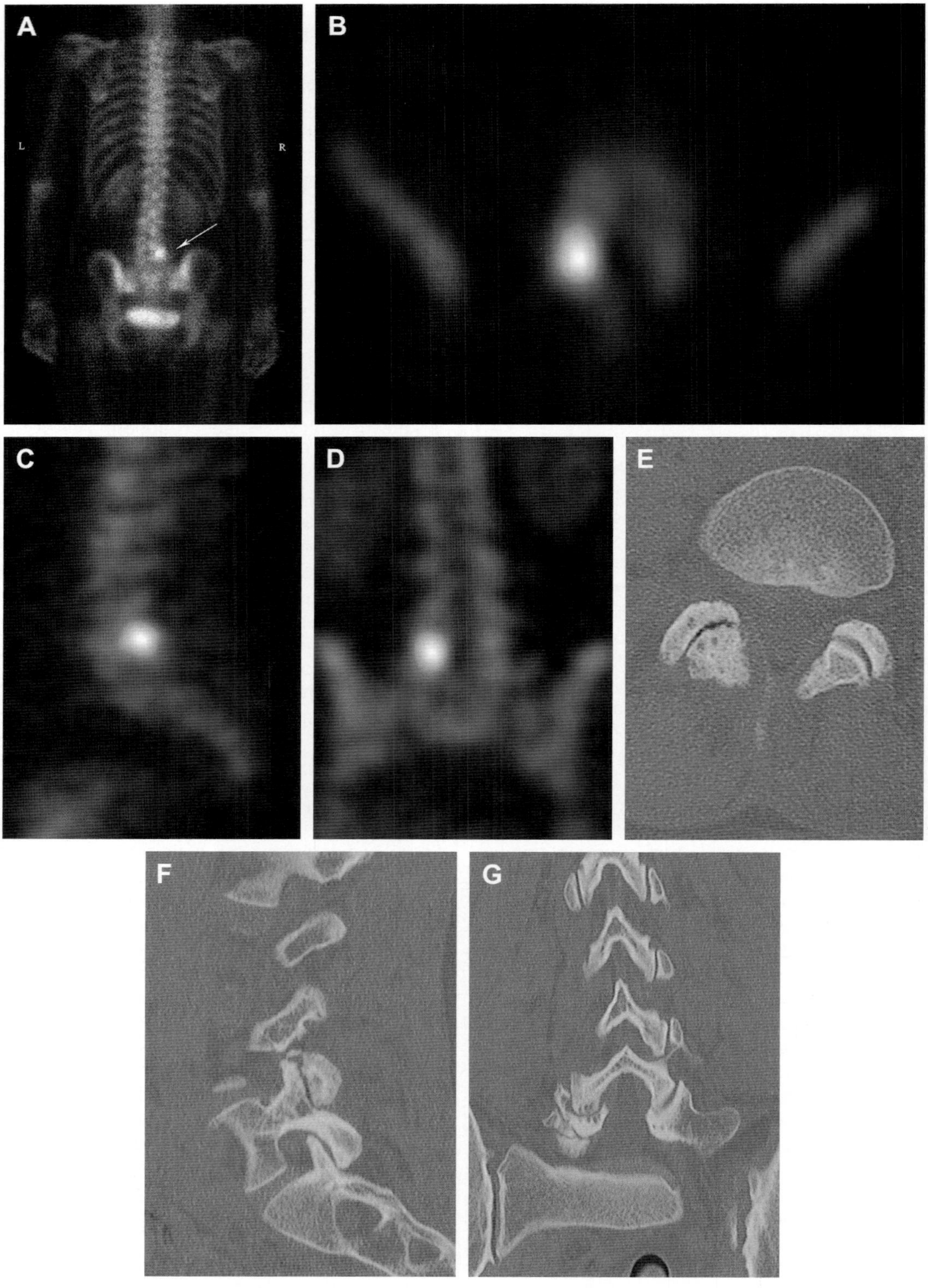

Fig. 5. Nuclear medicine bone scintigraphy with SPECT for the same patient as in **Fig. 3**. Increased radionuclide uptake posteroanterior (PA) planar bone scan (*A*) in the lower lumbar spine on the right (*arrow*) more clearly localizes to the facet joint on axial (*B*), sagittal (*C*), and coronal (*D*) SPECT and corresponds to advanced osteoarthrosis on axial (*E*), sagittal (*F*), and coronal (*G*) CT.

This aspect has been studied, and no consistent evidence has emerged to support such a relationship. Schwarzer and colleagues[39] semiquantitatively scored the degree of facet degeneration on CT in patients with axial LBP; there was no correlation between the degree of degeneration and response to placebo-controlled intra-articular anesthetic blocks. In a more recent study, Cohen and colleagues[40] showed no relationship between MR-imaging structural evidence of facet hypertrophy or degeneration and the response to radiofrequency facet denervation. In a systematic review, the investigators noted no credible evidence that structural imaging can predict a painful facet joint. Physiologic imaging parameters are discussed later.

It is well established that facet abnormality may account for 15% to 30% of mechanical axial LBP.[37,38,40–42] Facet joint abnormality encompasses osteoarthrosis, joint effusions, ligamentous laxity, inflammatory facet synovitis, and synovial cysts. Facet-mediated pain can be radicular, and may result from mass effect and central or lateral recess stenosis related to hypertrophic degeneration and osteophytes, ligamentum flavum redundancy, or synovial cysts. Alternatively, an intrinsic inflammatory process of the facet, facet synovitis, can result in axial neck and back pain (**Box 3**).

Osteoarthrosis

Age-related disc changes may result in loss of disc height and load-bearing capacity, shifting a greater burden to the posterior column. The alteration in spatial relationships caused by the loss of disc height leads to malalignment of facet joints, increased biomechanical stress, and subsequent facet joint osteoarthrosis. Both disc degeneration and facet osteoarthrosis lead to increased stress on the posterior ligaments, with subsequent ligamentous laxity and buckling. Facet joint degeneration leads to further disc degeneration, facet osteoarthrosis, ligamentous buckling, and a continued positive feedback cycle.[2] As a result the facet joints are rarely the only, and often not the primary, source of LBP.

Anatomic changes of facet osteoarthrosis include erosion of the articular cartilage associated with joint-space narrowing, periarticular hyperostosis with marginal osteophyte formation, subchondral eburnation/sclerosis, subchondral erosions and cysts, intra-articular bony fragments ("joint mice"), intra-articular gas (vacuum phenomenon), joint subluxation, and joint effusions (**Fig. 6**). Hypertrophy, redundancy, thickening or buckling, and calcification of the ligamentum flavum may also be seen.[16,43] Facet osteoarthrosis alone, or in combination with buckling of the ligamentum flavum, can result in spinal stenosis (**Fig. 7**).

Osteophytes develop at the site of greatest stress on the joint, more frequently involving the superior facet of the lower vertebral body as the inferior facet is covered by the ligamentum flavum.[43] This hypertrophy can result in spinal stenosis, narrowing of the lateral recess, or narrowing of neural foramina, with a resultant mass effect on adjacent spinal nerve roots and radicular symptoms (**Fig. 8**). Subluxation of the facet joint can also result in compression of the nerve root in the lateral recess between the superior facet of the vertebral body below and pars interarticularis of the vertebral body above.

> **Box 3**
> **Facet joint–related back and limb pain**
>
> Radiculopathy: mass effect
> - Osteoarthrosis
> - Osteophytes
> - Joint effusions
> - Synovial cysts
> - Ligamentum flavum laxity/buckling
>
> Axial pain: intrinsic pathology
> - Facet synovitis

Synovial Cysts

Synovial cysts form from degenerated facet joints when synovium herniates through the facet joint capsule, which may result from facet joint effusion and and/or associated capsular inflammation. These cysts may be true synovium-lined cysts or fibrous tissue–lined pseudocysts. Ninety percent of synovial cysts occur in the lumbar region with 65% to 80% occurring at L4-L5.[44,45] Synovial cysts may narrow the neural foramen or central spinal canal and impinge on adjacent nerve roots. As a result, patients with synovial cysts most frequently present with radicular symptoms.[45,46] When symptomatic, these are seen as a cyst in the lateral or posterolateral extradural space or neural foramen arising from the facet joint (**Fig. 9**). Synovial cysts are difficult to detect on CT because the fluid density in the cyst is similar to that of cerebrospinal fluid (CSF) in the adjacent thecal sac. The presence of hemorrhage in the cyst increases conspicuity on CT secondary to the increased density associated with the hemorrhage. If present, facet joint gas may communicate with the synovial cyst. On MR imaging, synovial cysts are also similar in signal to CSF, being hypointense on T1-weighted and hyperintense on

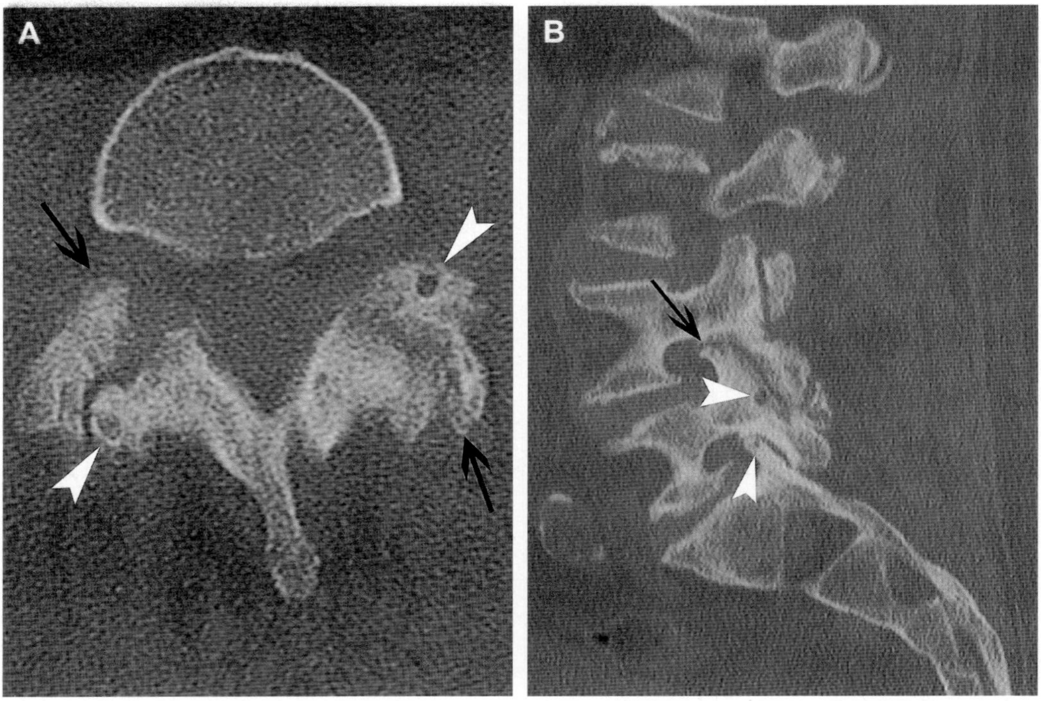

Fig. 6. Facet joint osteoarthrosis. A 77-year-old man imaged for thoracic spine trauma. Axial (*A*) and sagittal (*B*) CT images demonstrate joint space narrowing, marginal osteophyte formation (*arrows*), subchondral sclerosis, and subchondral cysts (*arrowheads*).

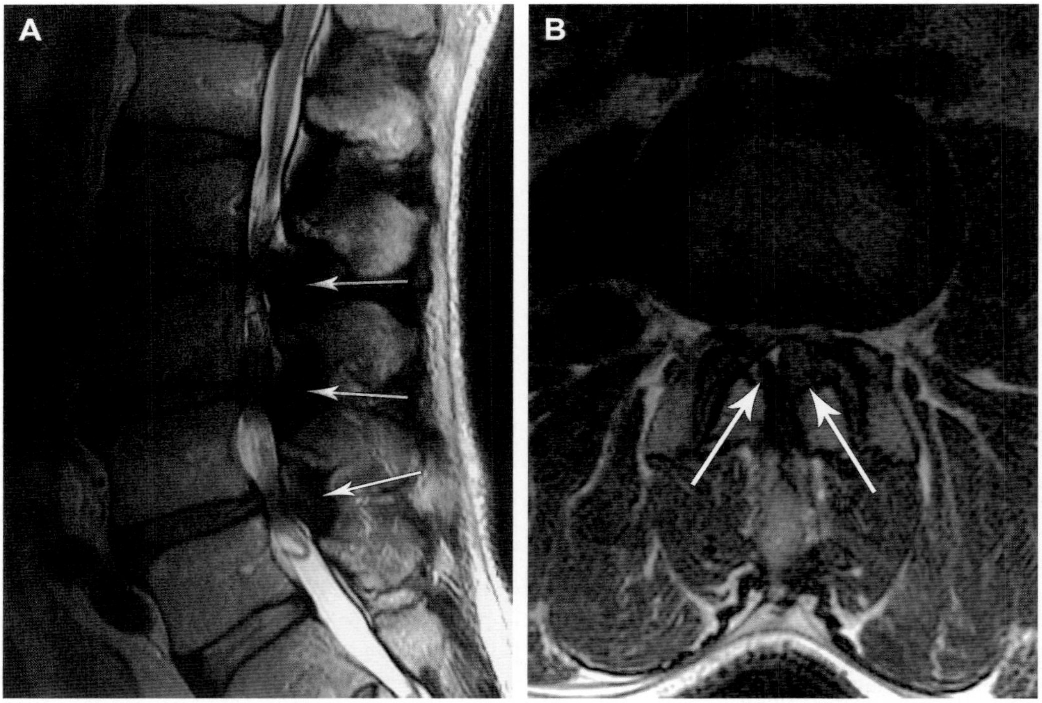

Fig. 7. Facet joint osteoarthrosis and spinal stenosis. A 67-year-old man with low back pain and weakness in both legs exacerbated with walking. Sagittal (*A*) and axial (*B*) FSE T2-weighted MR images demonstrate multilevel loss of disc space height with resultant redundancy of the ligamentum flavum (*arrows*), causing severe spinal stenosis at each level.

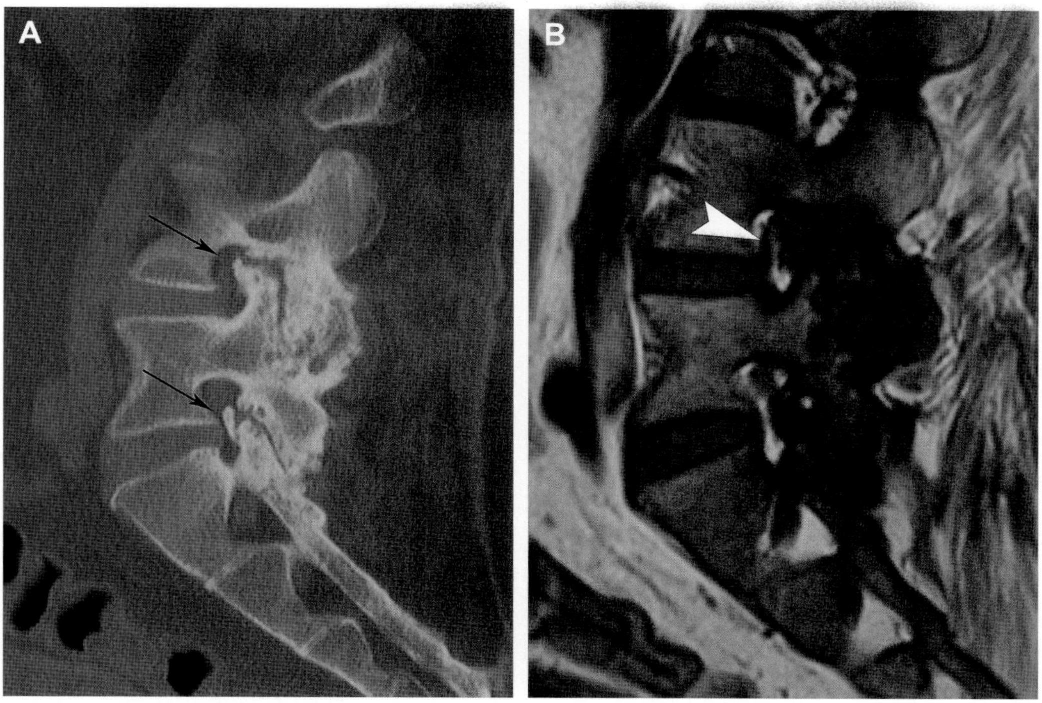

Fig. 8. Superior articular facet osteophytes. A 47-year-old man imaged for right-sided radiculopathy. Sagittal CT (*A*) and sagittal FSE T2-weighted MR (*B*) images demonstrate osteophytes from the right superior articular facets at L5 and S1 (*arrows*) with impingement of the exiting L4 nerve root (*arrowhead*).

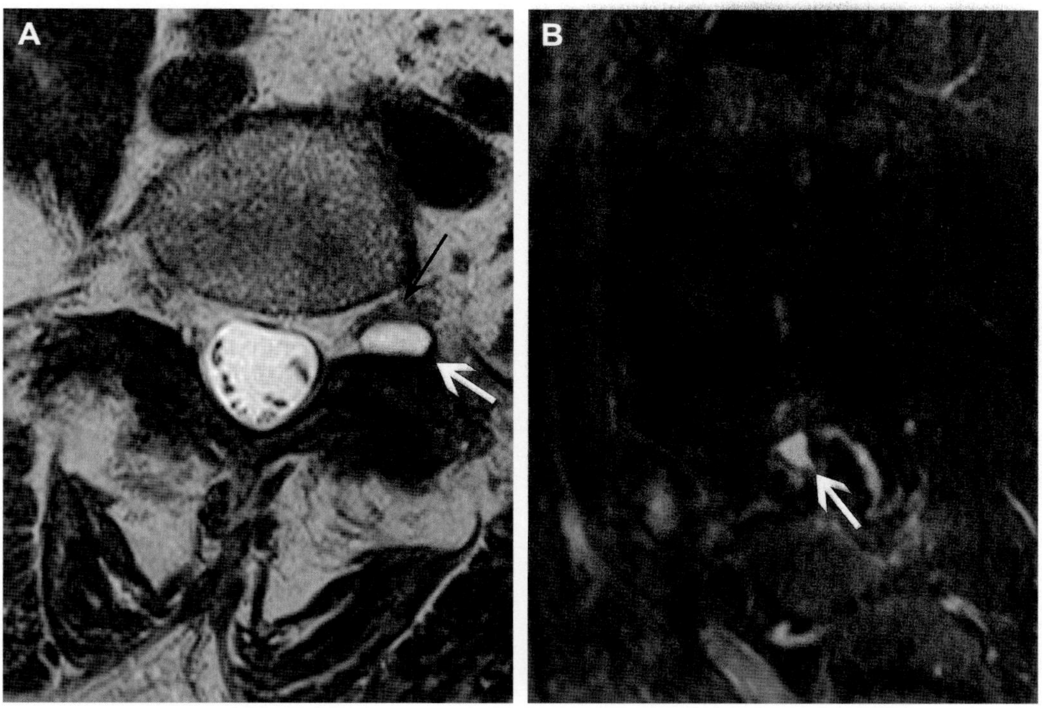

Fig. 9. Synovial cyst in the neural foramen. A 50-year-old woman presents with LBP radiating down the left leg to the foot. Axial FSE T2-weighted sequence (*A*) shows a cystic structure in the left L5 neural foramen (*white arrow*) compressing the exiting nerve root (*black arrow*). Sagittal STIR sequence (*B*) more clearly demonstrates that the cyst (*white arrow*) arises from a degenerated facet joint with associated synovial effusion, pedicle and periarticular soft-tissue edema.

T2-weighted imaging. Acute hemorrhage into a synovial cyst may result in rapid enlargement of the cyst with impingement of neural structures and acute radicular symptoms. In these cases, the cyst may then be isointense or hyperintense on T1-weighted imaging, and hypointense on T2-weighted imaging, with occasional identification of blood/fluid levels (**Fig. 10**). A low-intensity rim related to the fibrotic reaction and enhancement related to the associated inflammatory process may also be seen. With chronic inflammation, synovial cysts may calcify.

Ligamentum Flavum Laxity

The ligamentum flavum normally contributes to spinal stability. Alteration in biomechanics with excessive lumbar lordosis, loss of disc-space height, or facet osteoarthrosis can result in degeneration of the ligamentum flavum. Intrinsic degeneration of the ligamentum flavum may manifest as edema, inflammation, calcification, and/or bone proliferation at attachment points on anatomic imaging (**Fig. 11**).

As the disc space narrows or facet subluxation progresses, the ligamentum flavum becomes redundant, buckling anteriorly into the spinal canal and resulting in narrowing of the canal from a posterior vector.[17] This spinal stenosis may result in symptoms of neurogenic intermittent claudication or radiculopathy. Symptoms may be exacerbated with weight bearing. In these cases, functional imaging with weight bearing or axial loading may demonstrate increased spinal stenosis (**Fig. 12**).[32]

Facet Synovitis

Active facet inflammatory arthropathy or facet synovitis is a noninfectious inflammatory osteoarthropathy. Nociceptors in the facet joint capsule may be sensitized by inflammatory mediators.[47] Patients with facet synovitis may present with morning stiffness, pain to palpation over the affected facet joints, and aggravation with rotation or extension; in these cases an inflammatory cause should be sought on imaging studies. Inflammatory changes are difficult to detect on standard T1 and FSE T2 sequences because of increased intensity of both marrow fat and edema/enhancement. Edema is much more conspicuous on fat-suppressed FSE T2-weighted or fat-suppressed CE T1-weighted images. Imaging findings in facet synovitis include T2 hyperintensity

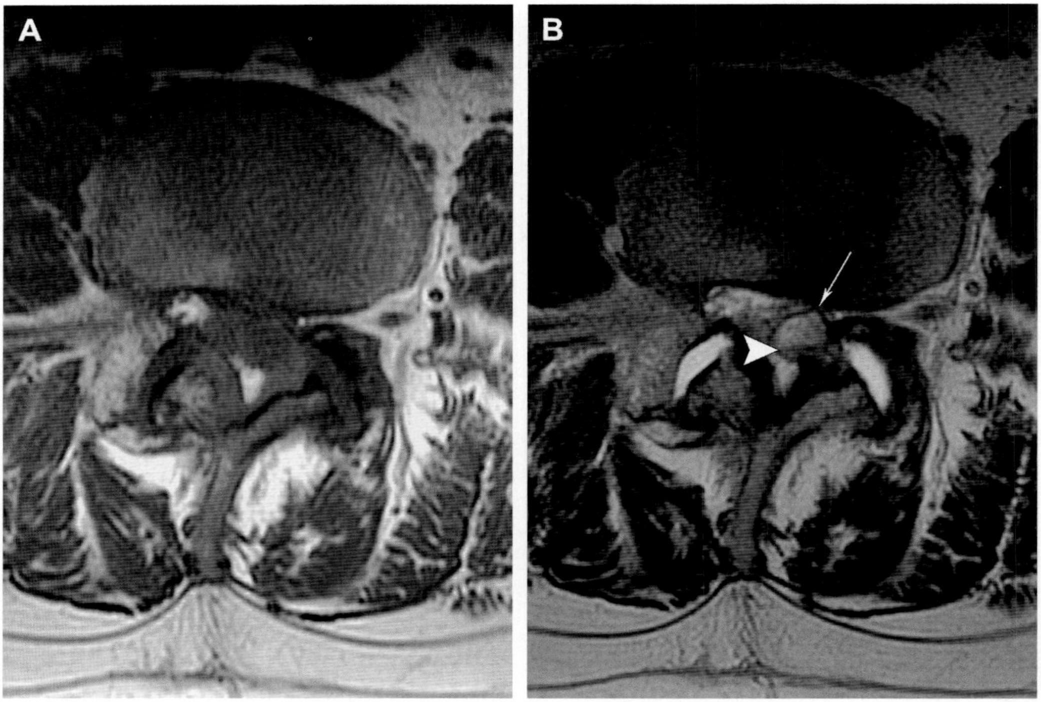

Fig. 10. Hemorrhagic synovial cyst. A 56-year-old man presents with acute left leg and back pain. Axial T1-weighted (*A*) MR image demonstrates bilateral L4-L5 facet osteoarthrosis, but the synovial cyst is difficult to identify because it is isointense to cerebrospinal fluid. Axial T2-weighted MR image (*B*) clearly shows bilateral joint effusions and a well-defined synovial cyst (*white arrow*), with a fluid-blood level (*arrowhead*) arising from the left-sided joint and low-intensity fibrotic rim.

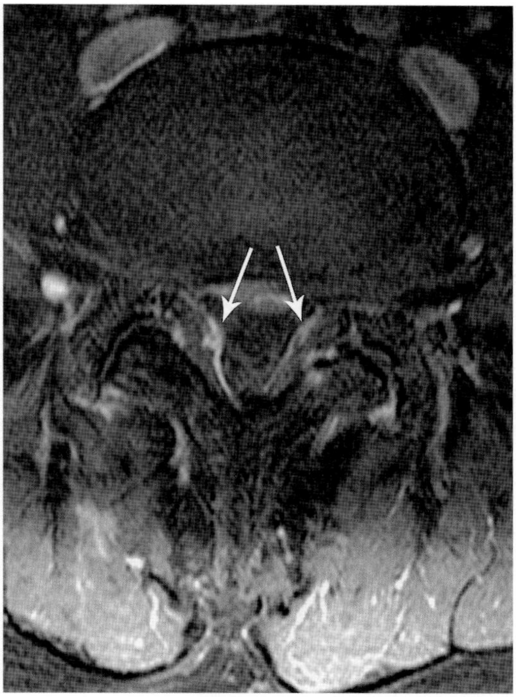

Fig. 11. Ligamentum flavum degenerative inflammation. A 84-year-old man presents with axial LBP. Axial fat-suppressed CE T1-weighted sequence demonstrates enhancement of bilateral ligamentum flavum (*white arrows*). Note bilateral facet osteoarthrosis and grade 2 facet synovitis.

or enhancement of the facet joint articular surfaces, joint capsule, and periarticular tissue on fat-suppressed images. Inflammatory soft-tissue changes are common and may appear aggressive, mimicking infection or neoplasm.[16]

Facet synovitis is a relatively common finding on MR imaging when appropriate fat-suppression techniques are used. In a retrospective review of 209 lumbar MR imaging examinations performed in 1 month at the Mayo Clinic, 41% of all lumbar spine studies demonstrated changes of synovitis as hyperintensity on fat-suppressed T2-weighted or CE T1-weighted images.[15] In this study, Czervionke and Fenton[15] proposed a grading system for facet synovitis using fat-suppressed MR imaging techniques (**Box 4**). In this same study, unilateral grade 3 or grade 4 imaging findings in a subset of 30 patients correlated with the side of pain in 100% (**Fig. 13**A).[15] In a subset of 9 patients with facet edema identified on STIR imaging, Friedrich and colleagues[48] found a correlation between increasing, stable or decreasing facet edema and a concurrent worsening, stability, or improvement in pain, respectively. Both groups concluded that facet synovitis is an underrecognized cause of back pain and radicular symptoms.[15,48]

Injection of local anesthetic into the facet joint is an imperfect gold standard for diagnosing facet joints as the source of axial LBP or neck pain; the false-positive rate for single intra-articular injections exceeds 30%.[14] Medial branch blocks under fluoroscopic guidance using a dual-block paradigm are considered the best available means of diagnosis of cervical or lumbar facet–mediated pain. Once the diagnosis is established, radiofrequency denervation of the painful facet joint is the only effective therapeutic intervention validated by high-quality literature.[49] The monetary costs, time, and risks associated with a multistep invasive diagnostic procedure (dual medial branch blocks) are not insignificant, and a noninvasive method to diagnose facetogenic pain would be preferred. To date, no controlled study of response to diagnostic injection of local anesthetic has been performed to confirm facet synovitis as the cause of axial pain in patients with MR imaging findings consistent with facet edema, inflammation, or hyperemia.

Several studies have suggested an association with inflammatory facet abnormality identified on nuclear medicine bone scintigraphy with SPECT.[27,29,50] Furthermore, nuclear medicine bone scintigraphy has a high negative predictive value, 93% with planar imaging and 100% with SPECT, excluding facet joints with degenerative changes on anatomic imaging as the source of pain (**Fig. 13**B).[29]

Dolan and associates[27] studied 58 patients with LBP clinically thought to be facetogenic, that is, their pain was exacerbated with extension and sitting and was relieved with rest. Twenty-two patients had increased radionuclide uptake localized to a facet joint on SPECT imaging, and 36 did not demonstrate focal radionuclide uptake. All patients were treated with intra-articular facet injection, those with positive scans at the level of the imaging abnormality and those without at the level suggested by clinical examination. The SPECT-positive patients had significantly greater response to injection at 1 and 3 months. There was no difference between the two groups at 6 months. SPECT-positive patients had more anatomic findings of degenerative facet osteoarthrosis than did SPECT-negative patients, but there was no correlation between the level of most severe morphologic degenerative osteoarthrosis and SPECT-positive level. Furthermore, the level of tenderness to palpation did not correlate with the level of SPECT positivity. The investigators concluded that SPECT could identify the facet joints most likely to

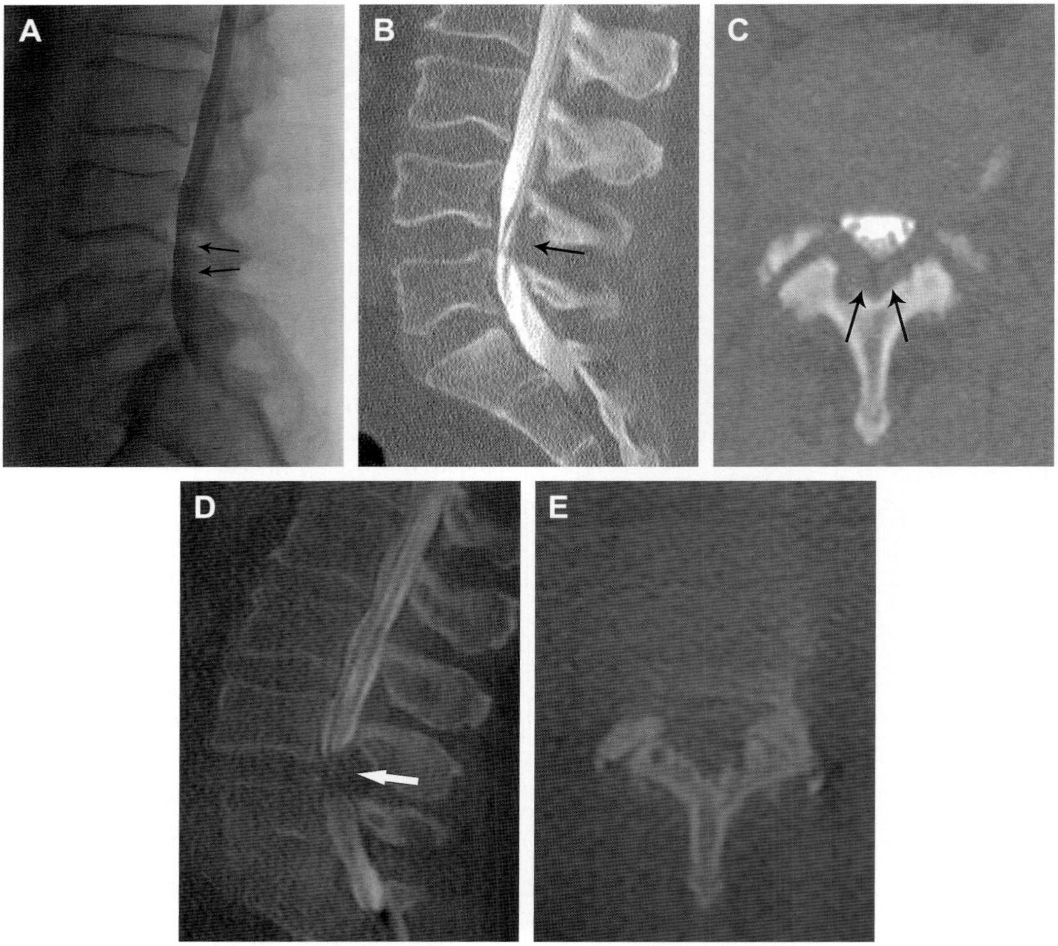

Fig. 12. Ligamentum flavum redundancy on upright myelography. A 66-year-old man imaged for LBP and burning sensation extending down both legs, worse with standing or walking. Conventional lateral myelogram in the lateral plane with the patient in the prone position (*A*) and postmyelogram sagittal (*B*) and axial (*C*) CT with the patient in the supine position show minimal redundancy of the ligamentum flavum (*black arrows*) and spinal stenosis at the L4-L5 level. Three-dimensional rotational myelography with the patient in the upright position demonstrates a marked increase in ligamentous redundancy (*white arrow*) on the sagittal reconstruction (*D*), and complete effacement of the thecal sac on the axial reconstruction (*E*). (*Courtesy of* Kent Thielen, MD, Mayo Clinic, Rochester, MN; with permission.)

have short-term benefit from facet injection therapy.[27]

Facet joints with increased activity on SPECT are often not those with the greatest degree of degenerative change on anatomic imaging studies such as CT and conventional MR imaging.[14,27,51] However, whereas SPECT imaging findings have been correlated with MR imaging, fat-suppressed MR imaging techniques have not been routinely used and inflammatory changes and edema have been likely overlooked.[51]

Pneumaticos and colleagues[50] prospectively studied 47 patients divided into 3 groups: SPECT-positive patients treated at the level of increased radionuclide uptake, SPECT-negative patients treated at levels ordered by the referring clinician, and patients that did not have SPECT imaging who received injections at levels requested by the ordering clinician. Improvement in the pain score was significantly higher in the patients treated at facet levels of positive SPECT radionuclide uptake than in either the SPECT-negative patients or those not evaluated with SPECT. Furthermore, it was found that SPECT imaging decreased the number of levels treated in the SPECT-positive patients from 60, as requested by the ordering clinician, to 27. The use of SPECT imaging to select patients for level of injection therapy resulted in Medicare

Box 4
Grading facet synovitis

Grade: Signal Abnormality/Enhancement Criteria

0: None

1: Confined to join capsule

2: Periarticular <50% of joint perimeter

3: Periarticular >50% of joint perimeter

4: Extension to foramen, ligamentum flavum, pedicle, transverse process, or vertebral body

Adapted from Czervionke LE, Fenton DS. Fat-saturated MR imaging in the detection of inflammatory facet arthropathy (facet synovitis) in the lumbar spine. Pain Med 2008;9(4):400–6; with permission.

cost reduction from $2191 in the patients not imaged with SPECT to $1865 in the patients selected for injection based on positive SPECT imaging. The investigators concluded that "bone scintigraphy with SPECT can help identify patients with LBP who would benefit from facet joint injections."[50]

Case reports and small series have shown that the FDG-PET component of FDG-PET/CT examinations may also show foci of increased FDG uptake corresponding to facet osteoarthrosis, most commonly in the lumbar spine.[30,52,53] The degree of uptake correlates with the degree of inflammation and not necessarily with the severity of osteoarthritic change seen on the CT component (**Fig. 14**).[30] As with SPECT, this seems to indicate that the inflammatory component represents an early phase of disease, with changes on CT representing the end result of the degenerative process. No reports of controlled response to injection or ablation therapy have been reported in FDG-PET/CT–positive patients.

PEDICLES AND PARS INTERARTICULARIS

Signal abnormality in the pedicles on T2 and STIR sequences are not uncommon, occurring in 1.7% to 5% of patients imaged for LBP.[54,55] These changes are generally associated with either a fracture of the ipsilateral pars interarticularis or pedicle, or with ipsilateral facet degeneration, all potential pain generators in their own right.[55] In

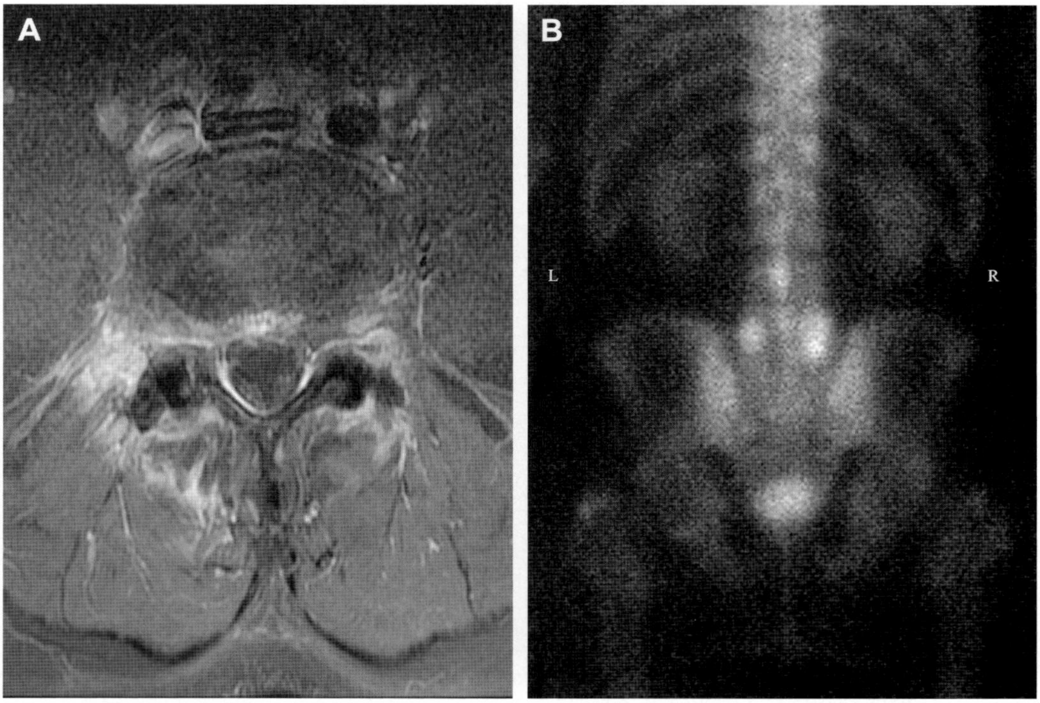

Fig. 13. Facet synovitis, grade 4. A 74-year-old man with a history of prostate carcinoma and right lower lumbar mechanical pain Axial fat-suppressed CE T1-weighted MR image (*A*) shows bilateral facet osteoarthrosis, and grade 4 synovitis on the right at the L4-L5 level, with extensive periarticular inflammatory enhancement extending into the right neural foramen. Grade 3 synovitis is present on the left. Radionuclide bone scan (*B*) in the PA projection demonstrates increased radionuclide uptake at the level of the L4-L5 facet joints, greater on the right. (*Courtesy of* Timothy Maus, MD, Mayo Clinic, Rochester, MN; with permission.)

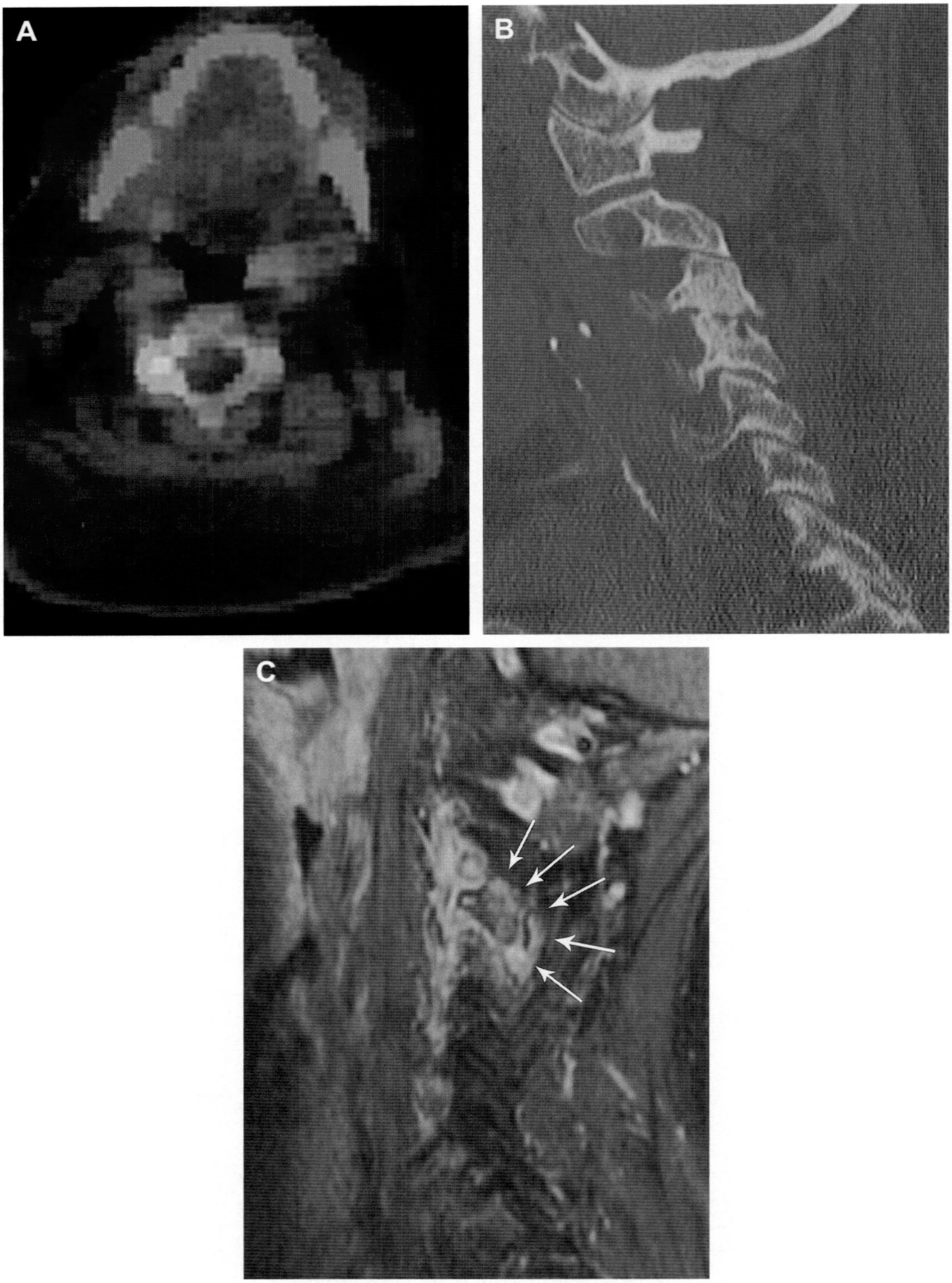

Fig. 14. FDG-PET/CT facet synovitis. A 68-year-old man with a history of small cell lung carcinoma presents with right neck pain. Axial FDG-PET/CT image (*A*) shows increased radiotracer uptake on the right at C4-C5. Sagittal CT (*B*) demonstrates facet osteoarthrosis with subchondral sclerosis and cysts. Fat-suppressed CE T1-weighted MR image (*C*) demonstrates facet synovitis with bone marrow edema and periarticular soft-tissue inflammation (*white arrows*).

these cases the increase in T2 signal is likely the manifestation of a stress reaction related to altered biomechanics. The intensity of the signal has been correlated with perceived patient pain and measures of function.[54] In the case of associated pedicle or pars interarticularis fracture, the changes in signal intensity may precede identification of a frank fracture line. These patients may also demonstrate increased T2 signal in adjacent structures such as facet joints, ligamentum flavum, and perispinal soft tissues (**Fig. 15**).

Continued repetitive microtrauma can progress to spondylolysis, or frank fracture through the pars interarticularis. Spondylolisthesis and edema of the pars and/or pedicle on T2-weighted MR imaging may be clues to the presence of spondylolysis but are nonspecific, as these findings are more commonly seen in cases of concurrent facet degeneration.[55] It can be difficult to detect the bony defect on MR imaging. CT may be necessary to clearly identify a fracture line in suspected cases. The bony defect may be bridged by fibrocartilage or a pseudarthrosis may occasionally develop.[16] Alternatively, T2 hyperintensity may resolve. It has been suggested that edema/inflammation on imaging may represent an acute phase to altered biomechanics and that their resolution suggests a stabilization phase.[54] SPECT imaging may be helpful in distinguishing chronic asymptomatic defects of the pars interarticularis from those that are the cause of the patient's pain.[25] This topic is more fully discussed elsewhere in this issue in the article by Murthy.

SPINOUS PROCESSES AND INTERSPINOUS LIGAMENTS

Baastrup disease, also termed kissing spines or interspinal bursitis, was first described in 1933, and results from close approximation of spinous processes and interspinal soft tissues.[56] This condition is thought to be more common in patients with lumbar hyperlordosis resulting in mechanical pressure between the apposing spinous processes,[57,58] but may also result from narrowing of the intervertebral disc space with resultant narrowing of the interspinous space, contact between apposing spinous processes and ligamentous tears, or fluid-filled pseudobursae or neoarthroses.[16,17] Baastrup disease is not uncommon in young gymnasts who perform repetitive hyperflexion and hyperextension maneuvers.[57] Baastrup disease maintains a controversial role as a spinal pain generator.[59–61] When symptomatic, Baastrup disease can result in midline lumbar pain that may be reproduced with palpation and exacerbated with extension. This pain may be relieved with flexion, interspinous injection of local anesthetic or, in severe cases, surgical excision of the affected spinous process(es).[61]

Imaging findings include contact between adjacent spinous processes, so-called kissing spines, with neoarthrosis formation. Radiographic findings of apposition, sclerosis, flattening, and enlargement of spinous processes are common and increase with increasing age, with 81% of patients older than 80 years affected in one study (**Fig. 16**).[60] There is no gender predilection. These findings are not specific and are often found in asymptomatic patients. Kwong and colleagues[60] found radiographic changes they termed "Baastrup phenomenon" in 41% of patients undergoing abdominopelvic CT for conditions unrelated to LBP. Of note, most patients in their series demonstrated imaging changes at only a single level.[60]

MR imaging, with its ability to depict physiology, may provide more specific identification of interspinal bursitis in symptomatic patients than CT. MR imaging may demonstrate edema and/or inflammation in adjacent spinous processes and in the interspinous or supraspinous ligaments, and frank fluid accumulation in an interspinous adventitial bursa or neoarthrosis on fat-suppressed FSE T2-weighted or CE T1-weighted images (**Fig. 17**).[61,62] Histologically these imaging changes are the result of disruption of the ligamentous fiber bundle, cellular proliferation, hypervascularity, and bursa or neoarthrosis formation.[63]

Findings of lumbar interspinous inflammation are not infrequent in patients undergoing MR imaging of the lumbar spine, most commonly occurring at the L4-L5 level.[60,62] Maes and colleagues[62] found lumbar interspinous fluid in 8.2% of symptomatic patients with back or leg pain undergoing lumbar MR imaging. In contrast to findings on CT, in this series almost half (47.7%) of the patients studied had involvement at more than 1 level. However, the prevalence of interspinous bursitis may be even higher, as not all of the patients in this study were evaluated with fat-suppressed T2-weighted imaging, which is likely more sensitive to hyperintense edema and fluid. In addition, they also excluded patients who had CE imaging, which may be even more sensitive to the edema and hyperemia associated with this condition. Associated disc pathology, degenerative end-plate changes, facet arthrosis, and spondylolysis were common.

In a small number of patients the interspinal bursal fluid may dissect centrally in a fashion analogous to that of synovial cyst formation, with a resultant midline posterior epidural fluid collection/cyst. This process may contribute to central canal stenosis and neurogenic claudication

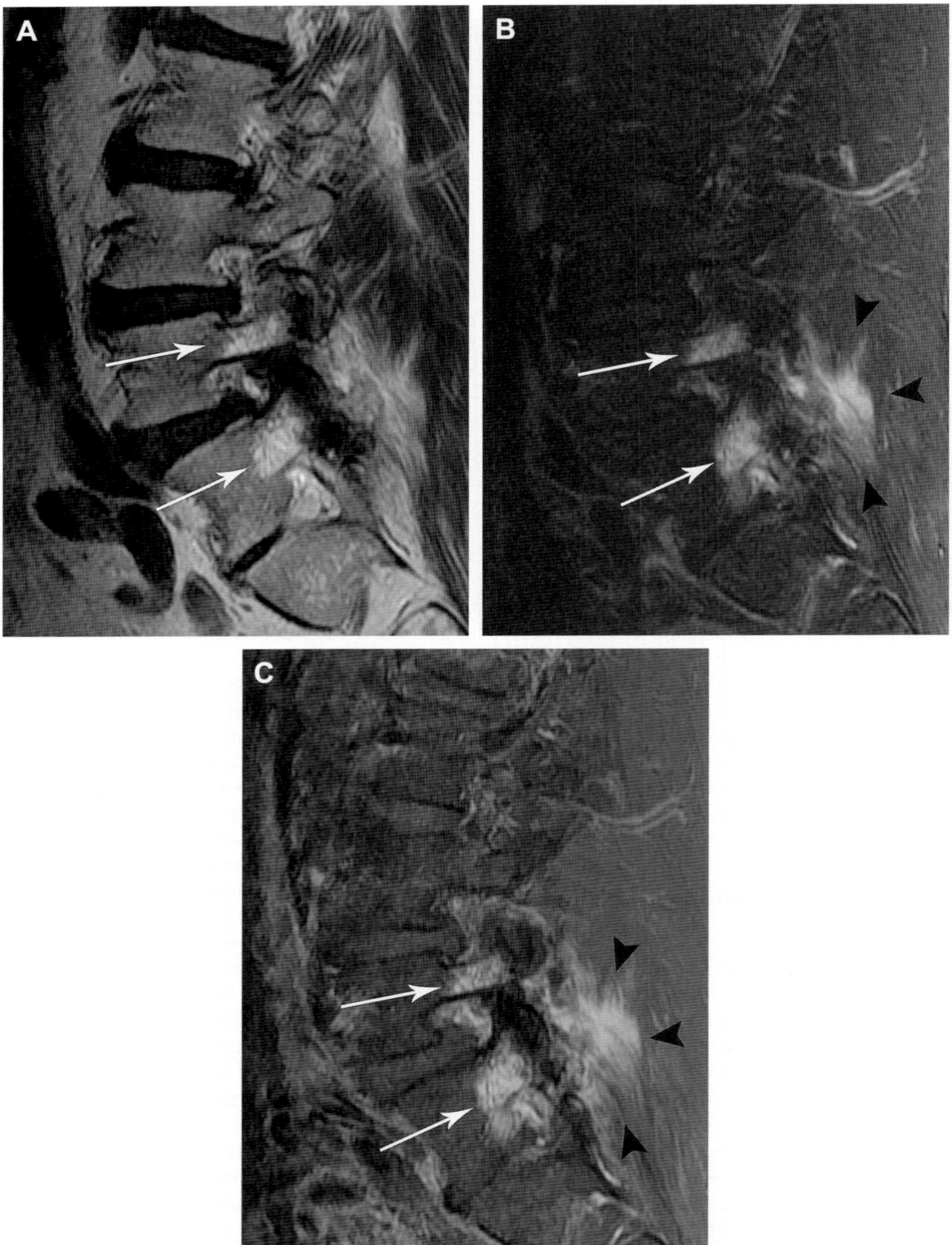

Fig. 15. Pedicle edema. A 74-year-old man (same patient as in **Fig. 13**) with a history of prostate carcinoma and right lower lumbar mechanical pain. Sagittal FSE T2-weighted image (*A*) demonstrates bone marrow edema in the right L4 and L5 pedicles (*white arrows*) without frank fracture line; facet synovitis is not appreciated. Sagittal fat-suppressed FSE T2-weighted (*B*) and CE T1-weighted (*C*) images also clearly demonstrate pedicle marrow edema (*white arrows*), but also clearly depict facet synovitis and extensive periarticular soft tissue inflammation and enhancement (*black arrowheads*).

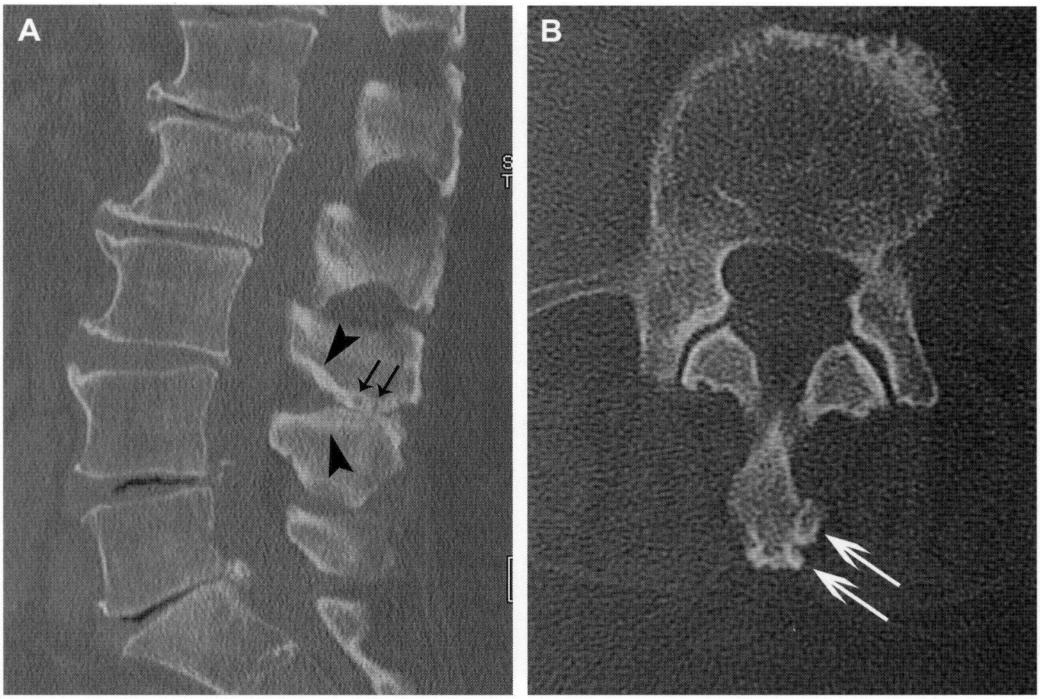

Fig. 16. Baastrup phenomenon. A 85-year-old man presents with chronic LBP and right leg pain. Sagittal (*A*) and axial CT (*B*) images demonstrate contact between the L3 and L4 spinous processes with subchondral sclerosis (*arrowheads*), erosions (*black arrows*), appositional flattening, and marginal osteophytes (*white arrows*).

(**Fig. 18**).[64] Fluid may track into the retroligamentous space of Okada, and from there communicate with one or both facet joints at the involved level or into associated pars defects.[9,64]

Baastrup disease with interspinal bursitis may demonstrate increased uptake on radionuclide bone scan or FDG-PET/CT scans.[65–67] These imaging findings are likely related to edema and inflammation associated with interspinous ligament degenerative inflammation and/or neoarthrosis formation, and should not be misinterpreted as neoplastic or infectious involvement of the spinous processes. These techniques may allow identification of degenerative changes of the spinous processes and interspinous ligaments more likely to account for the patient's pain.[66]

TRANSITIONAL SEGMENTS AND PSEUDOARTICULATIONS

Transitional spinal segments can occur in as many as 30% of patients, typically involving the last lumbar or first sacral segment.[68] The transitional segment demonstrates anatomic features of both lumbar-type and sacral-type vertebral bodies with frequent asymmetry from the left to the right side, particularly of the facet joints. Accurate counting of segments from C2 inferiorly is required to precisely define transitional anatomy, to prevent intervention at the wrong spinal level.[7,13] This topic is more fully addressed elsewhere in this issue in the article by Carrino and colleagues.

The relationship between LBP and transitional lumbosacral segments, called Bertolotti syndrome, is controversial. The incidence of symptoms in patients with transitional segments is similar to the incidence of LBP in the general population.[13] When symptoms occur, they may arise from neoarthrosis formation between the transitional segment and upper sacrum or iliac wing, from nerve root impingement by an enlarged transverse process, from the contralateral facet joint, or from early degeneration at the suprajacent lumbar segment. As each of these processes may be treated differently, it is important to both recognize the presence of a transitional lumbosacral segment and to identify the specific source of the patient's pain syndrome (**Fig. 19**).[13,35]

In most cases of transitional lumbosacral segments, symptoms are related to degenerative changes at the suprajacent lumbar level. There is thought to be increased stability at the transitional segment related to partial or complete fusion with the sacrum or ileum, which alters biomechanics at the lumbar level immediately above the transitional

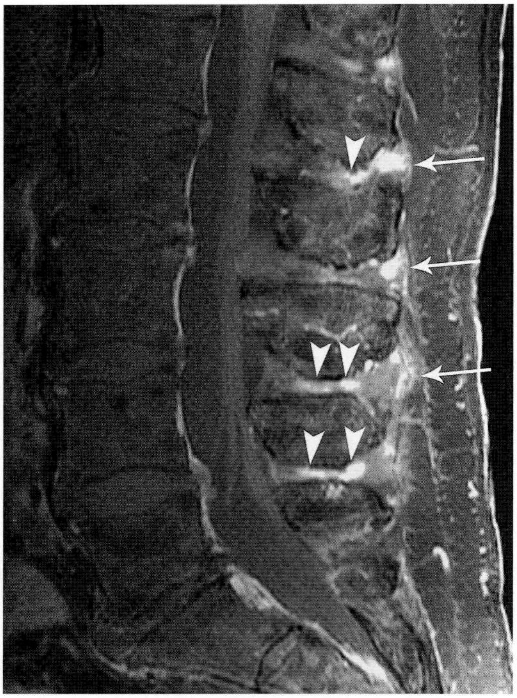

Fig. 17. Baastrup phenomenon and interspinal bursitis. A 84-year-old man presents with LBP and neurogenic claudication. Sagittal fat-suppressed T1-weighted MR image shows multilevel interspinous (*arrowheads*) and supraspinous (*arrows*) ligament degenerative inflammation and enhancement. (*Courtesy of* Timothy Maus, MD, Mayo Clinic, Rochester, MN; with permission.)

segment and predisposes this level to early degenerative change.[69]

In a small group of patients with unilateral transitional segments, the side of pain correlated with the side of the anomaly, and in most patients was relieved with injection of local anesthetic and/or resection of the anomalous articulation.[70] This pain was thought to be secondary to increased biomechanical stress at the pseudoarticulation or neoarthrosis. MR imaging with fat-suppressed sequences may demonstrate T2 hyperintensity related to marrow edema or enhancement related to hypervascularity at the neoarthrosis. Increased uptake on nuclear medicine bone scintigraphy may be also seen at the articulation of the anomalous spinal segment with the sacrum or ileum, and is best identified using SPECT (see **Fig. 19**B).[71] In cases of unilateral anomaly, the extraforaminal nerve root may be also impinged between the enlarged transverse process and sacral wing. This characteristic is best detected using a coronal MR imaging sequence.[13]

In cases of a unilateral or asymmetric anomaly, there may also be increased biomechanical stress on the contralateral facet, which may result in changes of facet osteoarthrosis and synovitis in the contralateral facet joint. In these cases imaging findings are as described previously, and are manifested by T2 hyperintensity and enhancement on fat-suppressed MR imaging sequences and increased uptake on nuclear medicine bone scintigraphy with SPECT or SPECT/CT.

Butterfly or hemivertebrae are rare spinal anomalies that are typically asymptomatic, incidental findings on imaging studies.[72] Occasionally anomalous articulations associated with these anomalies may be symptomatic and likely related to altered biomechanics and stress reactions, edema, or inflammation manifested as increased signal on fat-suppressed T2-weighted or CE T1-weighted images, or increased uptake on bone scintigraphy with SPECT (**Fig. 20**).

SACROILIAC JOINTS

SI joint pain accounts for 13% to 18% of patients with axial LBP.[42] Historical information and findings on physical examination, as with other posterior element pain generators, are unreliable in identifying the SI joints as the source of a patient's axial LBP. Factors that may predispose patients to SI joint–related back pain are pregnancy in women, spinal fusion to the sacrum, and leg-length discrepancies. Patients with seronegative spondyloarthropathies also have a high prevalence of SI joint–related inflammatory changes and associated SI joint pain.[11]

The ileal surface of the SI joint is lined by fibrocartilage. This cartilage may account for greater susceptibility of the iliac side of the joint to degenerative or age-related change, which is present in most individuals by the age of 40 years.[10] The posterior-superior one-third of the joint is a ligamentous connection.[73] Inflammatory and structural changes of the SI joints may result in LBP. Structural changes include those seen in joints elsewhere: sclerosis, juxta-articular erosions and cysts, osteophytes, and ankylosis.

Radiography, CT, and MR imaging can identify successive stages of SI joint involvement from subchondral bone marrow edema and inflammation with bone erosions, evolving to postinflammatory fatty infiltration, subchondral sclerosis, and finally osteophytes and ankylosis. CT is more sensitive than either MR imaging or radiography in detecting later chronic structural changes of erosions, sclerosis, and ankylosis (**Fig. 21**).[74] However, MR imaging best demonstrates both the structural changes and the early inflammatory component

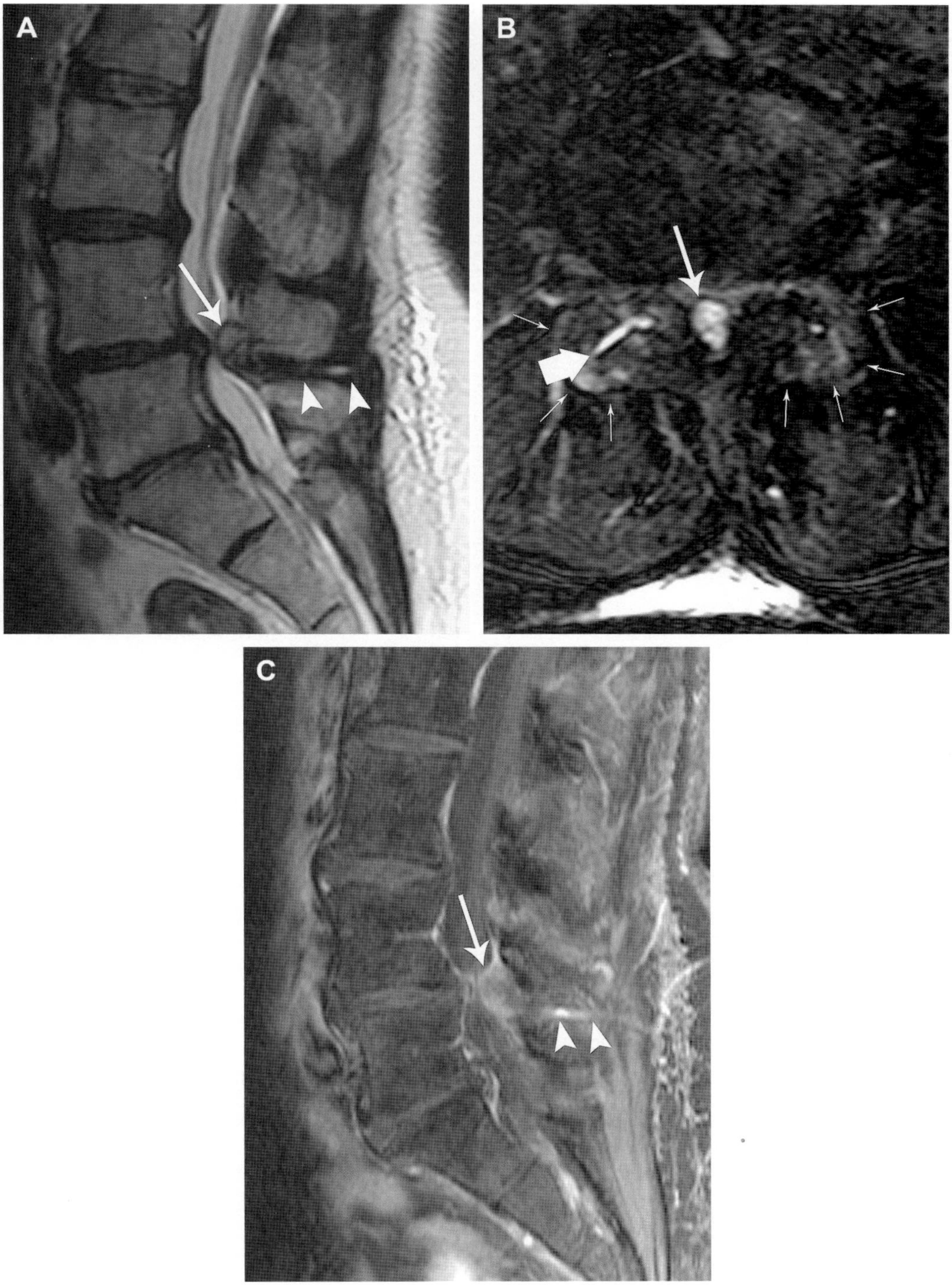

Fig. 18. Interspinal bursitis and midline epidural cyst. A 59-year-old woman with a history of breast cancer presents with back pain radiating to left buttock exacerbated in the upright position. Sagittal FSE T2-weighted image (*A*) shows fluid in the interspinous space (*arrowheads*) tracking to a poorly visualized midline posterior epidural cyst (*white arrows*). Axial fat-suppressed FSE T2-weighted image (*B*) better demonstrates the midline posterior epidural cyst (*arrow*), concurrent bilateral facet synovitis (*thick white arrow*), and right facet joint effusion (*small white arrows*). Enhancement in the interspinal space (*arrowheads*) and at the periphery of the midline epidural cyst (*arrow*) is well seen on the sagittal fat-suppressed CE T1-weighted image (*C*).

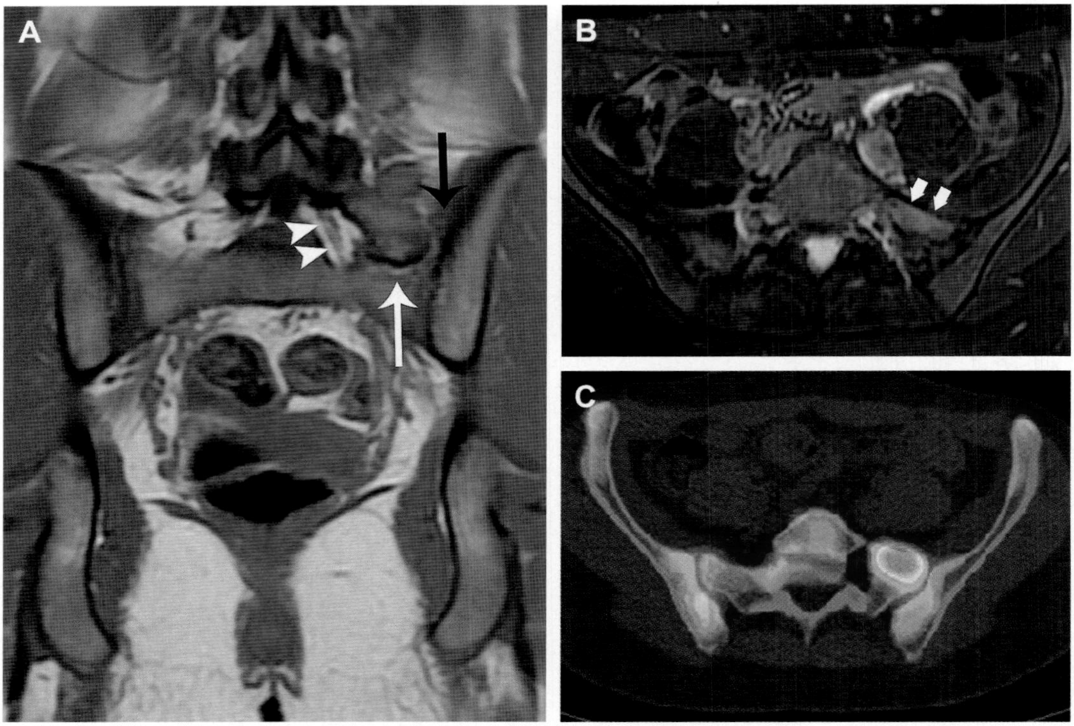

Fig. 19. Transitional lumbosacral segment. A 17-year-old female patient imaged for 1-year history of left-sided LBP. Coronal T1-weighted image (*A*) shows left-sided transitional lumbosacral segment articulating with both the sacrum (*white arrow*) and iliac wing (*black arrow*). The coronal plane clearly depicts the exiting nerve root (*white arrowheads*). Axial fat-suppressed FSE T2-weighted sequence (*B*) demonstrates marrow edema in the enlarged transverse process at the transitional level (*thick white arrows*), and there is increased radiotracer uptake in this region on radionuclide SPECT fused with CT (*C*). (*Courtesy of* Timothy Maus, MD, Mayo Clinic, Rochester, MN; with permission.)

associated with SI joint pain. MR imaging is significantly more sensitive to subchondral bone marrow edema and synovial, capsular, and ligamentous enhancement using STIR, fat-suppressed T2-weighted, and/or CE fat-suppressed T1-weighted imaging, and may identify changes in the SI joints even in patients with structurally normal radiographs.[74–76]

One consideration when imaging the SI region with CT or MR imaging is the parasagittal orientation of the joint surface and narrow anteroposterior dimension of the joint space, which may cause volume-averaging artifacts on sagittal or oblique coronal imaging. Therefore, transaxial imaging should always be used to better assess the articular surfaces and joint space.[77]

Makki and colleagues[78] found increased uptake localized to the SI joints on nuclear medicine bone scintigraphy with SPECT in 5.7% of patients with LBP. Most of these patients were eventually diagnosed with inflammatory spondyloarthropathy. These investigators suggest that SPECT may be able to diagnose this condition at an early phase, allowing for more prompt treatment. The imaging findings of inflammatory spondyloarthropathies are described in detail elsewhere in this issue by Amrami.

IMPORTANCE OF CLINICAL CONTEXT

In patients with LBP it is common to encounter multiple degenerative or age-related changes (often at multiple vertebral levels) on conventional anatomic imaging. In such cases, it is impossible to determine from imaging alone which, if any, of the structural changes are possibly responsible for causing the patient's symptoms. The literature is quite clear that the vast majority of structural age-related changes identified on imaging bear no relationship to axial or radicular pain syndromes. In this context, to perform an appropriate imaging examination and to provide useful information to the referring clinician, the imager must understand the nature of the patient's pain syndrome. Only

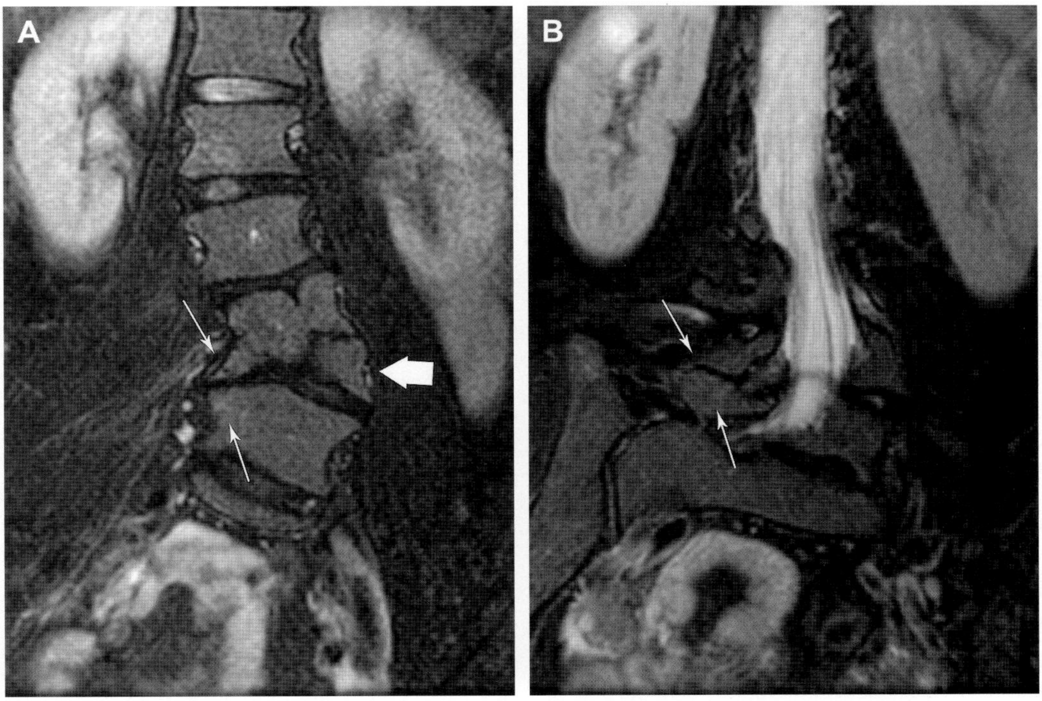

Fig. 20. Transitional lumbosacral segment. A 50-year-old woman with long history of scoliosis presents with increasing right back, buttock, and hip pain, worse with sitting and forward flexion. Coronal FSE T2-weighted sequences (*A*) at the level of the left L4 hemivertebra (*thick white arrow*) and (*B*) at the level of the pseudoarticulation between the right L3 and L5 vertebral bodies and enlarged transverse processes demonstrate subtle bone marrow edema around the anomalous articulation (*thin white arrows*). (*Courtesy of* Naveen Murthy, MD, Mayo Clinic, Rochester, MN; with permission.)

a clear concordance of the pain syndrome and imaging findings can suggest causality (**Box 5**).

The intervertebral disc is the single most common source of LBP in adults, but taken as a group posterior element structures may be responsible for nearly half of all axial LBP. DePalma and colleagues[42] studied 358 patients with chronic LBP and found facetogenic pain in 31%, SI joint pain in 18%, and interspinous bursitis in 2%. In their study population, discogenic pain was more

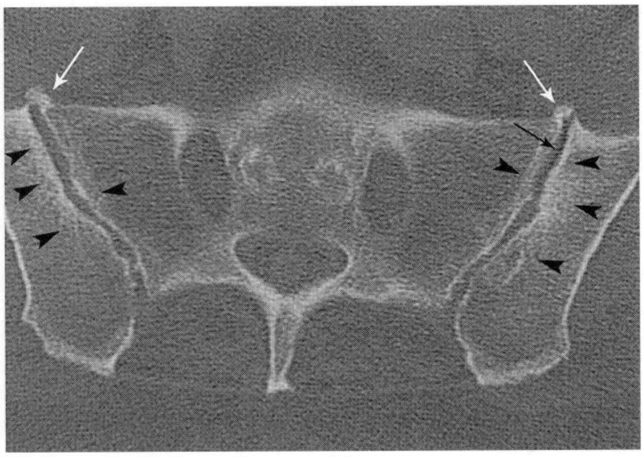

Fig. 21. Sacroiliac joint osteoarthrosis. An 85-year-old man presents with chronic LBP and right leg pain. Axial CT shows subchondral sclerosis (*black arrowheads*), marginal osteophytes (*white arrows*), and interarticular gas (vacuum phenomenon) (*black arrow*). Note the subchondral sclerosis is more severe on the iliac side of the joint.

Box 5
Importance of clinical context

Axial, nonradicular pain → seek out a posterior element cause

Additional suggestive findings:

- Morning back stiffness
- Decreased range of motion
- Mechanical pain with extension, flexion, or rotation maneuvers
- Pain to palpation over facet joints and spinous processes

Patient age

- Young → more likely discogenic
- Older → more likely posterior elements

prevalent in younger patients and posterior element pain more common in older adults.

In patients with axial, nonradicular pain, the imager should seek out a posterior element cause. While morning back stiffness, decreased range of motion, and pain with extension, flexion, or rotation maneuvers and pain to palpation over facet joints and spinous processes are nonspecific findings, they may also suggest a posterior element source of pain.[16,37,38,42,61,79] To best identify posterior element pain generators, the imager must look beyond meaningless structural changes to the physiologic clues of edema, hypervascularity, and inflammation, to identify a possible cause of pain. This course of action implies guiding the referring physicians in choosing appropriate imaging tests, and conducting those studies so as to maximize conspicuity of inflammatory imaging findings.

SUMMARY

Facet joints, pedicles, ligaments, spinous processes, transitional lumbosacral segments, and SI joints have all been implicated as sources of nonradicular axial back pain. Imagers should be aware of these causes and tailor imaging examinations to identify these sources of back pain. Posterior element causes of back and neck pain may remain underrecognized secondary to use of MR imaging techniques which fail to demonstrate the bone marrow edema, soft-tissue inflammation, and hypervascularity often associated with posterior element pain generators. Fat-suppressed FSE T2-weighted and/or fat-suppressed CE T1-weighted sequence should be performed in at least one imaging plane in all MR examinations of the lumbar spine. Radionuclide bone scanning with SPECT, SPECT/CT, and FDG-PET/CT are additional imaging techniques that add specificity to the diagnosis of posterior element pain generators.

ACKNOWLEDGMENTS

The author would like to thank Mr Carl Clingman for preparation of anatomic drawings, and Drs Timothy Maus, Naveen Murthy, and Kent Thielen for image contributions.

REFERENCES

1. Denis F. The three column spine and its significance in the classification of acute thoracolumbar spinal injuries. Spine (Phila Pa 1976) 1983;8(8):817–31.
2. Schellinger D, Wener L, Ragsdale BD, et al. Facet joint disorders and their role in the production of back pain and sciatica. Radiographics 1987;7(5): 923–44.
3. Farfan HF, Sullivan JD. The relation of facet orientation to intervertebral disc failure. Can J Surg 1967; 10:179–85.
4. Lee DY, Ahn Y, Lee SH. The influence of facet tropism on herniation of the lumbar disc in adolescents and adults. J Bone Joint Surg Br 2006;88(4): 520–3.
5. Bogduk N, Wilson AS, Tynan W. The human lumbar dorsal rami. J Anat 1982;134(Pt 2):383–97.
6. Pederson HE, Blunck CF, Gardner E. The anatomy of lumbosacral posterior rami and meningeal branches of spinal nerves (sinuvertebral nerves). J Bone Joint Surg Am 1956;38(2):377–91.
7. Harnsberger HR, Osborn AG, Ross J, et al. Diagnostic and surgical imaging anatomy: brain, head and neck, spine. Salt Lake City (UT): Amirsys; 2006.
8. Okada K. Studies on the cervical facet joints using arthrography of the cervical facet joint. Nihon Seikeigeka Gakkai Zasshi 1981;55(6):563–80 [in Japanese, author's transl.].
9. Murthy NS, Maus TP, Aprill C. The retrodural space of Okada. Am J Roentgenol 2011;196(6): W784–9.
10. Bowen V, Cassidy JD. Macroscopic and microscopic anatomy of the sacroiliac joint from embryonic life until the eighth decade. Spine (Phila Pa 1976) 1981;6(6):620–8.
11. Cohen SP. Sacroiliac joint pain: a comprehensive review of anatomy, diagnosis, and treatment. Anesth Analg 2005;101(5):1440–53.
12. Yin W, Willard F, Carreiro J, et al. Sensory stimulation-guided sacroiliac joint radiofrequency neurotomy: technique based on neuroanatomy of the dorsal sacral plexus. Spine (Phila Pa 1976) 2003;28(20): 2419–25.
13. Konin GP, Walz DM. Lumbosacral transitional vertebrae: classification, imaging findings, and clinical relevance. AJNR Am J Neuroradiol 2010;31(10): 1778–86.
14. DePalma M. iSpine: evidence-based interventional spine care. 1st edition. New York: Demos Medical Publishing; 2011.
15. Czervionke LF, Fenton DS. Fat-saturated MR imaging in the detection of inflammatory facet arthropathy (facet synovitis) in the lumbar spine. Pain Med 2008;9(4):400–6.
16. D'Aprile P, Tarantino A, Jinkins JR, et al. The value of fat saturation sequences and contrast medium administration in MRI of degenerative disease of the posterior/perispinal elements of the lumbosacral spine. Eur Radiol 2007;17(2):523–31.
17. Jinkins JR. Acquired degenerative changes of the intervertebral segments at and suprajacent to the lumbosacral junction. A radioanatomic analysis of

the nondiscal structures of the spinal column and perispinal soft tissues. Eur J Radiol 2004;50(2): 134–58.
18. Fleckenstein JL, Archer BT, Barker BA, et al. Fast short-tau inversion-recovery MR imaging. Radiology 1991;179(2):499–504.
19. Bydder GM, Young IR. MR imaging: clinical use of the inversion recovery sequence. J Comput Assist Tomogr 1985;9(4):659–75.
20. Keller PJ, Hunter WW, Schmalbrock P. Multisection fat-water imaging with chemical shift selective presaturation. Radiology 1987;164(2):539–41.
21. Hauger O, Dumont E, Chateil JF, et al. Water excitation as an alternative to fat saturation in MR imaging: preliminary results in musculoskeletal imaging. Radiology 2002;224(3):657–63.
22. Gerdes CM, Kijowski R, Reeder SB. IDEAL imaging of the musculoskeletal system: robust water fat separation for uniform fat suppression, marrow evaluation, and cartilage imaging. AJR Am J Roentgenol 2007;189(5):W284–91.
23. Hardy PA, Hinks RS, Tkach JA. Separation of fat and water in fast spin-echo MR imaging with the three-point Dixon technique. J Magn Reson Imaging 1995;5(2):181–5.
24. Delfaut EM, Beltran J, Johnson G, et al. Fat suppression in MR imaging: techniques and pitfalls. Radiographics 1999;19(2):373–82.
25. De Maeseneer M, Lenchik L, Everaert H, et al. Evaluation of lower back pain with bone scintigraphy and SPECT1. Radiographics 1999;19(4):901–12.
26. Collier BD, Kir KM, Mills BJ, et al. Bone scan: a useful test for evaluating patients with low back pain. Skeletal Radiol 1990;19(4):267–70.
27. Dolan AL, Ryan PJ, Arden NK, et al. The value of SPECT scans in identifying back pain likely to benefit from facet joint injection. Br J Rheumatol 1996; 35(12):1269–73.
28. Willick SE, Kendall RW, Roberts ST, et al. An emerging imaging technology to assist in the localization of axial spine pain. PM R 2009;1(1): 89–92.
29. Holder LE, Machin JL, Asdourian PL, et al. Planar and high-resolution SPECT bone imaging in the diagnosis of facet syndrome. J Nucl Med 1995; 36(1):37–44.
30. Rosen RS, Fayad L, Wahl RL. Increased ^{18}F-FDG uptake in degenerative disease of the spine: characterization with ^{18}F-FDG PET/CT. J Nucl Med 2006;47(8):1274–80.
31. Ido K, Shiode H, Sakamoto A, et al. The validity of upright myelography for diagnosing lumbar disc herniation. Clin Neurol Neurosurg 2002;104(1): 30–5.
32. Jinkins JR, Dworkin JS, Damadian RV. Upright, weight-bearing, dynamic-kinetic MRI of the spine: initial results. Eur Radiol 2005;15(9):1815–25.
33. Kufeld M, Claus B, Campi A, et al. Three-dimensional rotational myelography. AJNR Am J Neuroradiol 2003;24(7):1290–3.
34. Kau T, Rabitsch E, Celedin S, et al. Feasibility and potential value of flat-panel detector–based computed tomography in myelography after spinal surgery. J Neurosurg Spine 2009;10(1):66–72.
35. Wybier M. Imaging of lumbar degenerative changes involving structures other than disk space. Radiol Clin North Am 2001;39(1):101–14.
36. Ross JS, Brant-Zawadski M, Moore KR. Diagnostic imaging: spine. Salt Lake City (UT): Amirysis; 2004.
37. Schwarzer AC, Derby R, Aprill CN, et al. Pain from the lumbar zygapophysial joints: a test of two models. J Spinal Disord 1994;7(4):331–6.
38. Schwarzer AC, Aprill CN, Derby R, et al. Clinical features of patients with pain stemming from the lumbar zygapophysial joints. Is the lumbar facet syndrome a clinical entity? Spine 1994;19(10): 1132–7.
39. Schwarzer AC, Wang SC, O'Driscoll D, et al. The ability of computed tomography to identify a painful zygapophysial joint in patients with chronic low back pain. Spine (Phila Pa 1976) 1995;20(8):907–12.
40. Cohen SP, Bajwa ZH, Kraemer JJ, et al. Factors predicting success and failure for cervical facet radiofrequency denervation: a multi-center analysis. Reg Anesth Pain Med 2007;32(6):495–503.
41. Cohen SP, Raja SN. Pathogenesis, diagnosis, and treatment of lumbar zygapophysial (facet) joint pain. Anesthesiology 2007;106(3):591–614.
42. DePalma MJ, Ketchum JM, Saullo T. What is the source of chronic low back pain and does age play a role? Pain Med 2011;12(2):224–33.
43. Gallucci M, Limbucci N, Paonessa A, et al. Degenerative disease of the spine. Neuroimaging Clin N Am 2007;17(1):87–103.
44. Doyle AJ, Merrilees M. Synovial cysts of the lumbar facet joints in a symptomatic population: prevalence on magnetic resonance imaging. Spine (Phila Pa 1976) 2004;29(8):874–8.
45. Lyons MK, Atkinson JL, Wharen RE, et al. Surgical evaluation and management of lumbar synovial cysts: the Mayo Clinic experience. J Neurosurg 2000;93(1):53–7.
46. Howington JU, Connolly ES, Voorhies RM. Intraspinal synovial cysts: 10-year experience at the Ochsner Clinic. J Neurosurg 1999;91(Suppl 2): 193–9.
47. Igarashi A, Kikuchi S, Konno S, et al. Inflammatory cytokines released from the facet joint tissue in degenerative lumbar spinal disorders. Spine 2004; 29(19):2091–5.
48. Friedrich K, Nemec S, Peloschek P, et al. The prevalence of lumbar facet joint edema in patients with low back pain. Skeletal Radiol 2007;36(8): 755–60.

49. Bogduk N. ISIS Guidelines. Practice guidelines for spinal diagnostic and treatment procedures: Standards Committee of the International Spine Intervention Society. San Rafael (CA): International Spine Intervention Society; 2004.
50. Pneumaticos SG, Chatziioannou SN, Hipp JA, et al. Low back pain: prediction of short-term outcome of facet joint injection with bone scintigraphy. Radiology 2006;238(2):693–8.
51. Kim KA, Wang MY. MRI-|based morphological predictors of SPECT positive facet arthropathyin patients with axial back pain. Neurosurgery 2006;59(1):147–56.
52. Houseni M, Chamroonrat W, Zhuang H, et al. Facet joint arthropathy demonstrated on FDG-PET. Clin Nucl Med 2006;31(7):418–9.
53. Lin E, Sicuro P. FDG uptake in cervical facet subchondral cysts demonstrated by PET/CT. Clin Nucl Med 2008;33(4):268–70.
54. Borg B, Modic MT, Obuchowski N, et al. Pedicle marrow signal hyperintensity on short tau inversion recovery- and T2-weighted images: prevalence and relationship to clinical symptoms. AJNR Am J Neuroradiol 2011;32(9):1624–31.
55. Morrison JL, Kaplan PA, Dussault RG, et al. Pedicle marrow signal intensity changes in the lumbar spine: a manifestation of facet degenerative joint disease. Skeletal Radiol 2000;29(12):703–7.
56. Baastrup CI. On the spinous processes of the lumbar vertebrae and the soft tissue between them and on pathological changes in that region. Acta Radiol 1933;14:52–4.
57. Clifford PD. Baastrup disease. Am J Orthop (Belle Mead NJ) 2007;36(10):560–1.
58. Goobar JE, Clark GM. Sclerosis of the spinous processes and low back pain ("cockspur" disease). Arch Int Am Rheum 1962;5:587–93.
59. Beks JW. Kissing spines: fact or fancy? Acta Neurochir (Wien) 1989;100(3–4):134–5.
60. Kwong Y, Rao N, Latief K. MDCT findings in Baastrup disease: disease or normal feature of the aging spine? AJR Am J Roentgenol 2011;196(5):1156–9.
61. Lamer TJ, Tiede JM, Fenton DS. Fluoroscopically-guided injections to treat "kissing spine" disease. Pain Physician 2008;11(4):549–54.
62. Maes R, Morrison WB, Parker L, et al. Lumbar interspinous bursitis (Baastrup disease) in a symptomatic population: prevalence on magnetic resonance imaging. Spine (Phila Pa 1976) 2008;33(7):E211–5.
63. Fujiwara A, Tamai K, An HS, et al. The interspinous ligament of the lumbar spine. Magnetic resonance images and their clinical significance. Spine (Phila Pa 1976) 2000;25(3):358–63.
64. Chen CK, Yeh L, Resnick D, et al. Intraspinal posterior epidural cysts associated with Baastrup's disease: report of 10 patients. AJR Am J Roentgenol 2004;182(1):191–4.
65. Gorospe L, Jover R, Vicente-Bartulos A, et al. FDG-PET/CT demonstration of Baastrup disease ("kissing" spine). Clin Nucl Med 2008;33(2):133–4.
66. Hamlin LM, Delaplain CB. Bone SPECT in Baastrup's disease. Clin Nucl Med 1994;19(7):640–1.
67. Ho L, Wassef H, Seto J, et al. Multi-level lumbar Baastrup disease on F-18 FDG PET-CT. Clin Nucl Med 2009;34(12):896–7.
68. Luoma K, Vehmas T, Raininko R, et al. Lumbosacral transitional vertebra: relation to disc degeneration and low back pain. Spine (Phila Pa 1976) 2004;29(2):200–5.
69. Elster AD. Bertolotti's syndrome revisited. Transitional vertebrae of the lumbar spine. Spine (Phila Pa 1976) 1989;14(12):1373–7.
70. Jonsson B, Stromqvist B, Egund N. Anomalous lumbosacral articulations and low-back pain. Evaluation and treatment. Spine (Phila Pa 1976) 1989;14(8):831–4.
71. Connolly LP, d'Hemecourt PA, Connolly SA, et al. Skeletal scintigraphy of young patients with low-back pain and a lumbosacral transitional vertebra. J Nucl Med 2003;44(6):909–14.
72. Patinharayil G, Han CW, Marthya A, et al. Butterfly vertebra: an uncommon congenital spinal anomaly. Spine 2008;33(24):E926–8.
73. Resnick D. Degenerative diseases of the vertebral column. Radiology 1985;156(1):3–14.
74. Lacout A, Rousselin B, Pelage JP. CT and MRI of spine and sacroiliac involvement in spondyloarthropathy. AJR Am J Roentgenol 2008;191(4):1016–23.
75. Heuft-Dorenbosch L, Landewe R, Weijers R, et al. Combining information obtained from magnetic resonance imaging and conventional radiographs to detect sacroiliitis in patients with recent onset inflammatory back pain. Ann Rheum Dis 2006;65(6):804–8.
76. Heuft-Dorenbosch L, Weijers R, Landewe R, et al. Magnetic resonance imaging changes of sacroiliac joints in patients with recent-onset inflammatory back pain: inter-reader reliability and prevalence of abnormalities. Arthritis Res Ther 2006;8(1):R11.
77. Puhakka KB, Melsen F, Jurik AG, et al. MR imaging of the normal sacroiliac joint with correlation to histology. Skeletal Radiol 2004;33(1):15–28.
78. Makki D, Khazim R, Zaidan AA, et al. Single photon emission computerized tomography (SPECT) scan—positive facet joints and other spinal structures in a hospital-wide population with spinal pain. Spine J 2010;10(1):58–62.
79. Schwarzer AC, Aprill CN, Bogduk N. The sacroiliac joint in chronic low back pain. Spine 1995;20(1):31–7.

Imaging the Postoperative Spine

Rashmi S. Thakkar, MD[a,*], John P. Malloy IV, DO[b],
Savyasachi C. Thakkar, MD[c], John A. Carrino, MD, MPH[d],
A. Jay Khanna, MD, MBA[e]

KEYWORDS

• Postoperative spine • Imaging • Complications • Surgery

KEY POINTS

- Imaging plays an important role in the preoperative and postoperative evaluation of patients undergoing spinal surgery.
- Appropriate imaging techniques and knowledge of their advantages and limitations are essential for optimal evaluation of the postoperative spine.
- Postoperative imaging examinations allow for the evaluation of implant positioning, adequacy of decompression, fusion status, and potential complications.
- This article provides an overview of the normal and abnormal postoperative appearances of the spine via various modalities, with an emphasis on postoperative complications.

INTRODUCTION

Imaging assessment of the spine after surgery is complex and depends on several factors, including the age and anatomy of the patient, indication for and type of surgery performed, biomaterials used, time elapsed since the surgical procedure, and (most importantly) the duration and the nature of the postsurgical syndrome.[1]

Imaging plays an important role in the preoperative and postoperative evaluation of patients undergoing spinal surgeries. Postoperative imaging examinations evaluate the position of implants, adequacy of decompression fusion status, and potential complications. For the optimal evaluation of patients who have had previous spinal instrumentation, proper adoption of the appropriate imaging techniques and knowledge of their advantages and limitations are essential.

This article provides a review of various imaging techniques, with their advantages and disadvantages, for the evaluation of the postoperative spine. It also gives an overview of normal and abnormal postoperative appearances of the spine via various modalities, with an emphasis on postoperative complications.

(Tags: imaging, spine, surgery, postoperative, complications).

The authors have no conflicts of interest to disclose. No funding was received in support of this study.

[a] The Russell H. Morgan Department of Radiology and Radiological Sciences, The Johns Hopkins University School of Medicine, 601 North Caroline Street, JHOC 4240, Baltimore, MD 21287, USA; [b] Alexander Orthopaedic Associates, 12416 66th Street North, Suite A, Largo, FL 33773, USA; [c] Department of Orthopaedic Surgery, The Johns Hopkins University School of Medicine, 601 North Caroline Street, JHOC 5161, Baltimore, MD 21287, USA; [d] Musculoskeletal Radiology, The Russell H. Morgan Department of Radiology and Radiological Sciences, The Johns Hopkins University School of Medicine, 601 North Caroline Street, JHOC 5165, Baltimore, MD 21287, USA; [e] Department of Orthopaedic Surgery, The Johns Hopkins University School of Medicine, 6410 Rockledge Drive, 309, Bethesda, MD 20817, USA

* Corresponding author.
E-mail address: rthakka4@jhmi.edu

Radiol Clin N Am 50 (2012) 731–747
doi:10.1016/j.rcl.2012.04.006
0033-8389/12/$ – see front matter

SURGICAL PROCEDURES

Goals

Surgical procedures in the spine are typically performed with the following goals in mind[2]:

- Decompression of neural elements via removal of herniated disk material or decompression of a stenotic spinal canal or neural foramen
- Stabilization and fusion of motion segments for existing instability or deformity (such as spondylolisthesis, scoliosis, or posttraumatic injury) or after iatrogenic instability (such as facetectomy or multilevel laminectomies)
- Excision of tumor or debridement of infection.

Decompressive Surgeries

1. Laminotomy: the bone resection is limited to small segments of inferior margin of the cephalic lamina and the superior margin of the caudal lamina to decompress the neural structures. This procedure is often performed in conjunction with a diskectomy (**Fig. 1**).
2. Laminectomy: the bone resection is extended to include the entire width of a lamina, as well as a small segment of the margin of the adjacent lamina, to decompress a larger area. The primary purpose is to relieve central stenosis or to give greater exposure to a herniated disk during diskectomy (**Fig. 2**).
3. Laminectomy and facetectomy: the bone resection is extended to include a part of or

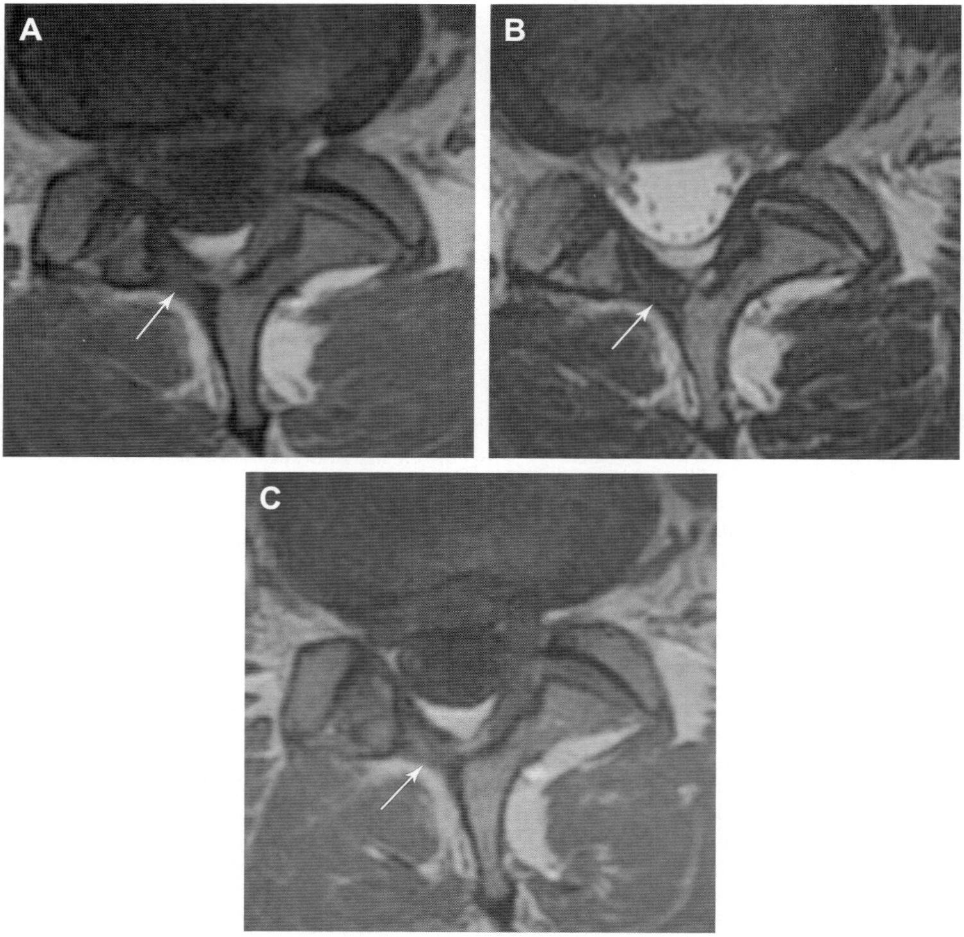

Fig. 1. Laminotomy of the lumbar spine. (*A*) An axial T1-weighted image (repetition time/echo time: 550/10.67), (*B*) an axial T2-weighted image (repetition time/echo time: 5966/118), and (*C*) an axial postcontrast T1-weighted image (repetition time/echo time: 550/10.67) show partial removal of the right-side lamina, identifying the laminotomy site (*arrows*).

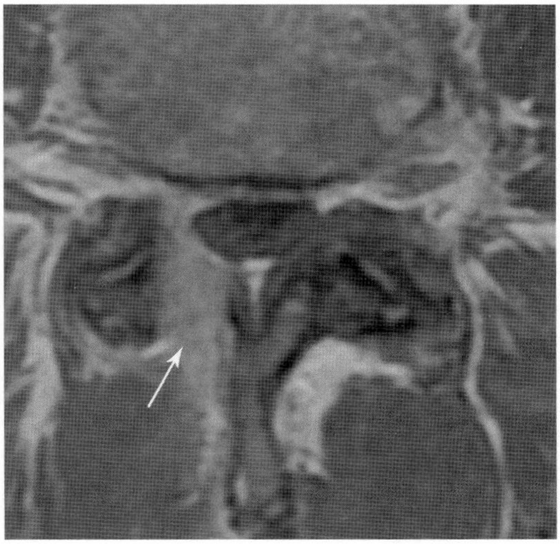

Fig. 2. Hemilaminectomy and partial diskectomy. T1-weighted axial postcontrast image (repetition time/echo time: 6116/10.9) shows evidence of right hemilaminectomy (*arrow*) and partial diskectomy.

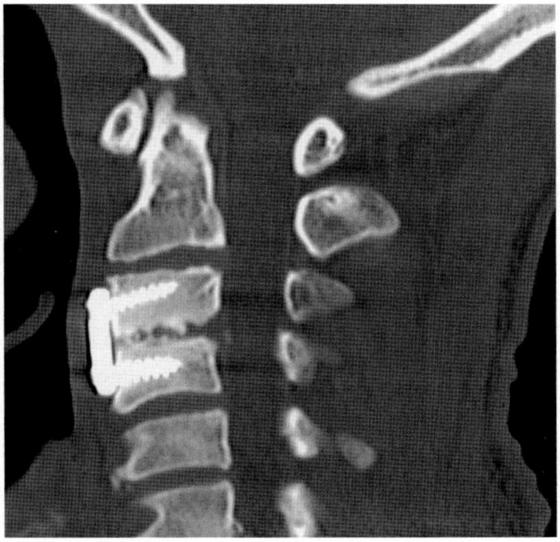

Fig. 3. CT sagittal reconstruction shows anterior cervical diskectomy and fusion with screws and plate at C3-4. Note the incomplete bone growth through the disk space between the vertebral bodies, which may be consistent with early postoperative changes or a failure of fusion (pseudarthrosis), depending on the time from surgery.

the complete facet joint in addition to the cephalic and caudal laminae to gain maximum exposure of the herniated disk and to relieve foraminal, lateral recess, and central stenoses.

4. Diskectomy: the herniated disk material that is causing compression on neural elements is removed.

Spinal Fusion

Surgical implants in spinal fusion surgeries are used to stabilize the spine, replace resected components (ie, vertebral body), and maintain anatomic alignment. Radiologists should be able to identify the devices most commonly used and understand the general rationale for their use.[3]

Commonly used devices are the following:

1. Rods and plates: rods can extend to single or multiple spine segments. They are attached to the spine most commonly by pedicle screws in the thoracic and lumbar spine and via lateral mass and other screws in the cervical spine. Hooks, sublaminar or interspinous wires, and cables can also be used. Various shapes and sizes of plates have been developed for anterior or posterior spinal fusion (**Figs. 3** and **4**).[4–6]
2. Translaminar or facet screws: these devices can be used when posterior elements are intact. They attach the laminae of 2 adjacent vertebrae.
3. Transpedicular screws: the use of pedicle screws in conjunction with plates or rods is generally well accepted as creating a primary stable construct, providing immediate postoperative stabilization without external support.[7,8] This allows early patient mobilization. Transpedicular screws are especially important for cases of posterolateral fusions of the lumbar spine performed for spondylolisthesis, degenerative disk disease, and scoliosis (**Fig. 5**).
4. Interbody spacers: interbody cages are available in various shapes and materials. After the removal of a disk, these spacers are inserted into the intervertebral space with or without additional screw and plate/rod fixation.[9] Cages are usually made of titanium, carbon fiber, polyetheretherketone (PEEK), or cortical or corticocancellous bone graft. Interbody cages are filled with bone graft material and inserted into the intervertebral space, or may be used to replace a vertebra after it is removed (ie, corpectomy). Most radiolucent cages contain 2 or more radiopaque markers to identify their position on radiographs and to enable their assessment. For a stand-alone interbody fusion cage, the interbody spacer is fixed to the adjacent vertebral body with screws to eliminate the need for additional instrumentation. Advantages of interbody devices include a larger surface area for fusion to occur and better restoration of spinal alignment through anterior column correction and support. Complications of interbody cages include retropulsion and cage subsidence. A distance of 2 mm or less between the posterior marker of the cage and the posterior margin of the vertebra should exist to provide reassurance that the cage is not invading the spinal canal.[4]

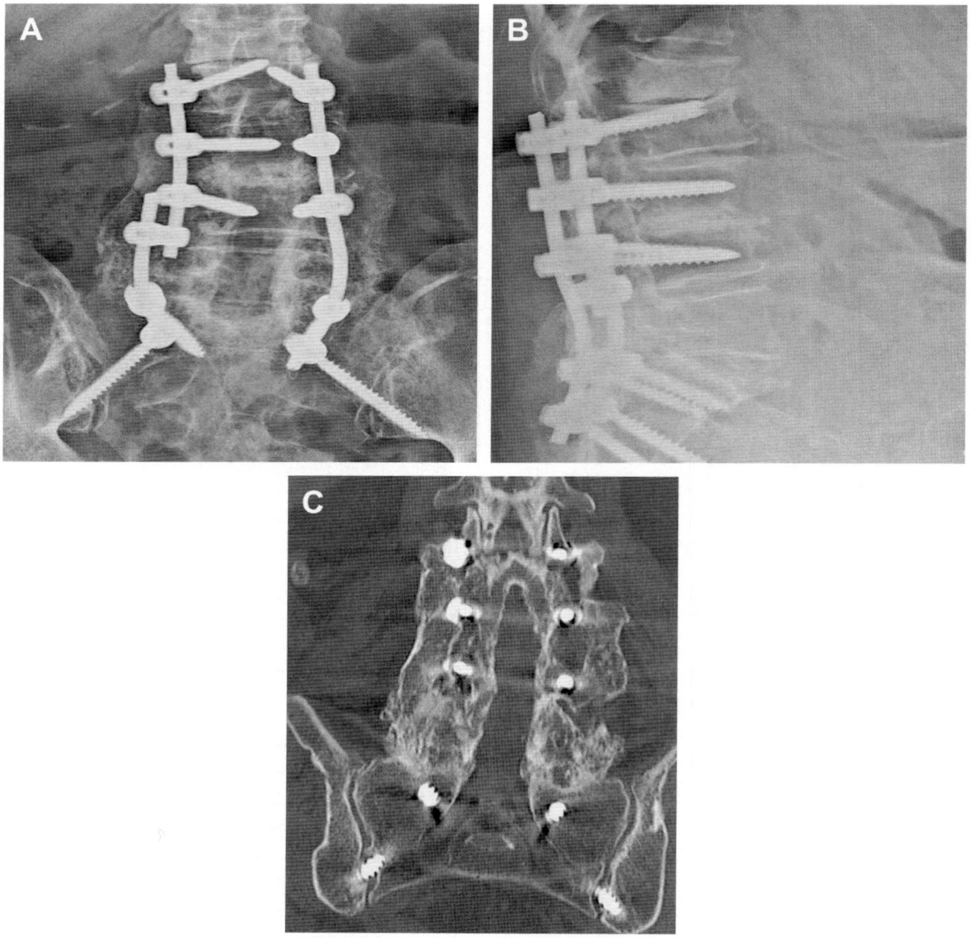

Fig. 4. Anteroposterior (*A*) and lateral (*B*) radiographs of a 73-year-old woman show posterior spinal fusion with bilateral rods and pedicle screws from L2 through S2. There has been posterior laminectomy from L3 through S1. There is evidence for posterior lateral osseous fusion at these levels in the intertransverse process space. (*C*) CT scan of the coronal section confirms a solid posterior spinal fusion with bilateral rods and pedicle screws from L2 through S2. There has been posterior laminectomy from L3 through S1.

Surgical methods can be divided into minimally invasive or traditional open procedures and by the vector from which the spine is approached (ie, anterior, posterior, or lateral).[10]

In interbody fusion, the intervertebral disk or a complete vertebra is removed and replaced with a bone graft. This procedure can be performed via an anterior approach (anterior interbody fusion) or a posterior approach (posterior interbody fusion). With anterior lumbar interbody fusions, the advantage is a broader access to the disk space. However, it is limited by potential injury to major vessels and the sympathetic nerve chain.[11] Oskouian and Johnson[12] reported an incidence of 5.8% for vascular complications in patients who underwent anterior thoracolumbar spine reconstruction procedures.

Direct lateral interbody fusion is a newer surgical technique performed transpsoas to fuse L1 to L5 and to minimize the disadvantages of conventional retroperitoneal anterior lumbar interbody fusions. Direct lateral interbody fusions allow for access to the anterior spine through the retroperitoneal space and can also be performed in the thoracic spine. It is a less invasive alternative to traditional anterior retroperitoneal or thoracoabdominal approaches.

With posterior lumbar interbody fusions, bilateral laminectomies are performed, and bone graft material with a cage or spacer is inserted into the disk space after the disk is removed. The disadvantages of this approach are potential injury to the nerve roots and retrograde migration or retropulsion of the graft or cage.[13]

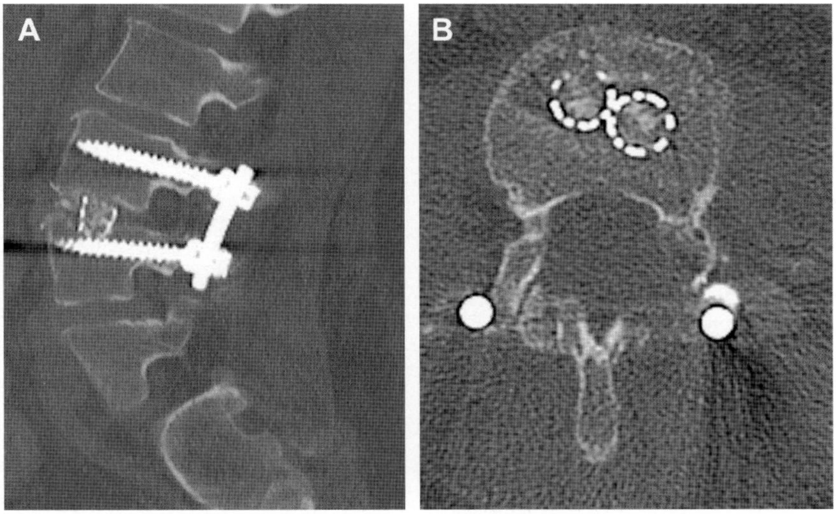

Fig. 5. (*A*) Sagittal CT image in a 52-year-old woman shows transpedicular screw fixation at the L3-4 level with intervertebral cage device containing bone graft material. On the axial section (*B*), the interbody cages and a partial laminectomy are noted.

Transforaminal interbody fusion is a modified posterior lumbar interbody fusion technique that uses a more lateral approach and thus leaves the midline bony structures intact. Min and colleagues[14] showed that anterior and posterior interbody fusion can produce good outcomes in treating lumbar spondylolisthesis, but anterior interbody fusion is more advantageous in preventing the development of adjacent segment degeneration.

Posterolateral fusion can be performed alone or in conjunction with interbody fusion. In this approach, the adjacent vertebrae are fused together by placing bone graft material between the transverse processes and facet joints.[15]

Disk Arthroplasty (Also Known as Total Disk Replacement)

This procedure includes removal of the diseased disk and insertion of a disk prosthesis to alleviate diskogenic pain and to restore normal disk height. The main goal of disk arthroplasty is to relieve pain while restoring or maintaining normal or near-normal disk space motion in an effort to decrease the potential for adjacent segment disease.[16]

(Tags: surgeries, implants, spine).

IMAGING

Radiography

Various radiographic modalities are used in the evaluation of the postoperative spine. Baseline radiographs are essential for evaluating implant position and serve as a starting point for evaluation of future studies, should patients develop symptoms suggesting possible complications.[17] With the help of serial radiographs, one can assess changes in component position, bony alignment, implant fractures, and changes in the bone-implant interface.[18,19] Radiographs are cost effective and accessible, which combined with their ability to obtain positional information with relatively low exposure to radiation compared with that of computed tomography (CT), makes them an indispensable tool for the assessment of the postoperative spine (**Fig. 6**). Anteroposterior (AP), lateral, oblique, and motion images (flexion, extension, or lateral bending) are usually adequate. Radiographic evidence of instability includes translation of 3 mm or more in L1 to L4 vertebrae, 5 mm at the L5 to S1 interspace, or more than 10° of angulation between adjacent vertebrae.[20] On occasion, however, fluoroscopically positioned images may provide better alignment of the implant or osseous structures to identify subtle changes more optimally.[21] The time to solid radiographic fusion is typically 6 to 9 months after surgery. Ray[22] defined 6 criteria to verify a solid fusion radiographically:

1. No motion or less than 3° of intersegment position change on lateral flexion and extension views
2. Lack of a lucent area around the implant
3. Minimal loss of disk height
4. No fracture of the implant, bone graft, or vertebrae
5. No sclerotic change in the bone graft or adjacent vertebrae
6. Visible osseous formation in or around the cage.

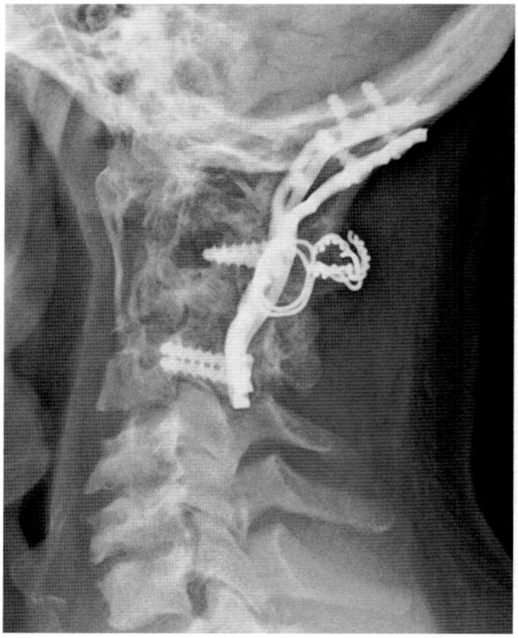

Fig. 6. Lateral radiograph in a 35-year-old woman with Down syndrome shows posterior fusion from occiput to C3 with plates, screws, and wire fixation. There is satisfactory alignment of the spine with a solid fusion mass.

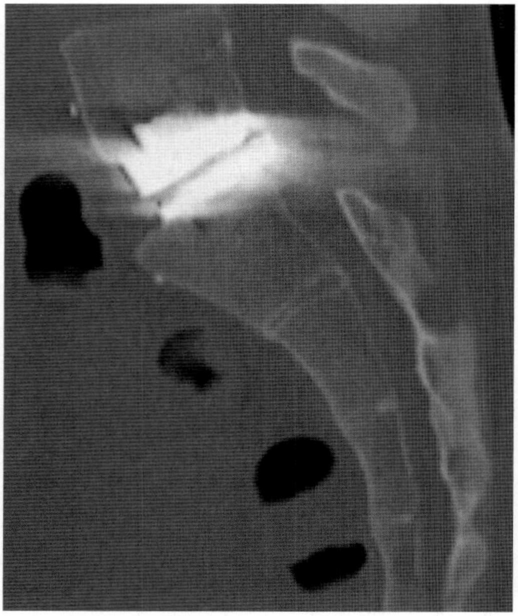

Fig. 7. A sagittal CT image of the lumbosacral spine of a 27-year-old woman showing metallic disk replacement at the L5-S1 level. The implant appears to be positioned posteriorly on the sacral end plate with slight overhang into the spinal canal.

Radiographs have a few limitations: they cannot evaluate soft tissue structures (such as neural elements, recurrent disk herniations, or scar tissue) and they are of little value in the noninstrumented postoperative spine.

Regarding disk arthroplasty, the midline placement, AP positioning, and the degree of vertebral body penetration or subsidence need to be identified by imaging. Disk arthroplasty is best evaluated with conventional radiography or CT. Ideally, the device is located in the midline between the 2 pedicles on AP radiographs or axial or coronal CT scans. There should be no penetration of the end plate. With respect to AP positioning, the center of rotation should be located in the posterior half of the disk space, but the implant should not extend beyond the posterior vertebral body line (**Fig. 7**).[23]

CT

The main role of CT in the postoperative spine is assessment after instrumentation or fusion surgery. At present, CT with multiplanar reconstruction is considered the modality of choice for imaging bony detail and assessing osseous formation and implant position despite artifact formation (**Fig. 8**). CT is also useful in showing the spinal canal and its alignment and is capable of detecting infection and pseudarthrosis.[18] Helical CT scans are useful for detecting and grading spinal and/or foraminal stenosis and can be used in the follow-up of stenosis after surgery. CT after intravenous contrast enhancement provides reliable differentiation between postoperative extradural fibrosis (scarring) and recurrent disk herniation.[24–26] Braun and colleagues[27] reported on a group of 98 postoperative patients, 22 of whom underwent re-exploration, and evaluated enhanced and unenhanced CT scans. CT scans with contrast enhancement were correct 74% of the time compared with surgery, whereas unenhanced CT scans were correct only 43% of the time. The investigators concluded that enhanced CT scans significantly increase the diagnostic accuracy in differentiating between scarring and recurrent disk herniation.

A limitation of CT scans is the beam-hardening artifact caused by the metallic prosthesis, which causes difficulty in soft tissue interpretation in the spinal canal.[28] Artifacts are the primary disadvantage of CT, although they are less common with titanium implants than with stainless steel because of the lower beam attenuation coefficient of titanium.[4] The x-ray beam should be positioned perpendicular to the orthopedic implant

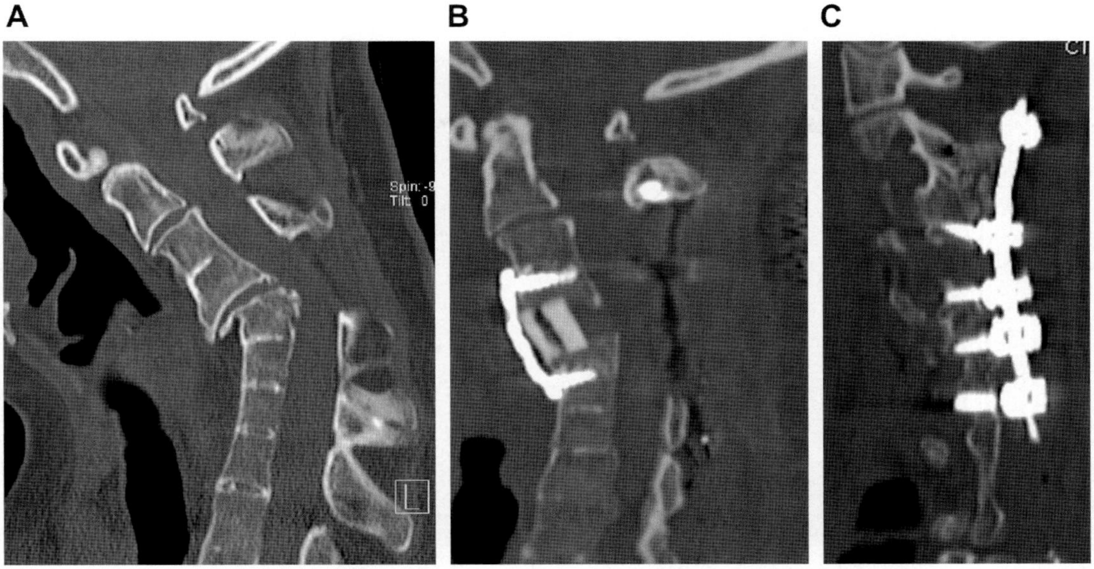

Fig. 8. A sagittal CT image in a 47-year-old woman with kyphosis and myelopathy demonstrates autofusion of C3-4 as well as C5 through the visualized levels of the thoracic spine consistent with ankylosing spondylitis. (*A*) At the C4-5 level, there is marked kyphotic deformity resulting in severe central canal stenosis. Postoperative CT sagittal images (*B*, *C*) show marked interval improvement in cervical kyphosis, partial C4 and C5 corpectomy and diskectomy with graft placement and anterior instrumentation from C4 to C6. Bilateral laminectomies from C3 to C6 with posterior spinal instrumentation from C2 to C7 are seen.

so that the beam traverses the metallic cross section with the smallest diameter.

Several factors can help reduce metallic artifact:

- During image acquisition
  1. Use of high peak voltage (kilovolts peak)
  2. Use of high tube current (milliampere-seconds)
  3. Use of narrow collimation
  4. Use of thin sections
- During image reconstruction
  1. Use of thick sections
  2. Use of lower kernel values.

The term kilovolt peak pertains to voltage across the tube, from anode to cathode, or the speed at which the electrons travel during x-ray production. Kilovoltage affects the penetrating ability of the x-ray beam or the average wavelength of the photon. Milliampere-seconds corresponds to the amount of energy used to create certain amounts of radiation. Reconstruction parameters can be expressed as standard (soft tissue) or high spatial (bone) frequency algorithms. Kernels (algorithms) are the reconstruction parameters that determine the image quality. As the kernel number increases, the image gets sharper and noisier. The high spatial frequency algorithms correspond to the higher kernel numbers.

CT provides better evaluation of fusion progression and status than dynamic radiography for patients who have undergone interbody fusion for lumbar spinal disorders.[29]

The use of myelography and postmyelography CT for the evaluation of patients with spinal abnormalities has been largely supplanted by the noninvasive modality magnetic resonance (MR) imaging. Despite this trend, myelography and postmyelography CT continue to play an important role in patients who have undergone a spine operation when MR imaging is contraindicated and in cases in which artifacts from surgical hardware may obscure the spinal canal and nerve roots on MR imaging (**Fig. 9**).[30]

Myelography can be helpful in depicting arachnoiditis, with thickening of the nerve roots causing blunting of the root sleeves. Commonly, myelography and postmyelographic CT show nonspecific extradural defects at the surgical sites, but these studies cannot differentiate recurrent disk herniations from scar. Postmyelographic CT is, however, outstanding at defining the degree of facet arthrosis and subsequent foraminal stenosis Sagittal and coronal reconstructions of thin, overlapping axial acquisitions can exquisitely define the neural foramina.[31]

MR Imaging

MR imaging is the preferred imaging modality in the evaluation of the postoperative spine because

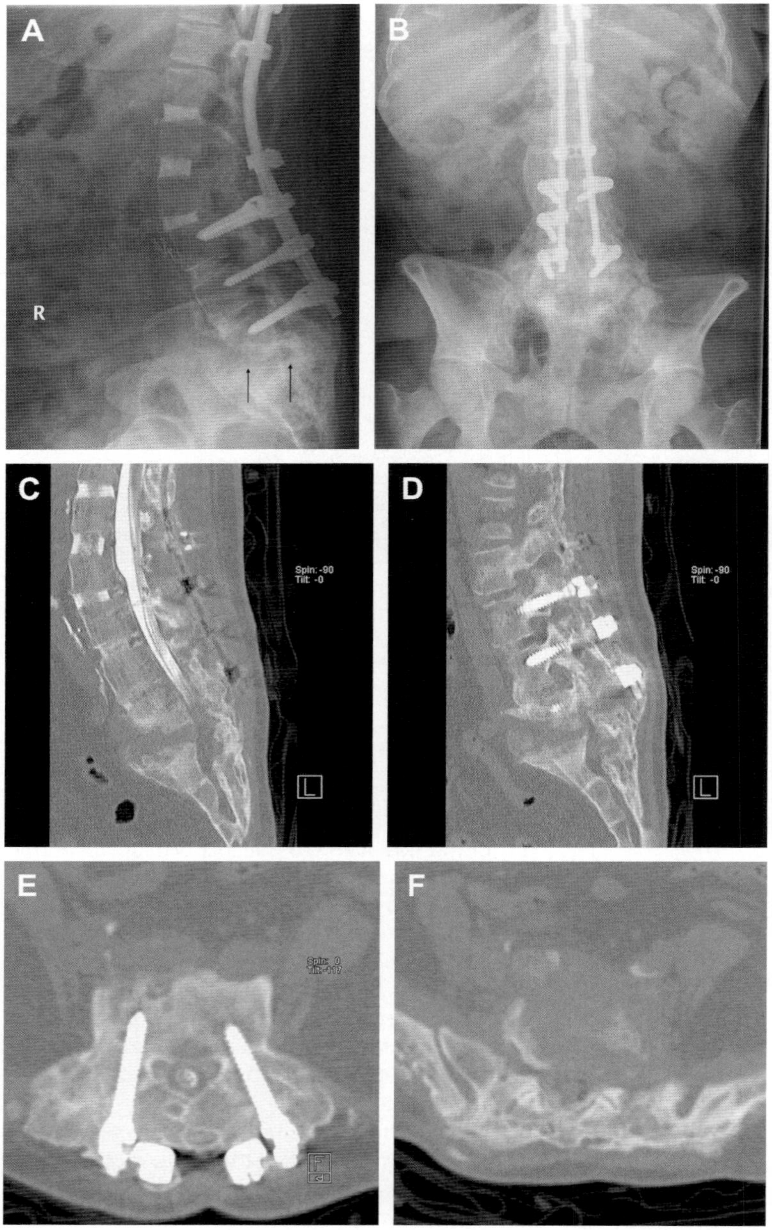

Fig. 9. CT myelography. This 71-year-old woman has undergone multiple spine surgeries and has an instrumented fusion from the upper thoracic region to L5. She presents with bilateral leg pain in an L5 radicular distribution. Radiographs (*A, B*) show lucency with surrounding sclerosis at the L5 level (*arrows in A*). CT myelography sagittal reconstructions (*C, D*) reveal a pseudarthrosis at L5 with Charcot or infectious features. Culture results were negative. Despite the instrumentation, the thecal sac is well demonstrated; it is patent at the L5 vertebral level (*E*) but obliterated at the L5 disk level (*F*).

of its superior soft tissue resolution.[32] Tissue enhancement is better evaluated on MR imaging than on CT,[33] allowing easier discrimination between recurrent disk herniation versus epidural fibrosis. Evaluation of bone marrow edema, soft tissue inflammation, nerve root enhancement, hemorrhage, facet joint inflammation, and spinal stenosis is much more accurate with MR imaging than CT or radiography. The high contrast between foraminal or epidural fat and disk material or osteophyte, coupled with multiplanar imaging, allows for accurate assessment of herniations and stenosis in the lumbar and cervical spine.[34,35]

In the past, MR imaging had limited use in imaging the instrumented spine because of commonly seen artifacts. However, with the introduction of the titanium pedicle screws and specialized pulse sequences, there has been considerable improvement in the MR imaging evaluation of the postoperative spine.[36–38]

The parameters used to reduce metal artifact in MR imaging are[39–41]

- Positioning the patient with the long axis of metallic hardware parallel to B_0 (B_0 is the constant, homogenous magnetic field used to polarize spins, creating magnetization. It can refer to both the direction and magnitude of the field. The direction of B_0 defines the longitudinal axis.)
- Using the optimum sequence, that is, a fast-spin echo sequence (to maintain short echo spacing rather than a short echo train)
- Using inversion recovery fat suppression
- Swapping phase and frequency encoding direction[42]
- Using view-angle tilting
- Increasing the readout bandwidth
- Decreasing the voxel size.

For routine imaging of the postoperative spine, sagittal and axial MR images are usually obtained. In the sagittal plane, T1- and T2-weighted images offer complementary information. Sagittal and axial T2-weighted images can depict the contour of the thecal sac and visualize focal areas of posterior expansion or for regions of compression of the thecal sac by scar tissue or recurrent/residual disk fragments. Axial T1-weighted images are useful for assessing the absence of osseous structures. Also, the normal epidural fat is very bright on T1-weighted images and contrasts well with the dural sac, as well as postoperative epidural fibrosis, which are dark. Additional axial spin echo T1-weighted images after enhancement with intravenous gadolinium are essential in postoperative studies because they can differentiate between scar tissue and recurrent disk herniation[43]; the latter is generally accepted to be a possible indication for additional surgery.[44]

In the immediate postoperative period, expected postdiskectomy changes cause significant alterations in the epidural soft tissue and intervertebral disk; caution must be used in interpreting MR imaging within the first 6 weeks after surgery. MR imaging may be used in the immediate postoperative period for a more gross view of the thecal sac and epidural space to exclude substantial postoperative hemorrhage at the laminectomy site, pseudomeningocele, or disk space infection. T1-weighted images show increased soft tissue signal anterior to the thecal sac and an indistinct posterior annular margin, which can mimic the appearance of preoperative disk herniation and produce mass effect. These changes within the anterior epidural space gradually involute 2 to 6 months after surgery.[45–47]

Other Modalities

Radionuclide scans are used mainly in the postoperative spine to evaluate for conditions such as pseudarthrosis, infection, or fracture of the fusion site, as well as an altered pattern of biomechanical stresses after a fusion.[48] Radionuclide scans may remain positive for 1 year or more in the region of the operative bed and instrumentation. In recent years, positron emission tomography has been useful for evaluating infection in the region of metal implants.[49]

Sonography is used to detect fluid collections and abscesses in the postoperative spinal fusion.[11]

(Tags: radiography, computed tomography, MR imaging, myelography).

POSTOPERATIVE COMPLICATIONS

Imaging plays a vital role in evaluating potential complications resulting from procedures that involve spinal instrumentation. The type of complication varies with the type of instrumentation, operative approach, and underlying clinical disorder.

Implant-Related Complications

Implant fractures generally occur secondary to metal fatigue from the repetitive stress of spinal movements. The fractured appliance may not be displaced, making its detection difficult. A fractured or dislodged appliance is frequently, but not always, associated with regional motion and instability, which may lead to or be the result of pseudarthrosis.[17] Prominence of the instrumentation can cause chronic tissue irritation, leading to pain, bursa formation, and even pressure sores with tissue necrosis, which occasionally can be indications for hardware removal (**Fig. 10**).

The pedicle screw is a commonly used implant that provides stabilization for posterior thoracolumbar fusion procedures. Screw placement is considered optimal when it traverses the central aspect of the pedicle and is aligned parallel to the superior end plate (neutral position).[4] Careful attention should be paid to pedicle screws because of their close proximity to neurovascular structures. Potential complications of the pedicle screw are fracture and abnormal screw orientation. The most common clinical complications are nerve root irritation (secondary to excessive medial angulation of the screw) and violation of the medial bony cortex.[50] Lateral position or migration should be carefully evaluated, especially in the cervical spine where the screw can breach the foramen transversarium and potentially damage the vertebral artery.

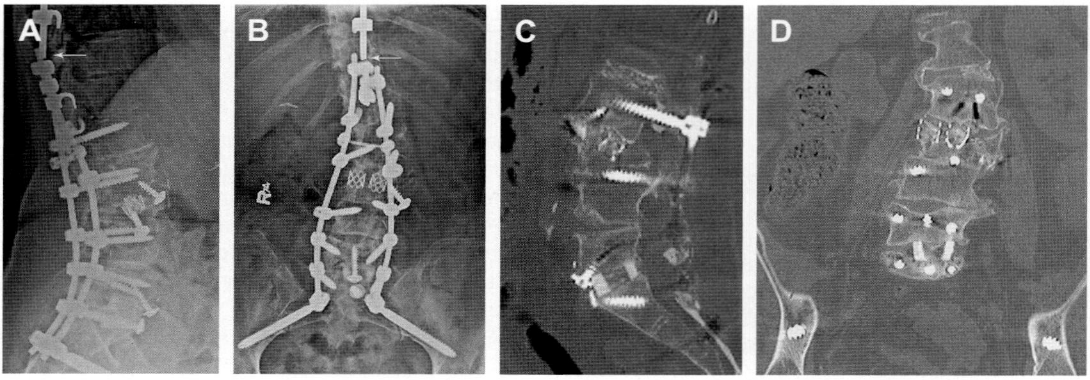

Fig. 10. Lateral (*A*) and AP (*B*) radiographs showing a rod fracture in a 68-year-old woman. Posterior segmental instrumentation is seen with hooks and pedicle screws connected by rods extending from the thoracic spine to the pelvis with transiliac screws. The rod is fractured at the level of T11-T12 (*arrow*). An intervertebral cage device at L2-L3 with moderate bridging bone is seen. Sagittal (*C*) and coronal sections (*D*) show incomplete bridging bone through the spacer, which is less than 25% of the cross-sectional diameter. At L5-S1, there is an intervertebral allograft held in place by anterior instrumentation; it appears well incorporated and fused.

Implant loosening can be caused by osseous resorption surrounding screws and implants. Loosening in turn allows movement, which causes further osseous resorption, increased mobility, and eventually catastrophic screw pullout or vertebral fractures.[51]

Restoration of disk height and achievement of anterior fusion are the major goals of interbody spinal surgery, and for this purpose, interbody spacers are used. Radiopaque markers are designed to allow sequential monitoring of cage position in otherwise radiolucent implants. Some degree of subsidence is expected and may facilitate fusion with the bone graft being loaded under compression. However, excessive subsidence leads to loss of disk height and may cause recurrent radicular symptoms secondary to foraminal height loss. Cage subsidence (defined as a migration of >3 mm into the adjacent vertebra) and lateral displacement are disadvantages of mesh and stand-alone cages (**Fig. 11**).[52–54]

Adjacent Segment Disease

Adjacent segment disease, or junctional stenosis, are terms used to designate the development of new clinical symptoms that correlate with radiographic changes adjacent to the level of previous spinal fusion.[55] Premature degenerative changes at the disk levels above or below the fused segments can occur because of the reduced number of mobile segments. This complication is reported in 10.2% of patients with posterior fusion and instrumentation[56] and even more frequently at long-term follow-up. It is more common in the lumbosacral spine than in the cervical spine, and it is rare in isolated thoracic fusion. It is markedly more common in the segment above the fusion because the rostral spine is levered against the fused caudal segment below (**Fig. 12**).

Stenosis

Stenosis may present years after a surgical procedure as a result of accelerated degeneration. It is best diagnosed with MR imaging. Bony stenosis may show a variety of changes on MR imaging because of the variability of the marrow content of the vertebral body and bony fusion masses and the degree of bony sclerosis. Sclerotic bone has low signal intensity on T1- and T2-weighted images and is recognized by the encroachment on the epidural and foraminal fat. Parasagittal images are most useful in defining bony foraminal stenosis, whether secondary to osteophyte formation or, more generally, secondary to disk degeneration.

Pseudarthrosis

Failure of fusion and the development of pseudarthrosis or fibrous union are the sequelae of ongoing low-grade mobility. Pseudarthrosis itself can be a source of pain, or it may provide a lead point for ongoing mobility leading to increased stress on hardware and inevitable failure. Radiographs should be evaluated for the presence of a lucent line or zone traversing the bone graft material with or without adjacent sclerosis. It is more common to use external braces than internal fixation. In asymptomatic patients, intervention may be deferred, and the patient's condition should be followed up.[57]

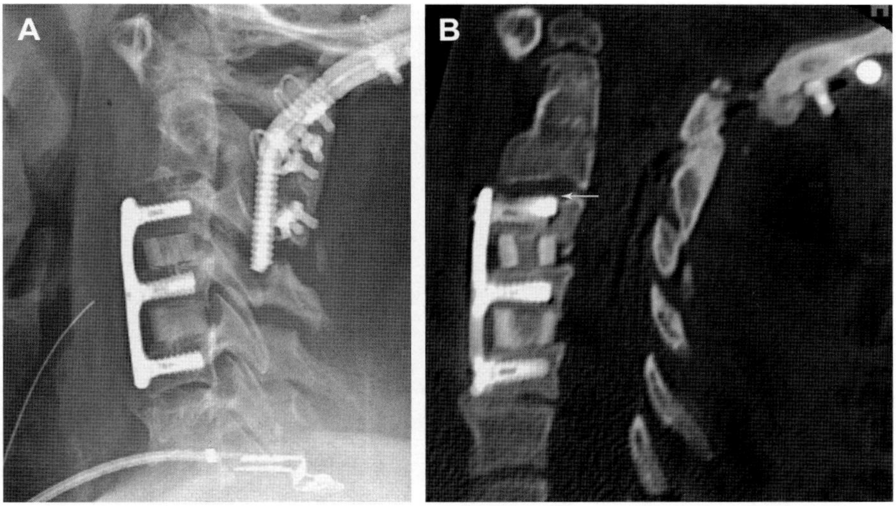

Fig. 11. (*A*) Lateral radiograph of a 27-year-old man after anterior fusion with screws and plate at C3-4 and C4-5 with interbody spacers placed at the C3-4 and C4-5 levels. 1.3-cm of soft tissue swelling anterior to the cervical spine is noted, which resolved. Soft tissue drain in the left anterior neck is seen. Healed posterior fusion from occiput to C3 with rod and cerclage wires is noted. (*B*) Six-month postoperative CT sagittal section scan shows anterior cervical diskectomy and fusion from C3 to C5. There are intervertebral disk spacers at C3-4 and C-5. The C3 anterior vertebral body screw enters into the C2-3 disk space (*arrow*). Superior migration of the anterior fusion plate is seen secondary to subsidence at the C3-4 level.

Complications Associated with the Type of Approach

In the cervical spine, complications of the posterior approach are mainly neurologic and include dural, nerve root, or cord injury. The anterior approach is associated with risks of injuring the vascular structures and damage to the recurrent laryngeal nerve or soft tissues, such as the esophagus, trachea, or lungs. In anterior plate and screw fixation, the screws may back out and impinge upon soft tissue structures or overpenetrate the posterior cortex and impinge on the cord. These complications can be minimized by using a cervical spine locking plate with screw caps and confirming screw position and length with intraoperative fluoroscopy.

Similarly, in the thoracolumbar spine, vascular injuries are more common with anterior procedures and neural injury is more common with the posterior approach. In addition, the use of iliac crest autograft carries with it the potential for donor site morbidity.[58]

Epidural Fibrosis and Recurrent Disk Herniation

Patients with recurrent disk herniation have complaints similar to those with primary disk herniation. Radiographs can be obtained to rule out other causes of back or sciatic pain, such as spondylolisthesis, fracture, and stenosis. Iatrogenic fracture through the pars interarticularis caused by previous laminectomy must be excluded. MRI is the imaging modality of choice to differentiate recurrent disk herniation from other soft tissue disease processes.[58] It is also very important to differentiate recurrent disk herniation from epidural fibrosis or scar formation. Recurrent disk herniation often presents as a polypoidal mass with smooth margins, has low signal on T1- and T2-weighted images, and shows no early enhancement after contrast administration. Epidural scar has intermediate signal intensity with irregular margins and shows early heterogeneous enhancement because of its vascularity.[59] A recent recurrent disk herniation initially shows no enhancement because it is devoid of any vascularization. However, it may be surrounded by epidural fibrosis that does show enhancement. Contrast material diffuses from the epidural scar into the disk material causing mild enhancement from outside in, late after contrast injection. Therefore, images after gadolinium administration should be acquired as quickly as possible (**Fig. 13**).[1] Exuberant epidural fibrosis is itself a risk factor for persistent radiculitis even in the absence of recurrent disk herniation.

Postoperative Infection

Postoperative infection may be the result of implantation at the time of surgery, or it may occur

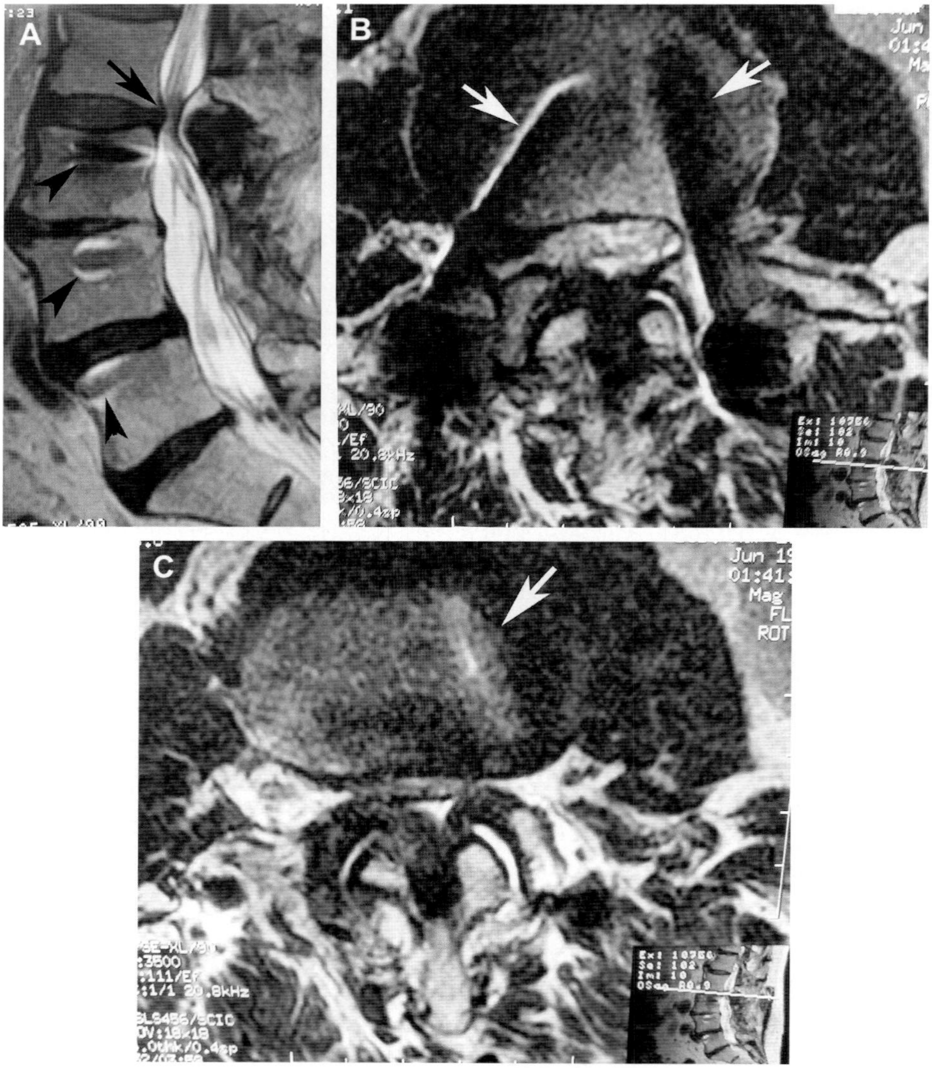

Fig. 12. Junctional lumbar stenosis above a previous instrumented fusion. (*A*) A sagittal T2-weighted image shows junctional stenosis (*arrow*) at the L2-3 level in a patient who has undergone prior L3-5 laminectomy and instrumented fusion. Note the minimal artifact from the pedicle screws (*arrowheads*). (*B*) An axial T2-weighted image at the level of the L3 pedicle screws shows moderate-severe stenosis and pedicle screw artifacts (*arrows*). Note the presence of the pedicle screws obscures the region of the lateral recess and foramen but does not prevent the evaluation of the central canal. (*C*) An axial T2-weighted image at the level of the L2-3 disk shows severe stenosis and only minimal residual artifact (*arrow*) from the pedicle screw below this level in the L3 vertebral body. Note the localizing sagittal image seen as an inset with each axial image (*B, C*). (*Reprinted from* Okubadejo GO, Daftary AR, Buchowski JM, et al. The lumbar and thoracic spine. In: MRI for orthopaedic surgeons. New York: Thieme; 2010. p. 309; Fig. 11.46; with permission.)

later in the course of recovery. Infection leads to bone destruction and resorption around the implant. On imaging, a lucent area around the implant implies a loose appliance and potential infection. Image-guided aspiration can be used to isolate the microorganisms. Radionuclide scans and MR imaging can be helpful in detecting infection in the early stages.[50] On MR imaging scans, the key features that point toward the presence of infection are the presence of peridiscal marrow changes (low signal intensity on T1-weighted images and high signal intensity on T2-weighted images), enhancement of the intervertebral disk space, and an enhancing soft tissue mass surrounding the affected spinal level in the perivertebral and epidural spaces.[60]

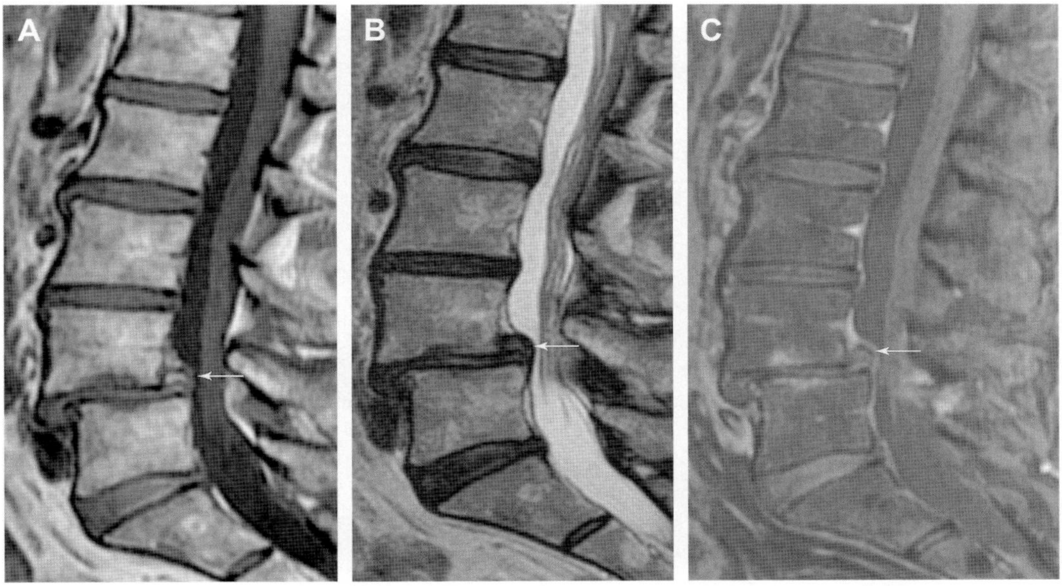

Fig. 13. For this 55-year-old woman, (*A*) a sagittal T1-weighted image (repetition time/echo time: 650/10.1), (*B*) a sagittal T2-weighted image (repetition time/echo time: 3600/121), and (*C*) a sagittal T1-weighted postcontrast image (repetition time/echo time: 550/10.1) show a soft tissue mass (*arrows*) with only peripheral enhancement in the anterior epidural space at the L4–L5 level. It is suggestive of recurrent disk herniation.

Arachnoiditis

Potential factors leading to arachnoiditis are the surgical procedure itself, the presence of intradural blood after surgery, treated perioperative spinal infection, and the previous use of myelographic contrast media. CT myelography and MR imaging can be used to diagnose these complications; however, MR imaging is superior and considered the imaging modality of choice. The 3 MR imaging patterns described in adhesive arachnoiditis are scattered groups of matted or "clumped" nerve roots, an "empty" thecal sac caused by adhesion of the nerve roots to its walls, and an intrathecal soft tissue "mass" with a broad dural base, representing a large group of matted roots that may obstruct the cerebrospinal fluid pathways. In most cases, there is little enhancement of arachnoiditis with gadolinium on MR imaging scans (**Fig. 14**).[61]

Sterile Radiculitis

On MR imaging scans, sterile radiculitis is seen as enhancement of the intrathecal spinal nerve roots of the cauda equina after contrast administration because a breach in the blood-nerve barrier occurs as a sequel to chronic neural trauma and ischemia. It is believed to be the cause of the abnormal neurophysiologic changes resulting in clinical radiculopathy that may continue long after the disk herniation has been surgically removed. It can extend cranially and caudally away from the surgical site in the chronic postoperative period (more than 6–8 months after the surgery).[62]

Postoperative Fluid Collections

Pseudomeningocele, a fairly common postoperative finding, results from a tear in the dura during the surgery. It is located posterior to the thecal sac and projects through posterior element surgical deformities. Pseudomeningoceles can be complex in signal intensity on MR imaging scans secondary to hemorrhage, and fluid-fluid levels can be present. In chronic cases, the fluid collection should follow cerebrospinal fluid on all sequences; however, the fluid signal characteristics can differ, depending on the amount of protein or blood (**Fig. 15**).[31]

Hematoma or seroma can also be formed in the epidural space or in the postoperative bed in the soft tissue posterior to the thecal sac. MR imaging is most sensitive in identifying the blood products. Hematomas may be hyperintense on T1-weighted images in the subacute phase because the signal is caused primarily by methemoglobin. Pure seroma should follow cerebrospinal fluid on all pulse sequences. Sterile fluid collections should resolve slowly over time; however, needle aspiration is necessary to rule out secondary infection (**Fig. 16**).

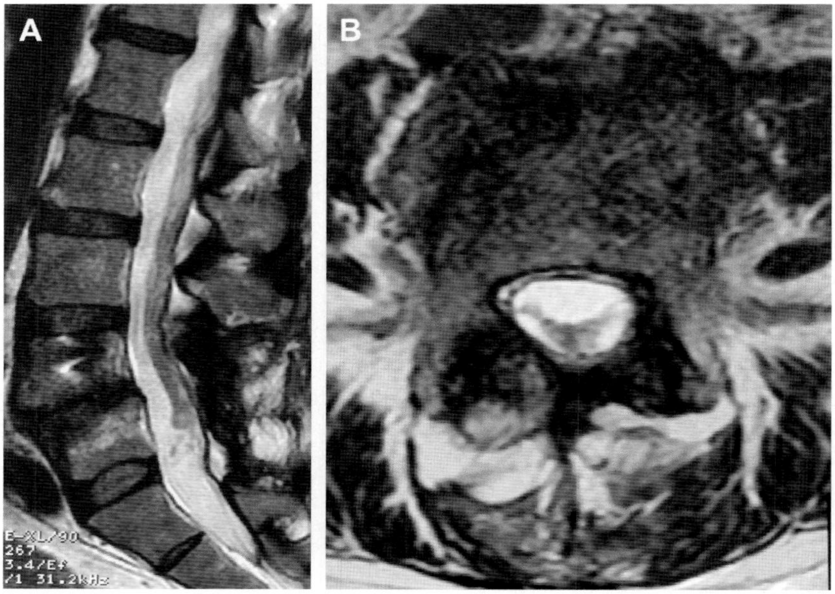

Fig. 14. Sagittal (*A*) and axial (*B*) T2-weighted images of a patient with arachnoiditis after L4-5 laminectomy and instrumented posterior fusion who had several previous decompressive surgeries. Note the central adhesion of the nerve roots within the thecal sac into a central clump of soft tissue signal (pseudocord) instead of their normal feathery appearance. The axial image (*B*) is at the L4-5 level. (*Reprinted from* Okubadejo GO, Daftary AR, Buchowski JM, et al. The lumbar and thoracic spine. In: MRI for orthopaedic surgeons. New York: Thieme; 2010. p. 312; Fig. 11.50; with permission.)

Miscellaneous

Ossification of the anterior longitudinal ligament and facet disease are common complications of anterior plating and posterior screw fixation.[5,11] Anterior plating can result in impingement of the adjacent segment vertebral body during flexion, contributing to adjacent segment disease. This complication can be avoided by selecting a plate length that results in the end of the plate being equal to or greater than 5 mm from the vertebral

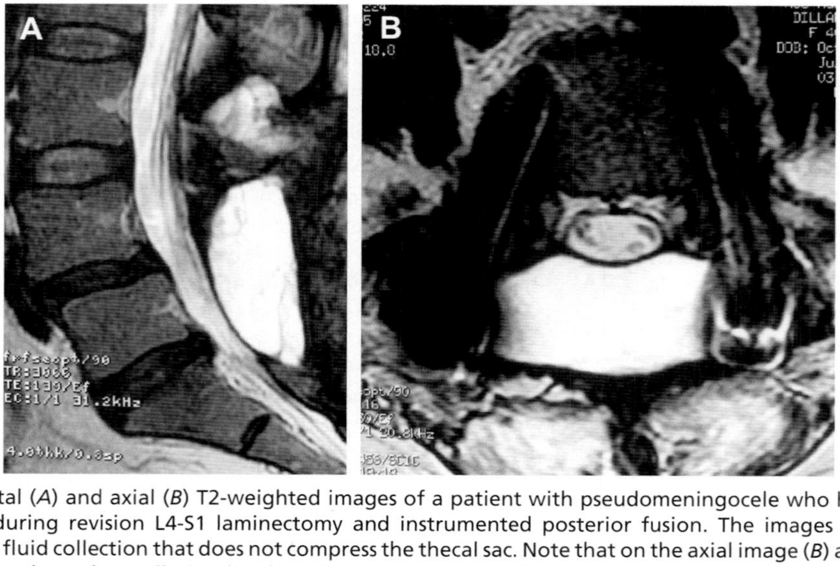

Fig. 15. Sagittal (*A*) and axial (*B*) T2-weighted images of a patient with pseudomeningocele who had sustained a durotomy during revision L4-S1 laminectomy and instrumented posterior fusion. The images show a well-circumscribed fluid collection that does not compress the thecal sac. Note that on the axial image (*B*) at the L5 level, the central canal can be well visualized in the presence of pedicle screws. (*Reprinted from* Okubadejo GO, Daftary AR, Buchowski JM, et al. The lumbar and thoracic spine. In: MRI for orthopaedic surgeons. New York: Thieme; 2010. p. 312; Fig. 11.49; with permission.)

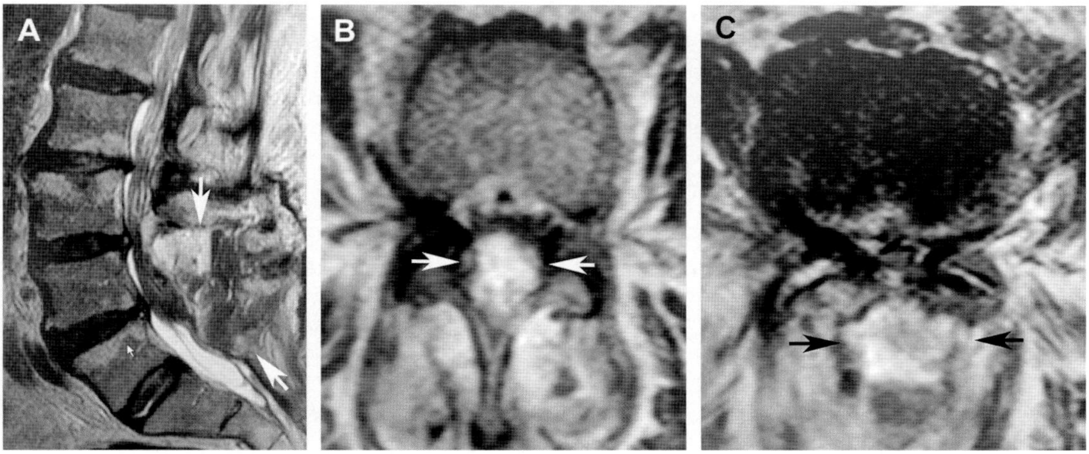

Fig. 16. (*A*) A sagittal T2-weighted image shows a large and compressive fluid collection (*between arrows*) at the L3-5 level in a patient with postoperative lumbar epidural hematoma after revision L4-5 laminectomies. Axial T2-weighted images at L3-4 (*B*) and L4-5 (*C*) levels show the hematoma (*between arrows on each*) and the associated compression of the thecal sac. (*Reprinted from* Okubadejo GO, Daftary AR, Buchowski JM, et al. The lumbar and thoracic spine. In: MRI for orthopaedic surgeons. New York: Thieme; 2010. p. 311; Fig. 11.48; with permission.)

margin.[63] Preservation of the facet capsule and avoidance of violating the adjacent segment facet joint during posterior instrumentation helps to minimize the potential for facet degeneration.

(Tags: complications, postoperative spine, imaging).

SUMMARY

Despite advances in imaging technology, imaging of the postoperative spine remains a challenging and difficult issue. Adequate understanding of various surgical techniques and instruments, coupled with an appropriate awareness of the possible complications, is vital when interpreting postoperative studies. To evaluate the postoperative spine optimally, it is essential that the radiologist knows the potential advantages and disadvantages of the various modalities.

REFERENCES

1. Van Goethem JW, Parizel PM, Jinkins JR. Review article: MRI of the postoperative lumbar spine. Neuroradiology 2002;44:723–39.
2. Okubadejo GO, Daftary AR, Buchowski JM, et al. The lumbar and thoracic spine. In: Khanna AJ, editor. MRI for orthopaedic surgeons. New York: Thieme; 2010. p. 269–315.
3. Hayeri MR, Tehranzadeh J. Diagnostic imaging of spinal fusion and complications. Appl Radiol 2009; 38:14–28.
4. Rutherford EE, Tarplett LJ, Davies EM, et al. Lumbar spine fusion and stabilization: hardware, techniques, and imaging appearances. Radiographics 2007;27:1737–49.
5. Slone RM, MacMillan M, Montgomery WJ. Spinal fixation. Part 1. Principles, basic hardware, and fixation techniques for the cervical spine. Radiographics 1993;13:341–56.
6. Slone RM, MacMillan M, Montgomery WJ, et al. Spinal fixation. Part 2. Fixation techniques and hardware for the thoracic and lumbosacral spine. Radiographics 1993;13:521–43.
7. Roy-Camille R, Saillant G, Mazel C. Internal fixation of the lumbar spine with pedicle screw plating. Clin Orthop Relat Res 1986;203:7–17.
8. Steffee AD, Brantigan JW. The variable screw placement spinal fixation system. Report of a prospective study of 250 patients enrolled in Food and Drug Administration clinical trials. Spine (Phila Pa 1976) 1993;18:1160–72.
9. Brantigan JW, Steffee AD. A carbon fiber implant to aid interbody lumbar fusion. Two-year clinical results in the first 26 patients. Spine (Phila Pa 1976) 1993; 18:2106–17.
10. Murtagh RD, Quencer RM, Castellvi AE, et al. New techniques in lumbar spinal instrumentation: what the radiologist needs to know. Radiology 2011;260: 317–30.
11. Slone RM, MacMillan M, Montgomery WJ. Spinal fixation. Part 3. Complications of spinal instrumentation. Radiographics 1993;13:797–816.
12. Oskouian RJ Jr, Johnson JP. Vascular complications in anterior thoracolumbar spinal reconstruction. J Neurosurg 2002;96:1–5.
13. McAfee PC. Interbody fusion cages in reconstructive operations on the spine. J Bone Joint Surg Am 1999;81:859–80.

14. Min JH, Jang JS, Lee SH. Comparison of anterior- and posterior-approach instrumented lumbar interbody fusion for spondylolisthesis. J Neurosurg Spine 2007;7:21–6.
15. Ekman P, Moller H, Tullberg T, et al. Posterior lumbar interbody fusion versus posterolateral fusion in adult isthmic spondylolisthesis. Spine (Phila Pa 1976) 2007;32:2178–83.
16. Murtagh RD, Quencer RM, Cohen DS, et al. Normal and abnormal imaging findings in lumbar total disk replacement: devices and complications. Radiographics 2009;29:105–18.
17. Venu V, Vertinsky AT, Malfair D, et al. Plain radiograph assessment of spinal hardware. Semin Musculoskelet Radiol 2011;15:151–62.
18. Berquist TH. Imaging of the postoperative spine. Radiol Clin North Am 2006;44:407–18.
19. Lonstein JE, Denis F, Perra JH, et al. Complications associated with pedicle screws. J Bone Joint Surg Am 1999;81:1519–28.
20. Zdeblick TA. The treatment of degenerative lumbar disorders. A critical review of the literature. Spine (Phila Pa 1976) 1995;20:126S–37S.
21. Whitecloud TS, Skalley TC, Cook SD, et al. Roentgenographic measurement of pedicle screw penetration. Clin Orthop Relat Res 1989;245:57–68.
22. Ray CD. Threaded fusion cages for lumbar interbody fusions. An economic comparison with 360-degree fusions. Spine (Phila Pa 1976) 1997;22:681–5.
23. Marshman LA, Trewhella M, Friesem T, et al. The accuracy and validity of "routine" X-rays in estimating lumbar disc arthroplasty placement. Spine (Phila Pa 1976) 2007;32:E661–6.
24. Cecchini A, Garbagna P, Martelli A, et al. CT of postoperative lumbar disk herniation. A multicenter study. Radiol Med 1988;75:565–76 [in Italian].
25. Kieffer SA, Witwer GA, Cacayorin ED, et al. Recurrent post-discectomy pain. CT–surgical correlation. Acta Radiol Suppl 1986;369:719–22.
26. Teplick JG, Haskin ME. Intravenous contrast-enhanced CT of the postoperative lumbar spine: improved identification of recurrent disk herniation, scar, arachnoiditis, and diskitis. AJR Am J Roentgenol 1984;143:845–55.
27. Braun IF, Hoffman JC Jr, Davis PC, et al. Contrast enhancement in CT differentiation between recurrent disk herniation and postoperative scar: prospective study. AJR Am J Roentgenol 1985;145:785–90.
28. Mall JC, Kaiser JA. The usual appearance of the postoperative lumbar spine. Radiographics 1987;7:245–69.
29. Williams AL, Gornet MF, Burkus JK. CT evaluation of lumbar interbody fusion: current concepts. AJNR Am J Neuroradiol 2005;26:2057–66.
30. Harreld JH, McMenamy JM, Toomay SM, et al. Myelography: a primer. Curr Probl Diagn Radiol 2011;40:149–57.
31. Ross JS. Magnetic resonance imaging of the postoperative spine. Semin Musculoskelet Radiol 2000;4:281–91.
32. Grane P. The post-operative lumbar spine. A radiological investigation of the lumbar spine after discectomy using MR imaging and CT. Acta Radiol Suppl 1998;39:2–11.
33. Bundschuh CV, Stein L, Slusser JH, et al. Distinguishing between scar and recurrent herniated disk in postoperative patients: value of contrast-enhanced CT and MR imaging. AJNR Am J Neuroradiol 1990;11:949–58.
34. Masaryk TJ, Modic MT, Geisinger MA, et al. Cervical myelopathy: a comparison of magnetic resonance and myelography. J Comput Assist Tomogr 1986;10:184–94.
35. Modic MT, Masaryk T, Boumphrey F, et al. Lumbar herniated disk disease and canal stenosis: prospective evaluation by surface coil MR, CT, and myelography. AJR Am J Roentgenol 1986;147:757–65.
36. Petersilge CA, Lewin JS, Duerk JL, et al. Optimizing imaging parameters for MR evaluation of the spine with titanium pedicle screws. AJR Am J Roentgenol 1996;166:1213–8.
37. Rudisch A, Kremser C, Peer S, et al. Metallic artifacts in magnetic resonance imaging of patients with spinal fusion. A comparison of implant materials and imaging sequences. Spine (Phila Pa 1976) 1998;23:692–9.
38. Viano AM, Gronemeyer SA, Haliloglu M, et al. Improved MR imaging for patients with metallic implants. Magn Reson Imaging 2000;18:287–95.
39. Lee MJ, Kim S, Lee SA, et al. Overcoming artifacts from metallic orthopedic implants at high-field-strength MR imaging and multi-detector CT. Radiographics 2007;27:791–803.
40. Suh JS, Jeong EK, Shin KH, et al. Minimizing artifacts caused by metallic implants at MR imaging: experimental and clinical studies. AJR Am J Roentgenol 1998;171:1207–13.
41. Vandevenne JE, Vanhoenacker FM, Parizel PM, et al. Reduction of metal artefacts in musculoskeletal MR imaging. JBR-BTR 2007;90:345–9.
42. Frazzini VI, Kagetsu NJ, Johnson CE, et al. Internally stabilized spine: optimal choice of frequency-encoding gradient direction during MR imaging minimizes susceptibility artifact from titanium vertebral body screws. Radiology 1997;204:268–72.
43. Jinkins JR, Van Goethem JW. The postsurgical lumbosacral spine. Magnetic resonance imaging evaluation following intervertebral disk surgery, surgical decompression, intervertebral bony fusion, and spinal instrumentation. Radiol Clin North Am 2001;39:1–29.
44. Suk KS, Lee HM, Moon SH, et al. Recurrent lumbar disc herniation: results of operative management. Spine (Phila Pa 1976) 2001;26:672–6.

45. Annertz M, Jonsson B, Stromqvist B, et al. Serial MRI in the early postoperative period after lumbar discectomy. Neuroradiology 1995;37:177–82.
46. Boden SD, Davis DO, Dina TS, et al. Contrast-enhanced MR imaging performed after successful lumbar disk surgery: prospective study. Radiology 1992;182:59–64.
47. Ross JS, Masaryk TJ, Modic MT, et al. Lumbar spine: postoperative assessment with surface-coil MR imaging. Radiology 1987;164:851–60.
48. Gates GF. SPECT bone scanning of the spine. Semin Nucl Med 1998;28:78–94.
49. Guhlmann A, Brecht-Krauss D, Suger G, et al. Chronic osteomyelitis: detection with FDG PET and correlation with histopathologic findings. Radiology 1998;206:749–54.
50. Young PM, Berquist TH, Bancroft LW, et al. Complications of spinal instrumentation. Radiographics 2007;27:775–89.
51. Tehranzadeh J, Ton JD, Rosen CD. Advances in spinal fusion. Semin Ultrasound CT MR 2005;26:103–13.
52. Barsa P, Suchomel P. Factors affecting sagittal malalignment due to cage subsidence in standalone cage assisted anterior cervical fusion. Eur Spine J 2007;16:1395–400.
53. Bartels RH, Donk RD, Feuth T. Subsidence of stand-alone cervical carbon fiber cages. Neurosurgery 2006;58:502–8.
54. Gercek E, Arlet V, Delisle J, et al. Subsidence of stand-alone cervical cages in anterior interbody fusion: warning. Eur Spine J 2003;12:513–6.
55. Lee CS, Hwang CJ, Lee SW, et al. Risk factors for adjacent segment disease after lumbar fusion. Eur Spine J 2009;18:1637–43.
56. Cho KJ, Suk SI, Park SR, et al. Complications in posterior fusion and instrumentation for degenerative lumbar scoliosis. Spine (Phila Pa 1976) 2007;32:2232–7.
57. Emami A, Deviren V, Berven S, et al. Outcome and complications of long fusions to the sacrum in adult spine deformity: Luque-Galveston, combined iliac and sacral screws, and sacral fixation. Spine (Phila Pa 1976) 2002;27:776–86.
58. Lee JK, Amorosa L, Cho SK, et al. Recurrent lumbar disk herniation. J Am Acad Orthop Surg 2010;18:327–37.
59. Babar S, Saifuddin A. MRI of the post-discectomy lumbar spine. Clin Radiol 2002;57:969–81.
60. Van Goethem JW, Parizel PM, van den Hauwe L, et al. The value of MRI in the diagnosis of postoperative spondylodiscitis. Neuroradiology 2000;42:580–5.
61. Ross JS, Masaryk TJ, Modic MT, et al. MR imaging of lumbar arachnoiditis. AJR Am J Roentgenol 1987;149:1025–32.
62. Jinkins JR, Roeder MB. MRI of benign lumbosacral nerve root enhancement. Semin Ultrasound CT MR 1993;14:446–54.
63. Park JB, Cho YS, Riew KD. Development of adjacent-level ossification in patients with an anterior cervical plate. J Bone Joint Surg Am 2005;87:558–63.

Imaging of Spine Neoplasm

John T. Wald, MD

KEYWORDS

• Spine • Neoplasm • Tumor • Pain • Intramedullary • Intradural • Innervation • MRI • CT

KEY POINTS

- The typical clinical history of spinal tumors can help direct advanced imaging in the evaluation of spinal pain syndromes.
- Innervation of the spine includes the ventral ramus, dorsal ramus, recurrent meningeal nerve, and the sensory fibers that course with the sympathetic nerves.
- Seventy-five percent of vertebral body lesions are malignant, whereas benign lesions predominate in the posterior elements (70%).
- Two-thirds of all spinal column lesions in children (<18) are benign, but this figure is reversed in adults.
- A multimodality approach (computed tomography, magnetic resonance imaging, positron emission tomography) is often necessary to define the characteristics and extent of extradural spine neoplasm.

The back and pain—these words have been linked since man began to walk upright. Although most often back pain is of benign origin, it can occasionally be a harbinger of a more serious spinal condition, including spine neoplasm. Knowledge of the typical clinical history of spinal tumors and an understanding of the innervation of the spine and surrounding supporting structures may allow us to better understand when to pursue advanced imaging in the evaluation of spinal pain syndromes.

Many radiologists have divided the differential diagnosis of neoplasms of the spine into compartments. These compartments include the extradural compartment, intradural/extramedullary compartment, and the intramedullary compartment. This division not only allows the clinician to evaluate neoplasms in a logical, concise manner but it also allows one to better understand the origin of pain associated with neoplasm based on the innervation of the spine and surrounding structures.

THE ORIGIN OF SPINE PAIN

There are 4 main sources of neural innervation to spinal structures: anterior primary division/ventral ramus, posterior primary division/dorsal ramus, recurrent meningeal nerve, and sensory fibers that course with the sympathetic nerves (**Fig. 1**).[1] The ventral ramus transmits afferent input from pain generators originating in the psoas muscles, intertransversarii muscles, quadratus lumborum muscle, and pain referred from the lumbar plexus.[1] Retroperitoneal tumors and tumors originating in the paraspinal soft tissues, including Ewing sarcoma, are possible pain generators in this region.

The dorsal ramus provides innervation to the deep muscles of the back, zygapophysial joints, interspinous ligaments, ligamentum flavum, and periosteum of the posterior vertebral arch. The recurrent meningeal (sinuvertebral nerve) nerve supplies the periosteum of the posterior vertebral body, epidural veins and basivertebral plexus, anterior epidural space, anterior spinal dura matter, and posterior longitudinal ligament.[1,2] There is sensory input from adjacent spinal levels, which can result in pain referred to adjacent spinal segments. The sympathetic trunk and the gray rami communicans innervate the periosteum of the anterior and lateral vertebral body, the intervertebral disks, and the anterior longitudinal ligament.[1]

Department of Radiology, Division of Neuroradiology, Mayo Clinic, 200 First Street Southwest, Rochester, MN 55901, USA
E-mail address: wald.john2@mayo.edu

Radiol Clin N Am 50 (2012) 749–776
doi:10.1016/j.rcl.2012.04.002

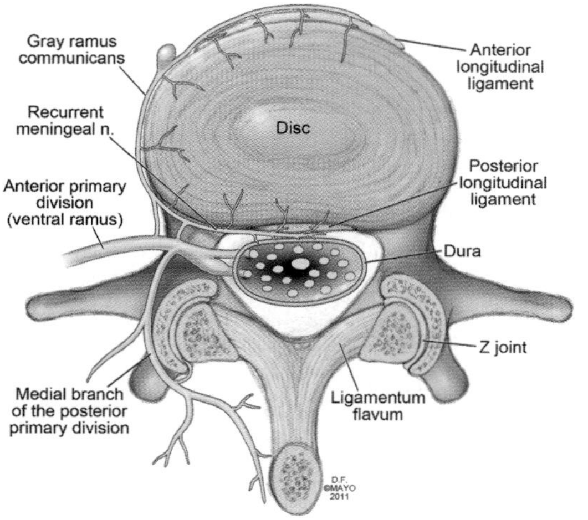

Fig. 1. Primary innervation of the spine and paraspinal soft tissues. Z, zygapophysial joint; n, nerve. (*Courtesy of* Mayo Clinic, Rochester, Minnesota; with permission.)

The interwoven relationship between the sympathetic trunk and the innervation of the anterior spinal structures can lead to pain syndromes characterized by the stimulation of the sympathetic system.[3]

Most neoplasms originating in the vertebral body and anterior paraspinal soft tissues will register pain through the ventral ramus, including branches of the sinuvertebral nerve and the gray rami communicates. Lesions in the vertebral body do not necessarily need to breech the periosteum to generate pain. Branches of the sinuvertebral nerve accompany basivertebral veins into the vertebral bodies and surround blood vessels in the spinal canal.[2] Thus, even small vertebral body lesions or spinal canal lesions can stimulate pain fibers.

Extradural Neoplasm

Axial pain is the most common presenting sign of extradural spinal tumors. Pain is more common (96%) and intense in malignant tumors compared with benign tumors (76%). Associated spinal cord compression is seen in 52% of malignant tumors, and greater than 90% of these patients will have pain.[4,5] Seventy-five percent of vertebral body lesions are malignant, whereas benign lesions predominate in the posterior elements (70%). Two-thirds of all spinal column lesions in children (<18 years of age) are benign, but this figure is reversed in adults.[5] Epidural tumors produce pain and dysfunction by compression, demyelination, ischemia, and tissue edema. The release of excitatory amino acids by injured neurons may promote further ischemia and pain.[6]

Metastatic Spine Disease

Autopsy studies have demonstrated an incidence of 30% to 90% of spinal metastasis in patients with a history of primary malignancy.[4] Metastasis to the spine most often involves the thoracic spine, followed by the lumbar and cervical spine.[7] Metastatic lesions to the spine are 3 to 4 times more common than primary spine neoplasms.[6] Virtually all patients with malignant epidural spinal cord compression present with pain. Fifty percent of patients presenting with epidural spinal cord compression do not carry a diagnosis of cancer at the time of presentation.[6]

Metastatic Spine Disease: Imaging

Magnetic resonance imaging (MRI) imaging is the preferred imaging modality in the evaluation of patients with suspected spinal metastasis. Metastatic disease is primarily a process of trabecular bone; radiography is a cortical bone imaging modality. There must be 50% to 75% bone destruction for plain radiographs to identify tumors.[4] Computed tomography (CT) scanning can demonstrate both lytic and blastic metastasis but lacks the sensitivity to identify marrow lesions, epidural tumor extension, and paraspinal or nerve root involvement (**Fig. 2**). Technetium (99mTc) bone scanning offers a high sensitivity for larger lesions, which typically involve bony cortex,[8] but it also lacks the specificity to define the extent of spinal bone involvement and the soft tissue extension of tumors. Single-photon emission CT (SPECT)/CT imaging improves specificity[9] but does not offer the lesion definition seen in MR imaging.

MR imaging with and without contrast allows imaging of the spine in one setting with greater sensitivity than bone scan for marrow-based lesions.[8] It can also delineate the soft tissue extension of neoplasm into the paraspinal and epidural soft tissues. The bilobed appearance or drawn-curtain sign of abnormal tissue within the ventral epidural space can be helpful in discriminating neoplasm from other pathological conditions in this location (**Fig. 3**).[10] Typical MR imaging multiplanar sequences include T1-weighted images with and without contrast and fast spin echo (FSE) T2 images, including fat saturation or short tau inversion recovery (STIR) techniques.[11] Inherent image contrast between low T1 signal tumor infiltration and high T1 marrow signal easily defines even subtle bone lesions without the use of intravenous contrast. Fat saturation and inversion recovery sequences are more helpful in defining tumors than simple FSE T2 sequences because the typical prolonged T2 signal of tumor infiltration blends into the prolonged T2 signal of marrow fat. By decreasing

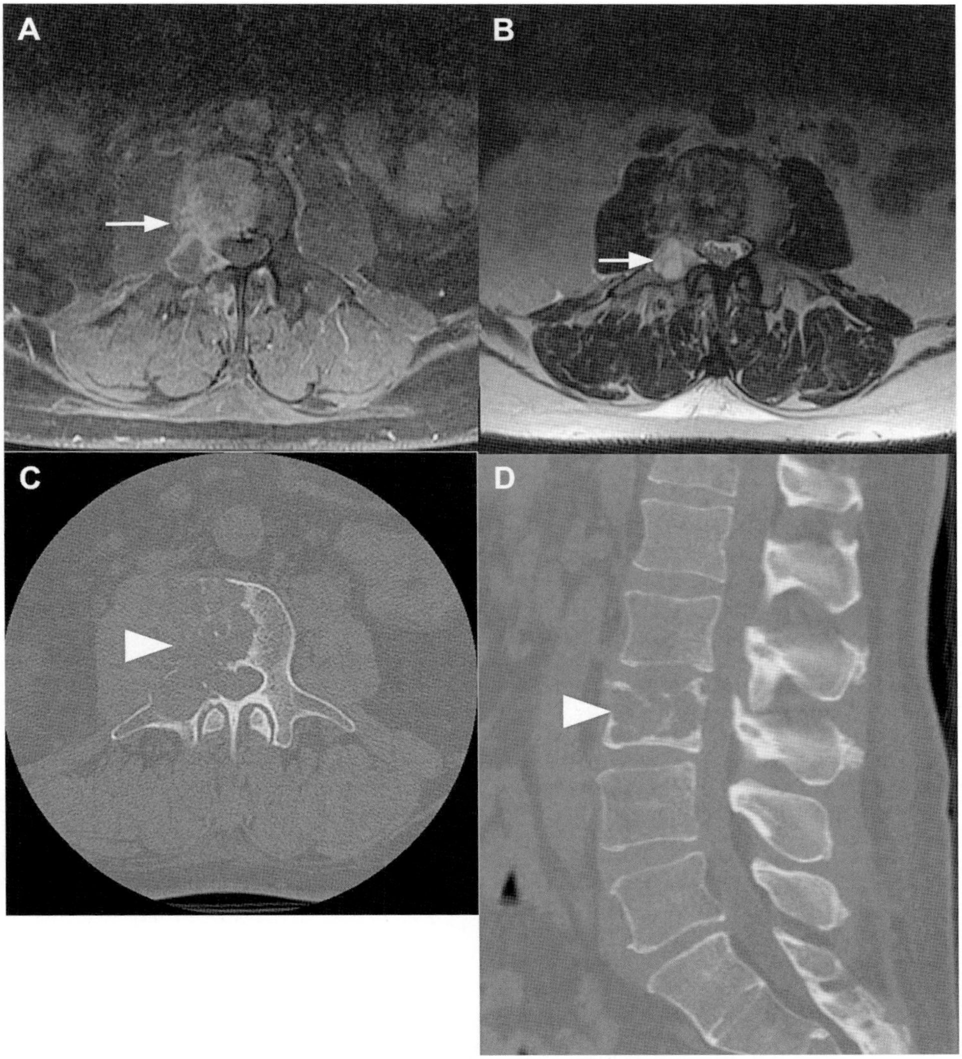

Fig. 2. A 50-year-old man with radicular back pain and weakness. Axial FSE T1 with contrast and fat saturation MR imaging sequence (*A*), and axial FSE T2 MR imaging sequence (*B*) demonstrate metastatic lesion within L3 (*arrows*). CT imaging, including axial image (*C*) and sagittal reformat image (*D*), defines lytic bone destruction (*arrow heads*) not clearly defined by MR imaging sequences.

the fat signal within the marrow, bone lesions are better defined (**Fig. 4**). Intravenous contrast is most helpful in imaging the soft tissue and epidural extension of metastatic lesions. Bone lesions typically enhance avidly. Therefore, after contrast administration, T1 sequences require fat-saturation techniques to maintain image/lesion contrast. The T1 shortening of tumors would be obscured by the short T1 of the marrow signal. Fat saturation allows the contrast-avid tumors to be defined on a low T1 background.

Primary Malignant Spine Tumors

Multiple myeloma

Multiple myeloma is a malignancy of monoclonal plasma cell proliferation in bone marrow. It is the second most common hematologic cancer, after non-Hodgkin's lymphoma, with an annual incidence of more than 50,000 cases in the United States.[12] The most common clinical symptoms at presentation include fatigue, bone pain, and recurrent infections. Bone pain is present at diagnosis in

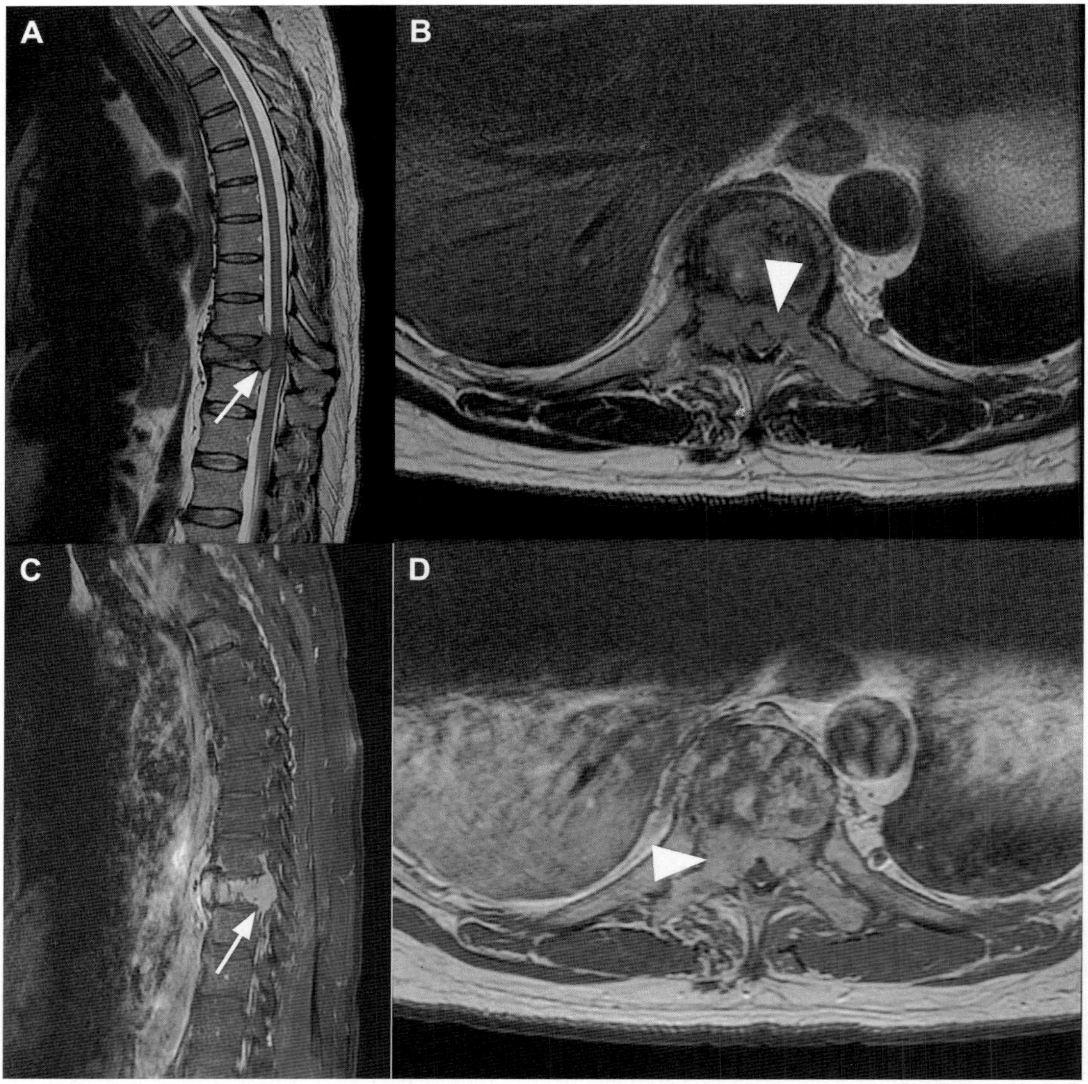

Fig. 3. A 59-year-old man with a several-month history of axial back pain and new-onset leg weakness and numbness. Pathologic compression fracture of T10 with epidural tumor extension, spinal cord compression (*arrow*), and drawn-curtain sign (*arrowhead*). (*A*) FSE T2 sagittal MR imaging sequence; (*B*) FSE T2 axial sequence; (*C*) FSE T1 plus fat saturation with contrast sagittal sequence; (*D*) FSE T1 plus fat saturation axial sequence with contrast.

58% of patients: mild in 29%, moderate in 20%, and severe in 9%. Pain had been present for 6 months or less in 73% of patients and for 12 months or less in 91% of patients in one review.[13] In approximately 5% of patients, the disease may manifest as a solitary plasmacytoma of bone, with a frequent site of presentation being the spine.[5] Two-thirds of these patients have been reported to go on to develop multiple myeloma.[5]

Myeloma imaging

Spine disease in multiple myeloma is characterized by diffuse osteopenia in 85% of cases and by multiple lytic lesions in 80% of cases. Twenty percent of patients do not manifest radiographic abnormalities.[14] Although standard bone scintigraphy has been reported to have a low sensitivity for multiple myeloma, fluorodeoxyglucose (FDG) positron emission tomography (PET) and 99mTc sestamibi have been demonstrated to be effective in the diagnosis and monitoring of bone disease.[15,16]

MR imaging is the preferred imaging modality for diagnosis. The abnormal T1 marrow pattern may be diffuse/speckled or focal. Lesion conspicuity is increased on T2 sequences by using fat saturation or STIR techniques. T1 images completed

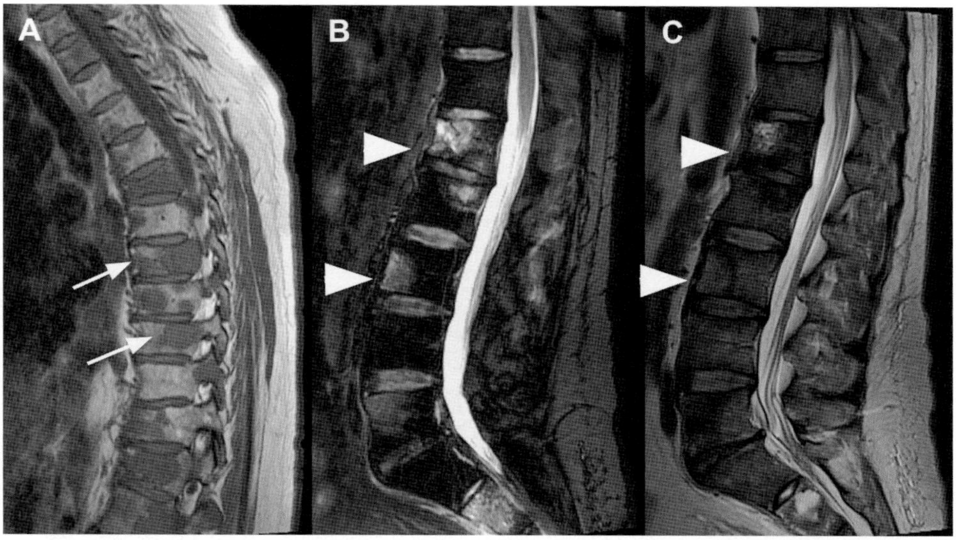

Fig. 4. A 53-year-old woman with history of breast carcinoma and metastatic spine disease. Note excellent delineation of circumscribed metastatic lesions (*arrows*) on T1 sagittal MR imaging without contrast (*A*). FSE T2 sagittal MR imaging sequence with fat saturation (*B*) also better defines multiple lesions with greater conspicuity than standard FSE T2 sequences (*arrowheads*) (*C*).

after contrast administration should include fat saturation. Focal myeloma lesions in the spine will image similarly to metastatic lesions on MR imaging, with pathologic fracture, marrow replacement, and epidural spread tumor (**Fig. 5**). Occasionally, acute to subacute pathologic spine fractures in myeloma may not demonstrate typical findings of increased FSE T2 signal abnormality (**Fig. 6**).[17] Eighty-seven percent of pathologic vertebral fractures in patients with myeloma are found between T6 and L4; this is similar to the distribution of fractures found in patients with osteoporosis.[18] Sixty-seven percent of these myelomatous fractures will have benign imaging characteristics.[18] CT examination without contrast is helpful in defining lytic bone lesions and cortical destruction that is not well demonstrated on MR imaging (See **Fig. 2**), which can be particularly helpful before surgical or percutaneous interventions, including vertebroplasty.[14]

Primary vertebral osteosarcoma

Primary vertebral osteosarcoma represents 4% of all osteosarcomas. Most of these occur at a single spinal segment but 17% involve more than one level. Lesions are typically seen in the posterior

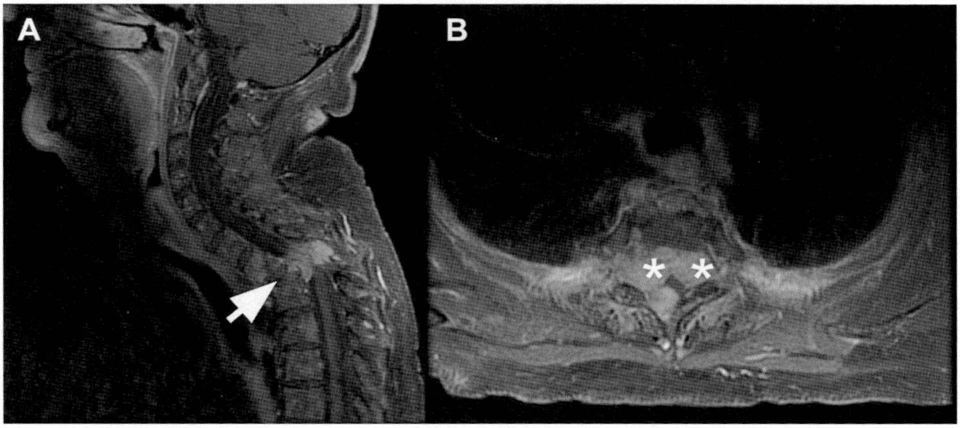

Fig. 5. Solitary plasmacytoma defined on FSE T1 MR imaging sequences with fat saturation (*A, B*). Note near complete loss of height of vertebrae (*arrow*) and prominent epidural tumor extension (*asterisks*).

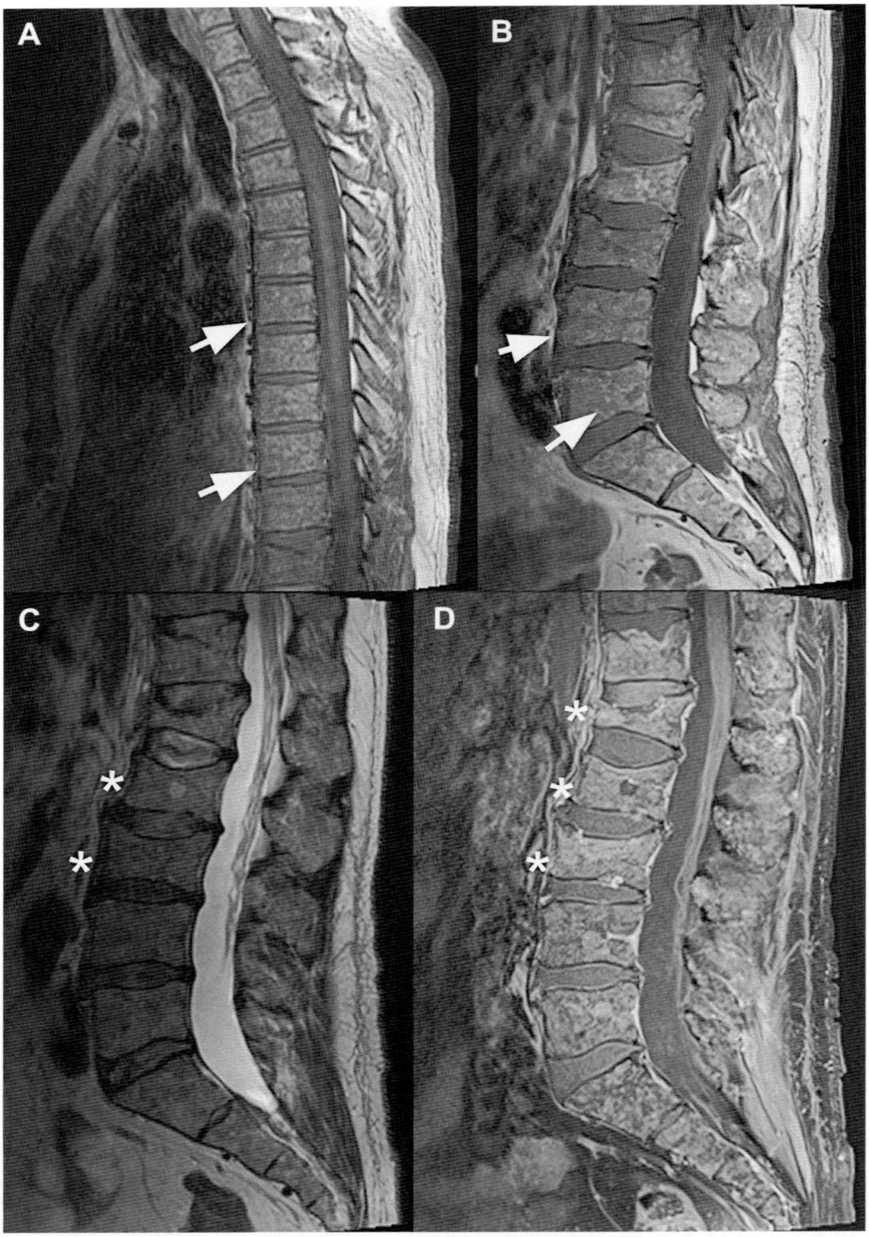

Fig. 6. A 56-year-old man with acute chronic back pain for many months. Note speckled appearance of vertebrae often seen in myeloma (*arrows*) and use of fat-saturation techniques to define pathologic lesions and associated compression fractures (***) (*A, B*). Sagittal FSE T1 MR imaging sequences without contrast (*C*). FSE T2 sagittal MR imaging sequence (*D*). Sagittal FSE T1 sequences with contrast and fat saturation. Note paucity of T2 signal abnormality of compression fractures on FSE T2 sequences (**).

elements, with only 17% of tumors, in one retrospective study, being completely confined to the vertebral body.[19] Other studies quote a significantly higher percentage of involvement of the vertebral body.[5] Most case demonstrate some form of mineralization. This includes an osteoid matrix in 28% of cases. Invasion of the spinal canal is frequent (up to 84% of cases), and a small percentage of cases will have a benign appearance similar to osteoblastoma.[19]

The most common presenting sign of primary spinal osteosarcoma is pain (90%). The duration of pain ranges from 2 months to 18 months. Pain, which intensifies at night, and radicular pain have also been reported. The next most common symptom is neurologic deficit, which was seen in 55% of one study cohort.[20] Although osteosarcoma, overall, has a peak incidence during the adolescent growth spurt, spinal osteosarcoma tends to occur in an older age group, with a mean age of 38 years.[20]

Osteosarcoma Imaging

A multimodality approach to imaging is vital in defining the presence and extent of spine osteosarcoma. The variable pathologic appearance, including osteoid matrix, marked mineralization, ivory vertebrae, primary lytic pattern, and a chondroblastic subtype, leads to a variety of imaging appearances (**Figs. 7** and **8**).[19]

Plain radiographs may demonstrate cortical destruction, a wide zone of transition, a permeative appearance, or bone matrix.[21] Noncontrast CT will better define plain film findings and is the best modality for defining matrix and bone destruction. The use of contrast on CT examinations may obscure bone matrix.[21] MR imaging findings are extremely variable, with the signal abnormality based on the pathologic subtype of the tumor.[5]

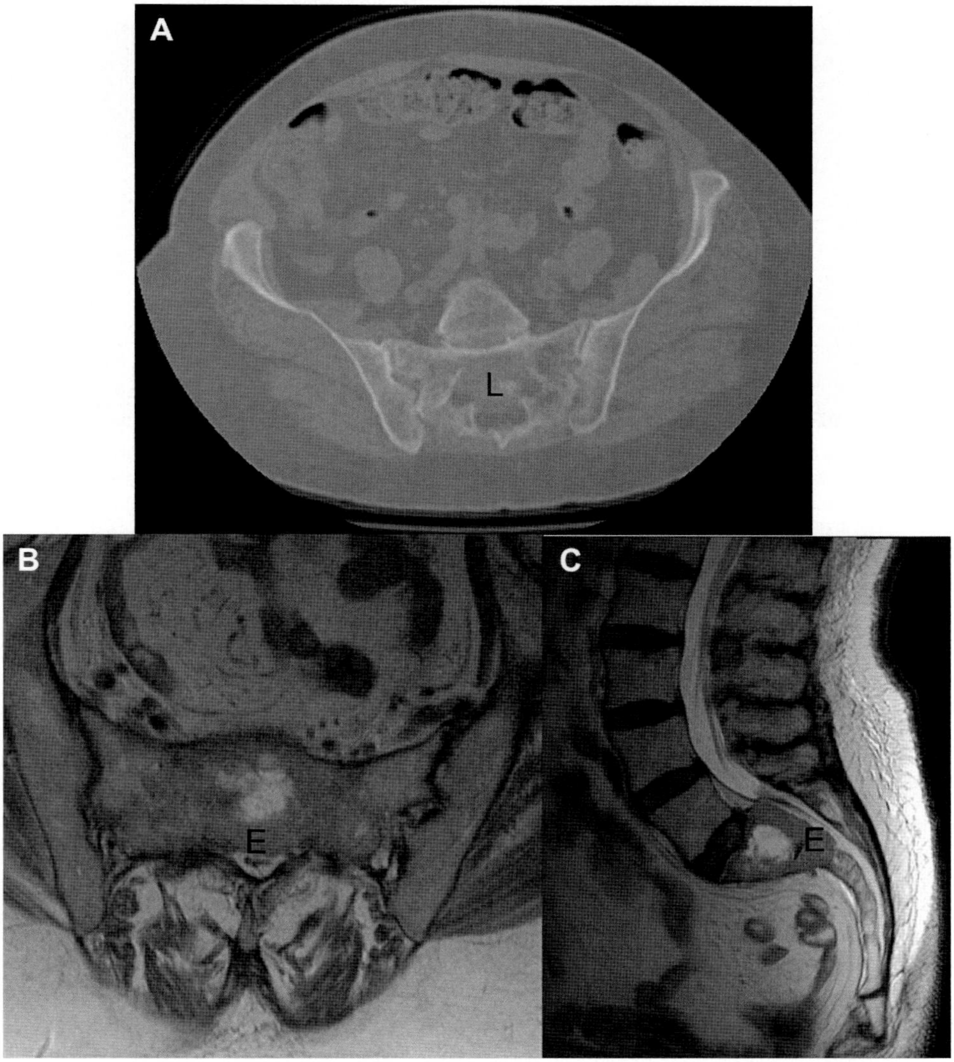

Fig. 7. A 82 year-old woman with sacral pain for many months and recent development of neurogenic bladder. (*A*) Axial CT image. (*B*) Axial FSE T2 MR imaging sequence. (*C*) Sagittal FSE T2 MR imaging sequence. Imaging demonstrates a central lytic lesion (L) of the sacrum with epidural extension (E). Note decreased T2 signal suggesting a cellular neoplasm. Osteogenic sarcoma.

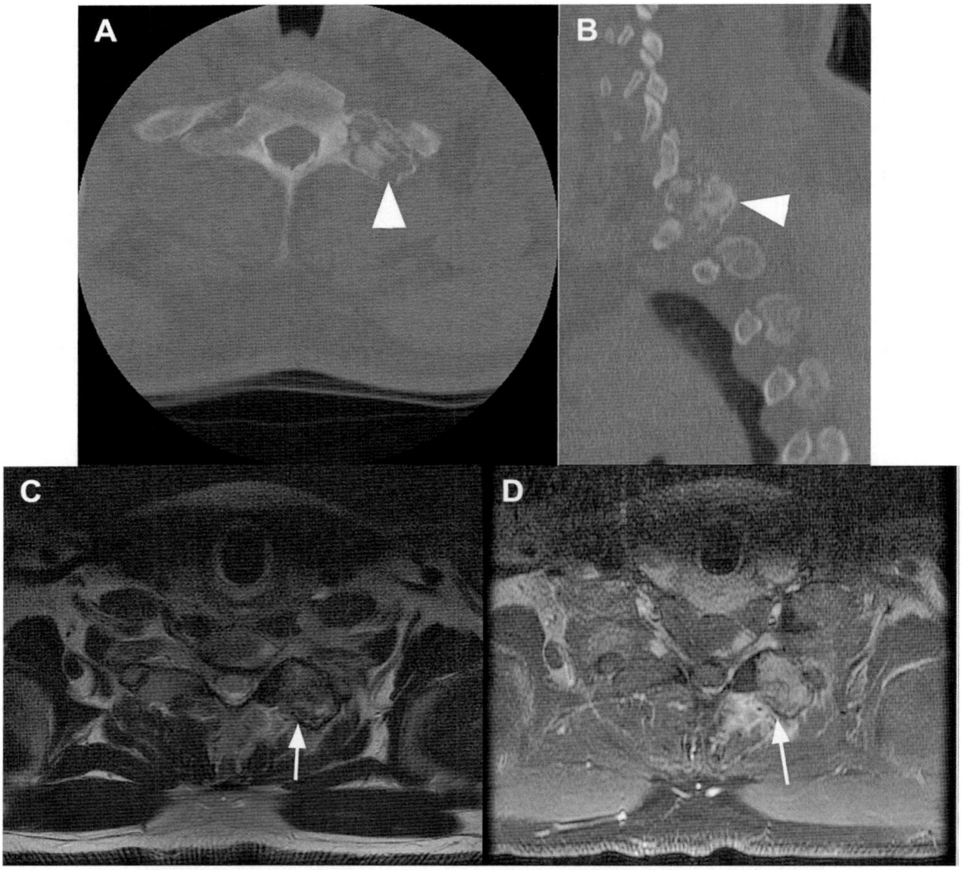

Fig. 8. Osteosarcoma centered within the transverse process (*arrowheads*) with central mineralized matrix. Excellent depiction of tumor using multimodality approach. Note decreased T2 signal within lesion on FSE T2 axial MR imaging sequence (*arrow*). (*A*) CT axial image; (*B*) CT sagittal reformatted image; (*C*) FSE T2 axial sequence with fat saturation; (*D*) FSE T1 axial sequence with contrast and fat saturation.

Nonmineralized tumors will typically have a low T1 signal and increased signal on T2 sequences. Densely mineralized tumors may demonstrate decreased signal on both T1 and T2 sequences. MR imaging with contrast enhancement is important to define the soft tissue extension of the tumor, particularly the intraspinal extension and the degree of central canal compromise. Nuclear medicine isotope scanning is helpful in defining remote lesions. PET/CT is the current standard of care to stage all patients with bone and soft tissue sarcomas. PET scanning is also used to monitor treatment response and conduct surveillance for recurrence.[5]

Ewing tumor of the spine

Ewing tumor of the spine is a rare diagnosis, with less than 30 cases diagnosed in the United States annually.[22] Localized pain is a common presenting sign in patients with Ewing sarcoma. In one series, 85% of patients with spine disease presented with local pain or radicular pain.[22] Pain may be accompanied by fever, leukocytosis, and an elevated sedimentation rate. In spinal lesions, early onset of neurologic symptoms associated with cord compression is common.[5] Up to 66% of patients may have neurologic symptoms at the time of presentation.[22] The median interval between onset of symptoms and time of presentation in one series was 2.3 months.[22] Diagnosis may be delayed in patients with sacral tumors (4 months vs 2 months).[23] Ninety percent of all Ewing sarcomas present before 20 years of age. There is a smaller second peak at approximately 50 years of age. Spine lesions tend to be seen in older patients than peripheral Ewing sarcoma.[21] The tumor occurs most often in the second decade of life and is rarely seen in patients of African or Asian decent.[5] The sacrum is a common location for spine lesions (30%), but extraosseous tumors are equally prevalent (30%). Thoracic, lumbar, and cervical sites are less common.[22] Metastatic disease is present at the time of diagnosis in 10% to 30% of patients.[24,25] Overall prognosis for patients with spine lesions is worse than patients with peripheral lesions secondary to limitations of surgical resection.[21]

Ewing tumor imaging

A permeative appearance mimicking osteomyelitis is the hallmark of Ewing tumor of the spine. This characteristic can be demonstrated on radiographs, but CT offers greater sensitivity.[25] Vertebra plana may be seen, and 2 or more adjacent vertebra may be involved. Fifty percent of tumors have a noncalcified soft tissue mass.[21] MR imaging, with its superb contrast resolution, is the study of choice for local tumor staging (**Fig. 9**).[25] The MR imaging appearance can be extremely variable on all sequences, depending on matrix formation and the degree of bone and soft tissue involvement.[26] MR imaging is the best modality for defining tumor boundaries, local and extracompartmental extension, and the involvement of the spinal canal and neurovascular bundles (**Fig. 10**).[25] FDG PET/CT is the standard for initial staging and the detection of recurrence or new metastatic disease.[5,25] The initial standardized uptake value of the primary tumor has been shown to correlate with tumor aggressiveness.

Both MR imaging and FDG PET/CT can be helpful in monitoring the tumor response to therapy. However, FDG PET offers greater utility in defining scar versus residual tumor in tumor surveillance.[5,25]

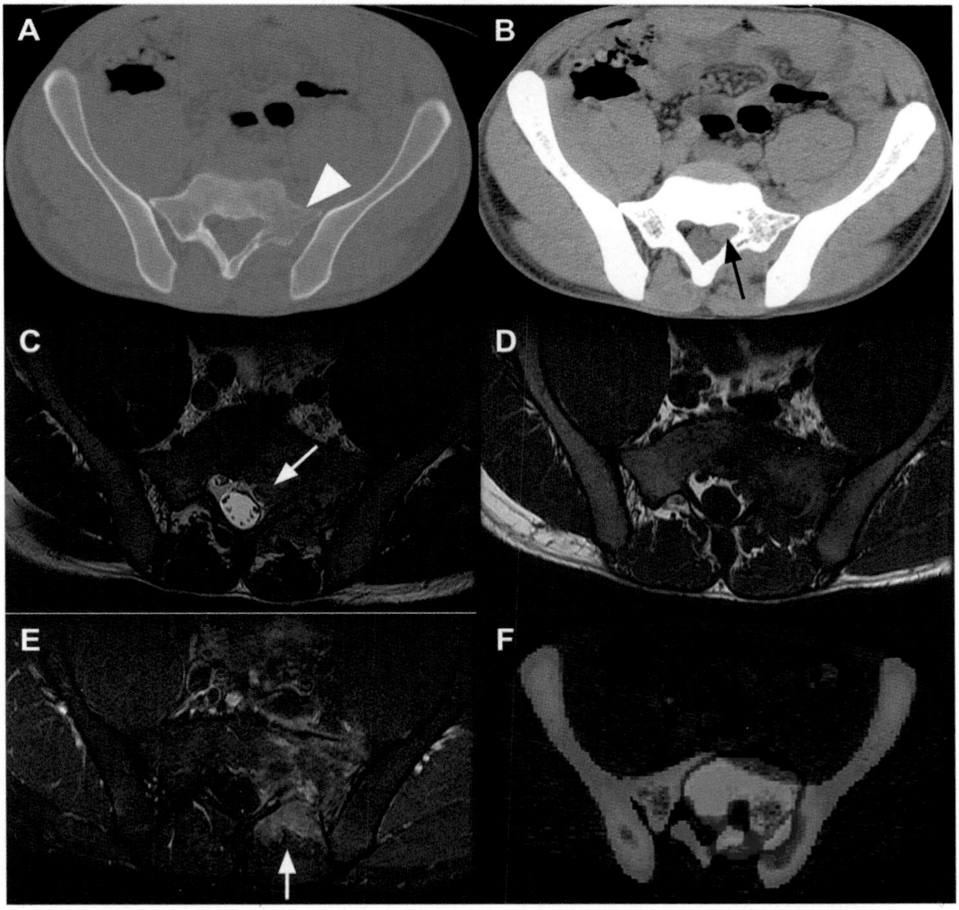

Fig. 9. A 30-year-old woman with back and leg pain and weight loss for several months. (*A, B*) CT without contrast defining permeative sacral bone lesion (*arrowhead*) and high-attenuation soft tissue extension into epidural space indicating cellular neoplasm (*arrow*). (*C*) MR imaging axial FSE T2 sequence demonstrates decreased signal of epidural tumor suggesting cellular neoplasm (*arrows*). (*D, E*) MR imaging axial FSE T1 sequences before and after contrast administration demonstrating extent of lesion. (*F*) Marked FDG uptake on PET imaging. Small, round, blue cell tumor. Imaging consistent with Ewing sarcoma.

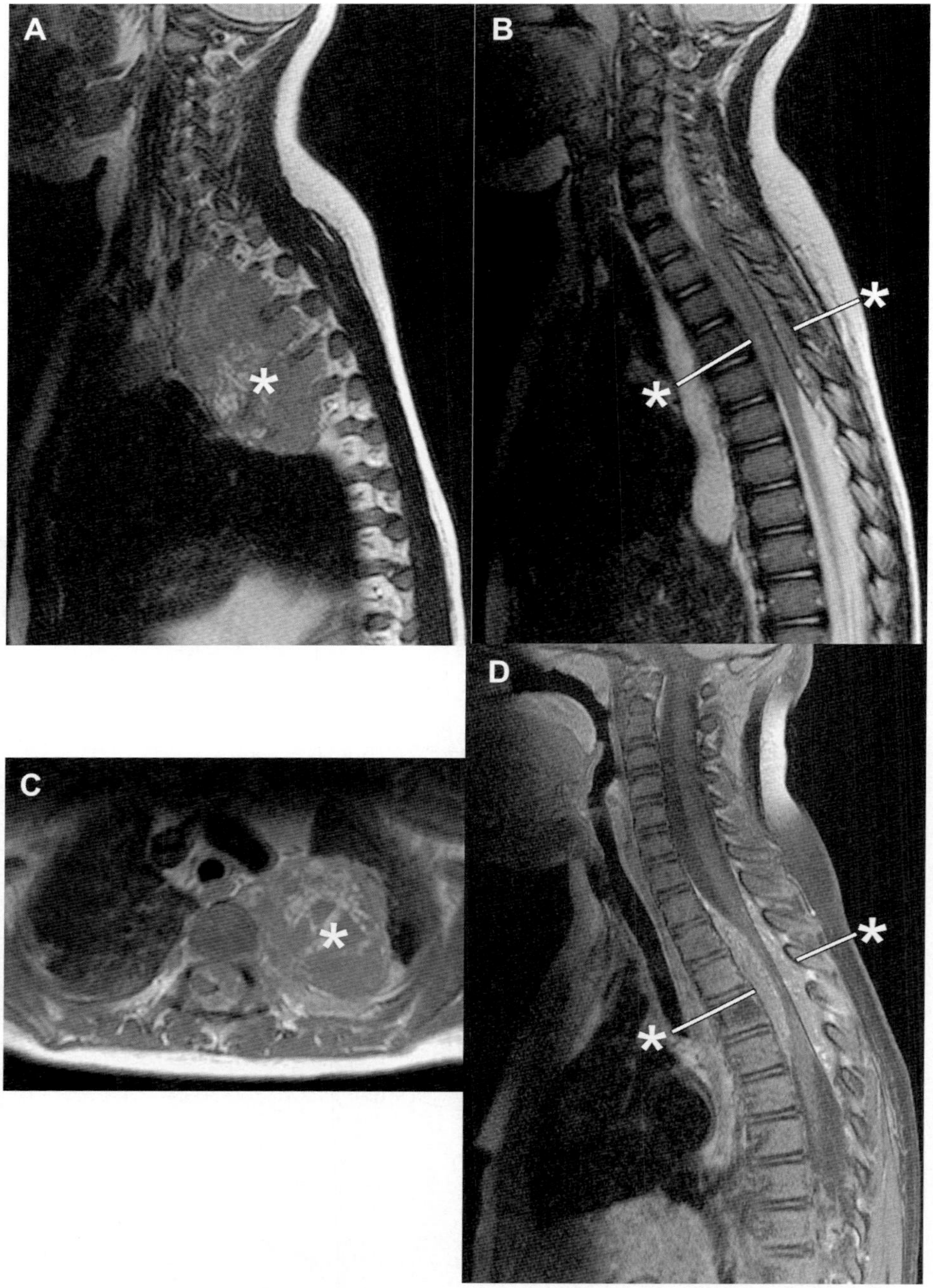

Fig. 10. A 3-year-old girl with inability to walk. Prominent paraspinal Ewing sarcoma (*asterisks*) with epidural extension. (*A, B*) Sagittal FSE T2 MR imaging sequences; (*C*) axial FSE T1 sequence with contrast; (*D*) sagittal FSE T1 sequence with contrast and fat saturation.

Chordoma

Chordomas are primary bone tumors thought to arise from notochordal remnants; the pathologic hallmark is the presence of physaliphorous cells.[5,27] Although rare, with an overall incidence of 1/1,000,000, chordomas represent the most common malignant tumor of the sacrum and the most common primary malignant tumor of the mobile spine.[27] The tumor occurs more frequently in men than woman, is rare in African Americans, and is rare before 40 years of age.[5] The tumor is most common in the sacrococcygeal area (45%–50%), followed by the spheno-occipital region (35%–40%) and the mobile spine (10%–15%).[28]

Presenting signs and symptoms of chordomas are location dependent, with any combination of pain, weakness, sensory abnormalities, or bowel or bladder dysfunction.[29] Because these tumors are slow growing, presentation is often delayed for many months or years before diagnosis.[30] The duration of symptoms ranged from 4 to 24 months in one review.[27] Nonspecific low back pain is the typical presenting feature of sacral lesions. In addition, up to 40% of patients describe symptoms of rectal dysfunction. A palpable tumor is typically present.[5] Symptoms are usually present for a shorter duration in tumors found in the mobile spine.[5,27] Almost all of these patients present with neck or back pain, often with a radicular component.[5] Neurologic symptoms are present more frequently in tumors of the mobile spine. More than two-thirds of patients may present with weakness or neurologic deficit.[5,27]

Chordoma imaging

CT scanning will demonstrate the soft tissue and bone components of the neoplasm. Typically, there is a central lytic process associated with a soft tissue mass, and calcification is present in 30% to 70% of cases.[31] Unlike other tumors of the vertebral column, chordomas may infiltrate the intervertebral disk and involve adjacent segments.[27] Multiplanar MR imaging is vital, in conjunction with CT scanning, to define the full extent of these tumors (**Fig. 11**). Compared with skeletal muscle, these tumors are

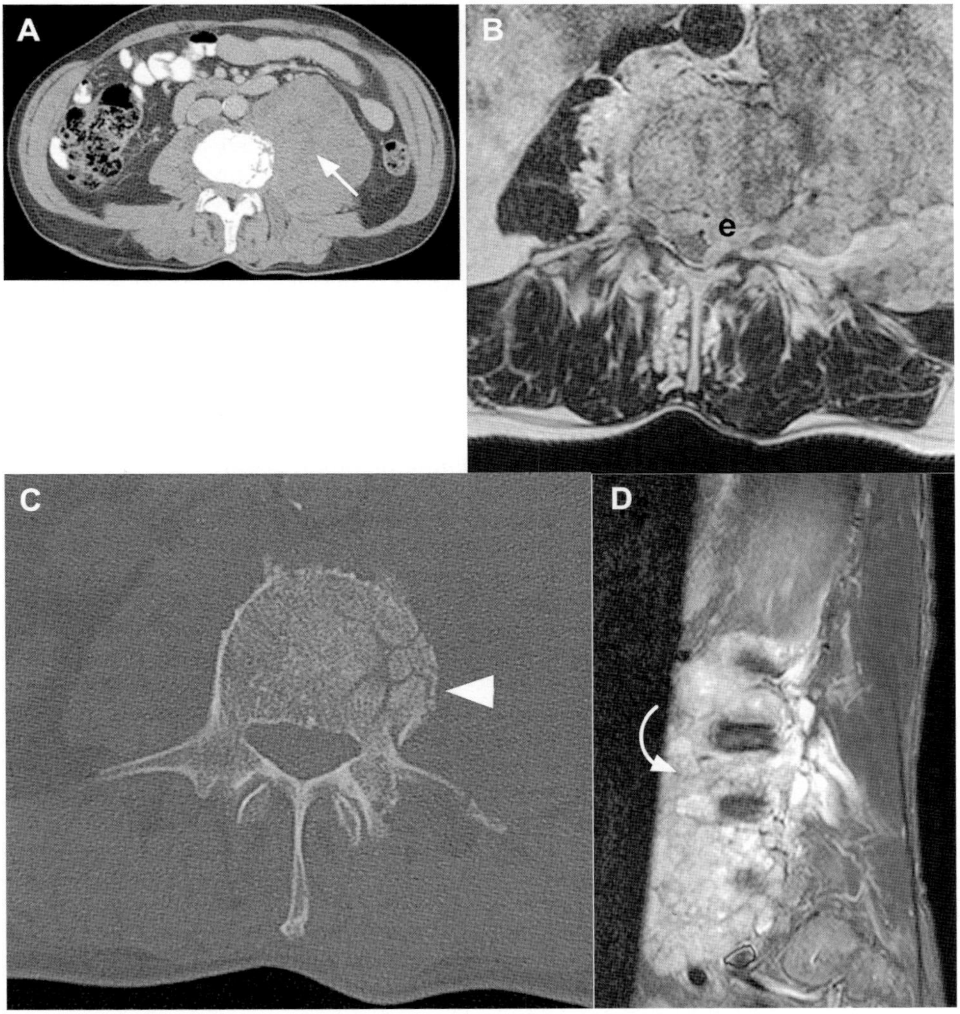

Fig. 11. A 70-year-old man with a 5-month history of left thigh pain and recent onset of leg weakness. L3 chordoma with prominent paraspinal component (*arrow*), epidural extension (e), sclerosis of vertebral body, and pathologic fracture (*arrowhead*). Note bubbly T2 signal often seen in chordoma (*curved arrow*). (*A*) Axial CT image without contrast; (*B*) FSE T2 axial MR imaging sequence; (*C*) axial CT image using bone algorithm; (*D*) sagittal FSET2 MR imaging sequence.

isointense to slightly hypointense on T1-weighted sequences. The soft tissue components of these tumors classically demonstrate hyperintense T2 signal, which typically correlates with the intratumoral accumulation of mucin.[31] MR imaging enhancement is variable, from a faint blush to intense enhancement.[21] Although chordomas rarely present with distal metastases, roughly 30% of sacrococcygeal tumors eventually metastasize.[27] PET/CT has been reported to demonstrate heterogeneous mildly increased uptake[32] and may be helpful in tumor surveillance.

Chondrosarcoma

Chondrosarcoma is a malignant tumor of bone in which the neoplastic tissue is fully developed cartilage without tumor osteoid matrix. The tumor may contain myxoid elements, calcification, or elements of ossification. Tumors may develop in normal bone or arise in preexisting benign cartilage tumors.[5] These tumors are rare, with only 21 chondrosarcomas reported at the MD Anderson Cancer Center over 43 years.[33] Chondrosarcomas compose 7% to 12% of all primary spine tumors and account for up to 25% of malignant spine tumors.[33] There is a 2:1 male-to-female predilection.[21,33] Sixty percent of tumors occur in the thoracic spine, with the remaining lesions distributed between the lumbar spine (20%–39%) and cervical spine (19%–20%).[34] The posterior elements are involved in 40% of cases, and the vertebral body alone in 15%.[21]

Slow and gradual onset of focal pain is the most common presenting sign (duration 4 weeks to 13 years, average 45 months) of chondrosarcoma, often associated with a neurologic deficit.[5,33,35] Pain, worse at night, has also been reported in these patients.[36] Neurologic symptoms may manifest as radiculopathy, myelopathy, or cauda equina syndrome.[33] Because of the indolent nature of these lesions, up to one-half of patients may have a neurologic deficit at the time of presentation.[33] A palpable mass may be present when these tumors arise from the posterior elements (34% in one series).[35]

Chondrosarcoma imaging

There are numerous types of primary chondrosarcomas, including conventional intramedullary, clear cell, juxtacortical, myxoid, mesenchymal, extraskeletal, and dedifferentiated. Chondrosarcomas are histologically graded from 1 to 4, with grade 4 lesions being the most aggressive and demonstrating metastasis in more than 50% of cases.[21,33] Imaging features directly reflect these pathologic subtypes, and the various subtypes often show distinctive characteristics.[36] Classically, imaging identifies the arc-and-ring appearance of the chondroid matrix mineralization. Although plain films may identify bone destruction and chondroid mineralization in up to 70% of cases,[36] cross-sectional imaging, including CT and MR imaging in combination, offers the best opportunity to define the tumor matrix and tumor extent (**Fig. 12**).

CT without contrast accurately identifies the bone destruction and chondroid mineralization. The extraosseous soft tissue mass will be defined to a variable degree.[21] MR imaging is the gold standard for demonstrating the soft tissue components of these tumors. In low-grade lesions, the high water content is seen in the nonmineralized components on both CT and MR imaging; prominent T2 hyperintensity reflects this water content on MR imaging.[36] Lower-grade lesions often demonstrate the classic arc-and-ring pattern of the matrix. Low-grade conventional chondrosarcomas represent 80% to 90% of tumor subtypes.[33] As the lesions increase in grade and aggressiveness, there is less chondroid matrix and an increase in myxoid material. MR imaging best demonstrates extraosseous lesions. MR imaging with contrast can define the enhancing periphery of the tumor and the internal septa. The nonenhancing components represent areas of hyaline cartilage, mucoid tissue, or necrosis.[21] Cross-sectional imaging can also demonstrate extension through the intervertebral disk, which has been reported in 35% of cases.[37]

Benign Spine Tumors

Osteoid osteoma/osteoblastoma

Osteoid osteoma and osteoblastoma are histologically similar benign neoplasms distinguished primarily by size, site of origin, and radiographic appearance.[38] Osteoid osteomas typically measure less than 1.5 cm and osteoblastomas measure greater than 1.5 cm (**Fig. 13**).[21] Microscopically, both neoplasms are comprised of interlacing trabeculae of woven bone surrounded by osteoblasts. The intervening stroma is loose vascular connective tissue containing variable numbers of giant cells.[38]

Osteoid osteoma is the classic spine tumor associated with a stereotypical pain at presentation. Night pain relieved by aspirin can be found in most medical literature describing this benign neoplasm. Despite these classic symptoms, this neoplasm may go undiagnosed for years, even in the setting of scoliosis.[39] The pain can be episodic and can increase at night or with physical activity.[40] The pain is presumed to be caused by the presence of nerve endings in the nidus that are stimulated by vascular pressure and the

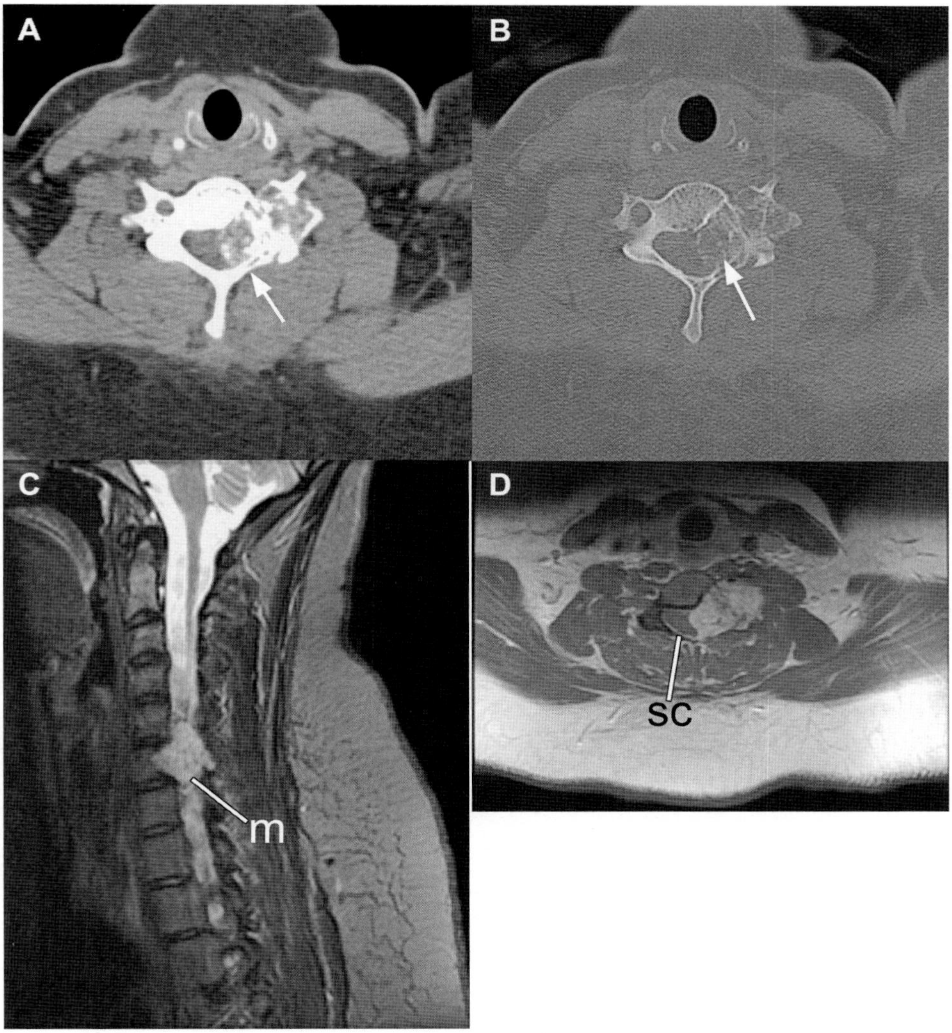

Fig. 12. Chondrosarcoma: 24-year-old woman with several-month history of localized neck pain. (*A*, *B*) CT without contrast defines bone destruction and chondroid matrix (*arrows*) of cervical lesion. (*C*, *D*) MR imaging without and with contrast demonstrates increased T2 signal in non mineralized component (m) and encroachment on spinal cord (SC). (*C*) MRI sagittal FSET2 sequence. (*D*) MRI axial T1 sequence with contrast.

production of prostaglandins,[41] which explains the clinical response of these tumors to nonsteroidal antiinflammatory drugs and aspirin.[40] Neurologic impairment is less common in benign spine neoplasms (28%) compared with malignant lesions (68%) and rarely occurs in osteoid osteoma.[40,42] However, osteoid osteoma may present with radicular pain either secondary to neural compression or secondary to tumorous inflammation.[43]

Osteoid osteoma is most common between the ages of 6 and 17 and is the most common vertebral tumor of children.[44] It accounts for 2% of all primary bone tumors of the axial skeleton.[24] Fifty-nine percent of these lesions occur in the lumbar spine, 27% in the cervical spine, and 12% in the thoracic spine. This lesion is a lesion of the posterior elements. Fifty percent of lesions arise in the lamina or pedicles and 20% occur in the articular processes. There is often a scoliosis associated with these lesions (70%),[21] with the apex of the scoliosis oriented away from the side of the lesion.[24] When back pain is associated with muscle spasm and painful scoliosis, osteoid osteoma of the spine must be suspected.[39]

Osteoid osteoma imaging

Plain radiographs will occasionally define reactive sclerosis about the obscured nidus and may demonstrate scoliosis with convexity of the curve

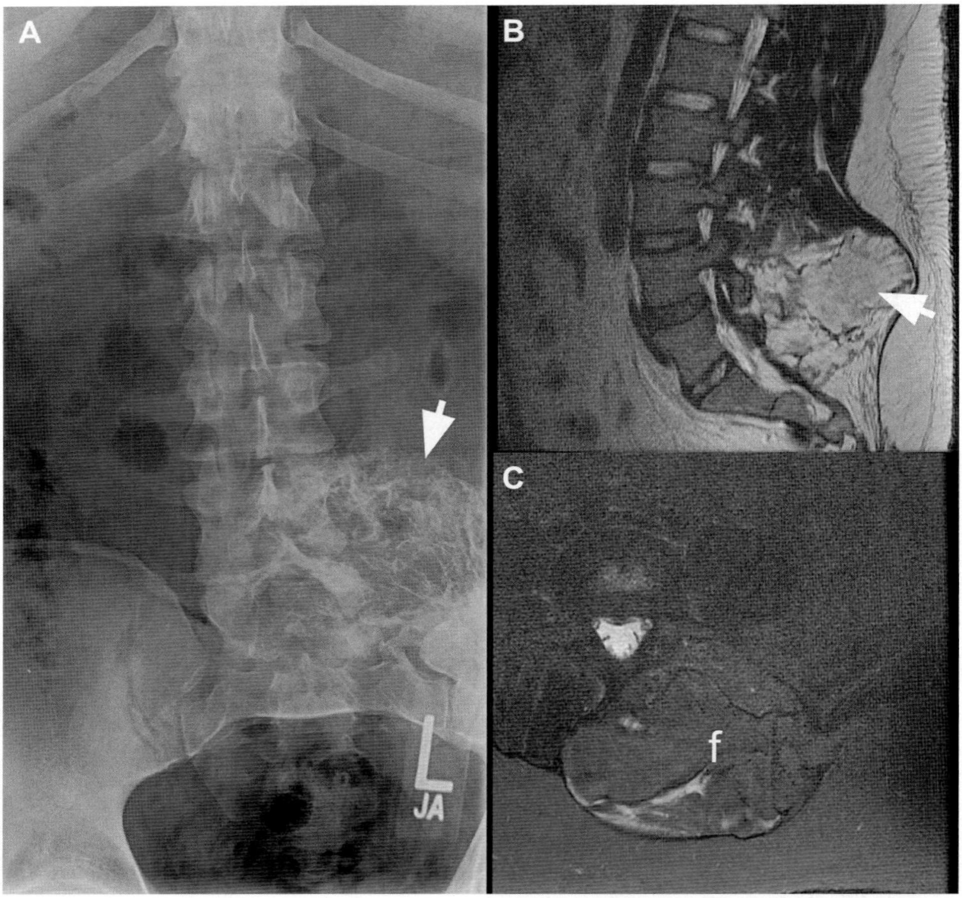

Fig. 13. Osteoblastoma: plain film (*A*), MR imaging sequences, including FSE T2 sagittal (*B*) and axial FSE T2 with fat saturation (*C*), demonstrate prominent L5 osteoblastoma (*arrow*) with prominent central fatty marrow component (f).

oriented away from the nidus.[21,43] Unlike most other spine tumor imaging, MR imaging plays a secondary role in the imaging of osteoid osteoma.[24] CT is the primary imaging modality used in diagnosis and can guide minimally invasive treatment.[45,46] CT without contrast demonstrates the less than 1.5-cm radiolucent nidus (lesions >1.5 cm are osteoblastomas) and the surrounding sclerosis. Occasionally, the nidus can be sclerotic. Periosteal reaction may be present.[21] Areas of calcification may be demonstrated by CT in the nidus.[24] Although early reports suggested a limited role for MR imaging in these lesions, current MR imaging techniques help to define this benign lesion. The central nidus typically demonstrates low signal intensity on T1-weighted sequences but will avidly enhance with contrast. MR imaging best defines the peritumoral inflammation associated with these lesions in both bone and soft tissues. This edema is demonstrated by increased STIR/T2 signal, low T1 signal, and avid gadolinium enhancement.[21,43] Bone scintigraphy using 99mTc invariably demonstrates the marked accumulation of tracer in the lesion in both blood pool and delayed imaging. SPECT aids image localization (**Fig. 14**).[21,24]

Aneurysmal bone cyst

Aneurysmal bone cyst (ABC) is a pseudotumoral hemorrhagic lesion of unknown cause.[47] The term aneurysmal bone cyst is purely descriptive; numerous researchers have failed to discover a genetic or neoplastic association to this lesion.[48] Many investigators describe both primary and secondary (arising from a preexisting lesion) subtypes.[49] ABCs usually occur between the ages of 10 and 20 years, with more than 85% of these lesions occurring in patients under 20 years of age. There is a slightly greater female-to-male predominance.[21,47,48] Approximately 20% to 35%

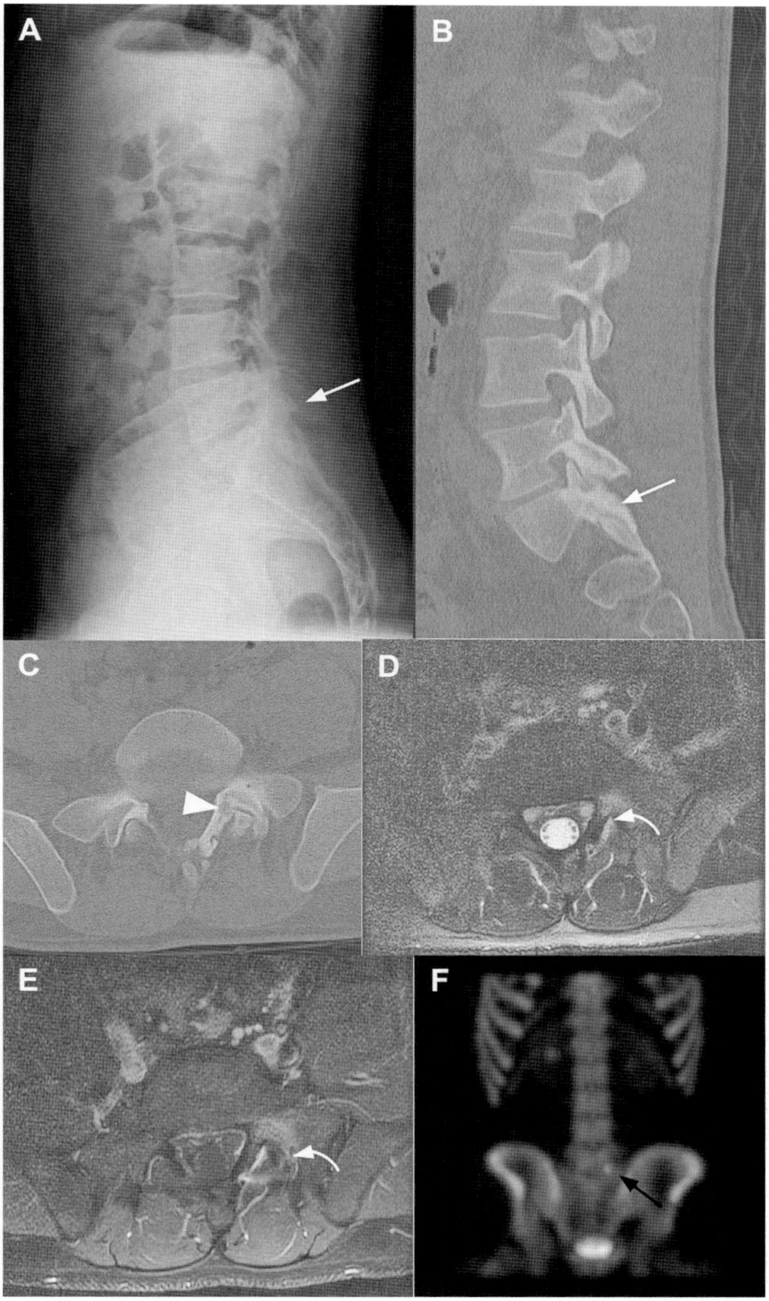

Fig. 14. Osteoid osteoma in a patient with a greater than 1-year history of focal back pain, worse at night. Plain film lumbar spine (*A*) and CT sagittal reconstructed image (*B*) demonstrate sclerosis of L5 posterior elements (*arrows*). Axial CT image (*C*) defines central nidus (*arrowhead*) with surrounding sclerosis. MR imaging sequences, including axial FSE T2 with fat saturation (*D*) and axial FSE T1 with contrast and fat saturation (*E*) poorly define the nidus, but demonstrate reactive signal and contrast enhancement (*curved arrows*). Increased uptake (*black arrow*) on 99mTc SPECT bone scan (*F*).

of these lesions occur in the spine, and ABCs represent 15% of all primary spine tumors.[24,47] Most of the lesions occur in the posterior elements. Seventy-five percent to 90% extend into vertebral body, and cysts may involve more than one vertebral segment.[21,24]

Common clinical signs are pain and swelling, and some patients may present with a pathologic fracture. Slow and gradual pain is often a presenting feature, with one study reporting a symptom range of 1 to 80 weeks (mean 20 weeks).[47] Patients often complain of disabling pain and tenderness over the site of the lesion.[48] Scoliosis has been reported in 10% of patients.[49] Neurologic involvement is rarely associated with these lesions but has been reported.[21,50,51]

ABC imaging

Imaging of these lesions recapitulates their underlying pathologic condition (**Fig. 15**). Plain films will demonstrate an eccentric lytic lesion with a remodeled, blown out, or ballooned contour of the host bone.[24,49] The lesions are typically well defined with geographic margins. CT without contrast will demonstrate uninterrupted cortex in many cases, better define the bone anatomy and extent of the lesion in the spine, and occasionally demonstrate fluid levels.[24,49,52] Scalloped ridges are often seen in the walls of the lesion, correlating with septations found on pathologic examination. Calcified tumor matrix is absent.[21] MR imaging demonstrates a peripheral rim of low T1 and T2 signal, reflecting the periosteum or pseudocapsule.[21] Fluid-fluid

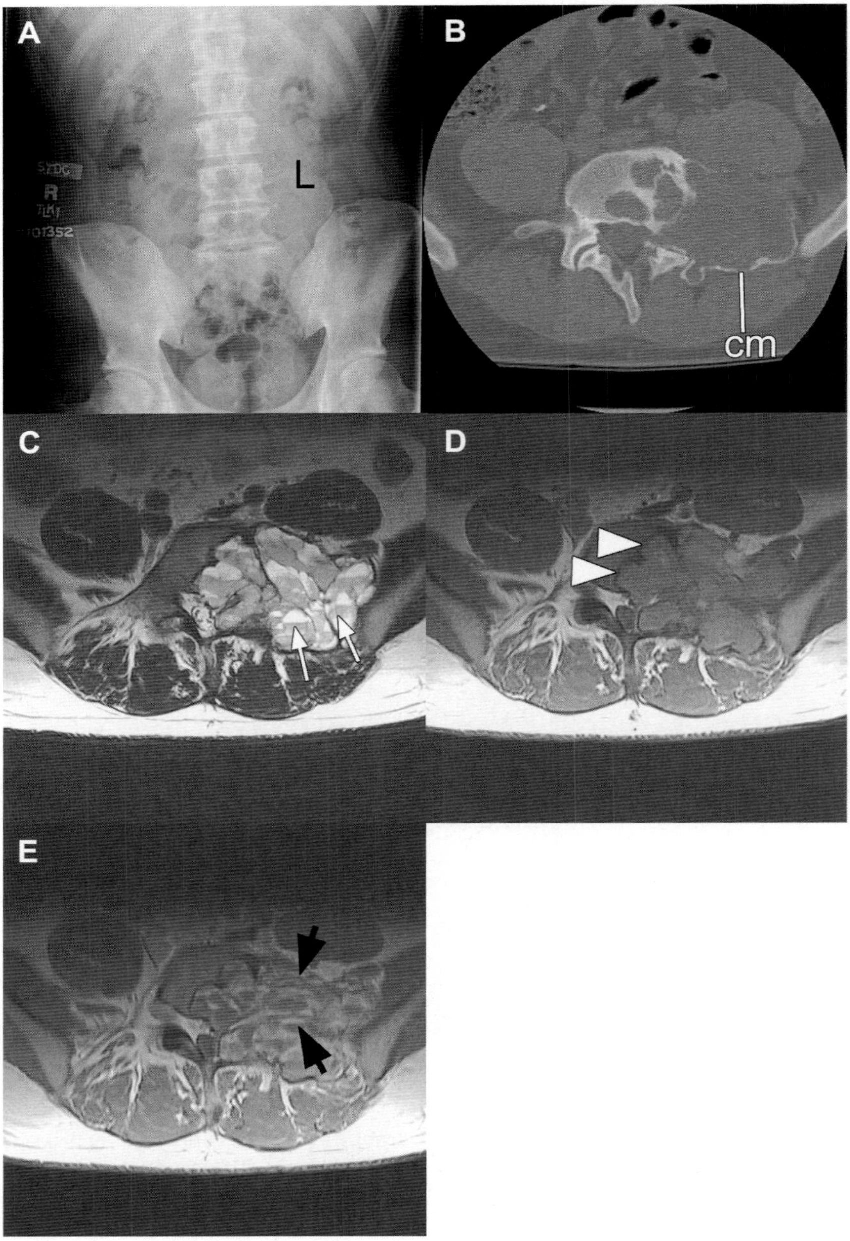

Fig. 15. A 25-year-old man with a greater than 1-year history of back pain with recent worsening of symptoms. Plain film (*A*) and CT (*B*) demonstrates eccentric blown out lesion (*L*) with intact cortical margin (cm). MR imaging, including axial FSE T2 (*C*), axial FSE T1 without (*D*), and with contrast (*E*), defines classic fluid/fluid levels (*arrows*), scalloped ridges (*arrowheads*), and enhancing septa (*black arrows*) ABC.

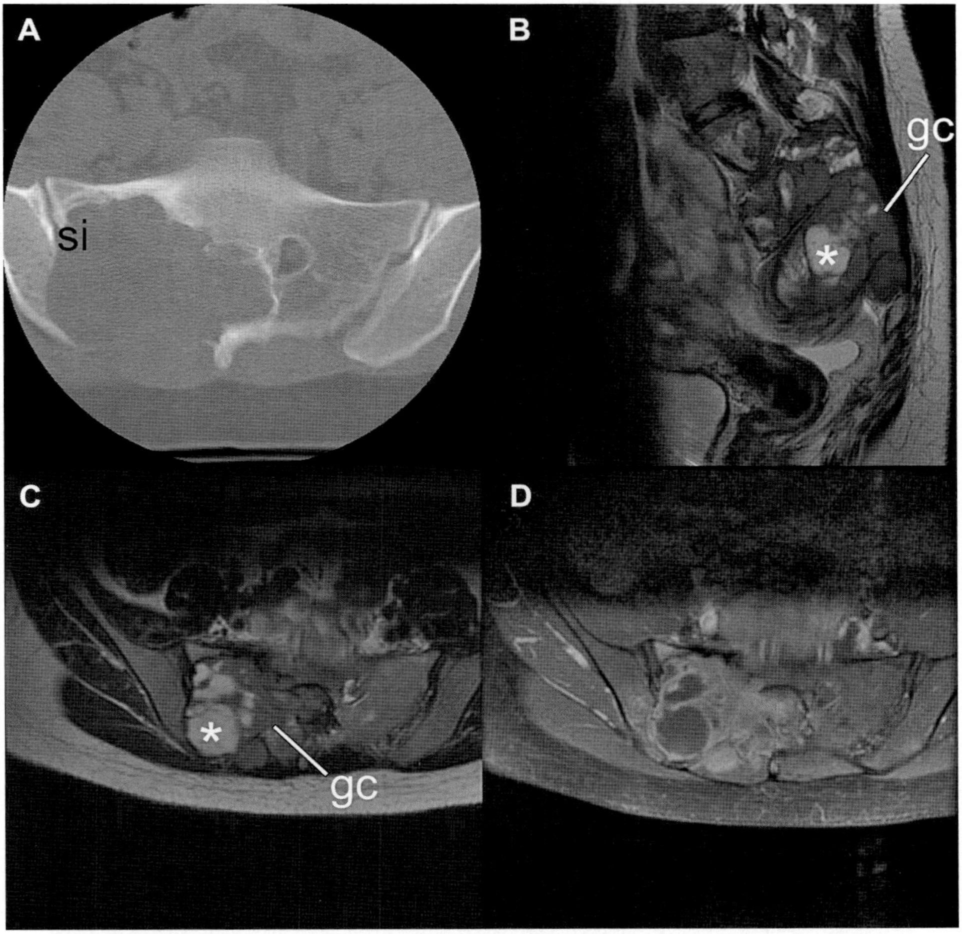

Fig. 16. GCT with ABC elements: CT axial image (*A*) defines a lytic lesion of sacrum that crosses sacroiliac joint (si). MR imaging sequences, including sagittal FSE T2 (*B*), axial FSET2 (*C*), and axial FSET1 with contrast and fat saturation (*D*), demonstrate low T2 signal associated with giant cell component (gc) and high T2 signal likely associated with ABC component (*asterisk*).

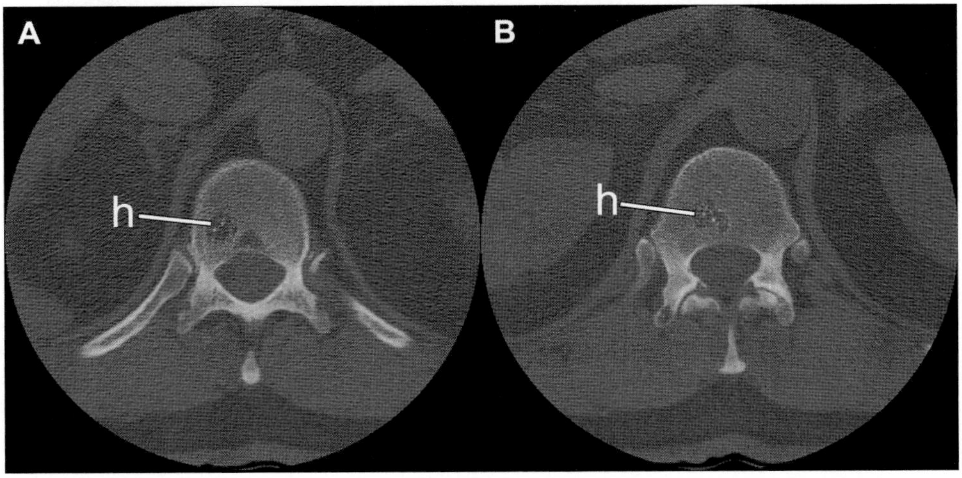

Fig. 17. A 52-year-old man with 3-month history of right back and increasing right leg pain. Benign and aggressive hemangiomas: CT axial images without contrast (*A*, *B*) showing the typical CT appearance of benign hemangiomas (h). Corollary MR imaging (Fig. 18*A–C*) demonstrates these lesions in the T11 and T12 vertebral bodies (h).

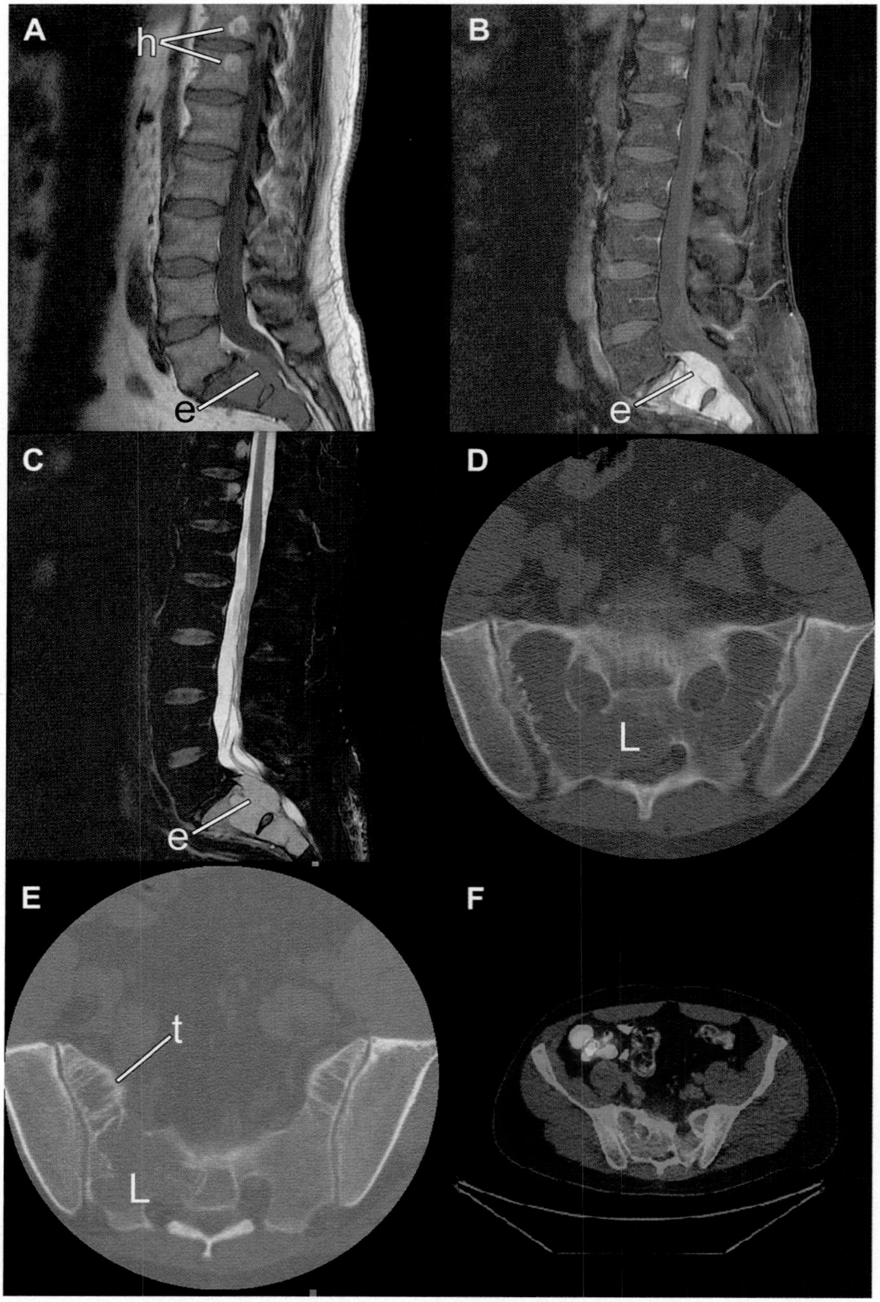

Fig. 18. MR imaging of patient described in **Fig. 17**. MR imaging: (*A*) FSE T1 sagittal sequence; (*B*) FSE T1 sagittal sequence with fat saturation after contrast; (*C*) FSE T2 sagittal sequence with fat saturation; (*D*, *E*) CT axial images without contrast; (*F*) FDG PET. Images demonstrate lytic lesion (L) with thickened trabeculae (t) on CT examination. Soft tissue component with epidural extension (e) best demonstrated on MR imaging sequences. Note no significant FDG uptake.

levels are often demonstrated in these lesions and may be better demonstrated on T1 sequences versus T2 sequences, secondary to the presence of methemoglobin.[24,49] Peritumoral edema is best defined on T2 and STIR weighted sequences and enhances with gadolinium. T1 images with gadolinium contrast also define the peripheral margins of lesions and the intervening septa.[21,24,49] Bone

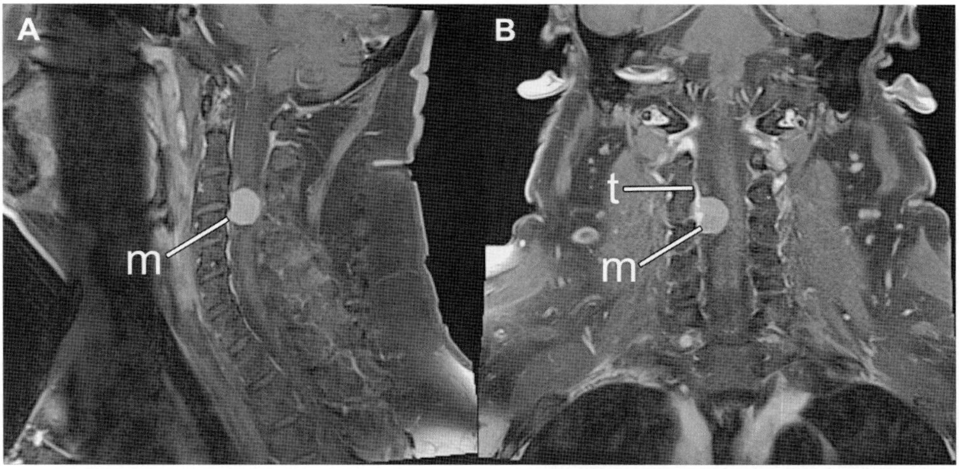

Fig. 19. Meningioma in a patient with chronic neck pain and recent onset of leg weakness. Sagittal (*A*) and coronal (*B*) MR imaging FSE T1 sequences with fat saturation after contrast administration define the classic appearance of this homogeneously enhancing meningioma (m) with dural tail (t).

scintigraphy is a sensitive examination for the detection of ABCs. The site of radiotracer uptake corresponds to the actual extent of the lesion.[24] In greater than 50% of cases, uptake will be localized to the periphery of the lesion.[49]

Giant cell tumors

Giant cell tumors (GCT) are rare neoplasms of the spine, representing less than 3% of all GCT. The Mayo Clinic reported only 24 patients with GCT of the spine over a 35-year period.[53,54] These tumors consist of osteoclastic giant cells within a spindle cell stroma. Ten percent to 15% will have an aneurysmal bone cyst-like component.[21,53] Reports vary regarding the spinal distribution of these lesions, with larger studies demonstrating an equal distribution throughout the spine and some studies demonstrating a sacral predominance. The typical age of onset is in the second to fourth decade of life.[53] Prolonged pain is the typical history at presentation, often associated with a neurologic deficit (>50%). Average duration of pain is approximately 5 months, with a range of 1.5 to 30.0 months.[54] Associated symptoms are related to the spinal segment of origin but may include hoarseness, focal back pain, radicular pain, extremity weakness, or sensory deficit.[53,54]

GCT imaging

Unlike most benign tumors of the spine, GCTs are found in greater frequency in the vertebral body (55%) but often involve the body and posterior elements (30%).[54] Plain films demonstrate a well-demarcated expansile lesion that often crosses the midline in the sacrum and may cross the sacroiliac joints (see **Fig. 16**). There is typically a narrow zone of transition.[21,53,54] These lesions are lytic lesions that almost always involve the cortex and do not contain mineralization.[54] CT better defines the characteristics identified on plain film images and better defines the bone architecture of the lesion. MR imaging typically demonstrates a heterogeneous lesion on all imaging sequences. MR imaging characteristics can be helpful in the diagnosis. Low to intermediate T2 signal is often seen within the lesion, which is thought to be secondary to the relative collagen content of fibrous components and hemosiderin within the lesion.[55] These lesions may also demonstrate curvilinear areas of low T1 and T2 signal, which may correspond to thickened trabeculae or fibrous septae.[53] GCTs demonstrate heterogeneous contrast enhancement with areas of nonenhancing tissue likely related to necrosis.[21] MR imaging also plays a critical role in the follow-up of these lesions. Although complete excision is the rule in tubular bones (85%–90%), axial skeletal lesions have a poorer prognosis secondary to the challenges of performing a complete resection.[53] MR imaging is the imaging modality of choice in monitoring these patients for local recurrence.

Vertebral hemangiomas

Vertebral hemangiomas are common benign lesions estimated to be present in 10% of autopsy specimens. Incidence increases with age, and there is a slight female predominance.[56] Twenty-five percent to 30% of cases involve multiple lesions.[21] Most vertebral hemangiomas are asymptomatic. However, when these lesions are symptomatic, the patients typically present with pain, myelopathy, and radiculopathy. In one series, greater than 50%

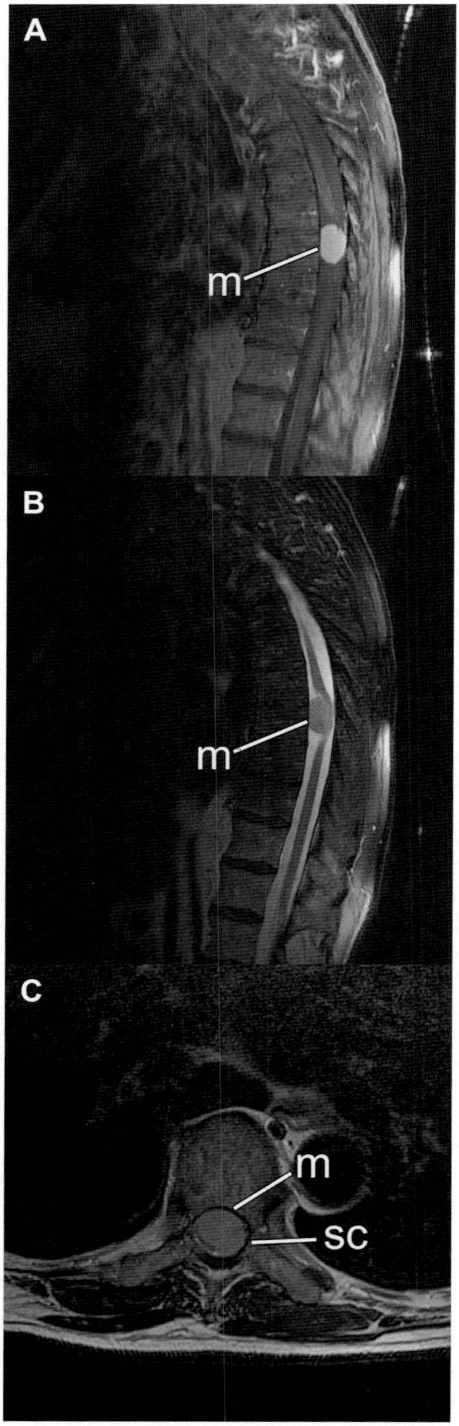

Fig. 20. A 70-year-old man with a 3-month history of progressive leg weakness and ascending numbness. (*A*) Sagittal FSE T1 MR imaging sequence with contrast and fat saturation. (*B*) Sagittal FSET2 MR imaging with fat saturation (*C*) and axial FSET2 with fat saturation demonstrate a midthoracic meningioma (m) with marked decreased T2 signal and severe mass effect on the spinal cord (sc).

of patients who presented with pain also presented with radiculopathy, myelopathy, or both.[57] Pathologically, vertebral hemangiomas consist of benign vascular proliferation of normal capillary and venous structures.[58] Two types of hemangiomas have been described: cavernous and capillary. The most common is the cavernous lesion, which is characterized by large sinusoidal spaces lined by a single layer of epithelium.[58] Smaller vascular channels define the capillary type of vertebral hemangioma.

Hemangioma imaging

Common hemangiomas are classically demonstrated on plain film or CT imaging as vertebral body lesions with coarsened trabeculae. Sparse thickened trabeculae surrounded by low-attenuation fat result in a "spotted or mottled"[56] appearance on axial CT images (see **Fig. 17**). Benign lesions on MR imaging are characterized by increased T1 and T2 signal (see **Fig. 18**). The fibroadipose tissue insinuated between the sinusoidal blood channels results in the increased T1 signal pattern of hemangiomas. These lesions will decrease in signal intensity on T2 imaging with fat saturation and will demonstrate gadolinium enhancement. Aggressive lesions will be characterized by a prominent soft tissue component that can invade the epidural space and encroach on the spinal cord.[59] The soft tissue component is often well demonstrated by MR imaging. The bone involvement of these lesions is best demonstrated by noncontrast CT imaging. Although the primary process within these lesions may be lytic, coarsened/thickened trabecular bone may also be seen (see **Fig. 18**). Posterior element involvement can be seen in the more aggressive variant of hemangioma.

Intradural-Extramedullary Tumors

Intradural-extramedullary tumors lie within the dura matter of the spinal canal but outside of the spinal cord. Lesions in this compartment include schwannoma, meningioma, neurofibroma, malignant nerve sheath tumors, hemangiopericytoma, paraganglioma, and metastasis. Tumors of the filum terminale are a unique subset of this tumor group. Clinical presentation and differential diagnosis can be challenging.

Schwannomas and meningiomas account for 45% of all intraspinal neoplasms.[60] The slow growth of these tumors tends to lead to vague symptoms and signs. Conti and colleagues[61] demonstrated an average duration of symptoms for schwannomas of 55 months, with a range of 1 to 360 months. The most common presurgical symptom was segmental pain, followed by radicular pain and variable motor deficits. Thirty-four

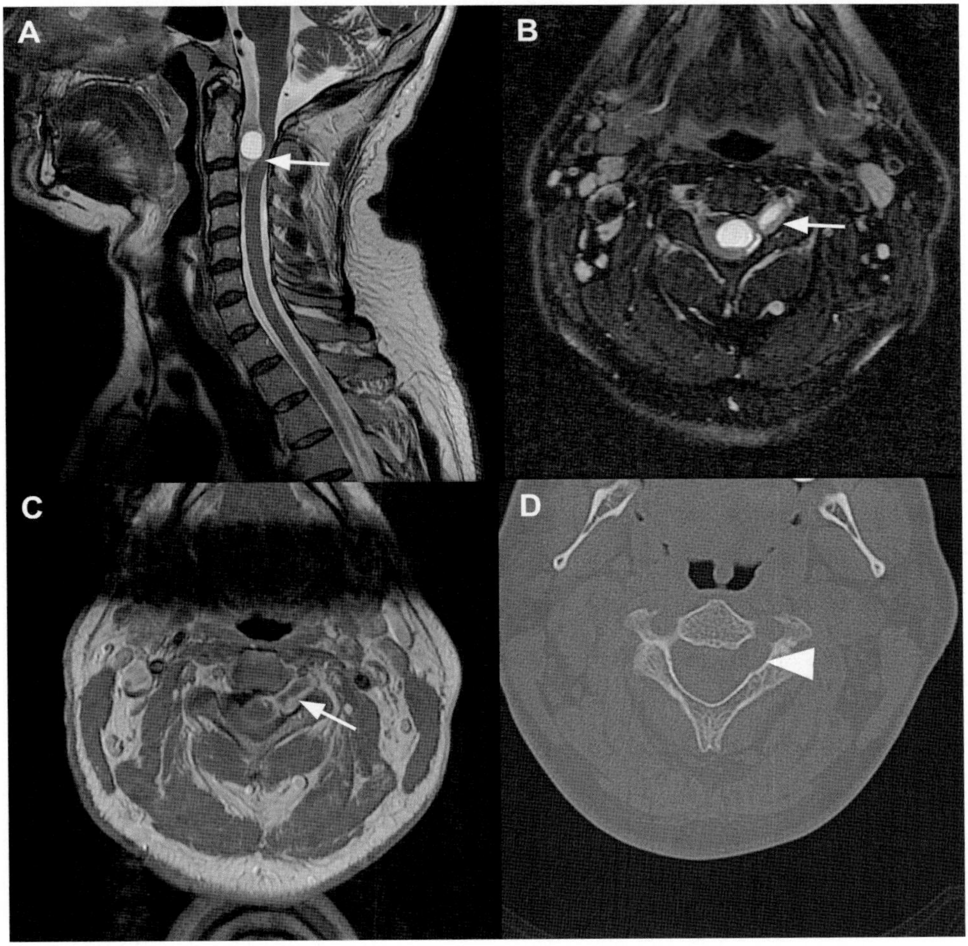

Fig. 21. Patient with chronic history of neck pain and 4-week history of cold sensation and stiffness in his left arm. (*A*) Sagittal FSE T2 MR imaging sequence; (*B*) FSE T2 axial sequence with fat saturation; (*C*) axial FSE T1 sequence with contrast; (*D*) axial CT image all demonstrating peripherally enhancing heterogeneous lesion (*arrows*) extending through the left C2-C3 neural foramen. Note expansion of neural foramen (*arrowhead*) on CT image. Schwannoma.

of 152 patients presented with paraplegia. There was a male predominance in this cohort.[61]

Women (between the fourth and fifth decades) account for approximately 85% of patients with spinal meningiomas and most of these lesions are in the thoracic spine. Meningiomas are much more common in the cervical spine in men.[62] Clinical presentation is often delayed secondary to the slowly progressive nature of meningiomas. One early study demonstrated a 6-month delay in diagnosis in 75% of their patients.[63] A more recent study demonstrated an average duration of symptoms of 23 months before diagnosis.[64] Regional pain and lower extremity paresthesias are the most common presenting features of spinal meningioma. Sensorimotor deficits are the next most prominent complaint leading to gait difficulty (83%).[21] The most common motor symptom is a spastic paraparesis secondary to the high frequency of thoracic lesions.[62,65] As opposed to schwannomas, meningiomas are less likely to present with radicular features.[63–65]

Paragangliomas are tumors of neural crest origin thought to arise in the filum terminale from peripheral neuroblasts.[21,66] Eighty percent to 90% of these tumors are associated with the carotid body or glomus jugulare. Spinal tumors are rare but are predominantly located in the intradural-extramedullary compartment of the lumbar spine at the level of the filum terminale.[67] These tumors typically present because of pain caused by the compression of neural structures.[67] The duration of pain symptoms can be extremely variable, but radicular or stenosis symptoms usually accompany

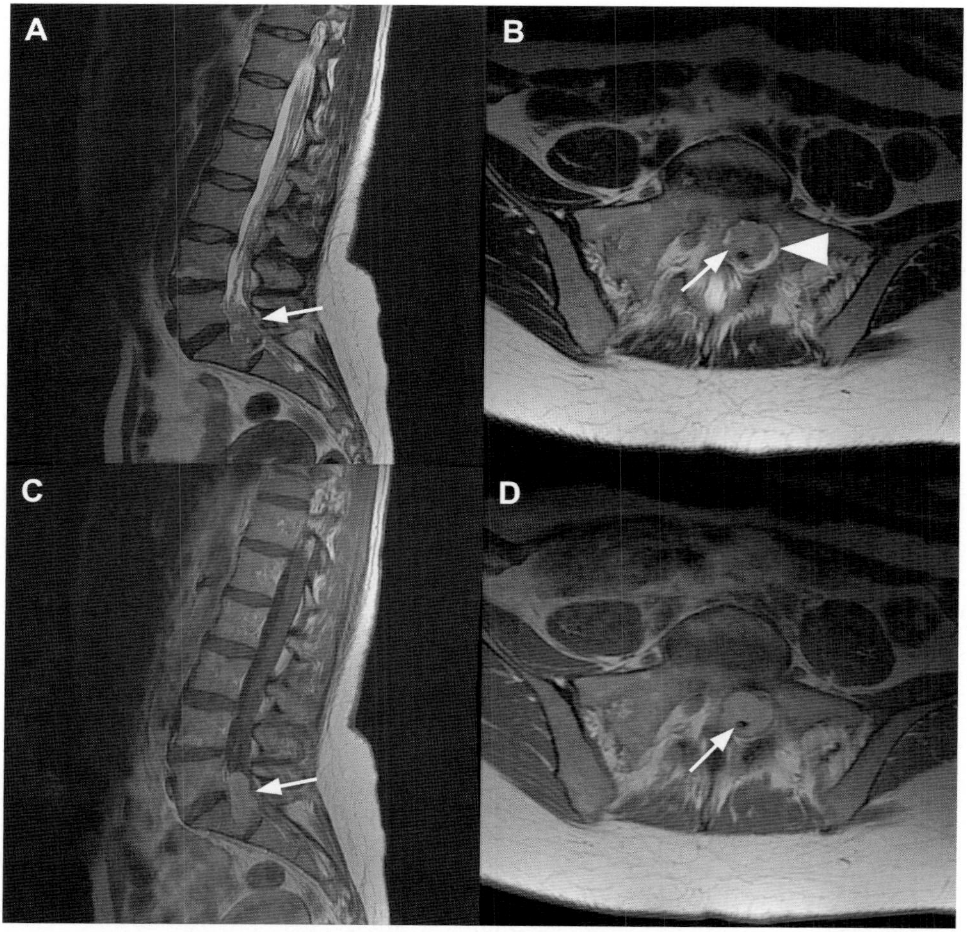

Fig. 22. FSE T2 sagittal sequence (*A*), FSE T2 axial sequence (*B*), FSE T1 sagittal (*C*), and axial (*D*) MR imaging sequences after contrast demonstrate a left S1 schwannoma (*arrow*) that extends through and expands the left S1 neural foramen (*arrowhead*).

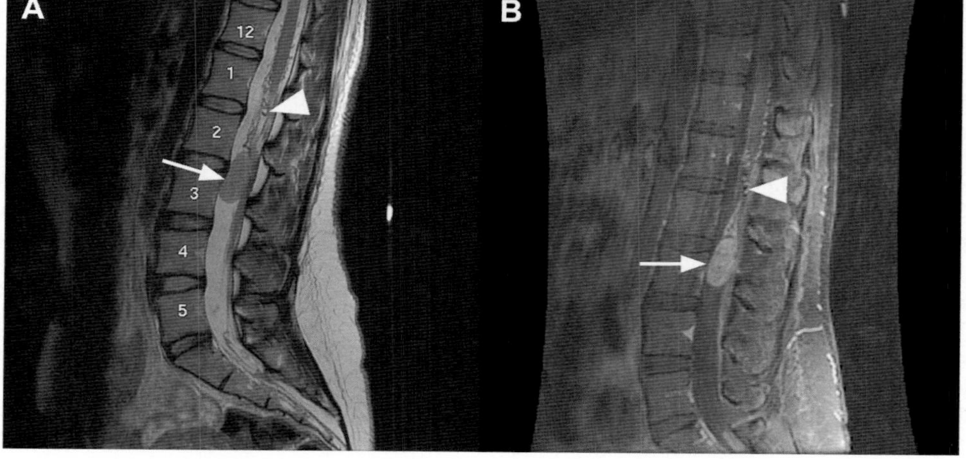

Fig. 23. A 37-year-old with a 5-month history of right hip pain, worse when reclining at night. Sagittal FSE T2 MR imaging sequence (*A*) and sagittal FSE T1 sequence with contrast and fat saturation (*B*) define this homogeneously enhancing lesion (*arrows*) of the filum terminale. Note prominent vascularity associated with this lesion (*arrowheads*). Paraganglioma.

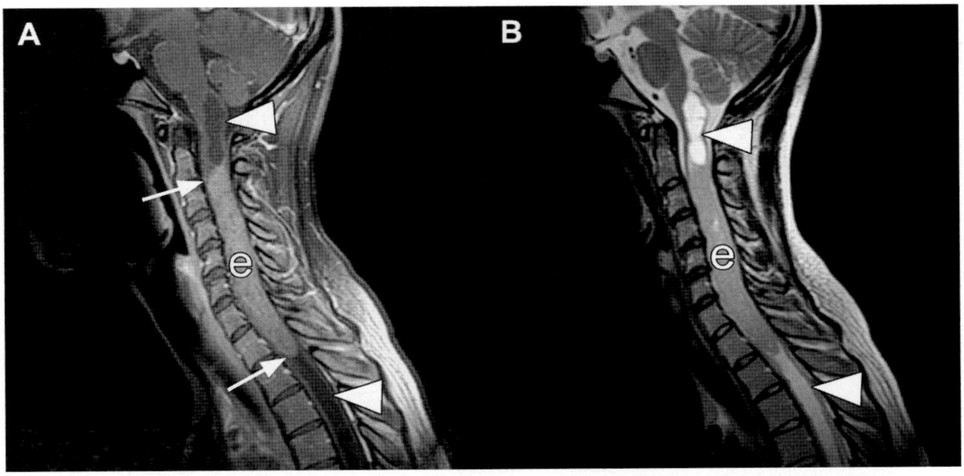

Fig. 24. A 22-year-old woman with a 6-month history of neck pain, followed by progressive upper-extremity weakness and incoordination. (*A*) FSE T1 sagittal MR imaging sequence after contrast with fat saturation. (*B*) FSE T2 sagittal sequence. Multilevel cervical ependymoma (e) with syrinx formation (*arrowheads*). Note sharp margins of enhancing tumor component (*arrows*).

back pain.[21] Recumbent pain has been reported in extramedullary tumors of the spine. Up to 50% of patients in reviews of lesions of the cauda equina have presented with pain when reclining.[68–70] Other investigators have described pain that awakens patients from sleep 4 to 6 hours after retiring or the necessity of sleeping in a recliner to relieve symptoms.[71,72]

Imaging of Intradural-Extramedullary Neoplasms

MR imaging is the modality of choice for defining intradural-extramedullary lesions. CT can be helpful in defining mineralization or bone remodeling[60] in these tumors, but MR imaging with contrast clearly better defines tissue characteristics and the multiple soft tissue planes surrounding these lesions. Radiologists have struggled to differentiate meningioma from schwannoma in the filum terminale and in other spinal locations. T1 and T2 signal characteristic are comparable on MR imaging, with schwannomas demonstrating slightly more heterogeneous increased T2 signal. Tumors that demonstrate a dural tail (**Figs. 19** and **20**) and contain calcification are predictors of meningioma, whereas lesions in the lumbar spine, lesions with rim enhancement, and lesions that result in vertebral scalloping or widening of neural foramen are predictors of schwannoma (**Figs. 21** and **22**).[60]

Paragangliomas typically demonstrate intense contrast enhancement and increased T2 signal. Occasionally, prominent vascularity may be associated with these lesions and may allow one to differentiate these lesions from other filum lesions (**Fig. 23**).[21,66,67]

Intramedullary Tumors

Ependymomas and Astrocytomas comprises 90% of intramedullary tumors.[66] Other intramedullary tumors include myxopapillary ependymoma, hemangioblastoma, metastasis, melanocytoma, and ganglioglioma. Because spinal cord astrocytoma and ependymoma account for the majority of intramedullary tumors, the clinical presentation and radiologic appearance of these intramedullary lesions are reviewed. Intramedullary ependymomas are the most common spinal cord tumor in adults, representing 60% of all intramedullary tumors.[73,74] These tumors are most frequent in middle age, men and woman are equally affected, and 68% of these lesions occur in the cervical spine.[73,74]

Clinical presentation can be extremely variable and depends on the site of the lesion. Symptom duration before diagnosis may extend for 3 to 4 years.[75] Sensory symptoms (dysesthesias) are typically the first to appear in approximately 70% of patients.[73,76] Painful aching sensations localized to the level of the tumor may also be present.[77] These symptoms are rarely radicular.[73] Upper extremity symptoms predominate in cervical lesions. Thoracic cord tumors produce spasticity and sensory disturbance in the lower extremities. Numbness is typical and usually begins distally in the legs with proximal progression.[75] Weakness

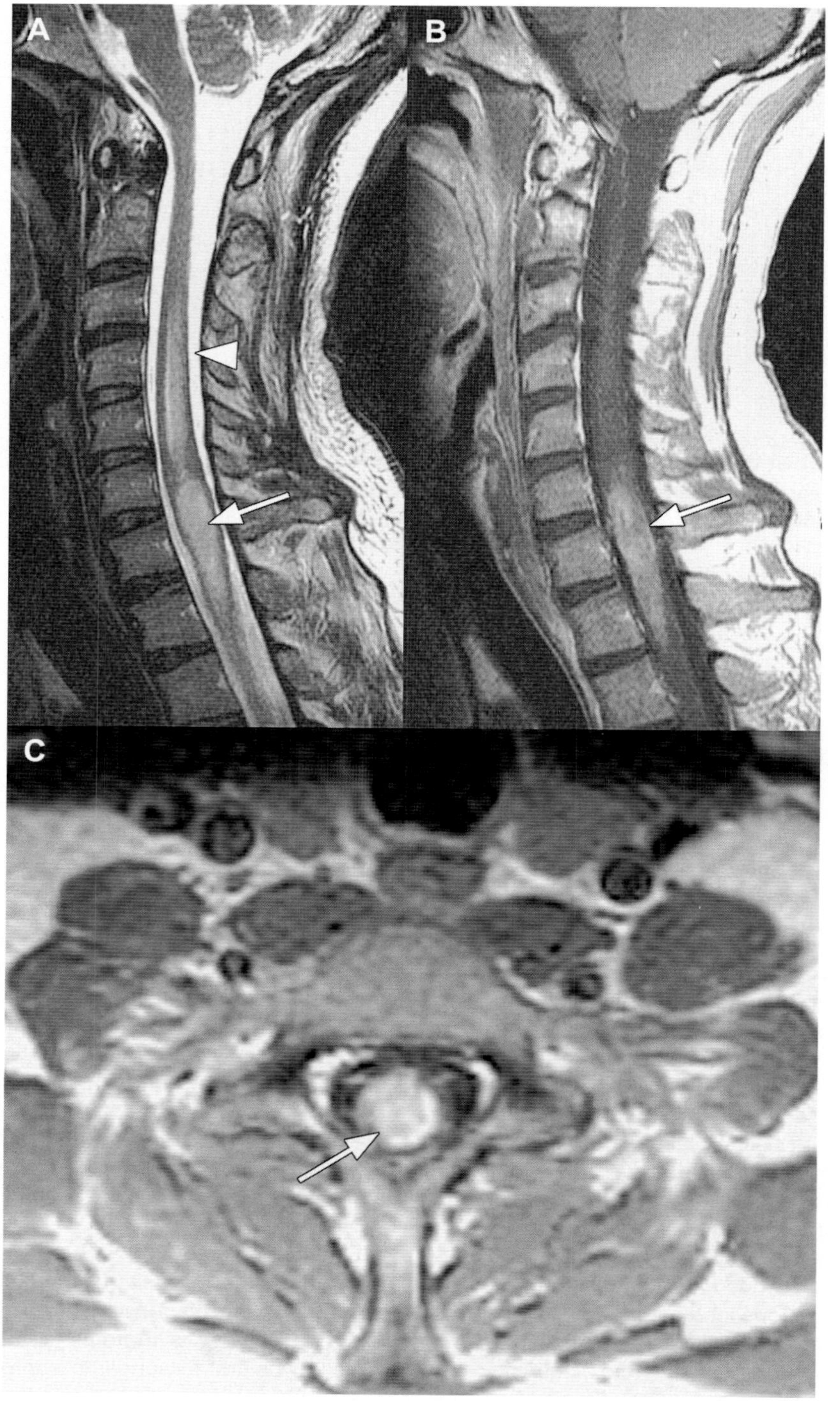

Fig. 25. A 37-year-old woman with neck pain and progressive myelopathy. (*A*) Sagittal FSE T2 MR imaging sequence; (*B*) sagittal FSE T1 sequence with contrast; (*C*) axial FSE T1 sequence with contrast. Poorly marginated, enhancing intramedullary lesion (*arrows*) with associated nonenhancing edema and cord expansion (*arrowhead*). Spinal astrocytoma.

usually occurs late and is usually associated with marked thinning of the cord.[76]

The clinical presentation of spinal cord astrocytomas parallels that of ependymomas. Variable presenting symptoms with a prolonged time to presentation over months to years is again the rule. Pain is the earliest presenting feature and it may be radicular. Sensory disturbance is common, including dysesthesias, and symptoms can be unilateral or bilateral. Spasticity and weakness are typically late features of presentation.[78] These tumors tend to be more centrally located. In young children, pain remains the most common early reported symptom; however, gait deterioration, motor regression, torticollis, and scoliosis are also significant findings.[78]

Imaging of Intramedullary Neoplasms

Prospectively, differentiating spinal astrocytomas from ependymomas is challenging. Some investigators do not think that imaging can reliably distinguish between these 2 tumors.[21,78] However, MR imaging characteristics, tumor location, age at presentation, and pathologic traits all offer clues to diagnosis. MR imaging with and without contrast is the modality of choice for evaluating these neoplasms. Spinal cord astrocytomas are more likely to be eccentrically located in the spinal cord.[78] Ependymomas are centrally located, possibly secondary to their origin from ependymal cells of the central canal. Ependymomas are rare in children, whereas astrocytomas are the most common spinal tumor of childhood.[79]

Spinal cord expansion, T1 and T2 signal abnormality, which can be homogeneous or heterogeneous, and tumor enhancement can be found in both astrocytoma and spinal ependymoma. Pathologically, ependymomas tend to be well-marginated lesions as opposed to astrocytomas, but this finding does not assure imaging diagnosis. T2 signal abnormality will encompass both the tumor margin and associated edema; hence, contrast enhancement is essential to define the true margin of the lesion. Nonenhancing ependymomas and astrocytomas exist but are rare entities.[79] Pathologically, hemosiderin is a frequent finding in ependymomas and this can be demonstrated on MR imaging, especially on gradient echo sequences.[79] In general, ependymomas are more likely to demonstrate heterogeneity on imaging with intratumoral hemorrhage, cysts, and syrinx found in greater frequency than in spinal astrocytomas (**Figs. 24** and **25**).[21]

Myxopapillary ependymoma occurs almost exclusively in the filum terminale or conus. Myxopapillary ependymomas represent more than 90% of filum terminale tumors. These soft tissue tumors consist of cellular elements in a papillary pattern with a characteristic intercellular mucinous matrix.[80] The lesion is typically well circumscribed, may fill the central canal, and may be associated

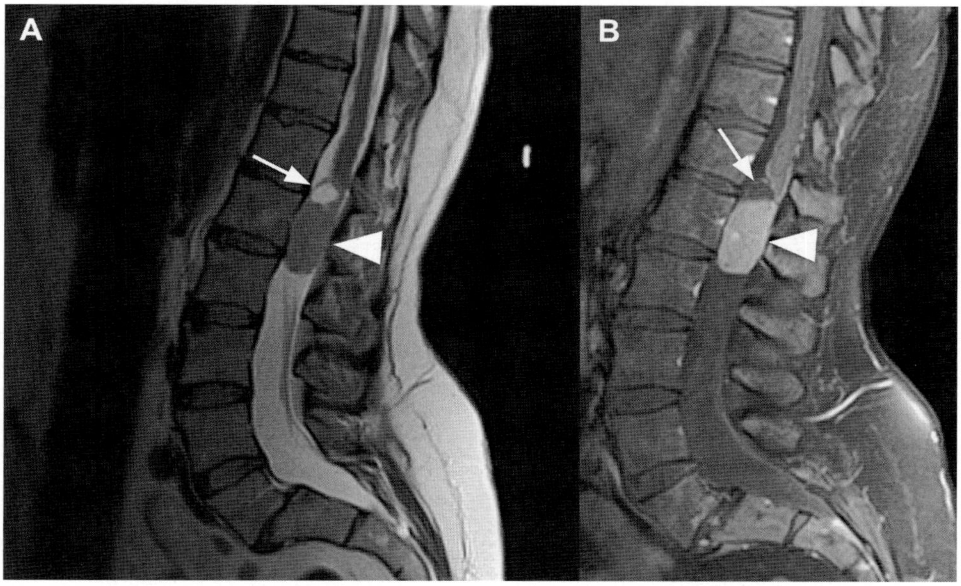

Fig. 26. A 47-year-old woman with a 6-month history of back pain with worsening pseudoclaudication symptoms and urinary incontinence. FSE T2 sagittal MR imaging sequence (*A*) and FSE T1 sagittal sequence with contrast and fat saturation (*B*). Heterogeneous enhancing mass of the filum (*arrowheads*) with cyst formation (*arrows*). Myxopapillary ependymoma.

with hemorrhage.[81] T2-weighted MR imaging sequences typically demonstrate a homogeneous hyperintense lesion unless hemorrhage is present. There is usually intense contrast enhancement (**Fig. 26**).[82]

SUMMARY

The spine is a complex organ comprised of multiple compartments. Tumors may arise from any of these compartments (extradural, intradural-extramedullary, or intramedullary) and patients may present with a wide range of clinical symptoms. Though the differential diagnosis of these spine lesions can be broad, a logical, concise differential diagnosis may be formed by defining these tumors by compartment, understanding the modality specific imaging appearance of these lesions and by considering the typical clinical presentation of these patients.

REFERENCES

1. Cramer GD, Darby SA. Basic and clinical anatomy of the spine, spinal cord and ANS. 2nd edition. St Louis (MO): Elesvier, Mosby; 2005.
2. Bogduk N. The innervation of the lumbar spine. Spine 1983;8(3):286–93.
3. Siddall PJ, Cousins MJ. Neurobiology of pain. Int Anesthesiol Clin 1997;35(2):1–26.
4. Donthineni R. Diagnosis and staging of spine tumors. Orthop Clin North Am 2009;40(1):1–7.
5. Sundaresan N, Rosen G, Boriani S. Primary malignant tumors of the spine. Orthop Clin North Am 2009;40(1):21–36.
6. Weinstein SM, Walton O. Management of pain associated with spinal tumor. Neurosurg Clin N Am 2004; 15(4):511–27.
7. Gasbarrini A, Cappuccio M, Mirabile L, et al. Spinal metastases: treatment evaluation algorithm. Eur Rev Med Pharmacol Sci 2004;8(6):265–74.
8. Taoka T, Mayr NA, Lee HJ, et al. Factors influencing visualization of vertebral metastases on MR imaging versus bone scintigraphy. AJR Am J Roentgenol 2001;176(6):1525–30.
9. Iqbal B, Currie GM, Wheat JM, et al. The incremental value of SPECT/CT in characterizing solitary spine lesions. J Nucl Med Technol 2011;39(3):201–7.
10. Kim DH, Rosenblum JK, Panghaal VS, et al. Differentiating neoplastic from nonneoplastic processes in the anterior extradural space. Radiology 2011; 260(3):825–30.
11. Scarabino T, Giannatempo GM, Popolizio T, et al. Fast spin echo imaging of vertebral metastasis: comparison of fat suppression techniques (FSE-CHESS, STIR-FSE). Radiol Med 1996;92(3): 180–5 [in Italian].
12. Kyle RA, Rajkumar SV. Multiple myeloma. N Engl J Med 2004;351(18):1860–73.
13. Kyle RA, Gertz MA, Witzig TE, et al. Review of 1027 patients with newly diagnosed multiple myeloma. Mayo Clin Proc 2003;78(1):21–33.
14. Mahnken AH, Wildberger JE, Gehbauer G, et al. Multidetector CT of the spine in multiple myeloma: comparison with MR imaging and radiography. AJR Am J Roentgenol 2002;178(6):1429–36.
15. Jadvar H, Conti PS. Diagnostic utility of FDG PET in multiple myeloma. Skeletal Radiol 2002;31(12):690–4.
16. Mele A, Offidani M, Visani G, et al. Technetium-99m sestamibi scintigraphy is sensitive and specific for the staging and the follow-up of patients with multiple myeloma: a multicentre study on 397 scans. Br J Haematol 2007;136(5):729–35.
17. Layton KF, Thielen KR, Cloft HJ, et al. Acute vertebral compression fractures in patients with multiple myeloma: evaluation of vertebral body edema patterns on MR imaging and the implications for vertebroplasty. AJNR Am J Neuroradiol 2006;27(8): 1732–4.
18. Lecouvet FE, Vande Berg BC, Maldague BE, et al. Vertebral compression fractures in multiple myeloma. Part I. Distribution and appearance at MR imaging. Radiology 1997;204(1):195–9.
19. Ilaslan H, Sundaram M, Unni KK, et al. Primary vertebral osteosarcoma: imaging findings. Radiology 2004;230(3):697–702.
20. Ozaki T, Flege S, Liljenqvist U, et al. Osteosarcoma of the spine: experience of the Cooperative Osteosarcoma Study Group. Cancer 2002;94(4):1069–77.
21. Ross JS, Moore KR, Borg B, et al. Diagnostic imaging: spine. 2nd edition. Salt Lake City (Utah): Amirsys; 2010.
22. Indelicato DJ, Keole SR, Shahlaee AH, et al. Spinal and paraspinal Ewing tumors. Int J Radiat Oncol Biol Phys 2010;76(5):1463–71.
23. Venkateswaran L, Rodriguez-Galindo C, Merchant TE, et al. Primary Ewing tumor of the vertebrae: clinical characteristics, prognostic factors, and outcome. Med Pediatr Oncol 2001;37(1):30–5.
24. Sty JR, Wells RG, Conway JJ. Spine pain in children. Semin Nucl Med 1993;23(4):296–320.
25. Mar WA, Taljanovic MS, Bagatell R, et al. Update on imaging and treatment of Ewing sarcoma family tumors: what the radiologist needs to know. J Comput Assist Tomogr 2008;32(1):108–18.
26. Resnick D. Diagnosis of bone and joint disorders. 4th edition. Philadelphia: Saunders; 2002.
27. Sciubba DM, Chi JH, Rhines LD, et al. Chordoma of the spinal column. Neurosurg Clin N Am 2008;19(1): 5–15.
28. McMaster ML, Goldstein AM, Bromley CM, et al. Chordoma: incidence and survival patterns in the United States, 1973-1995. Cancer Causes Control 2001;12(1):1–11.

29. Sciubba DM, Hsieh P, McLoughlin GS, et al. Pediatric tumors involving the spinal column. Neurosurg Clin N Am 2008;19(1):81–92.
30. Boriani S, Bandiera S, Biagini R, et al. Chordoma of the mobile spine: fifty years of experience. Spine 2006;31(4):493–503.
31. Llauger J, Palmer J, Amores S, et al. Primary tumors of the sacrum: diagnostic imaging. AJR Am J Roentgenol 2000;174(2):417–24.
32. Park SA, Kim HS. F-18 FDG PET/CT evaluation of sacrococcygeal chordoma. Clin Nucl Med 2008; 33(12):906–8.
33. McLoughlin GS, Sciubba DM, Wolinsky JP. Chondroma/chondrosarcoma of the spine. Neurosurg Clin N Am 2008;19(1):57–63.
34. Chow WA. Update on chondrosarcomas. Curr Opin Oncol 2007;19(4):371–6.
35. Boriani S, De Iure F, Bandiera S, et al. Chondrosarcoma of the mobile spine: report on 22 cases. Spine 2000;25(7):804–12.
36. Murphey MD, Walker EA, Wilson AJ, et al. From the archives of the AFIP: imaging of primary chondrosarcoma: radiologic-pathologic correlation. Radiographics 2003;23(5):1245–78.
37. Murphey MD, Andrews CL, Flemming DJ, et al. From the archives of the AFIP. Primary tumors of the spine: radiologic pathologic correlation. Radiographics 1996;16(5):1131–58.
38. Kumar V, Abbas AK, Fausto N, et al. Robbins basic pathology. Philadelphia: Saunders; 2007.
39. Sapkas G, Efstathopoulos NE, Papadakis M. Undiagnosed osteoid osteoma of the spine presenting as painful scoliosis from adolescence to adulthood: a case report. Scoliosis 2009;4:9.
40. Gasbarrini A, Cappuccio M, Bandiera S, et al. Osteoid osteoma of the mobile spine: surgical outcomes in 81 patients. Spine 2011;36(24):2089–93.
41. Greco F, Tamburrelli F, Ciabattoni G. Prostaglandins in osteoid osteoma. Int Orthop 1991;15(1):35–7.
42. Dreghorn CR, Newman RJ, Hardy GJ, et al. Primary tumors of the axial skeleton: experience of the Leeds Regional Bone Tumor Registry. Spine 1990;15(2): 137–40.
43. Zenmyo M, Yamamoto T, Ishidou Y, et al. Osteoid osteoma near the intervertebral foramen may induce radiculopathy through tumorous inflammation. Diagn Pathol 2011;6:10.
44. Afshani E, Kuhn JP. Common causes of low back pain in children. Radiographics 1991;11(2):269–91.
45. Cove JA, Taminiau AH, Obermann WR, et al. Osteoid osteoma of the spine treated with percutaneous computed tomography-guided thermocoagulation. Spine 2000;25(10):1283–6.
46. Gangi A, Alizadeh H, Wong L, et al. Osteoid osteoma: percutaneous laser ablation and follow-up in 114 patients. Radiology 2007;242(1): 293–301.
47. Boriani S, De Iure F, Campanacci L, et al. Aneurysmal bone cyst of the mobile spine: report on 41 cases. Spine 2001;26(1):27–35.
48. Mankin HJ, Hornicek FJ, Ortiz-Cruz E, et al. Aneurysmal bone cyst: a review of 150 patients. J Clin Oncol 2005;23(27):6756–62.
49. Kransdorf MJ, Sweet DE. Aneurysmal bone cyst: concept, controversy, clinical presentation, and imaging. AJR Am J Roentgenol 1995;164(3):573–80.
50. Chan MS, Wong YC, Yuen MK, et al. Spinal aneurysmal bone cyst causing acute cord compression without vertebral collapse: CT and MRI findings. Pediatr Radiol 2002;32(8):601–4.
51. Raftopoulos C, Hurrel A, Ticket L, et al. Total recuperation in a case of sudden total paraplegia due to an aneurysmal bone cyst of the thoracic spine. Childs Nerv Syst 1994;10(7):464–7.
52. Hudson TM. Fluid levels in aneurysmal bone cysts: a CT feature. AJR Am J Roentgenol 1984;142(5): 1001–4.
53. Kwon JW, Chung HW, Cho EY, et al. MRI findings of giant cell tumors of the spine. AJR Am J Roentgenol 2007;189(1):246–50.
54. Sanjay BK, Sim FH, Unni KK, et al. Giant-cell tumours of the spine. J Bone Joint Surg 1993; 75(1):148–54.
55. Aoki J, Tanikawa H, Ishii K, et al. MR findings indicative of hemosiderin in giant-cell tumor of bone: frequency, cause, and diagnostic significance. AJR Am J Roentgenol 1996;166(1):145–8.
56. Ropper AE, Cahill KS, Hanna JW, et al. Primary vertebral tumors: a review of epidemiologic, histologic and imaging findings. Part II: locally aggressive and malignant tumors. Neurosurgery 2011; 69(6):1171–80.
57. Acosta FL Jr, Sanai N, Chi JH, et al. Comprehensive management of symptomatic and aggressive vertebral hemangiomas. Neurosurg Clin N Am 2008; 19(1):17–29.
58. Pastushyn AI, Slin'ko EI, Mirzoyeva GM. Vertebral hemangiomas: diagnosis, management, natural history and clinicopathological correlates in 86 patients. Surg Neurol 1998;50(6):535–47.
59. Karaeminogullari O, Tuncay C, Demirors H, et al. Multilevel vertebral hemangiomas: two episodes of spinal cord compression at separate levels 10 years apart. Eur Spine J 2005;14(7):706–10.
60. Liu WC, Choi G, Lee SH, et al. Radiological findings of spinal schwannomas and meningiomas: focus on discrimination of two disease entities. Eur Radiol 2009;19(11):2707–15.
61. Conti P, Pansini G, Mouchaty H, et al. Spinal neurinomas: retrospective analysis and long-term outcome of 179 consecutively operated cases and review of the literature. Surg Neurol 2004;61(1):34–44.
62. Souweidane MM, Benjamin V. Spinal cord meningiomas. Neurosurg Clin N Am 1994;5(2):283–91.

63. Davis RA, Washburn PL. Spinal cord meningiomas. Surg Gynecol Obstet 1970;131(1):15–21.
64. Levy WJ Jr, Bay J, Dohn D. Spinal cord meningioma. J Neurosurg 1982;57(6):804–12.
65. Iraci G, Peserico L, Salar G. Intraspinal neurinomas and meningiomas. A clinical survey of 172 cases. Int Surg 1971;56(5):289–303.
66. Sousa J, O'Brien D, Crooks D. Paraganglioma of the filum terminale. J Clin Neurosci 2005;12(5): 584–5.
67. Sundgren P, Annertz M, Englund E, et al. Paragangliomas of the spinal canal. Neuroradiology 1999; 41(10):788–94.
68. Nicholas JJ, Christy WC. Spinal pain made worse by recumbency: a clue to spinal cord tumors. Arch Phys Med Rehabil 1986;67(9):598–600.
69. Fearnside MR, Adams CB. Tumours of the cauda equina. J Neurol Neurosurg Psychiatr 1978;41(1): 24–31.
70. Milnes JN. The early diagnosis of tumours of the cauda equina. J Neurol Neurosurg Psychiatr 1953; 16(3):158–65.
71. Allen IM. Tumours involving the cauda equina: a review of their clinical features and differential diagnosis. J Neurol Psychopathol 1930;11(42):111–43.
72. Rasmussen TB, Kernohan JW, Adson AW. Pathologic classification, with surgical consideration, of intraspinal tumors. Ann Surg 1940;111(4):513–30.
73. Schwartz TH, McCormick PC. Intramedullary ependymomas: clinical presentation, surgical treatment strategies and prognosis. J Neurooncol 2000; 47(3):211–8.
74. Helseth A, Mork SJ. Primary intraspinal neoplasms in Norway, 1955 to 1986. A population-based survey of 467 patients. J Neurosurg 1989;71(6):842–5.
75. Schwartz TH, McCormick PC. Non-neoplastic intramedullary pathology. Diagnostic dilemma: to Bx or not to Bx. J Neurooncol 2000;47(3):283–92.
76. Epstein FJ, Farmer JP, Freed D. Adult intramedullary spinal cord ependymomas: the result of surgery in 38 patients. J Neurosurg 1993;79(2):204–9.
77. McCormick PC, Stein BM. Intramedullary tumors in adults. Neurosurg Clin N Am 1990;1(3):609–30.
78. Houten JK, Cooper PR. Spinal cord astrocytomas: presentation, management and outcome. J Neurooncol 2000;47(3):219–24.
79. Lowe GM. Magnetic resonance imaging of intramedullary spinal cord tumors. J Neurooncol 2000;47(3): 195–210.
80. Sonneland PR, Scheithauer BW, Onofrio BM. Myxopapillary ependymoma. A clinicopathologic and immunocytochemical study of 77 cases. Cancer 1985;56(4):883–93.
81. Hanbali F, Fourney DR, Marmor E, et al. Spinal cord ependymoma: radical surgical resection and outcome. Neurosurgery 2002;51(5):1162–72 [discussion: 72–4].
82. Yamada CY, Whitman GJ, Chew FS. Myxopapillary ependymoma of the filum terminale. AJR Am J Roentgenol 1997;168(2):366.

Imaging of Spine Infection

Felix E. Diehn, MD

KEYWORDS

• Spine infection • Pyogenic spondylodiscitis • Pyogenic • Granulomatous • Epidural abscess • Facetitis • Pyomyositis

KEY POINTS

- Spinal infections are increasing, and the radiologist plays a critical a role in both image interpretation and image-guided sampling.
- Magnetic resonance imaging is the modality of choice for imaging spinal infection.
- Pyogenic spondylodiscitis is typically centered about a disc space and when possible, should be differentiated on imaging from Modic type 1 endplate changes.
- Spinal epidural abscesses and the rare subdural abscesses are emergencies.
- Tuberculous spondylitis can be suggested over pyogenic spondylodiscitis on the basis of several characteristic imaging features.

This article reviews the imaging and relevant clinical details of infection of the extradural spine. Radiologists play an important role in diagnosing spinal infection. Due to the aging and more globally mobile population, the increase in predisposing comorbid factors such as diabetes and intravenous drug use, the increase in spinal instrumentation, elevated awareness, and the increased use and diagnostic performance of advanced imaging, spine infections are increasing in incidence and in frequency of diagnosis. They are clinically important despite their relative rarity, because they may be life-threatening, and because early diagnosis leads to improved outcomes. The focus is on pyogenic spondylodiscitis, the most common type of spine infection encountered in routine clinical practice. The also typically pyogenic conditions of epidural abscess and subdural abscess, facet joint infection, and pyomyositis are discussed. Nonpyogenic, granulomatous infections are also addressed. Magnetic resonance imaging (MRI) is emphasized, as it is generally the most sensitive and specific diagnostic modality for these entities. The radiologist's role in performing minimally invasive sampling procedures is highlighted. With the exception of subdural (intradural) abscess, infections and inflammatory conditions of the spinal cord, spinal nerve roots, and spinal meninges are not considered. The extremely rare parasitic spinal infections are also beyond the scope of this article. The imaging of these conditions has been reviewed elsewhere, including recently in this journal.[1–3]

PYOGENIC SPONDYLODISCITIS

Background

Pyogenic spondylodiscitis is a bacterial infection of the bony spinal column, the intervertebral discs, and/or the ligaments of the extradural spine. The most common cause of pyogenic spondylodiscitis is hematogenous spread of infection from a remote site. This is typically via the arterial route, although the paravertebral venous plexus has also been implicated. Urinary tract infections are the most frequent culprit. Other etiologies include direct inoculation, such as in the postoperative setting, discography, and therapeutic spinal injections,[4] and contiguous spread from adjacent infected sites. The infection is usually unimicrobial. *Staphylococcus aureus* is the most frequent causative organism, accounting for at least one-third of cases in multiple studies.[5,6] Diabetic patients in their 50s and 60s are frequently affected, and

Division of Neuroradiology, Department of Radiology, Mayo Clinic, 200 First Street SW, Rochester, MN 55905, USA
E-mail address: Diehn.felix@mayo.edu

Radiol Clin N Am 50 (2012) 777–798
doi:10.1016/j.rcl.2012.04.001
0033-8389/12/$ – see front matter

the disease is more common in men. Additional predisposing factors include chronic disease, such as renal failure and cirrhosis, other immunosuppressed states, and intravenous drug use.

Clinically, patients with pyogenic spondylodiscitis often pose a diagnostic dilemma, because the presentation may be subtle, insidious, and nonspecific. The time course can range from acute to chronic. Typically the patients present with focal back pain, often with associated muscle spasm and tenderness to palpation. There may be limited range of motion, neurologic deficit, weight loss, and malaise. Fever is relatively common but inconsistently present. The symptoms are often progressive, as the disease is frequently diagnosed relatively late in its course, even up to several months after symptom onset. Laboratory evaluation is not reliable, although elevated erythrocyte sedimentation rate (ESR) and elevated C-reactive protein (CRP) are often present. Leukocytosis is less commonly observed.[7–9]

Anatomically, the lumbar spine is most frequently affected, while the cervical spine is the least common subsite. The vertebral bodies and the intervertebral discs in the adult have a tenuous vascular supply, as both the rich network of intraosseous anastomoses and the profuse capillary network at the vertebral margins of the discs involute by adolescence. The most widely accepted pathophysiologic hypothesis is that an infected embolus causes infarction and subsequent infection in the vertebral body metaphysis. Infection typically begins in the anterior aspect of the vertebral bodies. It can spread to the remainder of the body, the opposite endplate, and particularly and early, the adjacent disc. Spread into the paraspinal and/or epidural spaces is common. Infection can also extend more deeply into the subdural or subarachnoid spaces. In children, the still highly vascular disc is often the primary site of infection, as the robust intraosseous arterial anastomoses protect the bone from substantial involvement.

Imaging Evaluation

Once a decision has been made to pursue spinal imaging in a patient with back pain, radiographs should be the first imaging modality obtained. However, radiographs are notoriously insensitive for discitis–osteomyelitis, particularly early in the course of the disease. They may in fact remain normal for several weeks after infection. Thus, findings such as endplate irregularity/destruction, loss of disc space height, and paraspinal bulging or loss of soft tissue planes typically lag behind the clinical evolution. But since the disease is often not diagnosed early, with at times months of symptoms before diagnosis, radiographs can be useful and are often positive (**Fig. 1**A, B). In a recent systematic review, radiographs demonstrated abnormal findings in 89% of cases.[5] Chronic phase findings include endplate sclerosis and ankylosis across an affected interspace.

MRI is the most useful modality for imaging spine infection, and the findings of pyogenic spondylodiscitis have been well described and reviewed in the literature (see **Figs. 1**C–G; **2**A–F, H–L, **3**C, D; **Box 1**). A screening study when clinical suspicion exists should evaluate the entire neuroaxis. Regarding MRI protocol, fat-suppressed T2-weighted sequences are useful, and postgadolinium T1-weighted imaging should include fat suppression to increase conspicuity of the findings.[10] In typical disease, infection begins in the anterior aspect of a vertebral body in the metaphyseal region and then spreads, often to involve the intervertebral disc and adjacent vertebral body. Bone marrow involvement manifests as an edema-type abnormality (T1 hypo-, T2 hyperintensity and contrast enhancement), and is classically most marked along the endplates at the infected level. Marrow T1 hypointensity and enhancement have each been found by some authors to be more common than marrow T2 hyperintensity.[11] Endplate erosions, and at later stages, vertebral body destruction, may be present. Disc involvement is evidenced by T2 hyperintensity, disc space height loss, loss of the normal T2 hypointense intranuclear cleft, and enhancement. The enhancement pattern of the involved disc is highly variable. Involved paraspinal soft tissues may show an enhancing edema-type abnormality (see **Fig. 1**G, **2**E, F and K, L) or frank abscess (T1 hypo-, T2 hyperintense fluid collection with peripheral contrast enhancement). Overall, findings that have been shown to have particularly high sensitivity for the diagnosis of pyogenic spondylodiscitis include the presence of paraspinal or epidural inflammation, vertebral body T1 hypointensity, disc space T2 hyperintensity, and disc space enhancement. In contrast, findings with relatively low sensitivity include disc T1 hypointensity and height loss.[12] Radiologists should scrutinize cases of pyogenic spondylodiscitis for the presence of an epidural abscess. Epidural abscesses have relatively high associated morbidity and mortality, particularly when treatment is delayed. Note that this subsite of infection may also be involved primarily, as extension of infection from other sites (such as facets, paraspinal regions, or the retroperitoneum), or in cases of granulomatous infection. Epidural abscesses, including the MRI

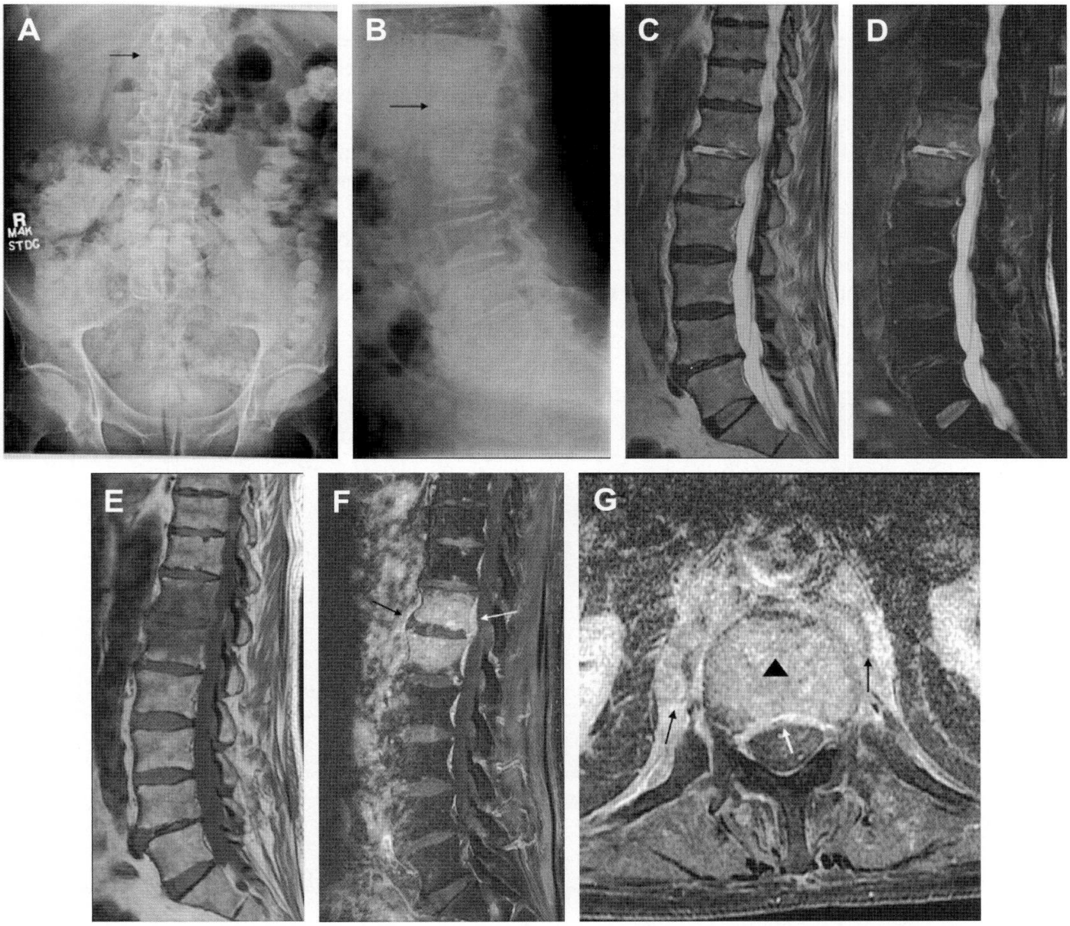

Fig. 1. Pyogenic spondylodiscitis. An 88-year-old man, with 1 month of back pain, presented with fever and *Escherichia coli* bacteremia. Anteroposterior (*A*) and lateral (*B*) views from standing radiographs demonstrate nonspecific loss of disc space height at T12-L1 (*arrows*). Radiographs are relatively insensitive. Even when findings are present, such as in this case, they are nonspecific. (*C*) T2-weighted sagittal MRI demonstrates T2 hyperintensity in the narrowed T12-L1 disc space. Note the relative lack of obvious T2 hyperintensity in the adjacent vertebral marrow. (*D*) T2-weighted, fat-saturated sagittal MRI demonstrates to much better advantage the abnormal T2 hyperintensity in the T12 and L1 vertebral bodies. (*E*) T1-weighted sagittal MRI demonstrates T1 hypointensity in the T12 and L1 vertebral bodies, centered about the T12-L1 interspace, with some sparing along the opposite endplates. Such marrow T1 hypointensity is a highly constant finding in spondylodiscitis. (*F*) Postgadolinium, fat-saturated T1-weighted sagittal MRI demonstrates avid enhancement corresponding to the abnormal vertebral marrow signal. Minimal disc space enhancement and mild ventral epidural (*white arrow*) and anterior paraspinal enhancement (*black arrow*) are evident. (*G*) Postgadolinium, fat-saturated T1-weighted axial MRI at the inferior T12 vertebral body level confirms the vertebral body (*black triangle*), ventral epidural (*white arrow*), and paraspinal contrast enhancement (*black arrows*). In this case, the epidural and paraspinal enhancement represents inflammation/phlegmon and/or venous engorgement in these spaces, without discrete abscess formation.

findings, are discussed in greater detail in a subsequent section.

The MRI-based diagnosis of pyogenic spondylodiscitis is not always straightforward. Indeed, pyogenic spondylodiscitis may have atypical appearances, including: lack of expected signal abnormalities and endplate erosive changes early in its course (see **Fig. 2**), involvement of a single vertebral body, involvement of 1 vertebral body and 1 disc, and involvement of 2 adjacent bodies without the intervening disc.[13] Occasionally, vertebral osteomyelitis may present as solitary or multiple discrete, enhancing bony spinal lesions without suspicious abnormalities of the intervertebral discs, mimicking metastatic disease.[14] In addition, when clinical information is not helpful or not available to the radiologist, confident diagnostic interpretation of equivocal cases can be difficult.

Although MRI is the modality of choice for imaging of pyogenic spondylodiscitis, it is not without shortcomings. MRI is not recommended for routine follow-up. It may lag behind the clinical picture, both at the onset of disease[15] and as the disease improves (see **Fig. 2**).[15–20] Several studies demonstrate that the MRI findings can worsen despite clinical improvement. Abnormal MRI findings, particularly of the involved bone and disc, and less so of the paraspinal soft tissues, may persist during the initial 4 to 8 weeks of antibiotic therapy[17] and even months after clinical cure has been achieved.[16,20,21] Therefore, MRI is not particularly useful in following patients who are clinically improving on antibiotic therapy. One study suggests that MRI at 4 to 8 weeks may be helpful in patients who are not demonstrating clinical or inflammatory biomarker evidence of improvement.[17] One sign that has been suggested to correlate with healing at MRI follow-up is focal development of marrow T1 hyperintensity (see **Fig. 2**M). This is thought to correspond with fatty

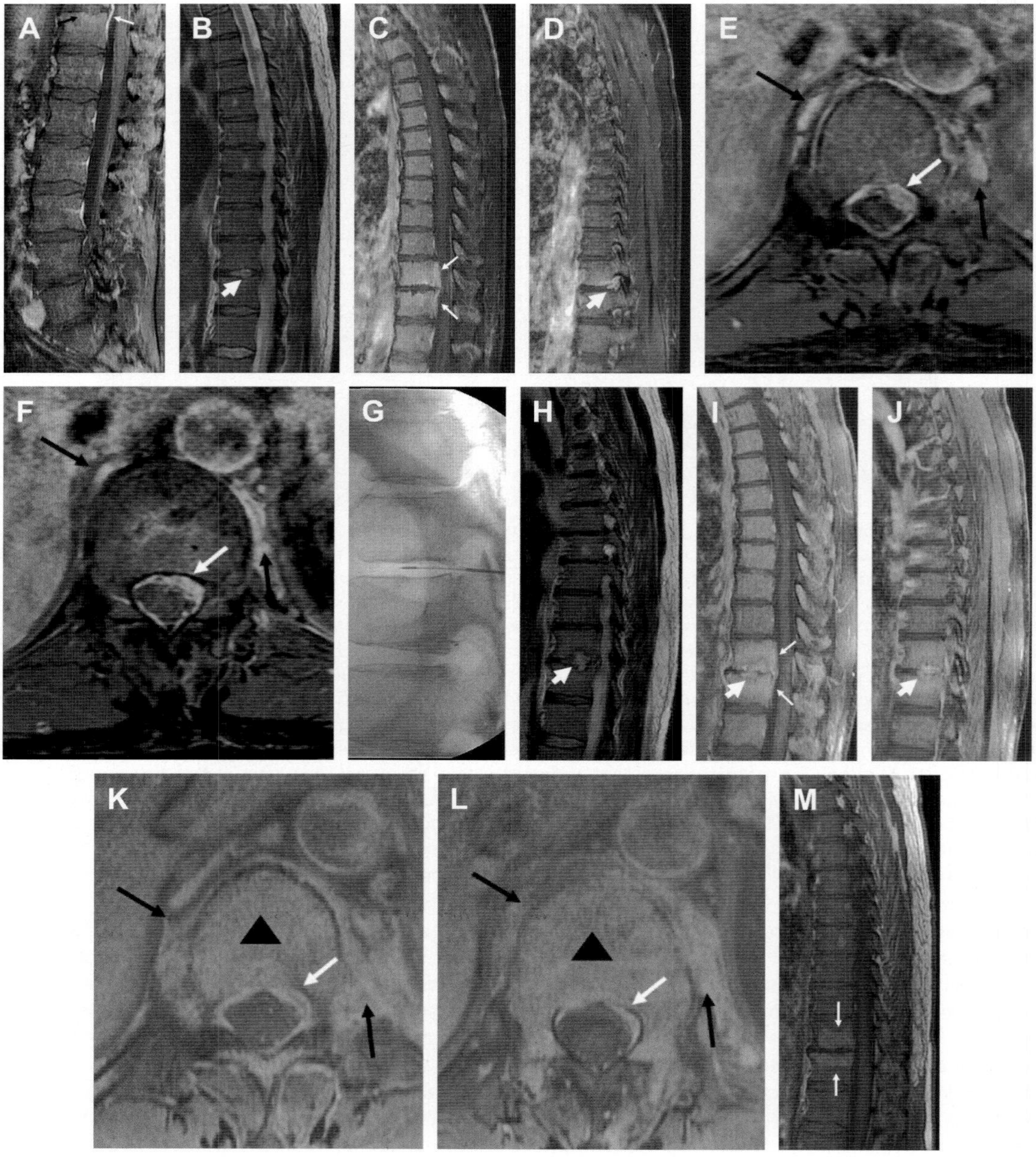

replacement of healed, previously abnormal bone marrow.[14,15]

MRI is also challenging in the setting of postoperative infection. Postoperative discitis and/or osteomyelitis is a relatively uncommon complication after lumbar spine surgery. MRI is less reliable in this setting, as even the normal postoperative spine may demonstrate disc or endplate signal changes/enhancement. MRI cannot reliably differentiate between pathology and expected postoperative evolution until at least 6 months after surgery.[22] One finding that may suggest postdiscectomy change rather than infection is 2 parallel thin bands of enhancement in the disc space; this is in contrast to the more amorphous enhancement generally seen with infection.[22] Paravertebral enhancement supports the diagnosis of infection, while the absence of enhancing, edema-type subendplate changes or disc space enhancement makes infection unlikely.[23]

Computed tomography (CT) is more sensitive than radiography, owing to its superior anatomic resolution. It can demonstrate many of the same findings as radiographs and even MRI, particularly when intravenous contrast is used to better evaluate the soft tissues. It is particularly useful where MRI is contraindicated, not available, or equivocal. In the author's experience, it can be especially helpful in confirming the suspicion of advanced degenerative (age-related) disc changes in patients who have been referred for biopsy to exclude infection (**Fig. 4**). Often, careful review of the CT (and any prior available imaging) may reveal evidence of advanced age-related disc changes, such as disc space vacuum phenomenon, which may obviate the need for biopsy. Image-guided biopsy will be discussed further, but it should be noted here that performing such a biopsy is not without risk. There are the inherent risks and costs of an invasive procedure, and perhaps more importantly, the imperfect sensitivity of biopsy sampling, which, if negative, obligates the clinician to at least consider ordering a repeat biopsy.

Despite relatively high sensitivity and specificity, nuclear medicine imaging is used only in select situations. This is primarily because of its limited spatial resolution and long examination time, as well as the availability, high spatial resolution, and excellent diagnostic performance of MRI. The nuclear study of choice in the author's center is sequential ^{99m}technetium-methylene diphosphonate and ^{67}gallium-citrate scintigraphy. Uptake that is greater and/or anatomically discordant on the gallium (inflammation detecting) than the technetium (metabolism detecting) portion of the study is the most accurate finding for spondylodiscitis. Select indications in the author's center include patients in whom MRI is contraindicated; MRI and CT are equivocal; multifocal infectious disease is suspected; or the clinical suspicion is high but the MRI is negative. Short-term follow-up MRI may also be helpful in the latter situation.

Fig. 2. MRI pitfalls in pyogenic spondylodiscitis: (1) initial findings may be subtle, especially when early and/or at edge of film if only 1 segment of spine is imaged, and (2) evolution of MRI findings is often discordant with clinical improvement. A 57-year-old man presented for lumbar spine MRI, for the indication of acute lumbar back pain. Initial lumbar spine MRI (*A*) postgadolinium, fat-saturated sagittal T1-weighted MR image was interpreted as negative. In retrospect, on the corner of the image is subtle thickening and enhancement in the ventral epidural space at T11-12 (*white arrow*) and less so subjacent to the T12 superior endplate (*black arrow*). 4 days later, thoracic spine MRI was obtained: sagittal T2-weighted (*B*), postgadolinium, fat-saturated T1-weighted sagittal (*C, D*) and axial (*E*) inferior T11 endplate, (*F*) superior T12 endplate MR images. The ventral epidural thickening and enhancement compatible with phlegmon is clearly demonstrated and has progressed (*white arrows* in *C, E, F*). Disc space T2 hyperintensity and enhancement are evident (*block white arrows* in *B* and *D*). Paraspinal inflammation is present (*black arrows* in *E, F*). A fluoroscopically guided disc space biopsy via discography approach was performed (*G*), yielding *Morganella morganii*, a gram-negative rod. Despite considerable clinical improvement with medical therapy, including improved symptoms and normalization of inflammatory markers, follow-up MRI 5 weeks later generally demonstrates progression of findings: sagittal T2-weighted (*H*), postgadolinium, fat-saturated T1-weighted sagittal (*I, J*) and axial (*K*) inferior T11 endplate, (*L*) superior T12 endplate MR images. There is interval increase in loss of disc space height and endplate erosion, T2 hyperintensity (*H*) and enhancement (*I, J*) of the disc space and adjacent endplates (*block white arrows* in *H–J*), enhancement of the vertebral bodies (*black arrowheads* in *K, L*) and paraspinal inflammation (*black arrows* in *K, L*). However, epidural thickening and enhancement has improved (*white arrows* in *I, K, L*). Some studies suggest soft tissue findings tend to improve before disc space and bony findings, but MRI is generally not useful to follow-up patients who are clinically improving. Sagittal T1-weighted MR image from a follow-up MRI performed 9 months later (*M*) demonstrates marrow T1 hyperintensity about the interspace (*white arrows*), corresponding with healed, fatty-replaced marrow. Note the otherwise diffuse marrow T1 hypointensity, which is related to the patient's known non-Hodgkin lymphoma and/or its treatment.

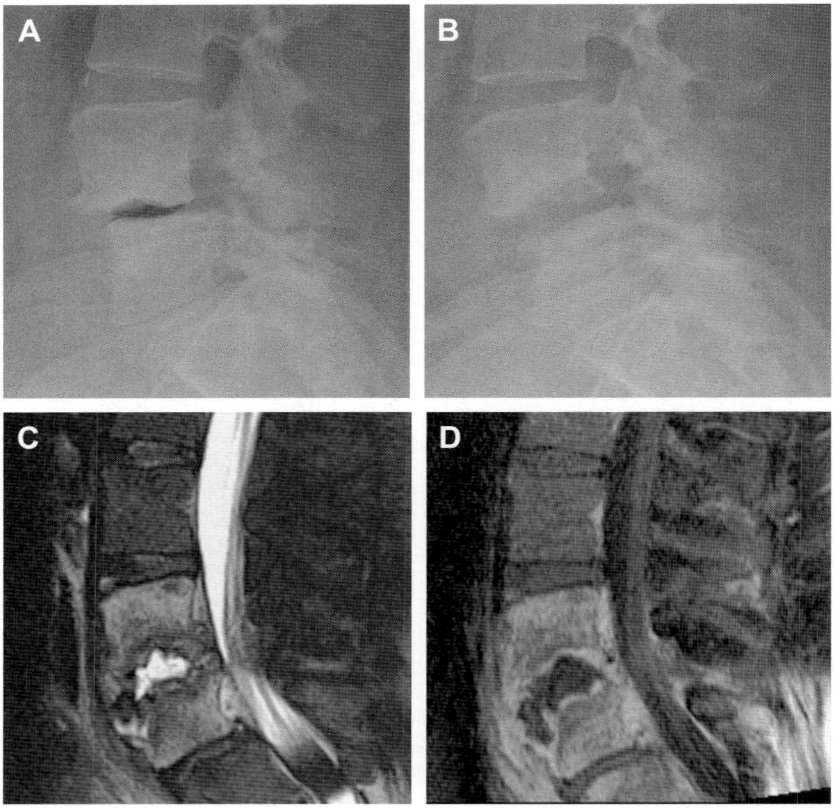

Fig. 3. Disappearing vacuum sign in pyogenic spondylodiscitis. A 46-year-old woman presented for lumbar spine radiographs for the indication of "back pain after a fall." Lateral radiograph (*A*) demonstrates a disc space vacuum phenomenon at L4-5. 3 weeks later, she presented with worsening back pain. Lateral radiograph (*B*) demonstrates loss of the vacuum sign, as well as endplate irregularity and apparent disc space widening at L4-5 suspicious for spondylodiscitis. Sagittal fat-saturated T2 (*C*) and T1 postgadolinium (*D*) MRI demonstrate findings of spondylodiscitis, with T2 hyperintense, fluid filled peripherally enhancing disc space, enhancing edema within the L4 and L5 vertebral bodies, and ventral epidural and paraspinal phlegmon/inflammation. Fluoroscopically guided aspiration of the disc fluid (not shown) was negative but patient had been on antibiotics. Given the imaging findings, clinical features (including elevated ESR and CRP), and risk factors (including morbid obesity and active bacterial external otitis), she was clinically presumed to have and treated for pyogenic spondylodiscitis. (*Courtesy of* K Schwartz, MD.)

Differential Diagnosis

The most common entity on the imaging differential diagnosis for pyogenic spondylodiscitis is degenerative or age-related disc change, more specifically, the Modic type 1, active endplate change (see **Fig. 4**). This distinction can be particularly challenging when clinical information is not supportive, as in an afebrile patient. Modic type 1 changes are characterized by edema-type (T1 hypo-, T2 hyperintense) signal abnormality along the vertebral endplates adjacent to a degenerating disc, and correlate with pain in at least some patients.[24] If gadolinium contrast is administered, these abnormally signaling areas, and occasionally the disc space itself, may enhance. If a herniated disc is present in association with the degenerating disc, some enhancement may be present at the periphery of the disc, which could potentially be confused with an epidural abscess[10] (see **Fig. 4**C, D).

In addition to a lack of clinical features supporting infection, several imaging features may help distinguish Modic type 1 changes and pyogenic

> **Box 1**
> **Pyogenic spondylodiscitis: classic imaging findings**
>
> Disc space: T2 hyperintensity, enhancement, height loss
>
> Adjacent vertebral bodies: endplate destruction, T1 hypo-, T2 hyperintensity, enhancement
>
> Paraspinal soft tissues: ill-defined inflammation/swelling, abscess
>
> Epidural space: reactive enhancement/venous plexus distention, phlegmon, abscess

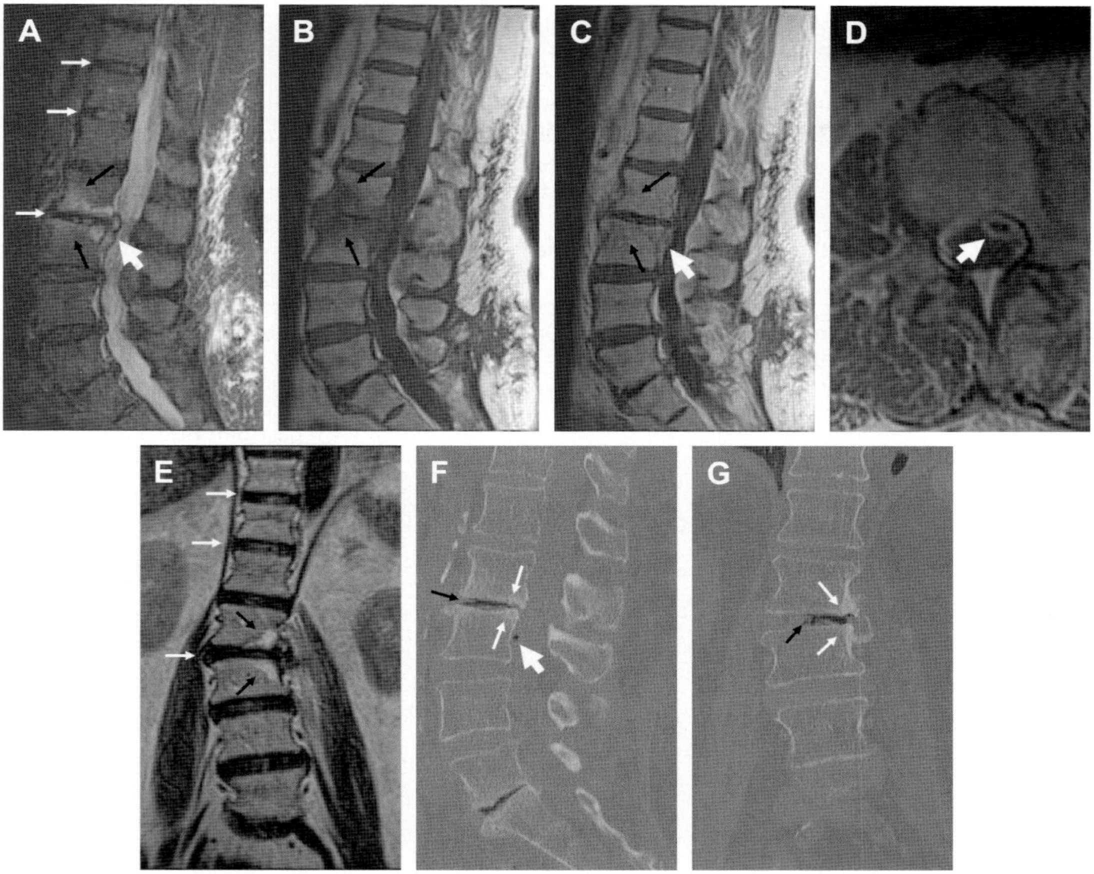

Fig. 4. Mimic of pyogenic spondylodiscitis, and utility of CT: advanced degenerative disc disease with Modic type 1 endplate changes and a disc extrusion. A 66-year-old woman with increasing back pain was referred from out-of-state for pathologic confirmation and treatment of spondylodiscitis. She presented to the neuroradiology service for biopsy at L2-3. However, the outside MRI was reviewed: sagittal fat-suppressed T2-weighted (*A*), sagittal T1-weighted (*B*), postgadolinium sagittal (*C*) and axial (*D*) T1-weighted, and coronal T2-weighted (*E*) images. T2 hyperintense, T1 hypointense, edema-type enhancing marrow signal abnormalities (*black arrows* in *A–C, E*) are present about the narrowed L2-3 interspace. The disc space T2 signal is similar to that of other levels (*white arrows* in *A, E*). There is no disc space enhancement. However, a left ventral epidural space mass is present, which was more T2 hyperintense than the disc space (*block white arrow* in *A*) and peripherally enhanced (*block white arrows* in *C, D*). This mimicks an epidural abscess, but a disc extrusion in setting of advanced degenerative disc disease with Modic type I changes, was suspected. A CT scan was performed: sagittal (*F*) and coronal (*G*) reformatted noncontrast images. This demonstrates loss of disc space height, extensive degenerative disc space vacuum phenomenon (*black arrows*), and associated sclerotic subendplate changes and hypertrophs (*white arrows*) at L2-3, which are all eccentric to the left, at the inner aspect of a convex right lumbar curve. The disc extrusion contains a small amount of gas also (*block white arrow* in *F*). Note the lack of erosive endplate changes. Laboratory evaluation confirmed normal inflammatory markers. The biopsy was therefore not performed; such procedures are not without risk and cost. (*Courtesy of* K Thielen, MD.)

spondylodiscitis (see **Box 1**; **Table 1**). Often, the degenerating disc associated with Modic type 1 changes demonstrates T2 hypointensity/lack of T2 hyperintensity, in contrast to the hyperintensity typically seen in discitis. This is not always the case, however, as a severely degenerated disc may be T2 hyperintense, and even signal isointense to fluid. Other useful MRI features that can suggest Modic type 1 changes over infection are: stability over time, lack of paraspinal or epidural involvement, lack of disc or endplate enhancement, lack of endplate destructive changes, and presence of a degenerative disc space vacuum sign. The vacuum sign is unlikely to be present in an infection; rare exceptions include an infection very early in its course, in case-reportable infections with gas-forming bacteria, or an infection due to fistula with the gastrointestinal tract. Occasionally

Table 1
Pearls and pitfalls: differentiating spondylodiscitis from Modic type 1 endplate changes

	Favoring Spondylodiscitis	Favoring Modic Type 1 Endplate Changes	Pitfall/Comments
Disc space signal	T2 hyperintensity	T2 hypointensity or lack of T2 hyperintensity	Severely degenerated discs can be T2 hyperintense (even fluid signal)
Disc space enhancement	Present	Absent	Rarely absent in infection; may be present in Modic 1
Disc space vacuum sign	Absent, only minimal, or "disappearing"	Often present	Gas may be present early in infection, in rare gas-forming bacterial infection, or in rare fistulas with gastrointestinal tract
Vertebral body endplates	Endplate destruction	Lack of endplate destruction	Modic 1 can have endplate irregularity CT is very useful here
Paraspinal, epidural spaces	Inflammation and/or abscess	Absent	Peripherally enhancing disc herniation can be confused for abscess
Location	Anteriorly eccentric	Laterally eccentric: at point of biomechanical stress (eg, inner aspect of curve)	Both spondylodiscitis and Modic 1 are often along entire endplate
Fever, elevated inflammatory markers	Present	Absent	Fever is only variably present in spondylodiscitis; inflammatory markers are nonspecific
Short-term follow-up	Progression	Stability	If remote comparison is available, even Modic 1 can show significant progression

disappearance of a previously visualized vacuum sign may be a clue to the presence of discitis (**Fig. 3**). Both the vacuum sign and the lack of destructive changes are often better appreciated with CT than MRI (see **Fig. 4**). In the author's center, CT is thus used liberally to further evaluate questionable discitis–osteomyelitis seen on MRI, especially when the MRI findings are not strongly suggestive, and a biopsy has been requested. Nuclear medicine imaging can also be helpful in such cases. However, active degenerative age-related disc change cannot always be confidently distinguished from infection by imaging. When the clinical impression, laboratory findings, and imaging do not allow exclusion of infection, biopsy may be performed.

Additional important differential considerations include granulomatous spine infections, which are the subject of a following section. Neuropathic arthropathy of the spine (Charcot spine) may also simulate disc space infection. Features of this destructive entity that are typically not present in pyogenic infection are: disc space vacuum phenomenon, facet joint involvement, exuberant bony debris about the arthropathic joint, joint disorganization with spondylolisthesis or dislocation, T2 hyperintensity and enhancement diffusely involving the vertebral body (rather than just adjacent to the endplates), and rim enhancement of the involved disc.[25,26] Acute Schmorl nodes may mimic spondylodiscitis, particularly as they may enhance and cause signal change and enhancement in the adjacent bone. However, such acute nodes are typically characterized by a concentric ring of edema-type signal around the node, involvement of only the endplate with the herniated node, and lack of diffuse abnormal signal changes within the disc.[13] Three-column fractures and/or resultant pseudarthrosis associated with ankylosing conditions (such as ankylosing spondylitis and diffuse idiopathic skeletal hyperostosis) may mimic pyogenic spondylodiscitis. The identification of fracture line(s) in the posterior elements can be helpful to suggest the former over infection.[13] Other entities that less commonly pose a diagnostic challenge include dialysis-associated spondyloarthropathy and tumors with propensity to cross the disc space, such as chordoma and myeloma.

Treatment

Antibiotic therapy is the mainstay of clinical management, but ideally is withheld or discontinued until after a sampling procedure has been performed.[7,27] Surgery is performed relatively commonly in patients who suffer complications, such as neural element compression, spinal deformity, or instability related to collapse of the discs or vertebral bodies. As mentioned previously, the clinical and imaging evolution may be discordant. The most important but not perfectly predictive feature indicating healing of discitis–osteomyelitis is decreasing clinical symptomatology, particularly pain and if initially present, fever. Laboratory markers such as improving leukocytosis and ESR can also be helpful. Persistently elevated or increasing ESR and CRP at week 4 of antibiotic therapy suggest a high rate of treatment failure.[6] Relapse risk is significant, and was found to occur in approximately one-third of patients in a recent systematic review,[5] although lower rates are reported elsewhere in the literature. The mortality rate is low, 6% in a recent systematic review.[5]

SPINAL EPIDURAL ABSCESS

Background

Although epidural abscesses may occur due to direct extension, such as from spondylodiscitis or facet joint infection, they are more commonly primary, related to either hematogenous spread or iatrogenic inoculation from an invasive spinal procedure.[28,29] An underlying infectious process is the most common comorbidity. Predisposing immunosuppressive conditions may be present, the most common being diabetes. As in pyogenic spondylodiscitis, men are more commonly affected; *S aureus* is the most common pathogen (~70% of cases).[28]

The clinical presentation of patients with spinal epidural abscess is variable. Middle-aged to elderly adults are most commonly afflicted. Back pain is the most common symptom and is often severe.[28,29] Fever and neurologic deficits are also common, and other features may be present, such as limited range of motion and tenderness. Elevations of ESR and CRP are more common than leukocytosis.[28,29]

Spinal epidural abscesses are most common in the thoracic spine, but can occur in any spinal segment and can even involve the length of the spine.[28] Some investigators have found that they more commonly complicate spondylodiscitis in the cervical than in the thoracic or lumbar spine.[8] The abscesses can be located either in the anterior or posterior epidural space. The cause of neurologic deficits can be direct mass effect or a vascular mechanism via thrombosis or thrombophlebitis.[30]

Imaging Evaluation

Some sources recommend emergent MRI of the entire spinal axis when spinal epidural abscess is clinically suspected.[29] MR images reveal a T1 hypo-, T2 hyperintense mass in the epidural space (**Figs. 5** and **7**). On postgadolinium T1-weighted imaging, this may enhance either homogeneously or heterogeneously in the stage of epidural plexus engorgement/phlegmon (see **Fig. 2**A, C, E, F) or peripherally with central fluid signal in the mature stage of a centrally pus-filled abscess (see **Figs. 5**C, E and **7**E).[11,21,31] Compared with neoplasms, more acute processes such as epidural abscess and hematoma more commonly violate the midline septum of the ventral epidural space.[32] There may be additional engorgement of the epidural plexus or basivertebral veins and/or prominent dural contrast enhancement. Thecal sac and even spinal cord (see **Fig. 5**D) or cauda equina (see **Fig. 7**D) compression are common. Diffusion weighted imaging may show the expected restricted diffusion within a spinal epidural abscess.[33]

On follow-up imaging, changes in an abscess do appear to correlate with clinical improvement or deterioration. However, findings of associated spondylodiscitis, when present, evolve in the unpredictable manner described previously.[21]

Differential Diagnosis

When associated with spondylodiscitis or facetitis, epidural abscess is not usually a diagnostic challenge on imaging. When an epidural abscess is primary, differential considerations include malignancy, particularly metastasis, and epidural hematoma. Clinical history is often most useful in distinguishing among such entities.

Treatment

The classic treatment of choice is emergent surgical decompression and abscess drainage, followed by antibiotic therapy. Select patients are managed medically. Antibiotic therapy may be delayed in the neurologically stable patient until emergent surgery with sampling has been

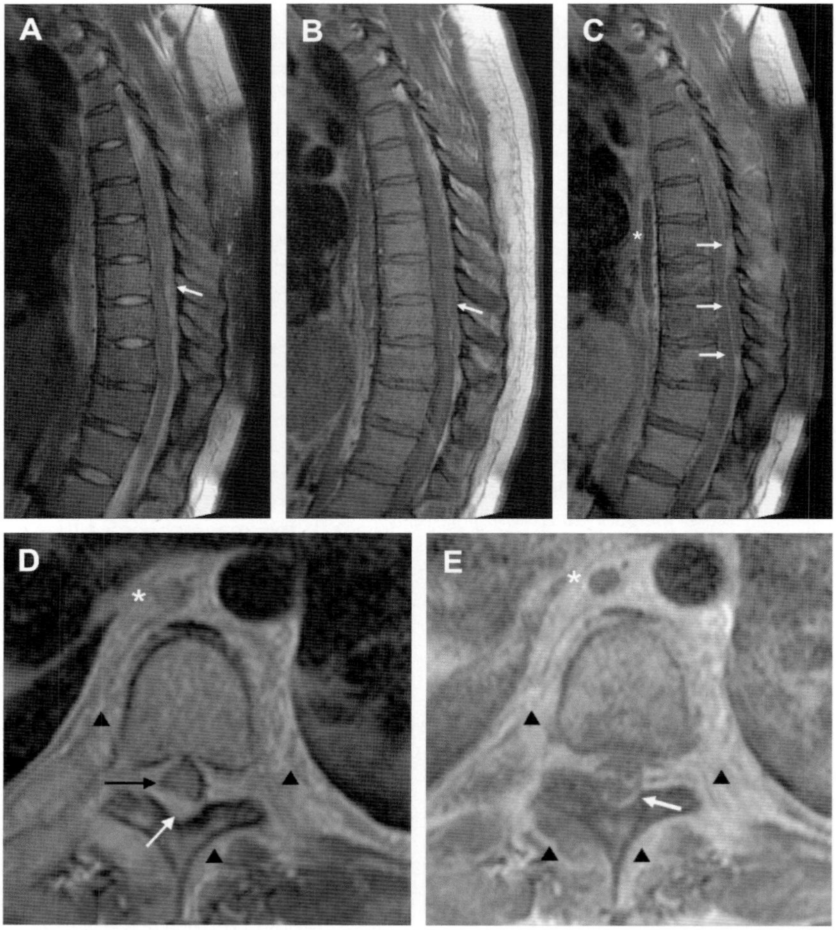

Fig. 5. Epidural abscess. A 28-year-old woman with a 10-day history of back pain presented with acute paraplegia. Sagittal T2-weighted (*A*), T1-weighted (*B*), postgadolinium, fat-saturated T1-weighted (*C*), and axial T2-weighted (*D*) and postgadolinium T1-weighted (*E*) MR images. A T2 hyperintense dorsal epidural fluid collection (*white arrows* in *A, D*) from the T7 through the T10 levels causes mass effect on the thecal sac and spinal cord (*black arrow* in *D*). The collection is T1 hypointense (*white arrow* in *B*), confirming its fluid nature. The collection peripherally enhances (*white arrows* in *C, E*), compatible with a frank dorsal epidural abscess. Ill-defined paraspinal inflammation is present (*black arrowheads* in *D, E*). The infection likely has thrombosed the azygous vein (*asterisk* in *C–E*). The patient underwent emergent surgical evacuation of the thoracic epidural abscess (*S aureus*) via a T7 to T10 decompressive laminectomy. At follow-up she had residual paraparesis and used a walker. (*Courtesy of* J Lane, MD.)

performed.[29] MRI findings may influence surgical approach, as a more phlegmonous collection may require a widespread decompressive approach with laminectomy, whereas a pus-filled abscess may be treated by limited laminotomies and catheter irrigation.[34] Even in some modern series, the mortality is relatively high (~10%–20%).[29,35]

SPINAL SUBDURAL ABSCESS

Primary subdural (intradural) abscess of the spine is an extremely rare, case-reportable condition. The most common location is the lumbar region. Risk factors and clinical features are similar to epidural abscess. *S aureus* is the most common organism. Treatment is typically emergent surgical drainage with subsequent antibiotic therapy.[36–38] The subdural location, deep to the epidural space, can be readily identified on MRI (see **Fig. 6**).

FACET JOINT INFECTION

Background

Facet joint infection (facetitis) is an uncommon condition, but like pyogenic spondylodiscitis, it is not rare.[39] It is being increasingly recognized and

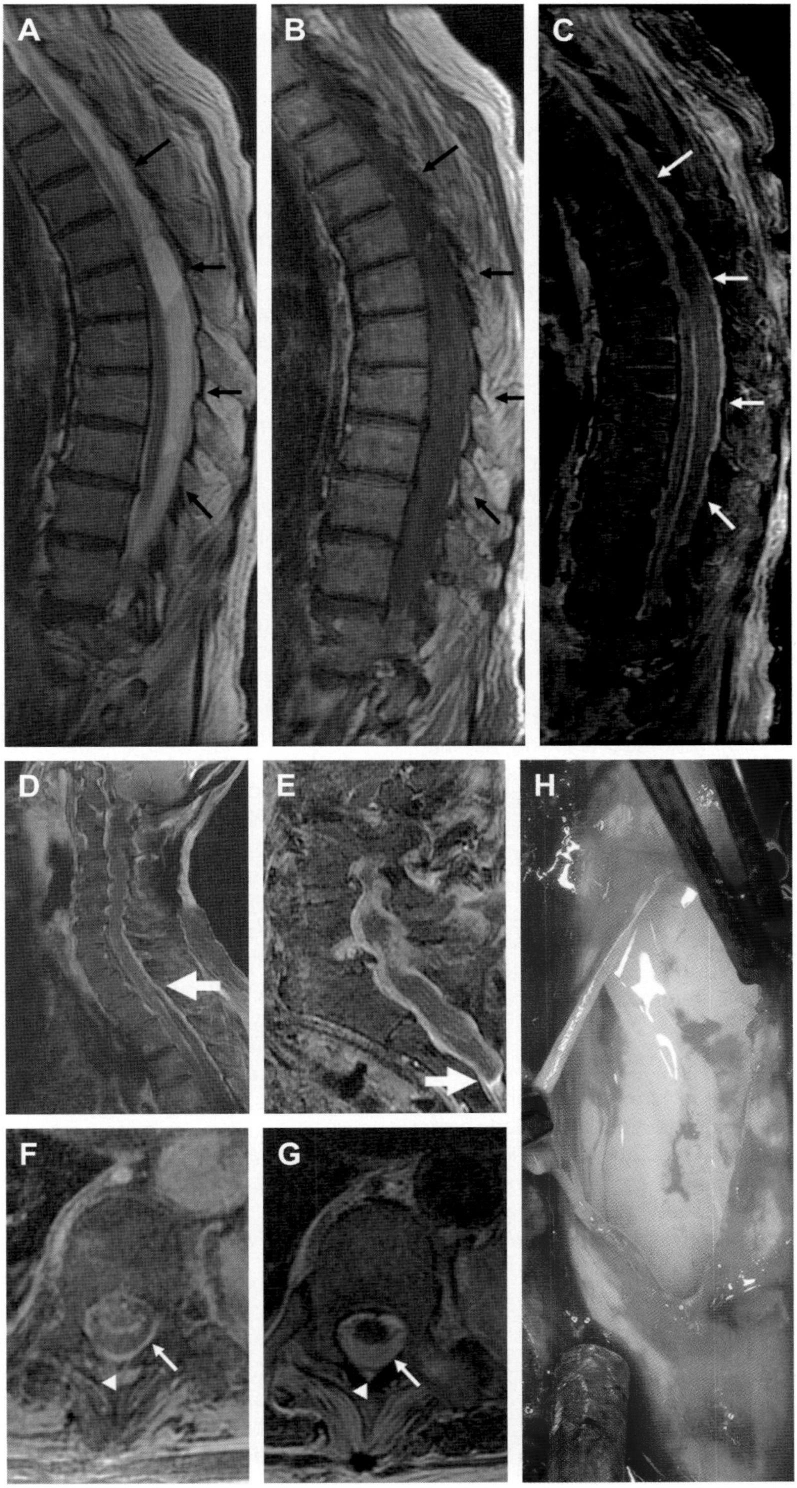

Fig. 6. Subdural abscess. An 82-year-old woman presented with acute severe back pain from the neck to the sacrum in the setting of a *S aureus* urinary tract infection. Sagittal T2-weighted (*A*), T1-weighted (*B*), postgadolinium fat-saturated T1 weighted (*C–E*), and axial (mid-thoracic level) postgadolinium fat-saturated T1-weighted (*F*) and T2-weighted (*G*) MR images. A large, extensive T2 hyper- (*A, G*), T1 hypointense (*B*), peripherally enhancing (*C–F*) fluid collection is located dorsally in the subdural (intradural) space (*small black/white arrows*). It contacts and ventrally displaces the spinal cord, and can be clearly delineated from the tiny, triangular, and more superficial dorsal epidural fat (*white arrowheads* in *F, G*). Its extent is from approximately T2 (*block white arrow* in *D*) to the sacrum (*block white arrow* in *E*). This was surgically evacuated (*H*), and *S aureus* was cultured. The patient's clinical status after 8 weeks of antibiotic therapy was excellent. (*Courtesy of* N Campeau, MD, A Nassr, MD.)

may be increasing in incidence. It may result from hematogenous dissemination of a pathogen,[40] most commonly *S aureus*, or be seen in patients without known predisposing recent infection.[41] Sources include cutaneous, respiratory, urinary, and catheter-related infections. The condition may also result as a direct complication of minimally invasive procedures, such as therapeutic facet joint injection.[42,43] Patients may have underlying immunosuppressed states, including diabetes mellitus, malignancies, and alcoholism.

The clinical picture of facet joint infection is similar to that of pyogenic spondylodiscitis. Patients tend to be over the age of 60.[39] They present with back pain that is typically unilateral and more acute and severe than that of pyogenic spondylodiscitis, and often is associated with muscle spasm.[39–41] Fever is common. Neurologic deficits are not uncommon, particularly when the condition is complicated by abscess formation.[44] ESR and CRP are typically elevated; leukocyte count is less frequently abnormal.[45]

Facet joint infection most commonly occurs in the lumbar spine, with rare reports in the cervical and thoracic spine.[39,45] It is usually unilateral, although at times it is bilateral at a single level.[40,41,46] Bilaterality suggests transmission through the retro-ligamentous space of Okada, an anatomic pathway more thoroughly described elsewhere in this volume by Kotsenas. In the author's anecdotal experience, bilaterality is more frequent than reported in the literature, and even multilevel involvement can be seen.

Imaging Evaluation

Despite the joint-centric nature, radiographs are of limited utility in facet joint infection, particularly early in the disease course. CT also tends to be low-yield early, but may demonstrate erosive or soft tissue inflammatory changes about the infected facet joint as the disease progresses (**Fig.** 7G).[39] As with other spine infections, MRI is the examination of choice (see **Fig. 7**). Inclusion of fat-suppressed T2-weighted and fat-suppressed postgadolinium T1-weighted imaging in the scan protocol is important. MRI typically demonstrates erosive changes and edema about a fluid-filled facet joint, with facet capsular enhancement (see **Fig.** 7C–E). Paraspinal and epidural inflammatory changes are common; complications such as frank paraspinal abscess (**Figs. 7** and **8**) and epidural abscess (see **Fig.** 7C–E) can occur.[40,41]

Treatment

Antibiotics are the mainstay of therapy. Image-guided drainage may result in significant, immediate, and prolonged pain relief.[40] Surgery is generally reserved for medical treatment failures or for some patients with epidural abscess.

PYOMYOSITIS

Background

Infections of the paraspinal muscles are most commonly due to spread from either an adjacent site of infection or hematogenous seeding from a remote site. Primary paraspinal pyomyositis is a rare, serious infection of the paraspinal musculature. Primary pyomyositis much more commonly involves the large muscles of the body, especially the thigh muscles. It is usually seen in tropical regions, where it is endemic, but it is being increasingly recognized in temperate zones. Any age group can be affected, but the classic tropical type is most common in children and young adults following muscle trauma.[47] *S aureus* is the pathogen in the majority of reported cases.

Patients present with fever, pain, and swelling of the involved region. Although inflammatory markers are typically elevated, blood cultures are frequently negative. Early recognition is critical, but delayed diagnosis is common. The condition is often initially misdiagnosed as a variety of conditions, such as hematoma, muscle strain/spasm/rupture, venous thrombosis, thrombophlebitis, cellulitis, osteomyelitis, septic arthritis, or tumor. Three classic stages are described: stage 1, diffuse muscle infection; stage 2, intramuscular abscess; and stage 3, myonecrosis with sepsis.

The condition is thought to occur most commonly due to a damaged muscle's compromised resistance to infection during concurrent transient bacteremia. However, a variety of predisposing factors causing immune-compromise may also be involved, particularly in older patients presenting in temperate zones.[47,48]

Imaging Evaluation

Radiographs have limited utility. Although they can help exclude a primary bone lesion, even when findings such as soft tissue prominence or loss of fat planes are demonstrated, they are nonspecific. Advanced cross-sectional imaging may demonstrate the replacement of muscle by fluid and inflammatory cells. On CT, hypoattenuation and swelling of the affected muscle group may be seen. Intramuscular accumulation of fluid can be seen in the abscess stage. Ultrasound may also be used to demonstrate the infected muscle or intramuscular abscess, particularly in children.[49]

MRI is the most sensitive and specific test (see **Fig. 8**). Findings in the early, invasive stage of

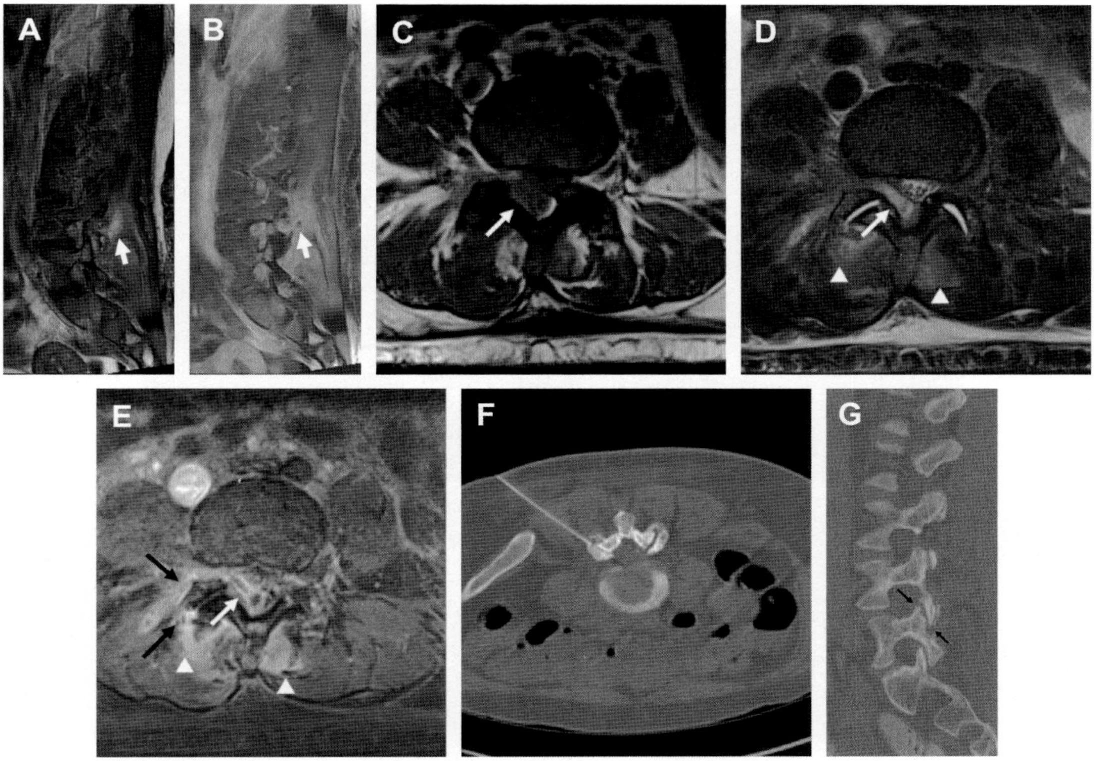

Fig. 7. Facet joint infection, complicated by epidural and paraspinal abscesses. A 48-year-old woman presented with fever, back pain, and an *E coli* pyelonephritis was diagnosed. MRI was performed for lower extremity radicular symptoms. Sagittal fat-saturated T2-weighted (*A*), postgadolinium, fat-saturated T1-weighted (*B*), and axial T1-weighted (*C*), fat-saturated T2-weighted (*D*), and postgadolinium fat-saturated T1-weighted (*E*) MR images. There is extensive facet and peri-facet T2 hyperintensity and enhancement at the fluid-filled right L4-5 facet joint, extending in the posterior paraspinal soft tissues to the left of midline (*white arrowheads* in *D*, *E*). The facet joint capsule enhances (*black arrows* in *E*). A small paraspinal abscess is present (*large white arrow* in *A*, *B*). Axial images demonstrate a T1 hypo-(*C*), T2 hyperintense (*D*), peripherally enhancing (*E*) right posterolateral epidural abscess adjacent to the involved joint (*small white arrows*), with mass effect on the thecal sac (*D*). CT-guided sampling (*F*) of the facet joint confirmed *E coli* (performed to exclude the possibility of concomitant second pathogen, as back pain had been present for several months). 1-month follow-up sagittal CT (*G*) demonstrates erosive changes of the facet joint (*black arrows*). (*Courtesy of* M Kiely, MD.)

infection are not as specific as when a frank abscess is demonstrated. This invasive stage is characterized primarily by T2 hyperintensity in the affected muscle. The abscess stage demonstrates a peripherally enhancing, centrally T2 hyperintense fluid collection, with variable central T1 signal intensity and mass effect (see **Fig. 8**). A peripheral T1 hyper-, T2 hypointense rim may be present. Lumbar paraspinal lesions can be so large that they cause mass effect on retroperitoneal structures.[50,51] Spread of inflammation/infection may occur from (see **Fig. 8**A, C) or to adjacent soft tissue, bone, or joints. Even associated epidural abscess formation has been reported.[48,52] When untreated or unrecognized, the disease progresses to its final stage of myonecrosis with sepsis; mass effect resolves and the central T2 hyperintensity decreases.[47]

Treatment

Treatment includes aggressive antibiotic therapy. Surgical or image-guided drainage is often required when the disease reaches the mature, suppurative abscess stage. The prognosis is good, unless cases are untreated or diagnosed late, in which case mortality can increase to approximately 15%.[50]

GRANULOMATOUS SPINAL INFECTION

Tuberculous Spondylitis

Background

Tuberculous spondylitis (Pott disease) is the most common nonpyogenic, granulomatous infection of the spine, and the most common overall cause of spine infection in the world. Tuberculosis

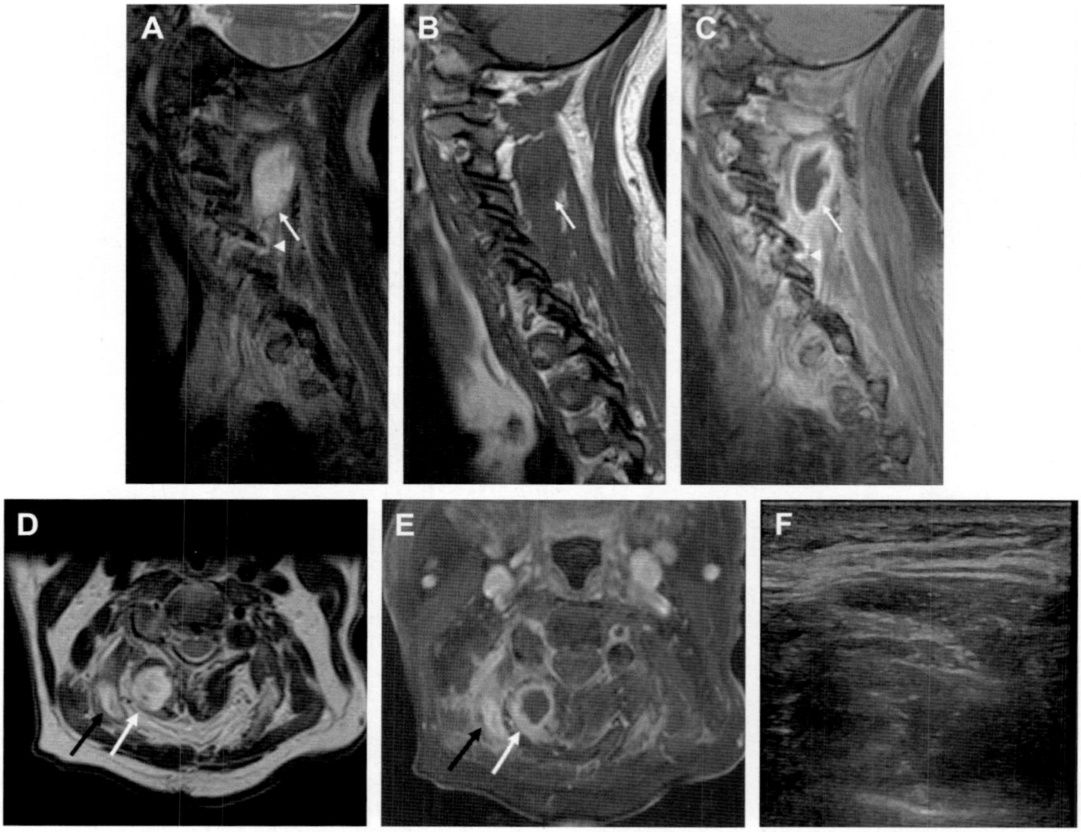

Fig. 8. Pyomyositis, with paraspinal abscesses, likely due to adjacent facetitis. 67-year-old man presented with methicillin resistant *S aureus* bacteremia and a screening spine MRI to search for a source was requested. Sagittal fat-saturated T2-weighted (*A*), T1-weighted (*B*), postgadolinium, fat-saturated T1-weighted (*C*), and axial T2-weighted (*D*), and postgadolinium fat-saturated T1-weighted (*E*) MR images. A nearly 3 cm T2 hyperintense (*A, D*), T1 hypointense (*B*), and peripherally enhancing (*C, E*), fluid collection (*white arrows*) is present in the left upper cervical paraspinal muscles. A second smaller, similar collection is present more posterolaterally (*black arrows* in *D, E*). Mild associated inflammation/poorly organized infection manifestes as ill-defined T2 hyperintensity (*A, D*) and enhancement (*C, E*) about the abscesses. The abscesses likely arises from the infected appearing left C5-6 facet joint, which is distended with fluid and exhibits facet/peri-facet edema and enhancement (*white arrowheads* in *A, C*). Ultrasound-guided drainage of the paraspinal abscess (*F*) yielded *S aureus*. (*Courtesy of* G Miller, MD.)

remains endemic in certain regions, and has been recently resurgent in developed countries due to increasing immigration of people from endemic areas, development of drug-resistant strains, and the human immunodeficiency virus (HIV) pandemic.[53] Among patients with tuberculosis, tuberculous spondylitis is much more common in HIV-positive than HIV-negative patients.[54]

Clinically, the classic presentation of tuberculous spondylitis is back pain, kyphotic deformity, and at times a cold abscess (a slowly forming abscess with little associated inflammation).[55] However, tuberculosis of the spine tends to have a more indolent and less painful course compared with pyogenic spondylodiscitis, with latency as long as several years.[56] Systemic symptoms such as weight loss, fever, and malaise may precede the spinal infection.[57]

Anatomically, tuberculous spondylitis is most common in the thoracic spine, particularly at the thoracolumbar junction. It classically begins in the anterior aspect of the vertebral body, from where it can spread in subligamentous fashion anteriorly in the paraspinal region or posteriorly in the epidural space. It is also prone to exhibit intradural involvement, including intradural abscesses and spinal cord myelitis; such spinal tuberculous meningitis will not be further considered here. *Mycobacterium tuberculosis* may seed the spine by hematogenous dissemination, typically from a clinically quiescent primary pulmonary focus.[56] Of note, chest radiographs commonly do not demonstrate evidence of pulmonary tuberculosis in patients with tuberculous spondylitis.[58]

Imaging evaluation

As for other spinal infections, MRI is the modality of choice in tuberculous spondylitis. The classic imaging appearance of tuberculous spondylitis is similar to pyogenic spondylodiscitis, with involvement of one or more adjacent vertebral levels, destruction of the interspace(s), and adjacent paraspinal soft tissue mass.[55] However, disc space involvement is often not present, not as severe, and/or more delayed when compared with bacterial spondylodiscitis. This atypical pattern of tuberculous spondylitis is reported by some authors to be quite common and increasing in frequency; in 1 large study, more than 50% of tuberculous spondylitis patients had only isolated vertebral lesions, mimicking metastases, without disc involvement.[59] Anecdotally, this is the most common pattern seen in the author's practice (**Figs. 9** and **10**). Sparing of the disc space has been ascribed to the fact that *Mycobacterium* lacks

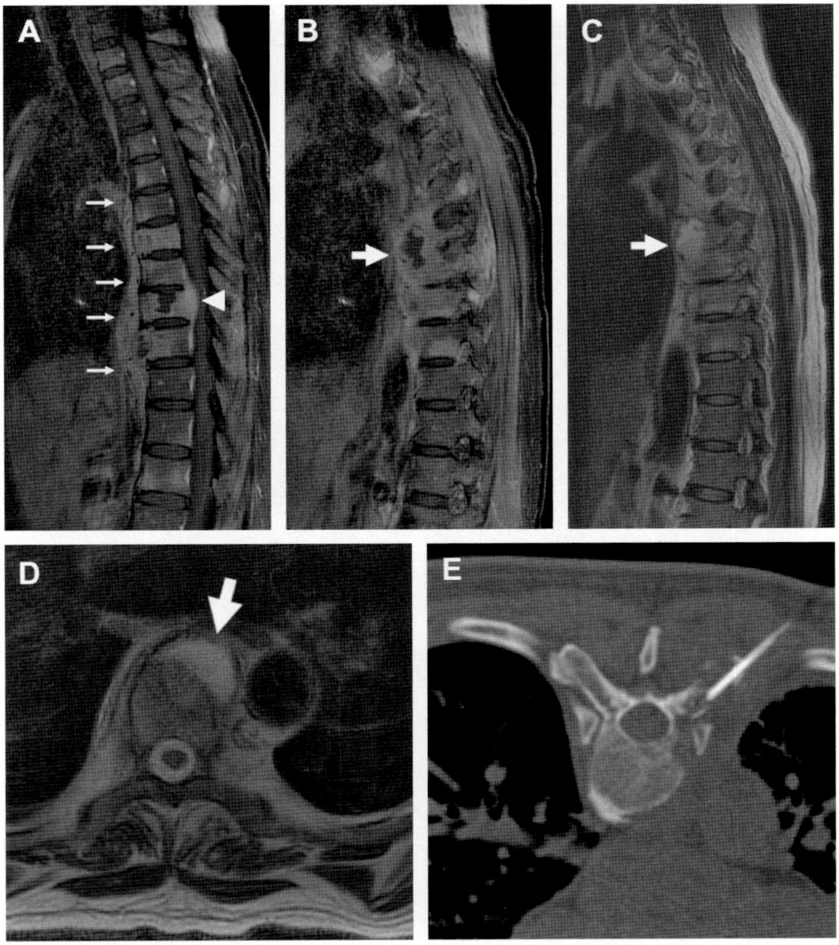

Fig. 9. Tuberculous spondylitis, with paraspinal abscesses and epidural phlegmon. A 53-year-old woman presented with several weeks of back pain and low-grade fevers. Postgadolinium, fat-saturated T1-weighted sagittal (*A*, *B*), and sagittal (*C*) and axial T2-weighted (*D*) MR images. There are multiple foci of abnormal marrow enhancement (*A*, *B*) and T2 hyperintensity (*C*) throughout the visualized spine. Prominent ventral paraspinal infection in the thoracic region (*small white arrows* in *A*) extends across multilevel levels along the anterior longitudinal ligament with relative preservation of disc spaces. A large, discrete peripherally enhancing, centrally T1 hypointense (*B*), T2 hyperintense (*C*, *D*) ventral paraspinal fluid collection is present (*large white arrow* in *B–D*), compatible with a paraspinal abscess. Subligamentous ventral epidural phlegmon along the posterior longitudinal ligament manifests as homogeneously enhancing epidural soft tissue (*arrowhead* in *A*). Percutaneous CT-guided sampling (*E*) yielded granulomatous inflammation on pathology, and *M tuberculosis* on microbiology. (*Courtesy of* J Wald, MD, J Morris, MD, G Miller, MD.)

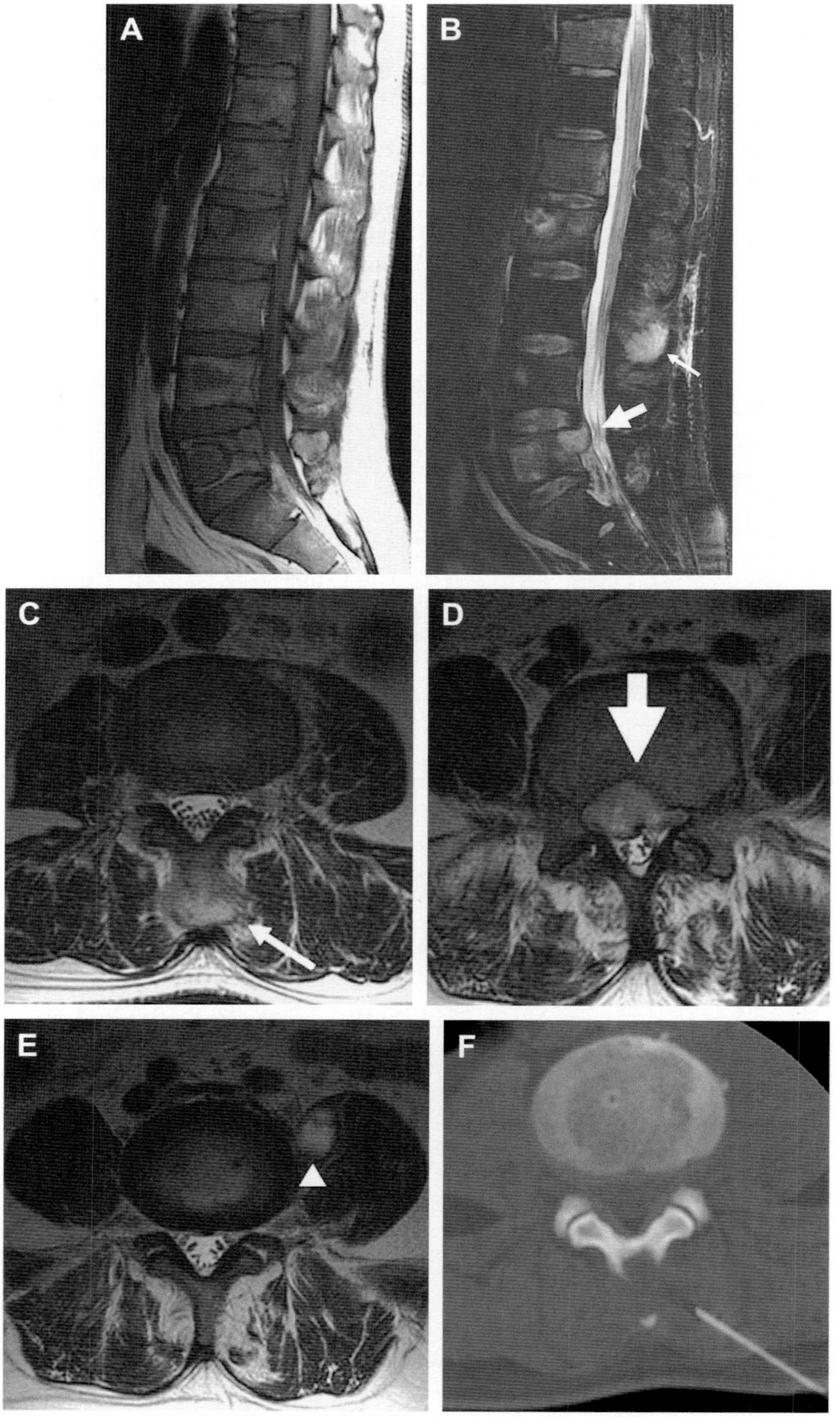

Fig. 10. Tuberculous spondylitis, with predominantly multilevel bony involvement, including of posterior elements. A 42 year-old man was referred for possible metastatic disease. Sagittal T1- (*A*) and fat-saturated T2- (*B*), and axial T2-weighted (*C–E*) MR images. There are multiple bony spinal lesions, including in the vertebral bodies (*A*, *B*). A prominent lesion is present in the L3 spinous process (*small white arrow* in *B*, *C*). At L5, a dorsal vertebral body lesion extends into the ventral epidural space and partially effaced the thecal sac (*large white arrow* in *B* and *D*). At L4, extension is seen into the left psoas muscle (*arrowhead* in *E*). Image from percutaneous CT-guided sampling (*F*) confirms the lytic nature of the L3 spinous process lesion. The biopsy yielded caseating granulomatous inflammation on pathology, and *M tuberculosis* on microbiology. (*Courtesy of* P McGough, MD, T Maus, MD.)

proteolytic enzymes. From this location, the infection may spread in subligamentous fashion across 1 or more levels beneath the anterior longitudinal ligament (see **Fig. 9**A). Spread in the epidural space may also occur (see **Figs. 9**A and **10**B, D) but is less common than in the anterior paravertebral regions (see **Fig. 9**A–D).[60] Contrast-enhanced studies often demonstrate thin, smooth enhancing walls of the paravertebral collections. The subligamentous spread may be much more extensive than the vertebral involvement (see **Fig. 9**A), and can lead to skip lesions of involved bones/discs with intervening normal levels.[61] In addition to subligamentous spread, spread to adjacent soft tissue is also common, particularly the anterolateral paraspinal soft tissues (see **Fig. 10**E). A tuberculous abscess of the psoas muscle occurs in approximately 5% of cases and may contain calcifications, best seen on CT.[62] CT can also be useful in demonstrating endplate erosive changes and bony lytic lesions. The posterior elements (see **Fig. 10**B, C) are more commonly involved than in pyogenic disease. A classic finding is gibbus deformity, due to preferential anterior column involvement causing collapse of a partially destroyed vertebral column. Similar to other spinal infections, radiographic findings tend to lag behind the pathologic changes of tuberculous spondylitis.[60]

In addition to disc space sparing, atypical appearances of tuberculous spondylitis include: single vertebral level disease (vertebra plana, ivory vertebra, neural arch involvement, or panvertebral involvement)[55] and multilevel disease (contiguous or noncontiguous).[55,63] Although considered atypical, several of these and some of the more typical features can suggest tuberculous spondylitis over pyogenic spondylodiscitis.

Differential diagnosis

As described previously, tuberculous spondylitis can appear identical to typical pyogenic spondylodiscitis when the disc space is involved. Imaging features that favor tuberculous spondylitis include: well-defined paraspinal signal abnormality; large (larger) inflammatory collections, including large paraspinal cold abscesses; thin, smooth abscess walls; sparing of the disc; subligamentous spread to three or more levels; multiple vertebral or entire-body involvement; skip lesions; and posterior element involvement (**Box 2**, **Table 2**).[13,60,64–66] An additional granulomatous disease that can mimic the appearance of tuberculous spondylitis is brucellar spondylitis, which will be discussed briefly. Solitary tumor or metastases may be misdiagnosed when tuberculous spondylitis demonstrates uni- or multilevel bony involvement with disc space sparing.

Box 2
Imaging clues: tuberculous spondylitis

Classic:

- Similar to pyogenic spondylodiscitis
- Disc space involvement less severe
- Large paraspinal abscess, smooth wall, ± calcifications
- Subligamentous spread

Atypical:

- Disc sparing, with either single or multilevel bony involvement only
- Multilevel involvement, contiguous or skip lesions
- Vertebra plana
- Posterior element involvement
- Panvertebral involvement

Treatment

Antituberculous medical therapy is the mainstay of treatment, and the duration is on the order of 6 to 12 months.[53] Surgery may be performed in select cases (eg, for complications, failure of medical therapy, neurologic compromise, palpable cold abscess, or occasionally, for prevention of new or worsening deformity or deficit).[53]

Brucellar Spondylitis

Background

Brucellosis is a zoonosis endemic in rural areas of Saudi Arabia and the Mediterranean basin. Those most at risk are farm workers, slaughterhouse workers, and veterinary personnel. It is caused by a gram-negative bacillus, and usually acquired by ingestion of raw meat or unpasteurized dairy products. The most common animals to harbor brucellosis are sheep, cattle, goats, pigs, and dogs.[61,67]

Some studies suggest high-grade fever is seen more commonly than with pyogenic spondylodiscitis or tuberculous spondylitis.[65] Blood cultures and serologic testing typically allow diagnosis, whereas percutaneous sampling of the spine is of little utility.[68] Treatment is medical therapy with antibiotics, with a typical duration of 3 to 6 months, but recurrences are not uncommon.[53]

Imaging evaluation, differential diagnosis

Brucellosis most commonly affects the lumbar and lumbosacral regions, unlike tuberculous spondylitis, which is more common in the thoracic spine. The MRI findings of brucellosis may be indistinguishable from those of tuberculous spondylitis. However, one study[69] suggests that brucellosis

Table 2
Pearls: differentiating pyogenic, tuberculous, and brucellar spine infections

	Pyogenic	Tuberculous	Brucellar
Preferential location	Lumbar	Thoracolumbar junction	Lower lumbar
Vertebral body	Endplate destruction	May have severe collapse	Relatively preserved
Posterior elements	Typically spared	May be involved	Typically spared
Disc space involvement	Present	Variable: from severe involvement to sparing; often less than bone destruction	Present
Paraspinal involvement	If present: small abscess with often thick, irregular rim enhancement	Large abscess, with often thin, smooth rim enhancement; may calcify (healing)	Relatively mild
Multilevel involvement	Uncommon	Common	Rare
Gibbus deformity	Uncommon	Common	Uncommon
Leukocytosis	Common	Less common	Less common
Neurologic deficits		Relatively more common	
Length of symptoms	Acute–subacute	Subacute–insidious	Acute-subacute
History	Recent bacterial infection	History of tuberculosis, originating from regions with high tuberculosis incidence	History of *Brucella* infection, travel to endemic regions

Data from James SL, Davies AM. Imaging of infectious spinal disorders in children and adults. Eur J Radiol 2006;58(1):27–40; Moorthy S, Prabhu NK. Spectrum of MR imaging findings in spinal tuberculosis. AJR Am J Roentgenol 2002;179(4):979–83; Turunc T, Demiroglu YZ, Uncu H, et al. A comparative analysis of tuberculous, brucellar and pyogenic spontaneous spondylodiscitis patients. J Infect 2007;55(2):158–63; Al-Sous MW, Bohlega S, Al-Kawi MZ, et al. Neurobrucellosis: clinical and neuroimaging correlation. AJNR Am J Neuroradiol 2004;25(3):395–401; Sharif HS, Clark DC, Aabed MY, et al. Granulomatous spinal infections: MR imaging. Radiology 1990;177(1):101–7.

tends to appear less aggressive than tuberculous spondylitis. Specific features that favor brucellosis over tuberculous spondylitis include: relatively intact vertebral body and even disc despite signal abnormality/enhancement, spared posterior elements, lack of paraspinal abscess, and lack of associated spinal deformity. A relatively low rate of abscess formation has been confirmed by other investigators.[70] The differentiating features among pyogenic, tuberculous, and brucellar spine infections are highlighted in **Table 2**.

Fungal Spondylitis

Fungal spondylodiscitis is uncommon, but the immunocompromised population susceptible to fungal infections is ever increasing. A wide variety of fungal organisms can cause spine infection, including *Candida* and *Aspergillus* species. An early report of the MRI findings in 3 cases of fungal spondylitis in immuoncompromised patients described lack of T2 hyperintensity in the disc spaces,[71] in contrast to pyogenic spondylodiscitis. A more recent report of 15 cases suggested that similar to tuberculous spondylitis, *Aspergillus* spondylitis should be suspected in immunocompromised patients when multiple vertebral levels are involved with skip lesions or subligamentous spread, or when a serrated appearance of the endplates and subchondral T2 hypointensity is present.[72]

IMAGE-GUIDED SAMPLING OF SPINAL INFECTION

The identification of a specific organism causing a spine infection is useful to direct antibiotic therapy. Blood or urine cultures are positive in some cases, but targeted sampling may be necessary even in some of these cases to definitively identify the pathogen. Thus, in many centers, radiologists play an additional important role in the diagnostic algorithm by performing image-guided percutaneous sampling procedures. If blood or urine cultures are positive, the risks of minimally invasive sampling need to be weighed against the likelihood that a separate concurrent infection is present. Either fluoroscopy (see **Fig. 2**G) or CT (see **Figs. 7**F, **9**E, **10**F) can be used for guidance. Ultrasound (see **Fig. 8**F) may also be used for relatively superficial paraspinal processes. For typical pyogenic spondylodiscitis, the author most often uses fluoroscopy and achieves sampling of the disc space and both adjacent endplates via an angled, caudocranial transpedicular approach.[73]

The reported diagnostic yield of image-guided sampling varies widely, but overall is relatively low. One of the most recent studies retrospectively assessing percutaneous image-guided (fluoroscopy or CT) needle biopsy in patients with vertebral osteomyelitis in routine clinical practice demonstrated a positive culture rate of 30% in 92 cases where clinical and imaging evaluation were consistent with infection. The yield was lower (16%) when imaging was indeterminate for infection.[74] False negatives may result for a variety of reasons, including fungal infections[75] and initiation of antibiotic therapy before sampling (eg, see patient in Fig. 3). In the appropriate patient, delaying the antibiotic therapy until this sampling has been performed is likely to increase the yield.[76,77] It is common to repeat the procedure in cases of suspected infection where the initial sampling is nondiagnostic. In fact, negative culture results are difficult to interpret. For example, the aforementioned study demonstrated a 5% positive culture yield even in cases where the probability of infection was considered low based on the radiographic appearance.[74] In some centers, surgical percutaneous endoscopic discectomy and drainage are performed, and at least 1 study suggests that the culture yield is higher compared with CT-guided biopsy.[78] In select patients, open biopsy is performed to attempt to establish the diagnosis.

The combination of histopathologic with microbiologic analysis of the biopsy specimen has been shown to improve the diagnostic performance of image-guided sampling.[14,75,79,80] This advantage stems from the potential for histology to distinguish pyogenic and granulomatous infections, diagnose culture-negative chronic osteomyelitis, and detect unsuspected neoplasm.[9,79] Typically, the microbiologic analysis includes aerobic, anaerobic, fungal, and mycobacterial tests and cultures. Some authors recommend drawing blood cultures within a few hours of the sampling procedure to further increase the chance of pathogen identification.[81]

SUMMARY

Spinal infections are increasing in incidence. Radiologists play a crucial role in the evaluation of these potentially life-threatening conditions. MRI is the modality of choice for imaging spinal infection. When extradural spinal infection is being considered, it is important to include fat-suppressed T2- and fat-suppressed, contrast-enhanced T1-weighted sequences. Pyogenic spondylodiscitis has characteristic imaging findings centered about an abnormal disc space, but may have atypical appearances. It can be difficult to distinguish pyogenic spondylodiscitis from other conditions, especially Modic type 1 endplate changes. MRI is critical in diagnosing both spinal epidural and the rare subdural abscess, which are both usually treated with emergent surgery. Facet joint infection and paraspinal pyomyositis are being increasingly recognized. Tuberculous spondylitis is the most common granulomatous spondylitis, and the most common spine infection worldwide. It has typical and atypical appearances. Features such as disc space sparing, multilevel subligamentous spread, and large abscesses are suggestive of this diagnosis. Brucellar spondylitis is most commonly seen in endemic regions. Although it can be indistinguishable from tuberculous spondylitis, it generally has a less aggressive appearance. Fungal spondylitis is rare and has a relatively nonspecific imaging appearance. Image-guided sampling is an important part of the diagnostic algorithm in spine infection.

REFERENCES

1. DeSanto J, Ross JS. Spine infection/inflammation. Radiol Clin North Am 2011;49(1):105–27.
2. Lury K, Smith JK, Castillo M. Imaging of spinal infections. Semin Roentgenol 2006;41(4):363–79.
3. Tali ET, Gultekin S. Spinal infections. Eur Radiol 2005;15(3):599–607.
4. Hooten WM, Mizerak A, Carns PE, et al. Discitis after lumbar epidural corticosteroid injection: a case report and analysis of the case report literature. Pain Med 2006;7(1):46–51.
5. Mylona E, Samarkos M, Kakalou E, et al. Pyogenic vertebral osteomyelitis: a systematic review of clinical characteristics. Semin Arthritis Rheum 2009;39(1):10–7.
6. Yoon SH, Chung SK, Kim KJ, et al. Pyogenic vertebral osteomyelitis: identification of microorganism and laboratory markers used to predict clinical outcome. Eur Spine J 2010;19(4):575–82.
7. Cottle L, Riordan T. Infectious spondylodiscitis. J Infect 2008;56(6):401–12.
8. James SL, Davies AM. Imaging of infectious spinal disorders in children and adults. Eur J Radiol 2006;58(1):27–40.
9. Gouliouris T, Aliyu SH, Brown NM. Spondylodiscitis: update on diagnosis and management. J Antimicrob Chemother 2010;65(Suppl 3):iii11–24.
10. Longo M, Granata F, Ricciardi K, et al. Contrast-enhanced MR imaging with fat suppression in adult-onset septic spondylodiscitis. Eur Radiol 2003;13(3):626–37.

11. Dagirmanjian A, Schils J, McHenry M, et al. MR imaging of vertebral osteomyelitis revisited. AJR Am J Roentgenol 1996;167(6):1539–43.
12. Ledermann HP, Schweitzer ME, Morrison WB, et al. MR imaging findings in spinal infections: rules or myths? Radiology 2003;228(2):506–14.
13. Hong SH, Choi JY, Lee JW, et al. MR imaging assessment of the spine: infection or an imitation? Radiographics 2009;29(2):599–612.
14. Hsu CY, Yu CW, Wu MZ, et al. Unusual manifestations of vertebral osteomyelitis: intraosseous lesions mimicking metastases. AJNR Am J Neuroradiol 2008;29(6):1104–10.
15. Gillams AR, Chaddha B, Carter AP. MR appearances of the temporal evolution and resolution of infectious spondylitis. AJR Am J Roentgenol 1996; 166(4):903–7.
16. Euba G, Narvaez JA, Nolla JM, et al. Long-term clinical and radiological magnetic resonance imaging outcome of abscess-associated spontaneous pyogenic vertebral osteomyelitis under conservative management. Semin Arthritis Rheum 2008;38(1): 28–40.
17. Kowalski TJ, Layton KF, Berbari EF, et al. Follow-up MR imaging in patients with pyogenic spine infections: lack of correlation with clinical features. AJNR Am J Neuroradiol 2007;28(4):693–9.
18. Carragee EJ. The clinical use of magnetic resonance imaging in pyogenic vertebral osteomyelitis. Spine (Phila Pa 1976) 1997;22(7):780–5.
19. Veillard E, Guggenbuhl P, Morcet N, et al. Prompt regression of paravertebral and epidural abscesses in patients with pyogenic discitis. Sixteen cases evaluated using magnetic resonance imaging. Joint Bone Spine 2000;67(3):219–27.
20. Zarrouk V, Feydy A, Salles F, et al. Imaging does not predict the clinical outcome of bacterial vertebral osteomyelitis. Rheumatology (Oxford) 2007;46(2): 292–5.
21. Numaguchi Y, Rigamonti D, Rothman MI, et al. Spinal epidural abscess: evaluation with gadolinium-enhanced MR imaging. Radiographics 1993;13(3): 545–59 [discussion: 59–60].
22. Ross JS, Zepp R, Modic MT. The postoperative lumbar spine: enhanced MR evaluation of the intervertebral disk. AJNR Am J Neuroradiol 1996;17(2): 323–31.
23. Van Goethem JW, Parizel PM, van den Hauwe L, et al. The value of MRI in the diagnosis of postoperative spondylodiscitis. Neuroradiology 2000;42(8): 580–5.
24. Zhang YH, Zhao CQ, Jiang LS, et al. Modic changes: a systematic review of the literature. Eur Spine J 2008;17(10):1289–99.
25. Lacout A, Lebreton C, Mompoint D, et al. CT and MRI of spinal neuroarthropathy. AJR Am J Roentgenol 2009;193(6):W505–14.
26. Wagner SC, Schweitzer ME, Morrison WB, et al. Can imaging findings help differentiate spinal neuropathic arthropathy from disk space infection? Initial experience. Radiology 2000;214(3):693–9.
27. Sobottke R, Seifert H, Fatkenheuer G, et al. Current diagnosis and treatment of spondylodiscitis. Dtsch Arztebl Int 2008;105(10):181–7.
28. Reihsaus E, Waldbaur H, Seeling W. Spinal epidural abscess: a meta-analysis of 915 patients. Neurosurg Rev 2000;23(4):175–204 [discussion: 5].
29. Tompkins M, Panuncialman I, Lucas P, et al. Spinal epidural abscess. J Emerg Med 2010;39(3):384–90.
30. Wang VY, Chou D, Chin C. Spine and spinal cord emergencies: vascular and infectious causes. Neuroimaging Clin N Am 2010;20(4):639–50.
31. Sandhu FS, Dillon WP. Spinal epidural abscess: evaluation with contrast-enhanced MR imaging. AJNR Am J Neuroradiol 1991;12(6):1087–93.
32. Kim DH, Rosenblum JK, Panghaal VS, et al. Differentiating neoplastic from nonneoplastic processes in the anterior extradural space. Radiology 2011; 260(3):825–30.
33. Eastwood JD, Vollmer RT, Provenzale JM. Diffusion-weighted imaging in a patient with vertebral and epidural abscesses. AJNR Am J Neuroradiol 2002; 23(3):496–8.
34. Parkinson JF, Sekhon LH. Spinal epidural abscess: appearance on magnetic resonance imaging as a guide to surgical management. Report of five cases. Neurosurg Focus 2004;17(6):E12.
35. Soehle M, Wallenfang T. Spinal epidural abscesses: clinical manifestations, prognostic factors, and outcomes. Neurosurgery 2002;51(1):79–85 [discussion: 6–7].
36. Vural M, Arslantas A, Adapinar B, et al. Spinal subdural *Staphylococcus aureus* abscess: case report and review of the literature. Acta Neurol Scand 2005;112(5):343–6.
37. Kulkarni AG, Chu G, Fehlings MG. Pyogenic intradural abscess: a case report. Spine (Phila Pa 1976) 2007;32(12):E354–7.
38. Saigal G, Donovan Post MJ, Kozic D. Thoracic intradural Aspergillus abscess formation following epidural steroid injection. AJNR Am J Neuroradiol 2004;25(4):642–4.
39. Narvaez J, Nolla JM, Narvaez JA, et al. Spontaneous pyogenic facet joint infection. Semin Arthritis Rheum 2006;35(5):272–83.
40. Muffoletto AJ, Ketonen LM, Mader JT, et al. Hematogenous pyogenic facet joint infection. Spine (Phila Pa 1976) 2001;26(14):1570–6.
41. Doita M, Nabeshima Y, Nishida K, et al. Septic arthritis of lumbar facet joints without predisposing infection. J Spinal Disord Tech 2007;20(4):290–5.
42. Weingarten TN, Hooten WM, Huntoon MA. Septic facet joint arthritis after a corticosteroid facet injection. Pain Med 2006;7(1):52–6.

43. Hoelzer BC, Weingarten TN, Hooten WM, et al. Paraspinal abscess complicated by endocarditis following a facet joint injection. Eur J Pain 2008; 12(3):261–5.
44. Okada F, Takayama H, Doita M, et al. Lumbar facet joint infection associated with epidural and paraspinal abscess: a case report with review of the literature. J Spinal Disord Tech 2005;18(5):458–61.
45. Michel-Batot C, Dintinger H, Blum A, et al. A particular form of septic arthritis: septic arthritis of facet joint. Joint Bone Spine 2008;75(1):78–83.
46. Doita M, Nishida K, Miyamoto H, et al. Septic arthritis of bilateral lumbar facet joints: report of a case with MRI findings in the early stage. Spine (Phila Pa 1976) 2003;28(10):E198–202.
47. Theodorou SJ, Theodorou DJ, Resnick D. MR imaging findings of pyogenic bacterial myositis (pyomyositis) in patients with local muscle trauma: illustrative cases. Emerg Radiol 2007;14(2):89–96.
48. Marshman LA, Bhatia CK, Krishna M, et al. Primary erector spinae pyomyositis causing an epidural abscess: case report and literature review. Spine J 2008;8(3):548–51.
49. Trusen A, Beissert M, Schultz G, et al. Ultrasound and MRI features of pyomyositis in children. Eur Radiol 2003;13(5):1050–5.
50. Hassan FO, Shannak A. Primary pyomyositis of the paraspinal muscles: a case report and literature review. Eur Spine J 2008;17(Suppl 2):S239–42.
51. Medappil N, Adiga P. A 31-year-old female with fever and back pain. J Emerg Trauma Shock 2011; 4(3):385–8.
52. Bowen DK, Mitchell LA, Burnett MW, et al. Spinal epidural abscess due to tropical pyomyositis in immunocompetent adolescents. J Neurosurg Pediatr 2010;6(1):33–7.
53. Skaf GS, Kanafani ZA, Araj GF, et al. Non-pyogenic infections of the spine. Int J Antimicrob Agents 2010; 36(2):99–105.
54. Moon MS. Tuberculosis of the spine. Controversies and a new challenge. Spine (Phila Pa 1976) 1997; 22(15):1791–7.
55. Pande KC, Babhulkar SS. Atypical spinal tuberculosis. Clin Orthop Relat Res 2002;(398):67–74.
56. Almeida A. Tuberculosis of the spine and spinal cord. Eur J Radiol 2005;55(2):193–201.
57. De Backer AI, Mortele KJ, Vanschoubroeck IJ, et al. Tuberculosis of the spine: CT and MR imaging features. JBR-BTR 2005;88(2):92–7.
58. Smith AS, Weinstein MA, Mizushima A, et al. MR imaging characteristics of tuberculous spondylitis vs vertebral osteomyelitis. AJR Am J Roentgenol 1989;153(2):399–405.
59. Pertuiset E, Beaudreuil J, Liote F, et al. Spinal tuberculosis in adults. A study of 103 cases in a developed country, 1980-1994. Medicine (Baltimore) 1999;78(5):309–20.
60. Sharif HS, Morgan JL, al Shahed MS, et al. Role of CT and MR imaging in the management of tuberculous spondylitis. Radiol Clin North Am 1995;33(4): 787–804.
61. da Rocha AJ, Maia AC Jr, Ferreira NP, et al. Granulomatous diseases of the central nervous system. Top Magn Reson Imaging 2005;16(2):155–87.
62. Whiteman ML. Neuroimaging of central nervous system tuberculosis in HIV-infected patients. Neuroimaging Clin N Am 1997;7(2):199–214.
63. Polley P, Dunn R. Noncontiguous spinal tuberculosis: incidence and management. Eur Spine J 2009;18(8):1096–101.
64. Moorthy S, Prabhu NK. Spectrum of MR imaging findings in spinal tuberculosis. AJR Am J Roentgenol 2002;179(4):979–83.
65. Turunc T, Demiroglu YZ, Uncu H, et al. A comparative analysis of tuberculous, brucellar and pyogenic spontaneous spondylodiscitis patients. J Infect 2007;55(2):158–63.
66. Jung NY, Jee WH, Ha KY, et al. Discrimination of tuberculous spondylitis from pyogenic spondylitis on MRI. AJR Am J Roentgenol 2004;182(6): 1405–10.
67. Al-Sous MW, Bohlega S, Al-Kawi MZ, et al. Neurobrucellosis: clinical and neuroimaging correlation. AJNR Am J Neuroradiol 2004;25(3):395–401.
68. Sharif HS, Clark DC, Aabed MY, et al. Granulomatous spinal infections: MR imaging. Radiology 1990;177(1):101–7.
69. Sharif HS, Aideyan OA, Clark DC, et al. Brucellar and tuberculous spondylitis: comparative imaging features. Radiology 1989;171(2):419–25.
70. Bozgeyik Z, Ozdemir H, Demirdag K, et al. Clinical and MRI findings of brucellar spondylodiscitis. Eur J Radiol 2008;67(1):153–8.
71. Williams RL, Fukui MB, Meltzer CC, et al. Fungal spinal osteomyelitis in the immunocompromised patient: MR findings in three cases. AJNR Am J Neuroradiol 1999;20(3):381–5.
72. Kwon JW, Hong SH, Choi SH, et al. MRI findings of *Aspergillus spondylitis*. AJR Am J Roentgenol 2011;197(5):W919–23.
73. Layton KF, Thielen KR, Wald JT. A modified vertebroplasty approach for spine biopsies. AJNR Am J Neuroradiol 2006;27(3):596–7.
74. Sehn JK, Gilula LA. Percutaneous needle biopsy in diagnosis and identification of causative organisms in cases of suspected vertebral osteomyelitis. Eur J Radiol 2012;81(5):940–6.
75. Chew FS, Kline MJ. Diagnostic yield of CT-guided percutaneous aspiration procedures in suspected spontaneous infectious diskitis. Radiology 2001; 218(1):211–4.
76. Enoch DA, Cargill JS, Laing R, et al. Value of CT-guided biopsy in the diagnosis of septic discitis. J Clin Pathol 2008;61(6):750–3.

77. Rankine JJ, Barron DA, Robinson P, et al. Therapeutic impact of percutaneous spinal biopsy in spinal infection. Postgrad Med J 2004;80(948): 607–9.
78. Yang SC, Fu TS, Chen LH, et al. Identifying pathogens of spondylodiscitis: percutaneous endoscopy or CT-guided biopsy. Clin Orthop Relat Res 2008; 466(12):3086–92.
79. White LM, Schweitzer ME, Deely DM, et al. Study of osteomyelitis: utility of combined histologic and microbiologic evaluation of percutaneous biopsy samples. Radiology 1995;197(3):840–2.
80. Lucio E, Adesokan A, Hadjipavlou AG, et al. Pyogenic spondylodiskitis: a radiologic/pathologic and culture correlation study. Arch Pathol Lab Med 2000;124(5):712–6.
81. Cherasse A, Martin D, Tavernier C, et al. Are blood cultures performed after disco-vertebral biopsy useful in patients with pyogenic infective spondylitis? Rheumatology (Oxford) 2003;42(7):913.

Imaging of Stress Fractures of the Spine

Naveen S. Murthy, MD

KEYWORDS

• Stress fracture • Insufficiency fracture • Vertebral body • Pars interarticularis • Pedicle • Sacrum

KEY POINTS

- The fluid sign on magnetic resonance (MR) imaging corresponds to the intravertebral vacuum cleft sign on computed tomography (CT) and can be seen in 40% of osteoporotic vertebral compression fractures.
- Secondary radiographic signs of spondylolysis include lateral deviation of the spinous process, unilateral pedicle sclerosis in cases of unilateral pars interarticularis defects, and spinal dysraphism.
- Combined single-photon emission CT (SPECT)/CT has been shown to be useful in the diagnosis of spondylolysis by assessing both metabolic activity and structural components.
- MR imaging with appropriate imaging sequences can be used as an effective and reliable first-line imaging modality for the diagnosis of juvenile spondylolysis with the advantage of not imparting ionizing radiation.
- MR imaging has a reported 100% sensitivity in detecting sacral stress fractures.

INTRODUCTION

Back or limb pain may result from a wide variety of etiology, which are described elsewhere in this issue on spine imaging. Etiology that should not be ignored are stress fractures, fatigue or insufficiency, which may present with minimal, unrecognized or repetitive trauma. The patient population usually determines the type of stress fracture and its location. On a basic level, younger patients typically suffer fatigue fractures as a result of repetitive trauma to bone with normal bone mineral density, whereas older patients typically suffer insufficiency fractures as a result of normal stresses applied to bone with reduced bone mineral density.

Stress fractures intrinsic to the spine that can manifest as back pain may involve the vertebral bodies, pars interarticularis, or the pedicles. Sometimes, stress fractures from the sacrum or bony pelvis may mimic low back pain and may be overlooked. The imaging workup of patients with suspected back pain from stress fractures can be challenging regarding selecting the most appropriate study that best depicts the area of interest and minimizes ionizing radiation and economic costs. This article reviews the relevant imaging literature and provides guidance in this evaluation.

SPINE: VERTEBRAL BODY

It was estimated in 2005 that more than 2 million osteoporotic (insufficiency) fractures occurred annually in the United States in patients older than 50 years; this results in a cost of least $17 billion dollars.[1] Of these fractures, 27% constitute vertebral fractures.[1] By 2025, these costs are expected to increase by 50%, with a rapid growth of fracture rates in individuals between 65 and 74 years of age and in non-White populations.[1] These figures are certainly underestimations, because there are many osteoporotic vertebral compression fractures

The author has nothing to disclose.

Division of Musculoskeletal Radiology, Department of Radiology, Mayo Clinic, 200 First Street Southwest, Charlton 2-290, Rochester, MN 55905, USA
E-mail address: murthy.naveen@mayo.edu

Radiol Clin N Am 50 (2012) 799–821
doi:10.1016/j.rcl.2012.04.009

that remain asymptomatic. Cooper and colleagues[2] in a population-based study from Rochester, MN, found that 59% of vertebral fractures occurred without a single traumatic episode. Although nonpainful fractures may not pose an immediate problem, the real potential of sustaining additional fractures or progression to painful fractures is of larger concern. Each compression fracture of a wedged configuration adds to kyphotic deformity and places additional stress on the anterior aspect of adjacent or regional vertebrae. One study found that women who had one or more age-indeterminate vertebral body compression deformity at baseline had a 5-fold increased risk of sustaining another vertebral fracture within 1 year.[3] The clinical consequences of osteoporotic vertebral fractures include, but are not limited to, a decrease in mobility, inability to perform activities of daily living, reduced pulmonary function, and chronic back pain.[4–6] For these reasons, it is imperative that an accurate and timely diagnosis be made to prevent further injury, morbidity, and socioeconomic costs.

Radiographs

Initial evaluation of suspected vertebral body compression fractures should include weight-bearing anterior-posterior (AP) and lateral radiographs. The radiographs allow for assessment of the spinal alignment and relative vertebral body height. They can also be used to follow a fracture with nominal radiation and monetary cost. Care must be taken to obtain a true lateral radiograph, especially in patients without a spine curvature or scoliosis, to avoid potential parallax error, which can falsely produce or falsely estimate a compression deformity. Another potential pitfall is recognizing normal developmental variants such a slight wedge morphology at the thoracolumbar junction and a Cupid's bow (**Fig. 1**), which is a biconcave deformity involving the posterior aspect of the inferior endplates of the lumbar spine best seen on the AP radiographs.

One classification that allows for semiquantitative differentiation of vertebral fractures is a method initially described by Genant and colleagues (**Fig. 2**).[7] This method has been shown to have excellent reliability between radiologists and is known to many clinicians dealing with metabolic bone disease.[8] In this method, a vertebral body between T4 and L4 with more than 20% loss of height and a reduction of area of more than 10% to 20% compared with a normal adjacent segment was considered fractured. Four fracture grades were established: grade 0 (no loss of vertebral body height); grade 1 (vertebral body loss of height 20%–25%); grade 2 (vertebral body loss of height 25%–40%); and grade 3 (vertebral body loss of height >40%). The anterior wedge deformity and the central, biconcave deformity can be seen with osteoporotic fractures. However, a posterior wedge deformity or crush fracture raises concern for a neoplastic etiology.[9] In one cadaveric study, 2 adjacent vertebral bodies from T9 to L4 were loaded to failure at 2° to 6° of flexion.[10] Approximately 89% of the resultant fractures involved the superior endplate in all specimen ages. Furthermore, the investigators found that the superior endplates were thinner than the inferior endplates, with the central most regions being the thinnest and supported by less dense trabecular bone.[10] These findings support the observation that an anterior or central vertebral compression deformity is the result of a more physiologic process, whereas a posterior vertebral deformity may be the result of a neoplastic process. Intervertebral disc age-related degeneration also plays a role in the location of a vertebral fracture. Another cadaveric study

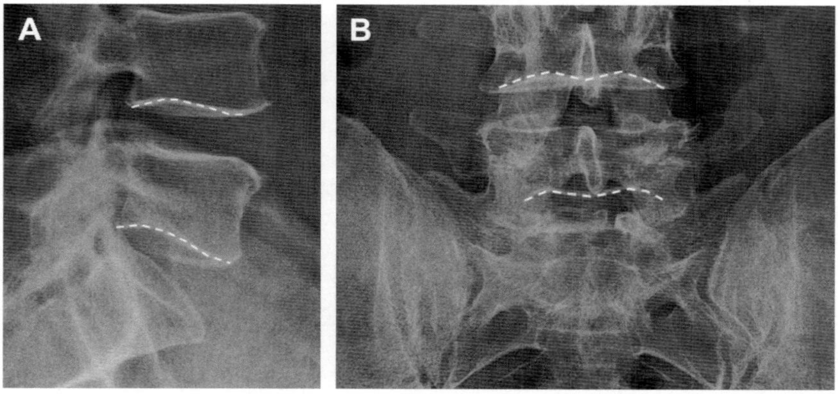

Fig. 1. Normal variant biconcave deformity involving the posterior aspect of the inferior endplates of the lumbar spine (*A, dashed white line*). This variant has the appearance of Cupid's bow on the AP radiograph and should not be confused with a vertebral fracture (*B, dashed white line,* bow pointing upward).

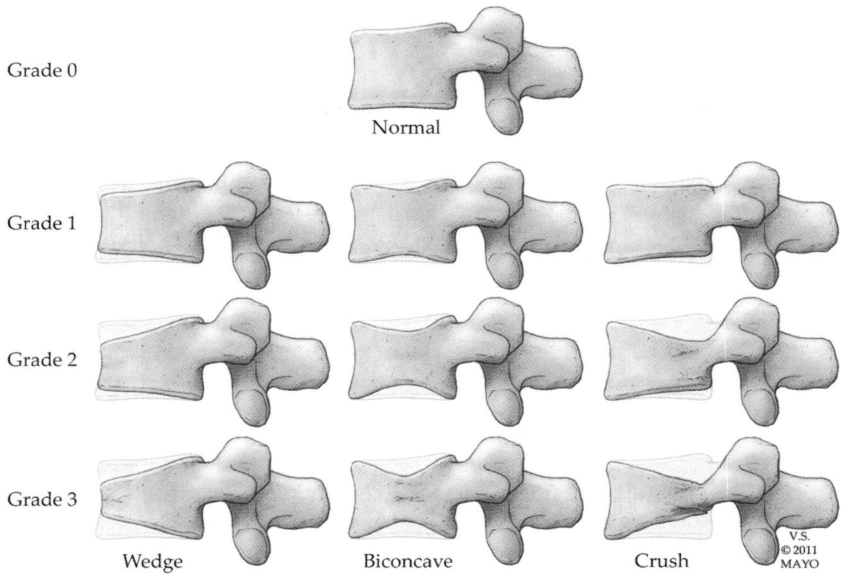

Fig. 2. Vertebral fracture grading by Genant and colleagues'[7]: grade 0 (no loss of vertebral body height); grade 1 (vertebral body loss of height 20%–25%); grade 2 (vertebral body loss of height 25%–40%); and grade 3 (vertebral body loss of height more than 40%). (*Courtesy of* Mayo Clinic, Rochester, Minnesota; with permission.)

showed that anterior vertebral bodies of thoracolumbar segments involved with intervertebral disc degeneration were associated with relatively less loading in an upright position.[11] The reduced load bearing of the anterior vertebral bodies resulted in locally reduced bone mineral density, which produced compression failure in flexion at reduced load levels.[11] It has been proposed that a concave posterior border of the vertebral body suggests a benign etiology, whereas a convex posterior border suggests a malignant etiology.[9,12] However, 20% of osteoporotic fractures have a posterior convex border.[12]

The acuity of the compression deformity may be challenging or impossible to ascertain without comparison radiographs taken in close temporal relationship. Acute factures may show increased density along the compressed endplate, whereas subacute fractures may show callus formation in addition to increased endplate density (**Fig. 3**).

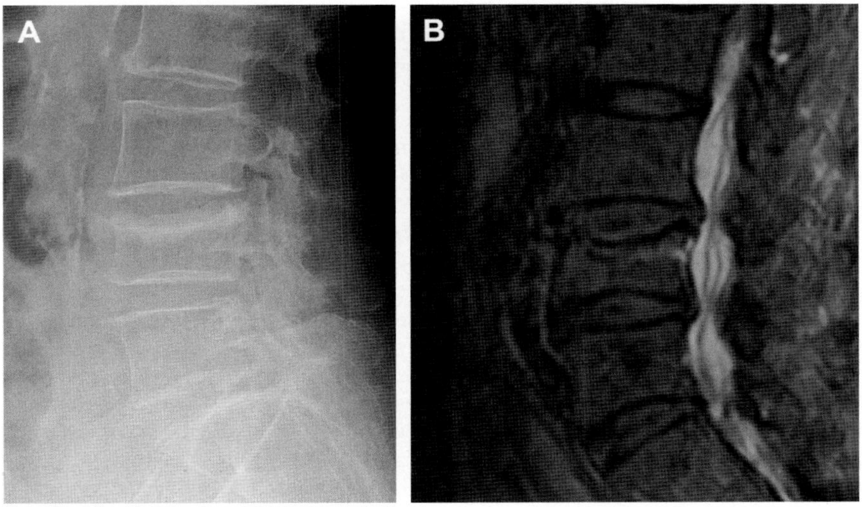

Fig. 3. Subacute L4 osteoporotic compression fracture. (*A*) Increased density along the compressed superior endplate of L4 in an 85-year-old woman who experienced the onset of low back pain 2 months earlier. (*B*) Corresponding sagittal STIR MR imaging taken at the time of the radiographs showing mild bone marrow edema and tiny fluid along the fracture also compatible with a subacute timeframe.

Chronic fracture deformities either from remote trauma or osteoporotic fracture may show remodeling of marginal osteophytes, if present. Although these findings are helpful, they are not pathognomonic. The degree of demineralization can make evaluation of subtle compression deformities, density changes, and callus formation difficult. As one retrospective study showed using nuclear medicine bone scans as the gold standard, osteoporotic vertebral fractures from T4 to L5 could be confidently diagnosed on radiographs only if the compression deformities were more than 3 standard deviations less than the normal mean vertebral height ratios, which were obtained from healthy women between 40 and 65 years of age without osteoporosis.[13] The sensitivity shortcomings of radiographs in diagnosing occult symptomatic osteoporotic vertebral fractures was further shown by Pham and colleagues.[14] These investigators presented a retrospective review of 21 vertebral fractures in 16 patients with no noteworthy vertebral compression deformities on radiographs but who all had positive magnetic resonance (MR) imaging examinations compatible with vertebral insufficiency fractures.

For those symptomatic individuals who have a visible deformity on radiographs, and no recent comparison examination to assess acuity, dynamic sitting and bolstered supine lateral radiographs may be helpful in identifying mobile osteoporotic vertebral fractures that may benefit from treatment (vertebroplasty or surgery).[15] Chen and colleagues[15] studied 105 patients (62–90 years of age) with 144 MR imaging-proven edematous osteoporotic vertebral compression fractures. These investigators found 126 (88%) of the fractures to be mobile on dynamic radiographs, with an average increase in anterior vertebral height from the sitting to bolstered supine position to be 8.5 mm. The overall sensitivity of this radiographic assessment for identifying painful, mobile osteoporotic vertebral compression fractures was 88%. Although this finding is helpful in identifying patients who would benefit from treatment, the investigators caution that this is not a substitute for MR imaging. Preprocedure MR imaging before vertebral augmentation has also been shown to be beneficial by changing the therapeutic plan in 57% of patients as a result of identifying malignancy, accurately localizing or excluding levels of treatment based on bone marrow edema, and finding alternate spatially related diagnoses.[16] The dynamic radiographs may be useful for screening and in the immediate preprocedure time period (if an MR imaging examination was not recently performed) to assist in detecting new fractures, estimating postprocedure height change, and to help determine the feasibility of vertebroplasty in vertebra plana.[15]

MR Imaging

As alluded to in the preceding paragraphs, MR imaging can be useful in evaluating age-indeterminate, occult, and pathologic vertebral fractures. Standard MR imaging sequences should include sagittal T1-weighted and T2-weighted fat-suppressed or short tau inversion recovery (STIR) and axial T2-weighted images. The latter sequence is helpful to assess for paravertebral soft tissue edema or mass. The presence and degree of bone marrow edema suggest the acuity and severity of the fracture. The bone marrow edema pattern is typically bandlike, paralleling the fractured endplate, with some preservation of marrow fat. The presence of a linear low-signal-intensity line within a zone of bone marrow edema can add confidence in the assessment of a fracture (**Fig. 4**).

MR imaging can also be helpful in aiding in the detection of other potential causes of back pain, such as the predictors of discogenic pain described elsewhere in this issue by Aprill and Maus, intervertebral disc herniation, and the less frequent, but most important, diagnosis of a neoplastic process. A malignant etiology should be considered when there is complete bone marrow replacement manifested as T1 hypointensity, involvement of the posterior elements, osseous destruction, surrounding soft tissue component, presence of additional lesions, and involvement of the upper cervical spine. A single finding in isolation may not be specific for malignancy, but when multiple of these imaging signs are present, the findings can be diagnostic.

One finding that seldom occurs with metastatic vertebral compression fractures, and strongly suggests a benign compression, is the fluid sign.[17] The fluid sign can be seen in 40% of osteoporotic vertebral compression fractures with bone marrow edema; it describes a typically linear zone of fluid signal intensity similar to that of cerebrospinal fluid adjacent to the fractured endplate (see **Fig. 4**B; **Fig. 5**).[17] It has been shown that this fluid sign on MR imaging corresponds to the intravertebral vacuum cleft sign seen occasionally with osteoporotic vertebral fractures on radiographs and CT (**Fig. 6**).[18] Lin and colleagues' explanation for the basis of this relationship is that in an upright position, the fracture cleft collapses and is mainly filled with fluid. As the spine is extended in the supine position, the distractive force produces negative pressure, pulling nitrogen gas into the cleft.

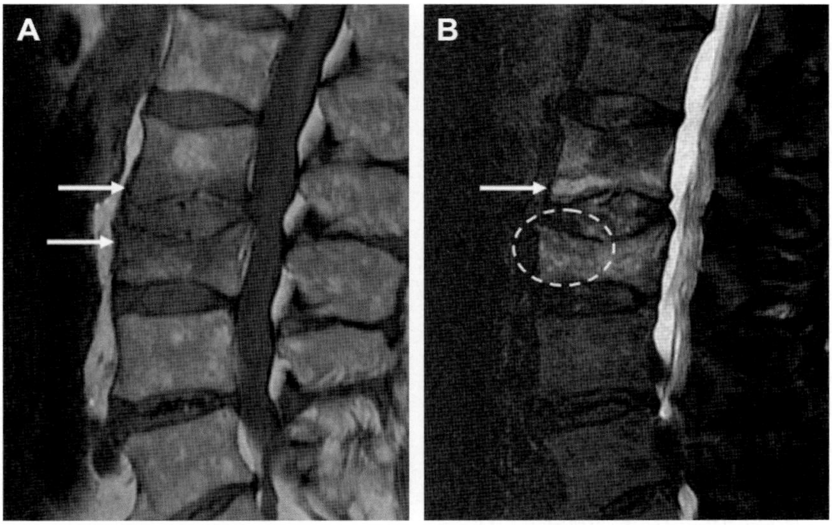

Fig. 4. L2 and L3 osteoporotic compression fractures. (*A*) T1-weighted MR imaging shows bands of decreased T1 signal within the fractured endplates of the vertebral bodies paralleling the L2 to 3 intervertebral disk (*white arrows*). There are small scattered areas of preserved marrow fat within these bands consistent with a benign etiology. (*B*) T2-weighted fat-saturated MR imaging reveals a horizontally oriented linear low signal abnormality within the anterior aspect of the L3 vertebral body paralleling the L2 to 3 intervertebral disk, representing the fracture line of the endplate (*dashed white oval*). Fluid signal cleft adjacent to the fractured endplate of L2, representing the fluid sign, which can be seen with osteoporotic compression fractures (*white arrow*).

Depending on the length of time this position is maintained, the cleft is slowly replaced with transudative fluid from the surrounding bone marrow edema.[18]

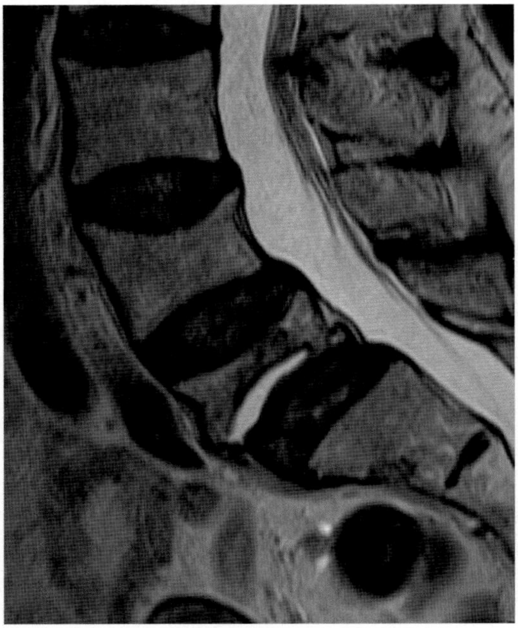

Fig. 5. T2-weighted MR imaging with a fluid signal cleft adjacent to the fractured inferior endplate of L5, representing the fluid sign, which can be seen with osteoporotic compression fractures.

If standard techniques cannot exclude a malignant etiology, advanced MR imaging sequences can be performed. These techniques include diffusion-weighted and chemical shift imaging. Diffusion-weighted imaging is based on the Brownian movement of water molecules. Extracellular water, which is mainly seen with osteoporotic fractures, has a higher diffusion capability than the

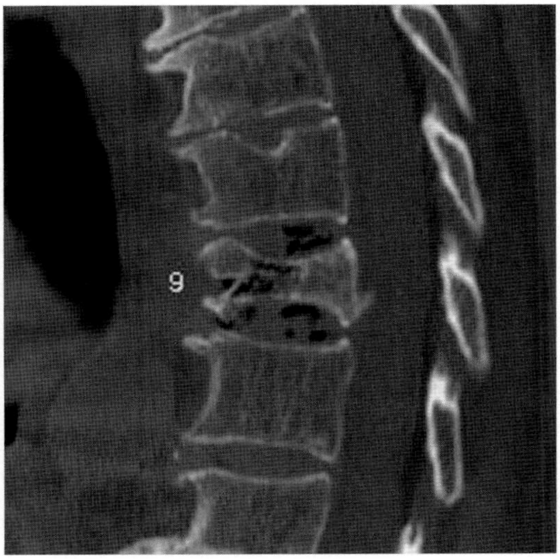

Fig. 6. Intravertebral vacuum cleft sign. Nitrogen gas within a benign, osteoporotic vertebral fracture of T9. (*Courtesy of* Louis Shulman, MD.)

increased intracellular water that occurs with neoplastic processes. Because of the ease of dispersion of extracellular water in osteoporotic vertebral fractures, there is relatively greater loss of signal of the extracellular water when compared with the intracellular water content of neoplastic processes. Tissues with prolonged T2 relaxation can manifest as increased signal on the diffusion-weighted images, simulating a neoplastic process. This phenomenon is known as T2 shine-through. To avoid this pitfall, the apparent diffusion coefficient maps must be assessed along with the diffusion-weighted images and conventional fast spin echo sequences to accurately assess for a neoplastic process.[19] Chemical shift imaging can detect the presence of microscopic fat, which should be preserved in osteoporotic fractures and replaced in pathologic fractures. Preserved microscopic fat shows a loss of signal on the out-of-phase images when compared with the in-phase images. A signal drop-out threshold of 35% has been shown to have a sensitivity of 95% and a specificity of 100%[20] for the presence of microscopic fat in a benign fracture.

Computed Tomography

For individuals unable to undergo an MR imaging examination, computed tomography (CT) may be a useful alternative. Although CT is less sensitive for assessing marrow disease, preservation of the trabeculae in nonfractured regions can be helpful in excluding an infiltrating neoplastic process (**Fig. 7**). The cortical margins are better depicted with CT than MR imaging, and therefore destructive processes and posterior convexity of the vertebral body suggestive of a neoplastic process can be assessed as on MR imaging. The intravertebral vacuum cleft discussed earlier, a sign of a benign process, is better depicted with CT (see **Fig. 6**).

Nuclear Medicine Imaging

Although the bone scan is sensitive for bone turnover, it is not specific for etiology. In regards to the acuity of an osteoporotic vertebral fracture, a comparison study was performed assessing planar nuclear medicine bone scan to MR imaging.[21] For a single level fracture, the bone scan correctly depicted 96% of the acute fractures. However, as the number of levels increased, the ability of the bone scan to correctly depict the acute fractures decreased precipitously. For three or more levels of activity, the rate of correctly depicting an acute fracture was only 36%.[21] The number and distribution of lesions seen on a bone scan may be helpful in predicting a benign versus malignant process, but it is often not diagnostic by itself (**Fig. 8**). Positron emission tomography (PET) may be helpful in distinguishing a benign from malignant vertebral fracture. In a recent study comparing MR imaging with PET/CT using a standard uptake value maximum of 4.25, the sensitivity and specificity for detecting a malignant process was 64% and 83% for MR imaging and 85% and 71% for PET/CT, respectively.[22]

SPINE: PARS INTERARTICULARIS

Pars interarticularis stress fractures, or isthmic spondylolysis (from the Greek *isthmic* [narrow], *spondylos* [vertebra], and *lysis* [defect]), are located between adjacent facet joints, where the pedicle, lamina, and facet joints coalesce. In a 45-year prospective study of 500 elementary school children using radiographs, the prevalence of pars interarticularis defects at 6 years of age

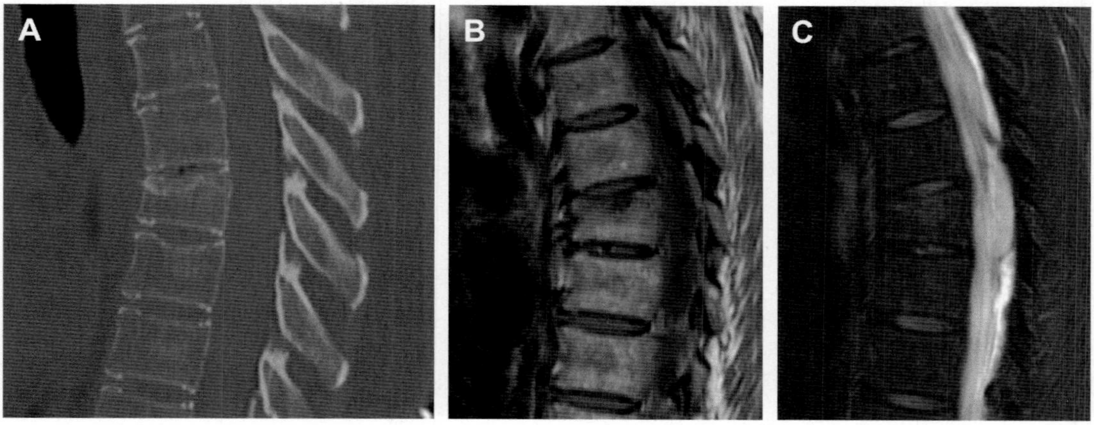

Fig. 7. (*A*) Osteoporotic compression fracture of a thoracic vertebral body. The CT image shows preservation of the vertically oriented trabeculae in the remainder of the body, suggestive of a nonneoplastic process. (*B, C*) Sagittal T1-weighted and T2-weighted fat-saturated MR images confirm a benign etiology.

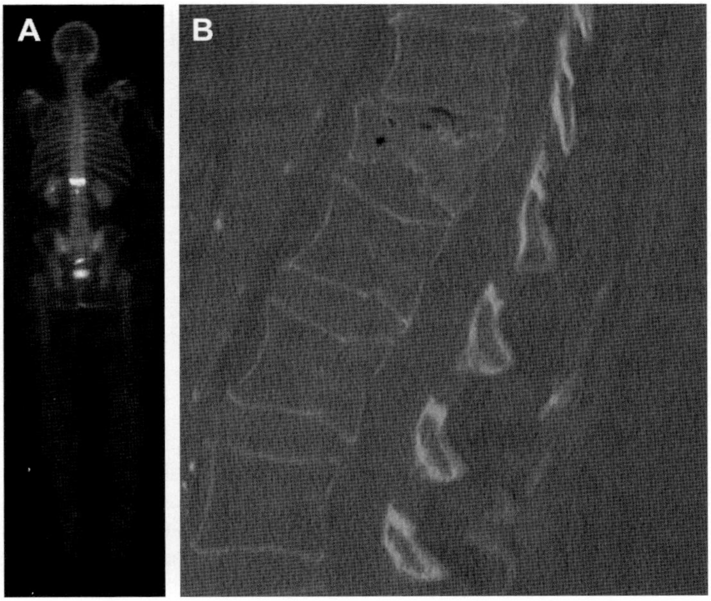

Fig. 8. (*A*) Nuclear medicine bone scan showing marked increased radiotracer activity at T12 consistent with an acute fracture. There are no other areas of increased radiotracer activity, which is not diagnostic for, but favors, a benign process. (*B*) CT examination has features compatible with an osteoporotic compression fracture.

was 4.4%, which increased to 6% at adulthood with a male/female ratio of 2:1.[23] Of the pars interarticularis defects, 73% were bilateral, and of these all occurred at the L5/S1 level.[23] All of the initial 500 children were asymptomatic at the start of the study; by the end of the study, their functional disability scores as measured by the Short Form (36) Health Survey were no different from the general population.[23] This study suggests that most spondylolytic defects are not symptomatic. In a more recent Japanese CT study of 2000 patients between the ages of 20 and 29 years, the prevalence in the general population was 5.9% with a male/female ratio of 2:1.[24] Of these patients, 90.3% occurred at L5; 5.6% at L4; and 3.2% at L3.[24] These studied populations are distinct from an athletic population, especially elite athletes. In an Italian retrospective review of 3505 athletes with low back pain, 13.5% of athletes had spondylolysis and 81% occurred at the L5/S1 level.[25] Furthermore, the incidence between different sports varies, with a higher occurrence in sports that include axial loading in extension. Another Italian study found 390 cases of lumbar spondylolysis in 3132 athletes with the highest percentages occurring in diving (43%), wrestling (30%), and weight lifting (23%).[26] In yet another study of the Japanese population, the incidence of lumbar spondylolysis was significantly higher in rugby and judo players, with an incidence of 20%, and higher still in soccer and baseball players, with an incidence of 30%.[27]

Spondylolysis is not limited to the lumbar spine but is rare in other spine segments. There have been approximately 100 cases of cervical spondylolysis reported in the literature without a clear, agreed compression fractures should include.[28] Forsberg and colleagues[29] described common imaging findings in a series of 12 patients. These findings include (1) a well-marginated cleft between the facets (**Fig. 9**), (2) a triangular configuration of the pillar fragments on either side of the spondylolytic defect, (3) posterior displacement of the dorsal triangular pillar fragment, (4) hypoplasia of the ipsilateral pedicle, (5) spinal dysraphism at the involved level (see **Fig. 9**), and (6) compensatory hyperplasia or hypoplasia of the ipsilateral articular pillars at the level above or below the defect.[29] Awareness of cervical spondylolysis is important to differentiate these findings from an acute fracture; these patients are also at an increased risk of developing neurologic compromise after relatively minor trauma.[28,29]

The etiology of spondylolysis remains controversial, but it is generally accepted that spondylolysis is multifactorial, with a combination of repetitive microtrauma related to flexion, extension, and rotation superimposed on congenital anatomic variations. In an anatomic study in 1951, Roche and Rowe[30] reported a varied incidence of spondylolysis among races and sex: White men, 6.4%; African American men, 2.8%; White women, 2.3%; African American women, 1.1%. This study supports a genetic component in the etiology of

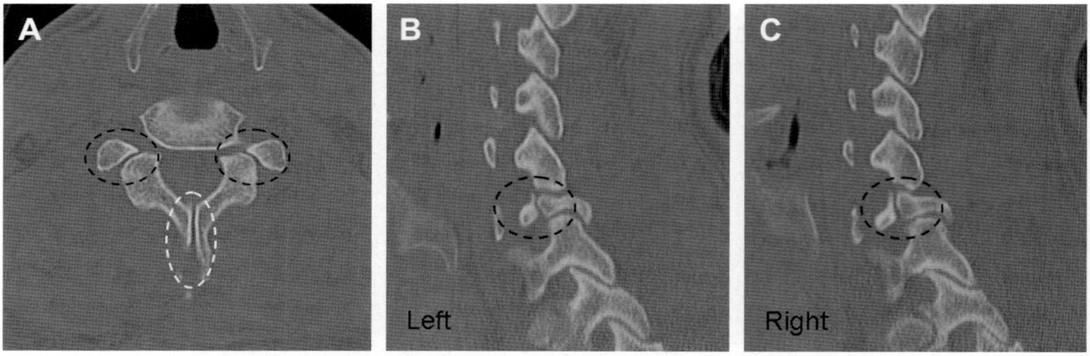

Fig. 9. CT of bilateral C6 spondylolysis. Well-marginated clefts between the facet joints (*A–C, dashed black ovals*). Associated spinal dysraphism at the affected level (*A, dashed white oval*). (*Courtesy of* Felix Diehn, MD.)

spondylolysis. Ward and colleagues[31] found that individuals with L5 spondylolysis had an inadequate increase in the transverse lumbar interfacet distance progressing caudally from L4 to S1 when compared with normal control individuals. The normal increase of the transverse interfacet distance progressing caudally in the lower lumbar spine allows the adjacent articular processes to slide by one another without exerting excessive pressure on the intervening pars interarticularis.[31] With the reduction of transverse interfacet distance progressing caudally, the inferior articular process of L4 and the superior articular process of S1 contact the same cross-section of the L5 pars interarticularis by a pinching mechanism first described by Capener in 1931 (**Fig. 10**).[31] These forces lead to bony resorption and weakening of the pars interarticularis. Ward and colleagues[31] concluded that these individuals were at higher risk of developing and maintaining a spondylolytic defect. Another contributing anatomic factor was described by Masharawi and colleagues,[32] who studied 115 cadaveric skeletons with L5 spondylolysis compared with 120 controls. These investigators found that greater degrees of coronal orientation, tropism, and asymmetry of the lower lumber facets was strongly associated with spondylolysis. They postulated that sagittally oriented facets allow for facilitated flexion and extension, whereas the more coronally oriented facets subject more force on the pars interarticularis as a result of increased surface area contact by the opposing articular processes.[32]

The imaging evaluation of spondylolysis may include radiographs, nuclear medicine imaging, CT, and MR imaging. Each modality has potential benefits and pitfalls that need to be considered when interpreting these images.

Radiographs

Radiographs are often obtained in the initial workup of low back pain related to spondylolysis. Common projections include AP, lateral, collimated lateral, and 45° oblique images. A displaced pars interarticularis defect can be seen on lateral views as a linear lucency with irregular or rounded margins, depending on the age of the defect. These fractures can also be seen on the 45° oblique views as a lucency traversing the neck of the Scotty dog likened to a collar (**Fig. 11**). One study consisting of 56 patients detected spondylolytic defects using a series of 6 radiographs including an AP, 30° up-angled AP, lateral, collimated

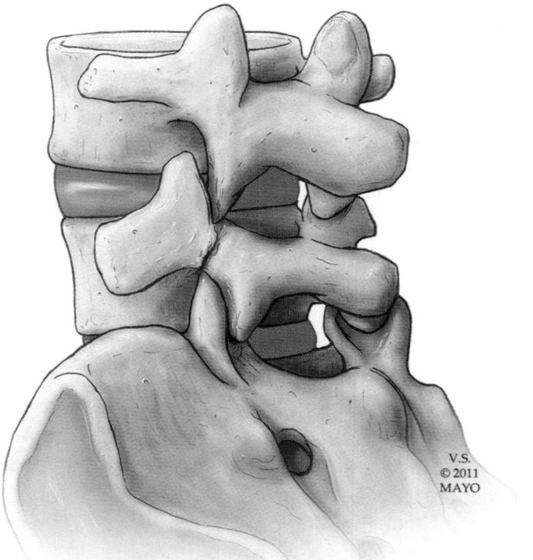

Fig. 10. The pincer mechanism as a proposed etiology of spondylolysis. The inferior articular process of the segment above and the superior articular process of the segment below contact the same cross-section of the intervening vertebra pars interarticularis by a pinching mechanism. (*Courtesy of* Mayo Clinic, Rochester, Minnesota; with permission.)

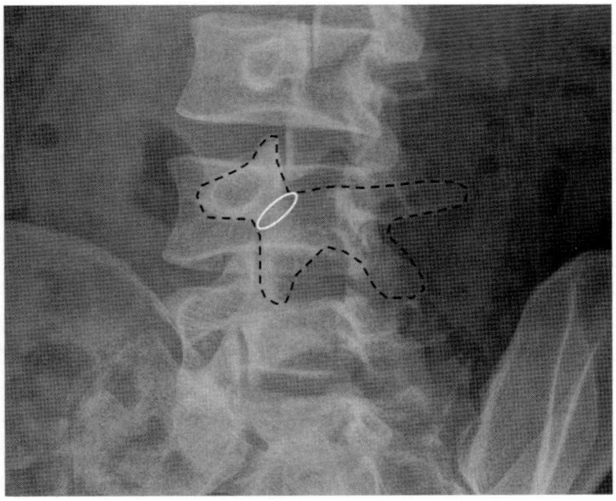

Fig. 11. Scotty dog appearance of a lumbar vertebra on a 45° oblique radiograph (*dashed black outline*). In the presence of a pars interarticularis defect, the collar (*white oval*) of the dog shows a linear lucency, representing the fracture line.

lateral, and two 45° oblique views.[33] This study found that 84% of the defects were detected on the collimated lateral view versus 77% detected on the 45° oblique views.[33] The oblique views have been considered to be important in the detection of the spondylolytic defects; however, in a CT study, the spondylolytic fracture plane was discovered to be oriented closer to the coronal plane rather than the 45° oblique plane.[34] This finding explains the higher sensitivity of detecting the spondylolytic defect with the collimated lateral view because it is more tangential to the radiograph beam (**Fig. 12**).[33,34] If a collimated lateral radiograph has already been obtained and a spondylolytic defect cannot be detected and is still suspected, oblique images only increase the radiation dose and do not necessarily offer greater diagnostic sensitivity. In this setting of clinical suspicion and negative AP and lateral radiographs, advancing imaging should be used, as discussed later.

Secondary radiographic signs of spondylolysis include lateral deviation of the spinous process, unilateral pedicle sclerosis in cases of unilateral pars interarticularis defects, and spinal dysraphism. Isolated lateral deviation and rotation of a spinous process toward the shorter lamina can occur in cases in which there is a unilateral defect or asymmetric bilateral defect.[35] The more distracted pars interarticularis defect is the more lengthened side. In cases of unilateral pars interarticularis defects, sclerosis and hypertrophy of the contralateral pedicle and neural arch have been described and attributed to a compensatory stress reaction (**Fig. 13**).[36,37] In the Japanese CT study of 2000 patients discussed earlier, spondylolysis was

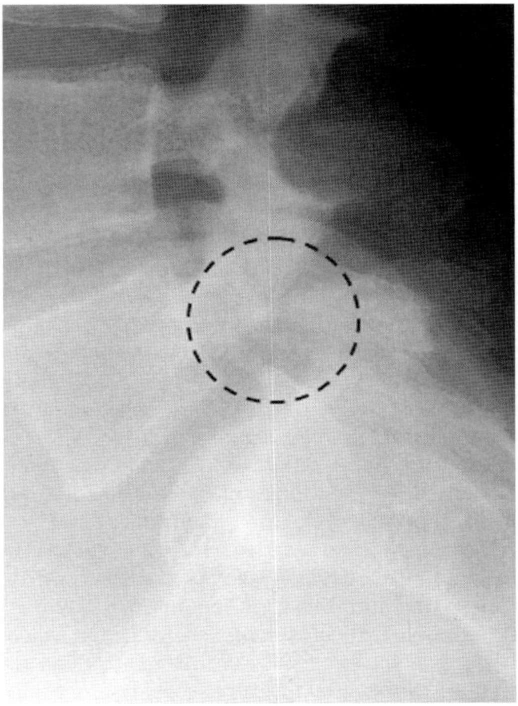

Fig. 12. Collimated lateral radiograph of the lower lumbar spine showing bilateral L5 spondylolytic defects (*dashed black circle*). (*Courtesy of* Timothy Maus, MD.)

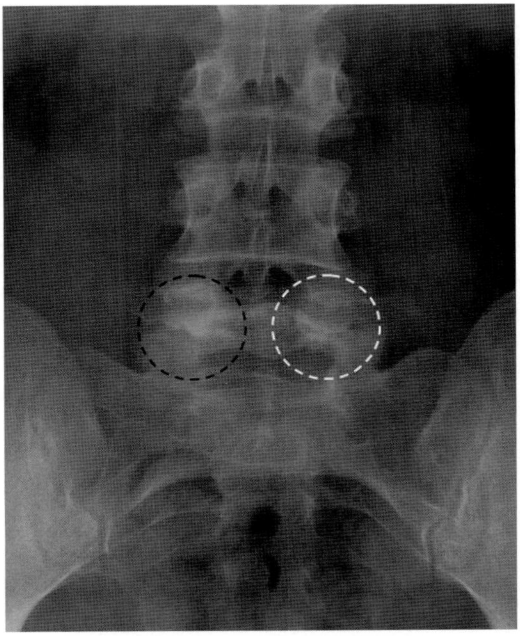

Fig. 13. Unilateral pars interarticularis defect of L5. Sclerosis and hypertrophy of the right pedicle and neural arch (*dashed black circle*) as a result of a compensatory stress reaction from the pars defect on the left (*dashed white circle*). (*Courtesy of* Timothy Maus, MD.)

found to be significantly greater in patients with spinal dysraphism as shown by an odds ratio of 3.7 (**Fig. 14**).[24] If a suspected spondylolytic defect cannot be detected on radiographs using primary and secondary signs, more advanced imaging techniques may be required.

Spondylolisthesis refers to the degree of anterior translation of the vertebral body with spondylolytic defects in relation to the vertebral body below and was originally classified by Meyerding.[38] The degree of spondylolisthesis is graded from I to V based on the percentage of anterior translation: grade I 0% to 25%; grade II 26% to 50%; grade III 51% to 75%; grade IV 76% to 100%; grade V >100% (spondyloptosis [falling off]) (**Fig. 15**).[34] Most isthmic spondylolistheses are grade I.[34] A trapezoidal appearance of L5 with a dome-shaped superior endplate of S1 can be seen with chronic spondylolysis with spondylolisthesis.[34]

A measure of motion and thus instability from the pars interarticularis defects can be obtained from flexion and extension radiographs. Although it has been extensively studied, absolute values to distinguish abnormal from normal motion are difficult to ascertain. Some investigators infer instability with sagittal rotation of more than 10° (**Fig. 16**) and sagittal translation of more than 4 mm on flexion-extension radiographs.[39–42]

CT

With the recent advances in multidetector CT, high-resolution, thin-section images can be rapidly obtained with isotropic voxels ideal for multiplanar two-dimensional reformations. In current clinical practice, CT provides the highest spatial resolution in characterizing a known or suspected spondylolytic fracture. Furthermore, CT is more sensitive than radiographs for identifying the primary and secondary radiographic findings, especially the sclerosis and hypertrophy of the contralateral pedicle and neural arch in unilateral spondylolysis (**Fig. 17**). This factor can be especially helpful in the diagnosis of osteoid osteoma (often in the differential diagnosis with unilateral spondylolysis) by confirming the presence of a nidus and the absence of a contralateral spondylolysis, which are unlikely to coexist (**Fig. 18**).

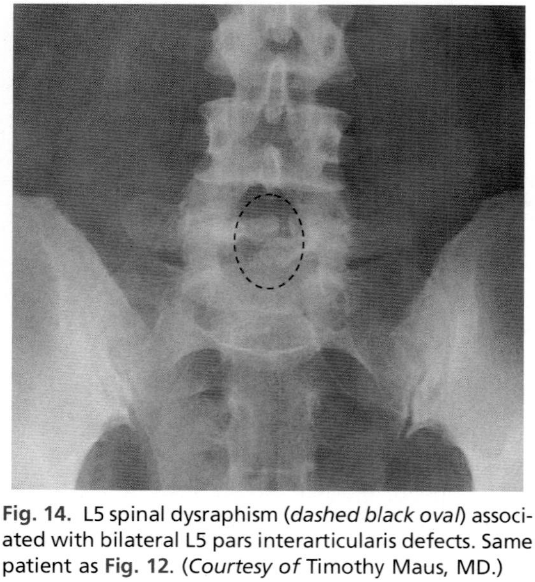

Fig. 14. L5 spinal dysraphism (*dashed black oval*) associated with bilateral L5 pars interarticularis defects. Same patient as **Fig. 12**. (*Courtesy of* Timothy Maus, MD.)

CT has been shown to be best at evaluating the size and extent of the fracture and is the best modality for fracture healing follow-up.[43,44] The reformatted sagittal plane and a plane parallel to the long axis of the articular pillar (also referred to as the reverse gantry technique) better depicts the spondylolytic defect distinct from the nearby facet joint. Fracture progression occurs from the inferior or inferomedial aspect of the pars interarticularis and propagates superiorly or superolaterally, whereas healing occurs in a reverse direction.[43] Fujii and colleagues[44] used CT to study the effect of prognostic variables in the healing of pars interarticularis defects with conservative measures, including a lumbar corset. These investigators found that the stage of the fracture at diagnosis was one of the predominant factors in predicting union. Three fracture stages were established: early, progressive, and terminal.[44] The early stage was defined as a narrow fissure through the pars with sharp margins (**Fig. 19**A). The progressive stage was a fissure that was still narrow but had slightly rounded margins (see **Fig. 19**B). The terminal stage was a wide defect with rounded margins and sclerosis (see **Fig. 19**C). A significantly greater proportion of defects achieved union at the early stage compared with the progressive and terminal stages.[44] None achieved union at the terminal stage.[44]

Nuclear Medicine Imaging

Whereas radiographs and CT may identify pars interarticularis defects, nuclear medicine imaging can provide information regarding metabolic activity, which can be inferred as necessary for the pars defect to be a pain generator. Planar bone scintigraphy and single-photon emission CT (SPECT) have been shown to identify symptomatic patients and sites of spondylolysis in patients with radiographic findings of spondylolysis.[45] SPECT imaging provides better sensitivity than planar bone scintigraphy by improved contrast and anatomic localization without increased radiation (**Fig. 20**).[45–47] A positive SPECT

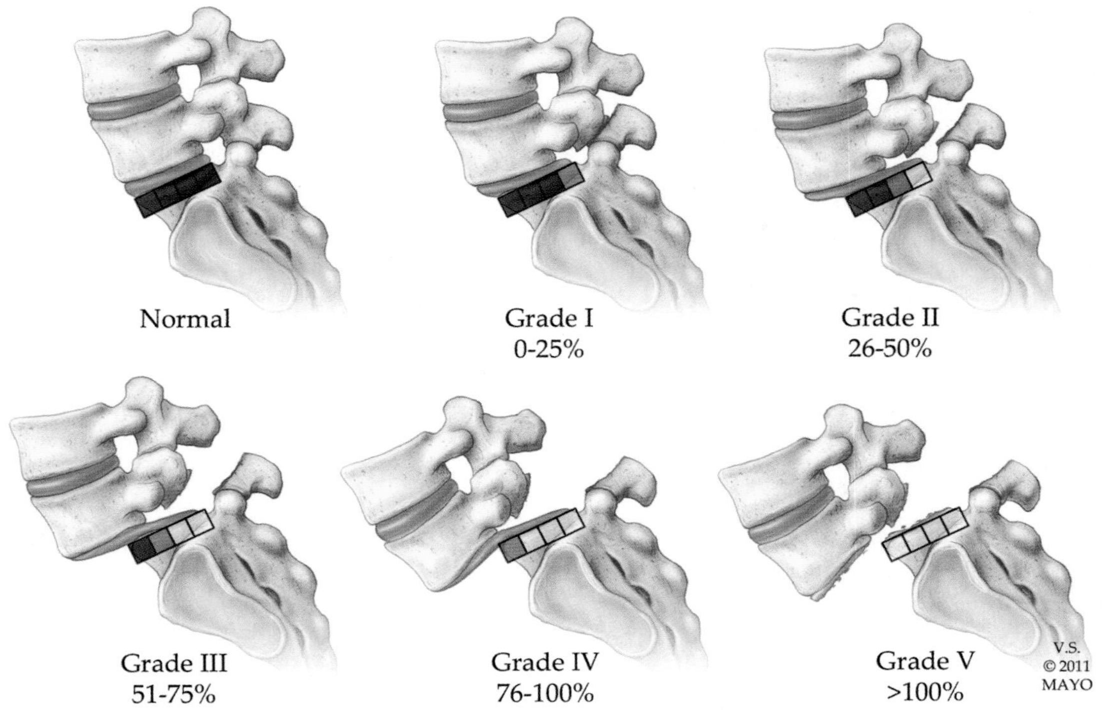

Fig. 15. Modified Meyerding classification of spondylolisthesis: grade I 0% to 25%; grade II 26% to 50%; grade III 51% to 75%; grade IV 76% to 100%; grade V greater than 100% (spondyloptosis [falling off]). (*Courtesy of* Mayo Clinic, Rochester, Minnesota; with permission.)

examination by itself cannot reliably distinguish a pars interarticularis defect from active facet synovitis, or in the unilateral cases, from a neoplastic process such as an osteoid osteoma, and infection.[42] Bellah and colleagues[47] stated that a negative SPECT examination virtually excludes a pars interarticularis defect as a etiology for back pain. In a more recent paper by Gregory and colleagues,[48] a negative SPECT examination translated into an 84.2% chance of not having spondylolysis or a 15.8% chance of having chronic pars defects that are unlikely to be pain generators. Gregory and colleagues assessed the diagnostic value of combining SPECT with CT in the

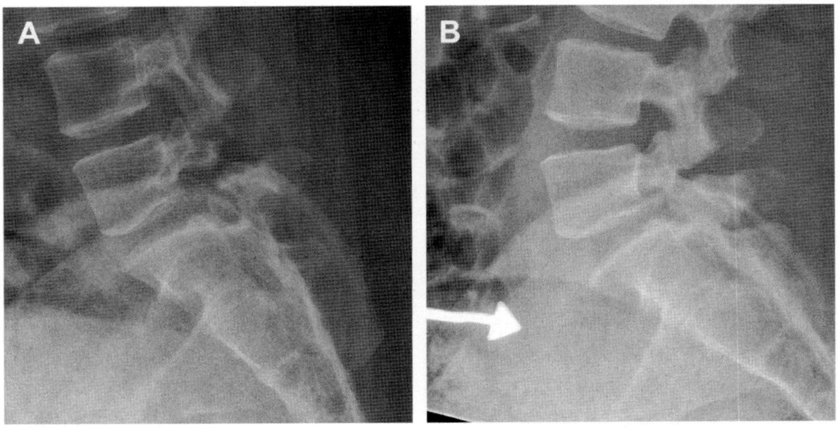

Fig. 16. L5 pars interarticularis instability with flexion (*A*) and extension (*B*) radiographs as measured by a sagittal rotation of 12°. Note the distraction of the pars defect in flexion. There is no sagittal translation with flexion and extension.

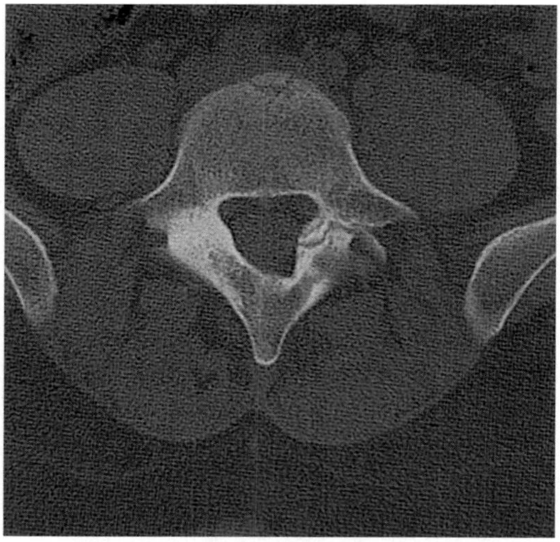

Fig. 17. CT of sclerosis and hypertrophy of the right pedicle and neural arch in unilateral spondylolysis seen with greater sensitivity than the radiographs depicted in the same patient in Fig. 13. (*Courtesy of* Timothy Maus, MD.)

evaluation of spondylolysis. They described 4 categories of patients: group A, (+) SPECT and (+) CT findings for spondylolysis; group B, (+) SPECT and (–) CT findings for spondylolysis ± sclerosis or the pars; group C, (–) SPECT and (+) CT findings for spondylolysis; and group D, (–) SPECT and (–) CT findings for spondylolysis. Group A and B patients were considered to have a healing potential. Group B patients were deemed to have a stress reaction, which could lead to a stress fracture without activity modification. Group C patients were considered to have chronic defects with no healing potential using conservative measures. Group D patients were generally found or considered to have an alternate pain generator other than a pars interarticularis defect. For this last group, the investigators recommended MR imaging for further evaluation. Of these group D patients who went on to have an MR imaging examination, 50% were diagnosed with discogenic pain as the etiology of their back pain.[48] SPECT combined with CT imparts a noteworthy amount of radiation to a relative young population. As a quantitative reference, the effective dose of background radiation in the United States is 3 mSv.[49] A CT examination of the lumbar spine delivers 6 mSv, whereas bone scintigraphy delivers 6.3 mSv.[49] Based on the radiation dose alone, nuclear scintigraphy may not be the best choice as a screening tool.[19] Combined SPECT/CT scanners can accomplish this evaluation with lower total radiation dose; the dose of the SPECT portion of the examination does not change but the dose of the CT portion does. At our institution, the CT portion of the combined SPECT/CT scanner delivers approximately half the dose (CTDIvol [CT dose index by volume]) of that of a routine lumbar spine CT. The trade-off is a modest reduction in CT image quality, which may not be relevant in this fusion of physiologic and anatomic data.

MR Imaging

MR imaging offers the distinct advantage of no ionizing radiation, which is of great importance in the relatively young population in whom spondylolysis occurs. High-resolution multiplanar techniques have been used to accurately identify pars interarticularis defects.[43,50] These sequences include oblique axial reverse gantry angled and sagittal T1-weighted images and STIR images, as well as sagittal three-dimensional spoiled gradient echo sequences.[43,50] To stratify the stress injuries, an MR imaging classification was developed by Hollenberg and colleagues (**Table 1**).[51]

This classification has been shown to have high intraobserver and interobserver reliability, as well as correlating well with CT and SPECT.[43,50,51] Grade 0 (normal) was assigned to the patients without signal abnormality of the pars interarticularis; grade 1 (stress reaction) denoted patients with T2 hyperintensity of the pars interarticularis with or without signal changes in the adjacent pedicle or articular process; grade 2 (incomplete fracture) identified the patients with T2 hyperintensity and thinning, fragmentation, or irregularity of the pars interarticularis visible on T1-weighted or T2-weighted images; grade 3 (complete active fracture) involved a visible complete unilateral or bilateral spondylolysis with associated abnormal T2 signal (**Fig. 21**); grade 4 (complete chronic fracture) was reserved for the cases of complete spondylolysis without abnormal T2 signal.[51]

In a study by Campbell and colleagues,[50] the aim was to evaluate whether MR imaging correlates with CT and SPECT imaging for the diagnosis of juvenile spondylolysis, and to determine whether MR imaging can be used as an exclusive image modality. These investigators found excellent agreement (κ >0.77) between MR imaging and SPECT. This study implies that MR imaging, with the addition of the oblique and STIR sequences, can replace SPECT in evaluating for metabolically active spondylolytic lesions. Furthermore, when comparing MR imaging with the combined CT and SPECT data, which was considered the gold standard, MR imaging correctly identified 73% of the pars defects but also showed some form of secondary signal change or morphologic abnormality in 98% of

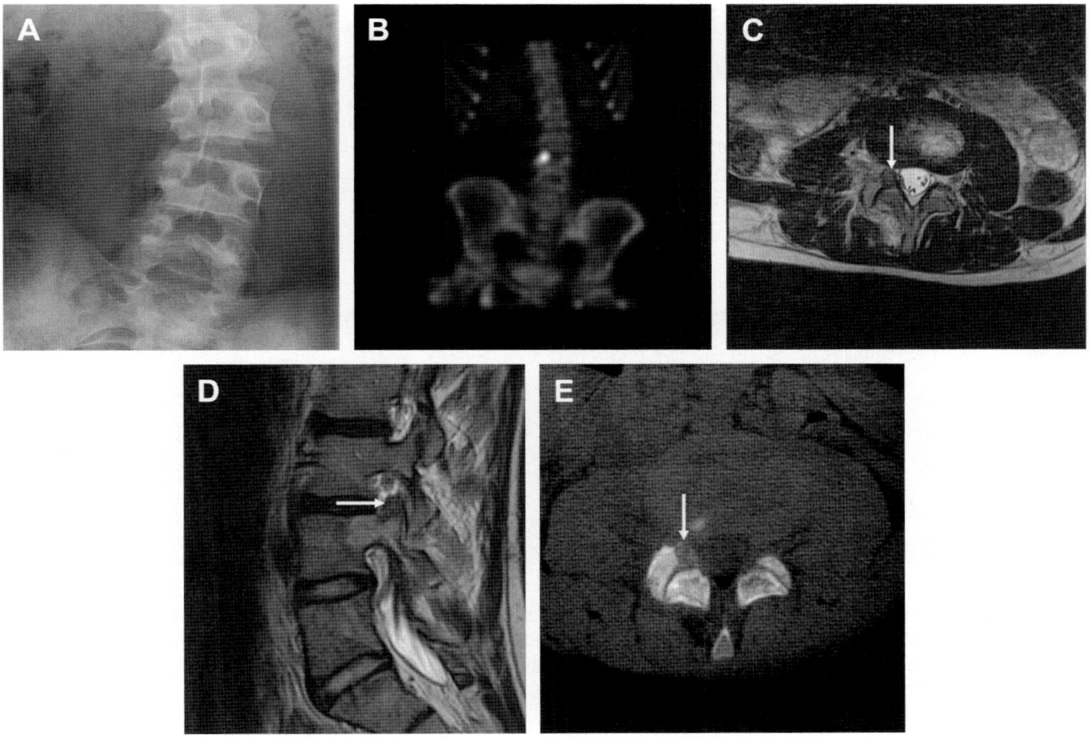

Fig. 18. 14-year-old boy with an osteoid osteoma. (*A*) AP radiograph of the lumbar spine reveals a levoscoliosis and L5 spinal dysraphism but no other findings to suggest an osteoid osteoma or spondylolysis. (*B*) Maximum intensity projection of a nuclear medicine SPECT study shows intense radiotracer activity about the right L4 pedicle, which is nonspecific and can be seen with either an osteoid osteoma or spondylolysis. (*C, D*) T2-weighted MR imaging confirms the presence of a low-signal-intensity nidus (*white arrows*) within the superior articular process of the right L4 vertebrae with surrounding reactive bone marrow edema. There are no findings for spondylolysis. (*E*) CT better depicts the relatively lower attenuation nidus (*arrow*) and absence of a pars defect, all consistent with an osteoid osteoma, which was eventually surgically excised. (*Courtesy of* Doris Wenger, MD.)

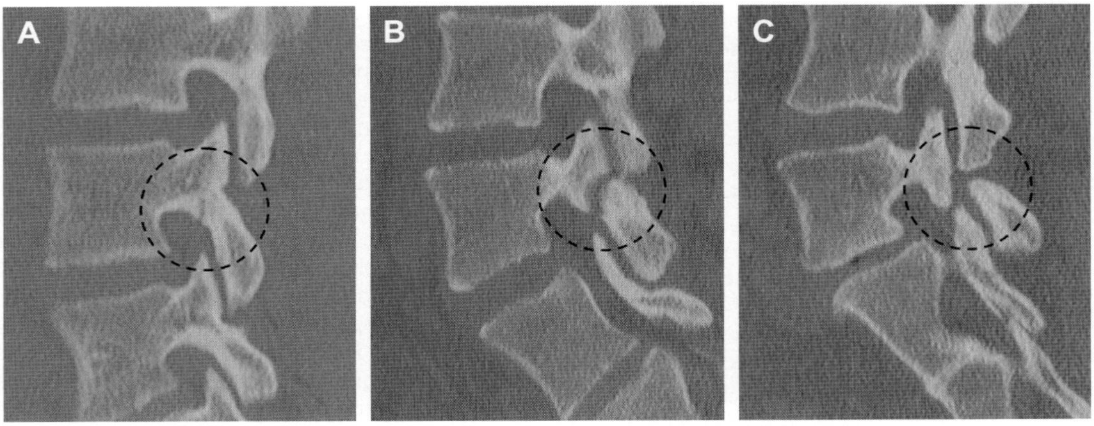

Fig. 19. Pars interarticularis fracture stages (*dashed circles*). (*A*) Early stage: narrow fissure through the pars with sharp margins. (*B*) Progressive stage: fissure that was still narrow but had slightly rounded margins. (*C*) Terminal stage: wide defect with rounded margins and sclerosis. (*Courtesy of* Timothy Maus, MD.)

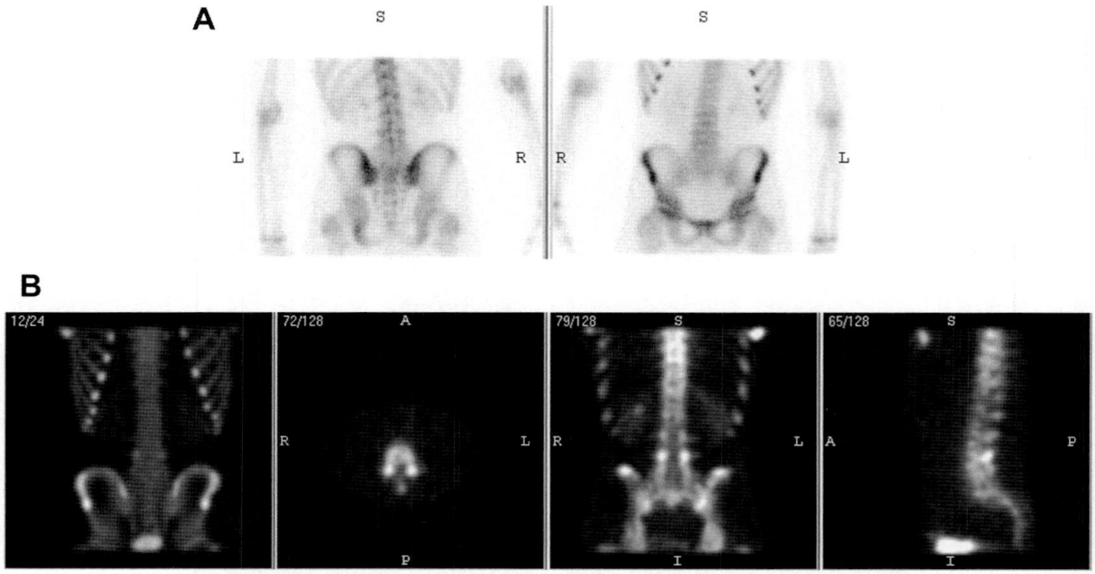

Fig. 20. (*A*) Nuclear medicine planar bone scan images of the lumbar spine. No discernible radiotracer activity at L4 in this same patient as **Fig. 19**A with early-stage CT findings of bilateral L4 pars interarticularis defects. (*B*) Nuclear medicine SPECT bone scan images of the lumbar spine in the same patient. Improved sensitivity in detection of the bilateral L4 pars interarticularis defects as a result of improved contrast and anatomic localization. (*Courtesy of* Timothy Maus, MD.)

the spondylolytic cases.[50] The use of secondary signs to identify spondylolysis was described for radiographs and CT earlier and can be equally useful in MR imaging. Ulmer and colleagues[52] described secondary findings present in 97% of 66 levels of lumbar spondylolyses studied. Theses findings included a widened sagittal spinal canal diameter (91% of cases), posterior wedging of the vertebral body bearing the defect (48% of cases), and reactive bone marrow edema in one or both of the adjacent pedicles (36% of cases).[52] Another study evaluated 36 pediatric and adolescent patients with 68 pars interarticularis defects using MR imaging and CT.[53] These investigators found that all the pars defects in the early stage on CT showed T2 hyperintensity in the ipsilateral pedicle (**Fig. 22**).[53] They also found that none of the pars defects in the terminal stage on CT showed T2 hyperintensity in the ipsilateral pedicle.[53] Of the 19 pars defects that showed T2 hyperintensity, 79% went on to heal with conservative management.[53] Of the 10 pars defects that did not show T2 hyperintensity, none went on to heal.[53] These investigators' conclusion was that T2 hyperintensity in the pedicle adjacent to a pars defect suggests an early diagnosis of spondylolysis and a greater potential for healing with conservative measures.[53] In a prospective study of 15 pediatric and adolescent patients with 22 early spondylolytic defects studied with CT and MR imaging and treated conservatively, most patients had resolution of the T2 hyperintensity at the 3-month follow-up; a longer period was needed for signal resolution in the few patients poorly compliant with therapy.[54] Nearly all the patients went on to heal and were symptom free with the resolution of the T2 hyperintensity.[54] These investigators concluded that follow-up MR

Table 1
MR imaging grading of spondylolysis

Grade	Description	MR Imaging Features
0	Normal	Normal bone marrow signal No cortical disruption
1	Stress reaction	Bone marrow edema No cortical disruption
2	Incomplete fracture	Bone marrow edema Incomplete fracture through the pars interarticularis
3	Acute complete	Bone marrow edema Complete fracture through the pars interarticularis
4	Chronic complete	No bone marrow edema Complete fracture through the pars interarticularis

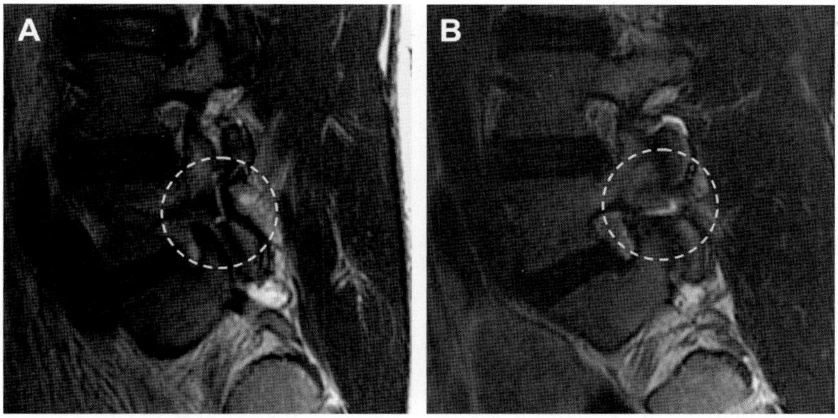

Fig. 21. Sagittal T2-weighted MR imaging images of complete left (*A*) and right (*B*) L5 pars interarticularis fractures (*dashed white circles*) containing tiny fluid signal with mild surrounding bone marrow edema, all compatible with MR imaging grade 3 spondylolysis. (*Courtesy of* Patrick Eiken, MD.)

imaging at 3 months after the initiation of conservative therapy can predict the success of treatment.[54]

Campbell and colleagues noted that the greatest discordance between MR imaging and CT was with grade 2 lesions in which the pars fracture is incomplete and cannot be reliably distinguished from the evolutionary or healing phase across all modalities at a single point in time.[42,50] This result was supported by Dunn and colleagues,[43] who evaluated grade 2 pars fractures with MR imaging and CT. These investigators concluded that MR imaging is limited in its ability to fully depict the cortical integrity of incomplete fractures of the pars, but the presence of marrow edema on the fluid-sensitive sequences (STIR and T2-weighted with fat saturation) is a useful means of detecting acute spondylolysis.[43] Of the CT-confirmed incomplete fractures, 77% showed a break in the inferomedial cortex of the pars interarticularis on MR imaging, whereas 92% showed reactive bone marrow edema about the pars.[43] Another more recent study by Ganiyusufoglu and colleagues[55] comparing the diagnostic accuracy of MR imaging with CT had similar results. These investigators found that MR imaging has a comparable diagnostic accuracy to CT in detecting complete fractures with or without accompanying

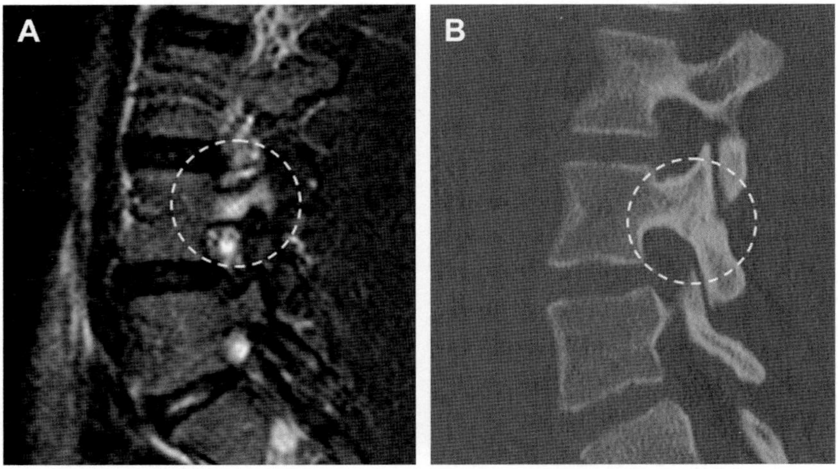

Fig. 22. (*A*) Sagittal STIR MR imaging in a 15-year-old girl with 9 months of right low back pain. There is increased T2 signal in the right L4 pedicle (*dashed white circle*). (*B*) Corresponding sagittal CT shows an early-stage right L4 pars interarticularis fracture with mild surrounding sclerosis (*dashed white circle*). These combined findings are compatible with an early spondylolytic fracture that has a good chance of healing with conservative measures. (*Courtesy of* Timothy Maus, MD.)

marrow edema and incomplete fractures with accompanying bone marrow edema, especially at the lower lumbar levels. The sensitivity of MR imaging in the detection of incomplete fractures was 75%, consistent with the findings presented by Ganiyusufoglu and colleagues.[55] Campbell and colleagues[50] concluded that MR imaging can be used as an effective and reliable first-line image modality for diagnosis of juvenile spondylolysis. Limited CT was recommended as an additional complementary examination in selected cases as a baseline for healing assessment, and for evaluation of indeterminate cases.

There are several other potential imaging pitfalls that one must be aware of when evaluating spondylolysis with MR imaging. Singh and colleagues[56] evaluated contiguous axial images compared with disc space targeted angled axial images and found a 50% decrease in detection of pars defects using the disc space targeted angled axial images compared with the contiguous axial images. The finding was not statistically significant because of the sample size. However, these investigators further observed that the disc space targeted angled axial images nearly excluded the pars interarticularis region. Furthermore, if a spondylolytic fracture was present, it was nearly parallel to the plane of the disc space targeted angled axial images, making detection even more difficult.[56] Potential false-positive findings of a spondylolytic defect on MR imaging may be the result of partial volume averaging of a marginal osteophyte from the adjacent superior facet, partial facetectomy, and sclerosis of the pars related to an osteoblastic metastasis.[57]

MR imaging can be used to evaluate the disc and nerve roots in cases of spondylolysis with and without spondylolisthesis as pain generators (**Fig. 23**). The lack of a structural connection between the anterior and posterior columns places significant shear stress on the intervertebral disc; it may develop internal disc disruption and be the etiology of axial pain (discogenic pain). Subsequent loss of disc space height and possible anterior translation of the vertebral body causes foraminal narrowing in a characteristic forward-leaning S shape, manifest clinically as radicular pain or radiculopathy. In cases in which no pars interarticularis defects are identified, MR imaging can potentially identify other causes of pain that may be difficult or impossible to evaluate with other modalities.

SPINE: PEDICLE

Pedicle stress fractures are less common than vertebral fractures and fractures of the pars interarticularis, as noted in a recent case report and literature review.[58] Aside from pedicle fractures related to trauma and previous surgery, the prevalence of pedicular stress fractures is difficult to ascertain. A study evaluating T2 hyperintensity of the pedicle on MR imaging and its relationship to symptoms in patients without acute trauma reported a pedicle fracture incidence of 7.6%.[59] When this subset of patients displaying T2 hyperintensity of the pedicle

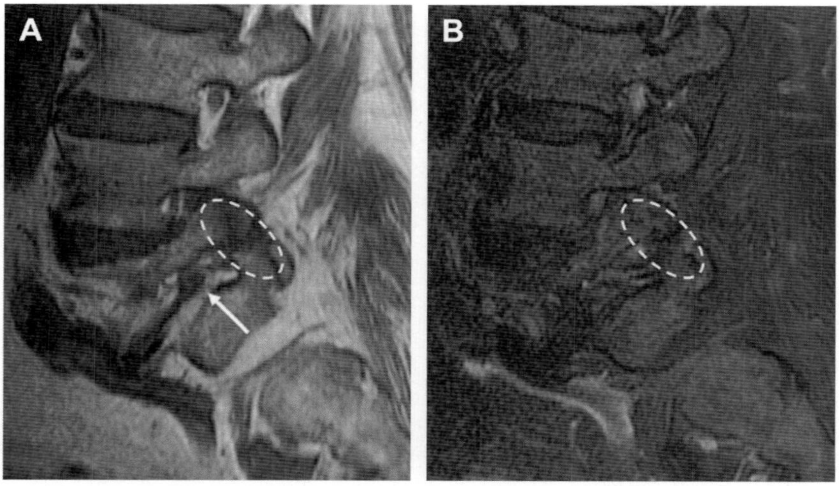

Fig. 23. Bilateral L5 spondylolysis with spondylolisthesis contributing to radiculopathy. (*A*) T1-weighted MR imaging showing marked L5 neuroforaminal narrowing with near complete obliteration of the epidural fat about the L5 nerve root (*white arrow*). Irregular low-signal intensity across the pars defect (*dashed white oval*). (*B*) T2-weighted MR imaging without bone marrow edema about the pars defect (*dashed white oval*) consistent with a chronic process. (*Courtesy of* Timothy Maus, MD.)

was broken down by age, 71% of the pedicle fractures occurred in patients less than 30 years of age.[59] These investigators did not report any association with pars interarticularis defects; however, it has been shown that pedicular stress fractures may be highly prevalent in cases of unilateral spondylolysis (**Fig. 24**).[60] In a study of 13 athletic patients younger than 20 years with unilateral spondylolysis diagnosed with MR imaging and CT, 46% showed a contralateral pedicle fracture or a chronic pedicle stress reaction in the form of sclerosis. None of the patients were in the early stage of spondylolytic fracture as seen on CT; nearly all were in the terminal stage.[60] The investigators also performed a finite element analysis of the stress imparted by a unilateral pars defect on the contralateral neural arch and found an increase in stress with all 6 tested lumbar motions, with the highest occurring in axial rotation.[60] The finite element analysis and the clinical findings of a unilateral pars defect support that cumulative stresses across the contralateral neural arch can lead to pedicle injuries and as the stage of the spondylolytic defect progresses so does the contralateral stress.[60]

Imaging

Imaging of pedicle stress fractures may be similar to imaging pars interarticularis defects. Radiographs are relatively insensitive in detecting pedicle stress fractures, as seen with vertebral fractures and pars defects.[13,33,34] Bone scintigraphy with SPECT was favored for initial assessment followed by CT for further evaluation in a 1991 publication.[61] As detailed earlier, SPECT combined with CT imparts a noteworthy amount of radiation to a relative young population and therefore may not be the best screening examination. MR imaging using standard sequences including T1-weighted and T2-weighted fat-saturated or STIR images may prove to be the best initial examination, because it does not impart ionizing radiation and uses physiologic imaging parameters of edema to identify early findings of a pedicle stress reaction (**Fig. 25**).[58] As with spondylolysis, limited CT may be used after MR imaging as an additional complementary examination in selected cases, and as a baseline for following fracture healing. If no pedicle injury is found, MR imaging is best able to identify other pain generators that may be difficult or impossible to evaluate with other modalities.

SACRUM

Sacral stress fractures can present as low back pain and the diagnosis can be elusive from both a clinical and imaging standpoint. These stress fractures can be seen in various patient populations. One is the young athlete presenting as a fatigue fracture. The prevalence of sacral fatigue fractures is unknown but this entity is believed to be uncommon and reported most often in female athletes, including distance runners.[62] Postmenopausal women with osteoporosis are another distinct population who are predisposed to sustaining sacral insufficiency fractures.[63] As with the younger patient, the prevalence is unknown but has been reported to be 1.8% of women older than 55 years in 1 series.[64] Sacral in sufficiency fractures can also be seen in patients with rheumatoid arthritis, those undergoing corticosteroid treatment, and after pelvic irradiation for gynecologic malignancy.[65] Sacral stress fractures may be

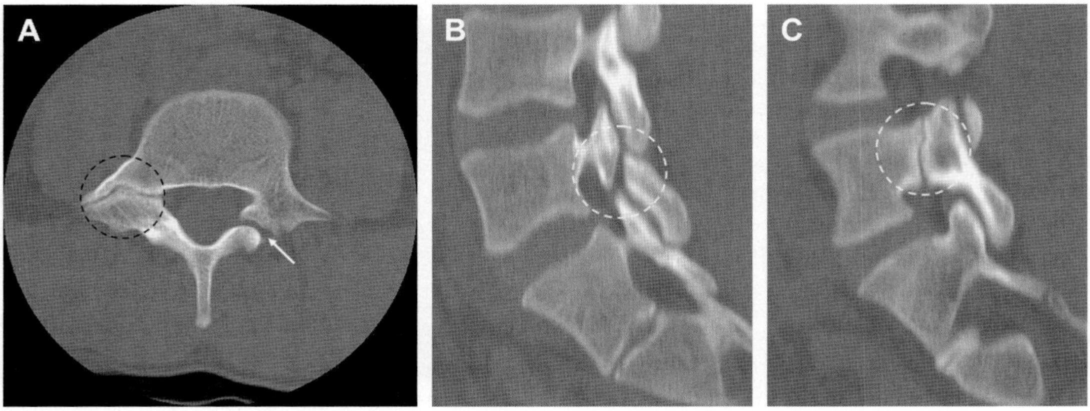

Fig. 24. (*A*) Axial CT scan of a left L5 terminal stage spondylolytic defect (*white arrow*) in a 29-year-old male athlete with a subacute to chronic contralateral pedicle stress fracture (*dashed black circle*). Sagittal CT images better showing the left (*B*) L5 pars defect and the right (*C*) pedicle fracture (*dashed white circle*). Incidental note is made of a lumbarized S1 segment. (*Courtesy of* Timothy Maus, MD.)

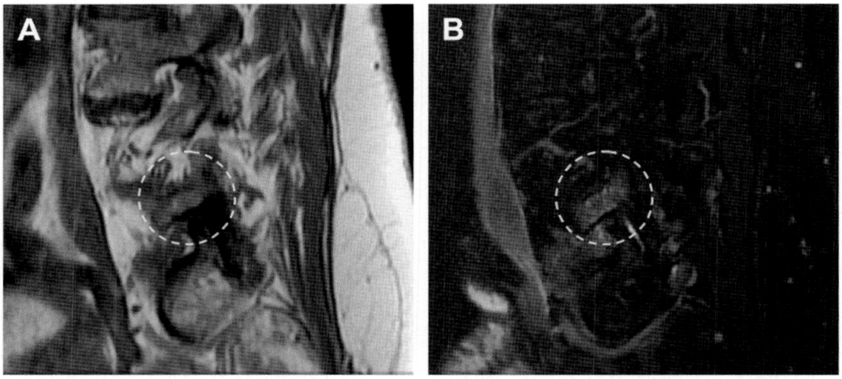

Fig. 25. T1-weighted (*A*) and T2-weighted with fat saturation (*B*) sagittal MR images through the right L5 pedicle (*dashed white circle*). There is increased T2 signal within the pedicle without a corresponding linear low-signal abnormality, compatible with the clinically concordant stress reaction of the pedicle without fracture.

imaged with radiographs, nuclear medicine imaging, CT, and MR imaging.

Radiographs

When evident on radiographs, sacral stress fractures can be seen as vertically oriented bands of sclerosis involving the ala paralleling the sacroiliac joints.[65] Sacral stress fractures can be difficult to appreciate on radiographs because of overlying bowel gas, arterial calcifications, and osteopenia, the latter two generally seen in older populations.[45,66–68] In a study comparing MR imaging with CT for the detection of insufficiency fractures, a subset of patients also had radiographs available. Of these patients, only 3.8% of the sacral insufficiency fractures could be detected using radiographs.[69]

Nuclear Medicine Imaging

Nuclear medicine bone scan can be sensitive in detecting sacral stress fractures. The classic finding of a sacral insufficiency fracture on a nuclear medicine bone scan is the Honda sign (**Fig. 26**). This sign occurs when the radiotracer activity appears as the letter H, with the vertical components along the sacral ala and the horizontal component crossing the sacral body. When the Honda sign and its variants (missing portions of the H) were identified, the sensitivity and positive predictive value were found to be 96% and 92%, respectively.[70] In 63% of these patients, a complete Honda sign was identified, whereas 33% showed variants of the Honda sign. The radiotracer activity can be variable at follow-up and may be present 8 to 10 months after the initial presentation.[63,66]

MR Imaging

MR imaging can also be used to detect sacral stress fractures, with a reported sensitivity of 100%.[69] MR imaging of the sacrum for this indication should include axial and coronal oblique T1-weighted and T2-weighted fat-suppressed or STIR images. The bone marrow edema is evident as increased signal on the T2-weighted and STIR images (**Fig. 27**), whereas the fracture line may be visible as a linear low-signal intensity following the pattern of the Honda sign or its variants.[69] A potential imaging pitfall is when a lumbar spine MRI examination is performed for back pain in patients who have an unsuspected sacral stress fracture. Routine lumbar spine MR imaging does not include all of the sacrum, and coronal oblique

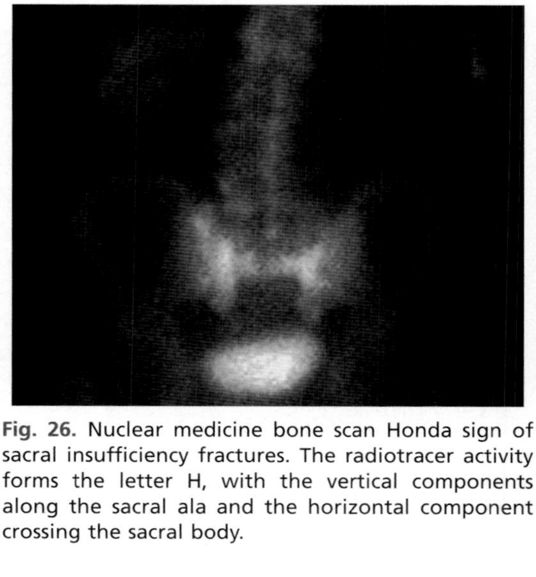

Fig. 26. Nuclear medicine bone scan Honda sign of sacral insufficiency fractures. The radiotracer activity forms the letter H, with the vertical components along the sacral ala and the horizontal component crossing the sacral body.

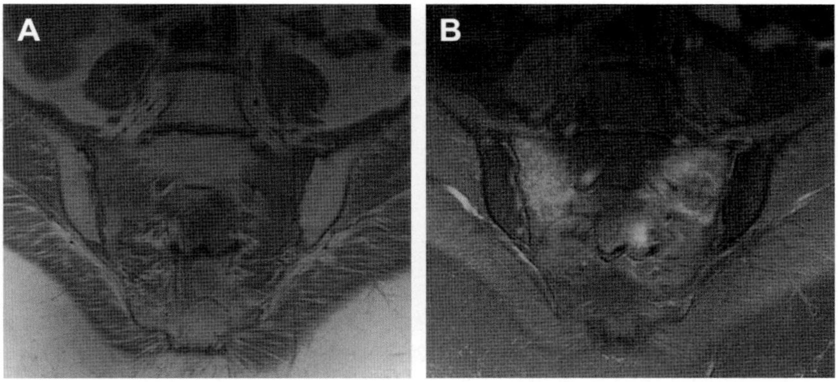

Fig. 27. MR imaging of sacral insufficiency fractures. The fractures form vertically oriented bands of decreased T1 (*A*) and increased T2 signal (*B*).

images of the sacrum are not routinely obtained (**Fig. 28**).[71] As discussed in the preface to this issue, the imager must know the location and character of the pain syndrome to appropriately image the patient.

CT

CT can depict the sclerosis and a fracture line with greater sensitivity than radiographs. MR imaging and CT were compared in the evaluation of

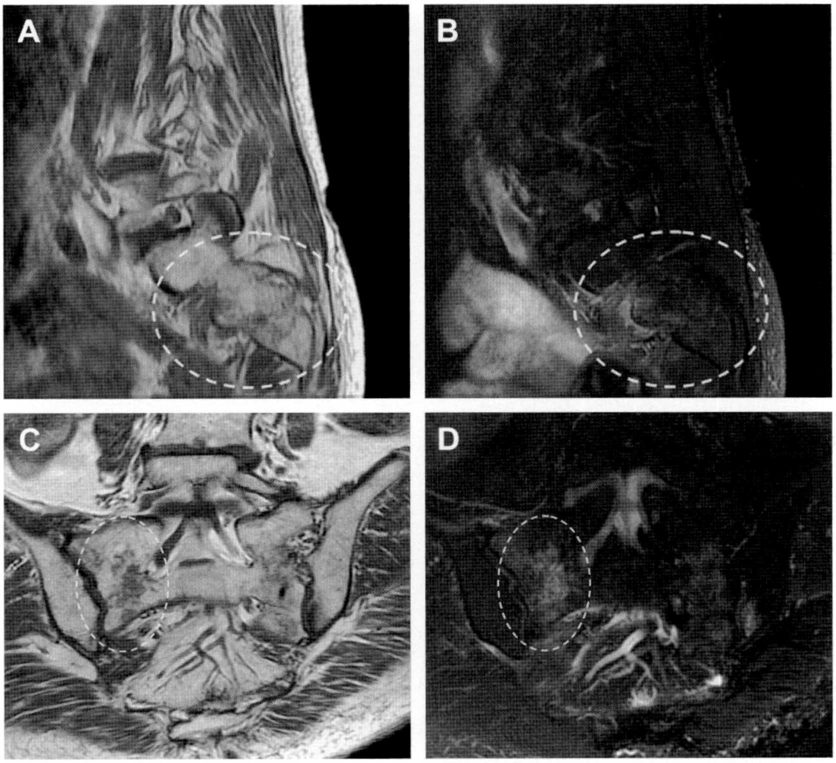

Fig. 28. Routine MR imaging examination of the lumbar spine. The rightmost sagittal image suggests a subtle decreased T1 (*A*) and increased T2 (*B*) signal abnormality of the sacral ala in a patient with back pain (*dashed white ovals*). Coronal oblique T1-weighted (*C*) and T2-weighted fat-saturated (*D*) sequences were added through the sacrum, which better depicts the new right sacral insufficiency fracture (*dashed white ovals*). The patient had undergone a sacroplasty of the left sacral ala 2 months previously, accounting for the signal changes in that region.

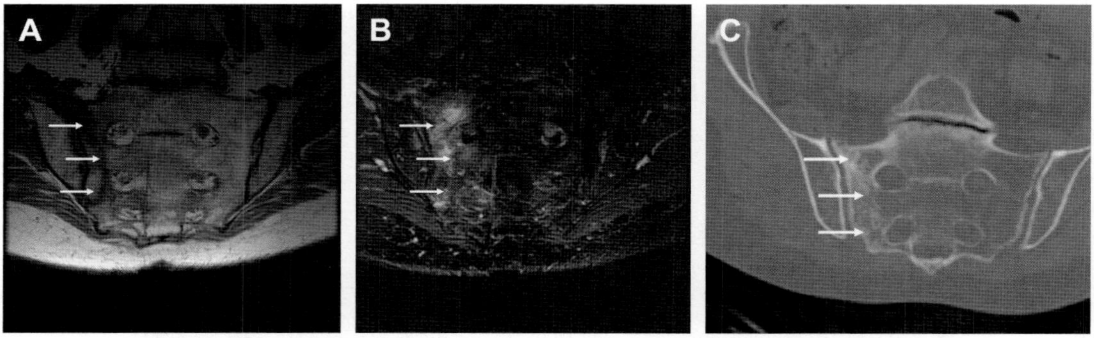

Fig. 29. Coronal oblique T1-weighted (*A*) and STIR (*B*) MR images of a vertically oriented right sacral ala insufficiency fracture (*white arrows*). The low-signal-intensity fracture line nears the S1 and S2 sacral neural foramina without definite extension into the foramina. (*C*) Corresponding coronal oblique CT of the same sacral insufficiency fracture (*white arrows*) taken immediately before sacroplasty confirms that there is no fracture extension into the sacral foramina, as shown by intact cortical margins.

insufficiency fractures about the pelvis, sacrum, and proximal femur.[69] MR imaging detected 100% of the sacral insufficiency fractures, whereas CT detected only 74.6%.[69] Although MR imaging and scintigraphy are more sensitive than CT in the detection of sacral insufficiency fractures, CT may provide complementary, detailed, high-resolution imaging of the cortical involvement of the fracture as it relates to neural foramina in patients being considered for sacroplasty, because they can be potential areas of cement leakage (**Fig. 29**).[71]

PELVIS

Sacral alar fractures are the most common of the pelvic fractures, but insufficiency fractures may occur at other pelvic sites, including the pubic rami, the pubic bone near the symphysis, and the periacetabular region. These fractures may present as hip or groin pain and may provoke an imaging investigation that begins in the spine. These lesions are also apparent as linear zones of sclerosis which are subtle on radiographs and more evident on CT. These lesions may have a bone marrow edema pattern, possibly accompanied by a low-signal fracture line, on MR imaging.[72] The presence of one insufficiency fracture should provoke careful scrutiny for other such lesions at sites of known predilection.

SUMMARY

As with many things in medicine, timely diagnosis is paramount in reducing morbidity from the afflicting condition. This goal is especially challenging in stress fractures of the spine, which can occur in both young and old patients, may be overlooked in the differential diagnosis, and can be difficult to detect without advanced imaging. Appropriate imaging of these conditions is a daunting task and is ever changing with the advances in technology and imaging techniques. As is seen elsewhere in this issue, the imager must be aware of the nature of the pain syndrome and the clinical suspicion to appropriately direct the imaging. Structural changes are difficult to detect until late in the process; early diagnosis depends on physiologic parameters of bone marrow edema or accelerated bone metabolism. Imaging must be undertaken with due regard to cost and radiation exposure, particularly in the adolescent spondylolysis population.

ACKNOWLEDGMENTS

The author wishes to thank Dr Timothy Maus for his mentorship and sharing his wealth of knowledge including case examples. Also, a special thanks to Mrs Jane Gagnon for her assistance in preparation of this article.

REFERENCES

1. Burge R, Dawson-Hughes B, Solomon DH, et al. Incidence and economic burden of osteoporosis-related fractures in the United States, 2005–2025. J Bone Miner Res 2007;22(3):465–75.
2. Cooper C, Atkinson EJ, MichaelO'Fallon W, et al. Incidence of clinically diagnosed vertebral fractures: a population-based study in Rochester, Minnesota, 1985-1989. J Bone Miner Res 1992;7(2):221–7.
3. Lindsay R, Silverman SL, Cooper C, et al. Risk of new vertebral fracture in the year following a fracture. JAMA 2001;285(3):320–3.
4. Cook DJ, Guyatt GH, Adachi JD, et al. Quality of life issues in women with vertebral fractures due to osteoporosis. Arthritis Rheum 1993;36(6):750–6.

5. Schlaich C, Minne HW, Bruckner T, et al. Reduced pulmonary function in patients with spinal osteoporotic fractures. Osteoporos Int 1998;8(3):261–7.
6. Nevitt MC, Ettinger B, Black DM, et al. The association of radiographically detected vertebral fractures with back pain and function: a prospective study. Ann Intern Med 1998;128(10):793–800.
7. Genant HK, Wu CY, van Kuijk C, et al. Vertebral fracture assessment using a semiquantitative technique. J Bone Miner Res 1993;8(9):1137–48.
8. Wu CY, Li J, Jergas M, et al. Comparison of semiquantitative and quantitative techniques for the assessment of prevalent and incident vertebral fractures. Osteoporos Int 1995;5(5):354–70.
9. Link TM, Guglielmi G, van Kuijk C, et al. Radiologic assessment of osteoporotic vertebral fractures: diagnostic and prognostic implications. Eur Radiol 2005;15(8):1521–32.
10. Zhao FD, Pollintine P, Hole BD, et al. Vertebral fractures usually affect the cranial endplate because it is thinner and supported by less-dense trabecular bone. Bone 2009;44(2):372–9.
11. Adams MA, Pollintine P, Tobias JH, et al. Intervertebral disc degeneration can predispose to anterior vertebral fractures in the thoracolumbar spine. J Bone Miner Res 2006;21(9):1409–16.
12. Moulopoulos LA, Yoshimitsu K, Johnston DA, et al. MR prediction of benign and malignant vertebral compression fractures. J Magn Reson Imaging 1996;6(4):667–74.
13. Ryan PJ, Fogelman I. Osteoporotic vertebral fractures: diagnosis with radiography and bone scintigraphy. Radiology 1994;190(3):669–72.
14. Pham T, Azulay-Parrado J, Champsaur P, et al. "Occult" osteoporotic vertebral fractures: vertebral body fractures without radiologic collapse. Spine 2005;30(12):2430–5.
15. Chen YJ, Lo DF, Chang CH, et al. The value of dynamic radiographs in diagnosing painful vertebrae in osteoporotic compression fractures. AJNR Am J Neuroradiol 2011;32(1):121–4.
16. Spiegl U, Beisse R, Hauck S, et al. Value of MRI imaging prior to a kyphoplasty for osteoporotic insufficiency fractures. Eur Spine J 2009;18(9):1287–92.
17. Baur A, Stabler A, Arbogast S, et al. Acute osteoporotic and neoplastic vertebral compression fractures: fluid sign at MR imaging. Radiology 2002;225(3):730–5.
18. Linn JM, Birkenmaier CM, Hoffmann RT, et al. The intravertebral cleft in acute osteoporotic fractures: fluid in magnetic resonance imaging-vacuum in computed tomography? [Miscellaneous Article]. Spine 2009;34(2):E88–93.
19. Khoo M, Tyler P, Saifuddin A, et al. Diffusion-weighted imaging (DWI) in musculoskeletal MRI: a critical review. Skeletal Radiol 2011;40(6):665–81.
20. Ragab Y, Emad Y, Gheita T, et al. Differentiation of osteoporotic and neoplastic vertebral fractures by chemical shift {in-phase and out-of phase} MR imaging. Eur J Radiol 2009;72(1):125–33.
21. Kim JH, Kim JI, Jang BH, et al. The comparison of bone scan and MRI in osteoporotic compression fractures. Asian Spine J 2010;4(2):89–95.
22. Cho WI, Chang UK. Comparison of MR imaging and FDG-PET/CT in the differential diagnosis of benign and malignant vertebral compression fractures. J Neurosurg Spine 2011;14(2):177–83.
23. Beutler WJ, Fredrickson BE, Murtland AM, et al. The natural history of spondylolysis and spondylolisthesis: 45-year follow-up evaluation. Spine (Phila Pa 1976) 2003;28(10):1027–35.
24. Sakai TM, Sairyo KM, Takao SM, et al. Incidence of lumbar spondylolysis in the general population in Japan based on multidetector computed tomography scans from two thousand subjects. Spine (Phila Pa 1976) 2009;34(21):2346–50.
25. Rossi F, Dragoni S. Lumbar spondylolysis and sports. The radiological findings and statistical considerations. Radiol Med 1994;87(4):397–400 [in Italian].
26. Rossi F, Dragoni S. Lumbar spondylolysis: occurrence in competitive athletes. Updated achievements in a series of 390 cases. J Sports Med Phys Fitness 1990;30(4):450–2.
27. Sakai T, Sairyo K, Suzue N, et al. Incidence and etiology of lumbar spondylolysis: review of the literature. J Orthop Sci 2010;15(3):281–8.
28. Ahn PG, Yoon DH, Shin HC, et al. Cervical spondylolysis: three cases and a review of the current literature. Spine (Phila Pa 1976) 2010;35(3):E80–3.
29. Forsberg DA, Martinez S, Vogler JB, et al. Cervical spondylolysis: imaging findings in 12 patients. Am J Roentgenol 1990;154(4):751–5.
30. Roche M, Rowe G. The incidence of separate neural arch and coincident bone variations; a survey of 4,200 skeletons. Anat Rec 1951;109(2):233–52.
31. Ward CV, Latimer BP, Alander DH, et al. Radiographic assessment of lumbar facet distance spacing and spondylolysis. Spine 2007;32(2):E85–8.
32. Masharawi YM, Alperovitch-Najenson DP, Steinberg NM, et al. Lumbar facet orientation in spondylolysis: a skeletal study. Spine 2007;32(6):E176–80.
33. Amato M, Totty WG, Gilula LA. Spondylolysis of the lumbar spine: demonstration of defects and laminal fragmentation. Radiology 1984;153(3):627–9.
34. Hu S, Tribus C, Diab M, et al. Spondylolisthesis and spondylolysis. J Bone Joint Surg Am 2008;90(3):656–71.
35. Ravichandran G. A radiologic sign in spondylolisthesis. Am J Roentgenol 1980;134(1):113–7.
36. Maldague B, Malghem J. Unilateral arch hypertrophy with spinous process tilt: a sign of arch deficiency. Radiology 1976;121(3 Pt 1):567–74.

37. Araki TM, Seiko-Harata MD, Nakano KM, et al. Reactive sclerosis of the pedicle associated with contralateral spondylolysis. Spine 1992;17(11):1424–6.
38. Meyerding H. Spondylolisthesis. Surg Gynecol Obstet 1932;54:371–7.
39. Leone A, Guglielmi G, Cassar-Pullicino VN, et al. Lumbar intervertebral instability: a review. Radiology 2007;245(1):62–77.
40. Hanley E. The indications for lumbar spinal fusion with and without instrumentation. Spine (Phila Pa 1976) 1995;20(Suppl 24):143S–53S.
41. Boden SD, Wiesel SW. Lumbosacral segmental motion in normal individuals. Have we been measuring instability properly? Spine 1990;15(6):571–6.
42. Leone A, Cianfoni A, Cerase A, et al. Lumbar spondylolysis: a review. Skeletal Radiol 2011;40(6): 683–700.
43. Dunn A, Campbell R, Mayor P, et al. Radiological findings and healing patterns of incomplete stress fractures of the pars interarticularis. Skeletal Radiol 2008;37(5):443–50.
44. Fujii K, Katoh S, Sairyo K, et al. Union of defects in the pars interarticularis of the lumbar spine in children and adolescents: the radiological outcome after conservative treatment. J Bone Joint Surg Br 2004;86(2):225–31.
45. Collier BD, Johnson RP, Carrera GF, et al. Painful spondylolysis or spondylolisthesis studied by radiography and single-photon emission computed tomography. Radiology 1985;154(1):207–11.
46. Zukotynski K, Curtis C, Grant F, et al. The value of SPECT in the detection of stress injury to the pars interarticularis in patients with low back pain. J Orthop Surg Res 2010;5(1):13.
47. Bellah RD, Summerville DA, Treves ST, et al. Low-back pain in adolescent athletes: detection of stress injury to the pars interarticularis with SPECT. Radiology 1991;180(2):509–12.
48. Gregory PL, Batt ME, Kerslake RW, et al. The value of combining single photon emission computerised tomography and computerised tomography in the investigation of spondylolysis. Eur Spine J 2004; 13(6):503–9.
49. Mettler FA, Huda W, Yoshizumi TT, et al. Effective doses in radiology and diagnostic nuclear medicine: a catalog. Radiology 2008;248(1):254–63.
50. Campbell RS, Grainger AJ, Hide IG, et al. Juvenile spondylolysis: a comparative analysis of CT, SPECT and MRI. Skeletal Radiol 2005;34(2):63–73.
51. Hollenberg GM, Beattie PF, Meyers SP, et al. Stress reactions of the lumbar pars interarticularis: the development of a new MRI classification system. Spine (Phila Pa 1976) 2002;27(2):181–6.
52. Ulmer JL, Mathews VP, Elster AD, et al. MR imaging of lumbar spondylolysis: the importance of ancillary observations. Am J Roentgenol 1997;169(1): 233–9.
53. Sairyo K, Katoh S, Takata Y, et al. MRI signal changes of the pedicle as an indicator for early diagnosis of spondylolysis in children and adolescents: a clinical and biomechanical study. Spine (Phila Pa 1976) 2006;31(2):206–11.
54. Sakai T, Sairyo K, Mima S, et al. Significance of magnetic resonance imaging signal change in the pedicle in the management of pediatric lumbar spondylolysis. Spine (Phila Pa 1976) 2010;35(14): E641–5.
55. Ganiyusufoglu AK, Onat L, Karatoprak O, et al. Diagnostic accuracy of magnetic resonance imaging versus computed tomography in stress fractures of the lumbar spine. Clin Radiol 2010; 65(11):902–7.
56. Singh K, Helms C, Fiorella D, et al. Disc space-targeted angled axial MR images of the lumbar spine: a potential source of diagnostic error. Skeletal Radiol 2007;36(12):1147–53.
57. Johnson D, Farnum G, Latchaw R, et al. MR imaging of the pars interarticularis. Am J Roentgenol 1989; 152(2):327–32.
58. Amari R, Sakai T, Katoh S, et al. Fresh stress fractures of lumbar pedicles in an adolescent male ballet dancer: case report and literature review. Arch Orthop Trauma Surg 2009;129(3):397–401.
59. Borg B, Modic MT, Obuchowski N, et al. Pedicle marrow signal hyperintensity on short tau inversion recovery- and T2-weighted images: prevalence and relationship to clinical symptoms. AJNR Am J Neuroradiol 2011;32(9):1624–31.
60. Sairyo K, Katoh S, Sasa T, et al. Athletes with unilateral spondylolysis are at risk of stress fracture at the contralateral pedicle and pars interarticularis: a clinical and biomechanical study. Am J Sports Med 2005;33(4):583–90.
61. Traughber PD, Havlina JM Jr. Bilateral pedicle stress fractures: SPECT and CT features. J Comput Assist Tomogr 1991;15(2):338–40.
62. Knobloch K, Schreibmueller L, Jagodzinski M, et al. Rapid rehabilitation programme following sacral stress fracture in a long-distance running female athlete. Arch Orthop Trauma Surg 2007;127(9): 809–13.
63. De Smet A, Neff JR. Pubic and sacral insufficiency fractures: clinical course and radiologic findings. AJR Am J Roentgenol 1985;145(3):601–6.
64. Weber M, Hasler P, Gerber H. Insufficiency fractures of the sacrum: twenty cases and review of the literature. Spine (Phila Pa 1976) 1993;18(16):2507–12.
65. Cooper KL, Beabout JW, Swee RG. Insufficiency fractures of the sacrum. Radiology 1985;156(1):15–20.
66. Blake SP, Connors AM. Sacral insufficiency fracture. Br J Radiol 2004;77(922):891–6.
67. Peh WC, Khong PL, Yin Y, et al. Imaging of pelvic insufficiency fractures. Radiographics 1996;16(2): 335–48.

68. White JH, Hague C, Nicolaou S, et al. Imaging of sacral fractures. Clin Radiol 2003;58(12):914–21.
69. Cabarrus MC, Ambekar A, Lu Y, et al. MRI and CT of insufficiency fractures of the pelvis and the proximal femur. Am J Roentgenol 2008;191(4): 995–1001.
70. Fujii M, Abe K, Hayashi K, et al. Honda sign and variants in patients suspected of having a sacral insufficiency fracture. Clin Nucl Med 2005;30(3): 165–9.
71. Lyders EM, Whitlow CT, Baker MD, et al. Imaging and treatment of sacral insufficiency fractures. AJNR Am J Neuroradiol 2010;31(2):201–10.
72. Otte MT, Helms CA, Fritz RC. MR imaging of supra-acetabular insufficiency fractures. Skeletal Radiol 1997;26(5):279–83.

Imaging of Dural Arteriovenous Fistula

Jonathan M. Morris, MD

KEYWORDS

• Dural arteriovenous fistula • Vascular malformations of the spine • MR imaging • MR angiography • Spinal angiography

KEY POINTS

- Because of their nonspecific clinical presentation, spinal dural arterial venous fistulas (SDAVFs) are often overlooked.
- SDAVFs should be considered and neuroimaging with gadolinium obtained in an elderly patient with slowly progressive myelopathic symptoms.
- Neuroimaging findings of SDAVF include an enlarged spinal cord with intramedullary enhancement and T2 hyperintensity associated with prominent flow voids along the dorsal aspect of the cord.
- Three-dimensional (3D) spinal magnetic resonance (MR) angiography as well as phase cycling-fast imaging employing steady state acquisition (PC-FIESTA), 3D-constructive interference steady state (CISS), or other myelographic sequences should be obtained before angiography to help localize the level of the fistula.
- After treatment of the fistula, the T2 hyperintensity, prominent flow voids, and enhancement should decrease with time, but can persist for up to a year.

INTRODUCTION

Spinal vascular malformations are rare. They are divided into shunting lesions, including spinal arteriovenous malformations (AVM) and arteriovenous fistulas (AVF), and nonshunting lesions, including capillary telangiectasia and cavernous malformations (cavernomas). There are numerous classification schemes based on arterial supply,[1] genetics,[2] inborn versus acquired,[3] or morphology and angioarchitecture (**Table 1**).[4–6] Dural AVF is the most common of the vascular malformations, accounting for 50% to 85% of all lesions.[7–10] Although it is the most common type of AVM, a delay in diagnosis of SDAVFs persists despite more widespread clinical and radiographic appreciation of this entity. This delay is largely caused by its nonspecific clinical presentation, which may mimic more prevalent conditions such as myelopathy or neurogenic claudication caused by central canal compromise, demyelinating disease, or neoplasm.[11–17] Most commonly, these patients are elderly men[12,14–19] who present with varied lower extremity motor and sensory myelopathic symptoms that slowly progress over several years. Patients are frequently subjected to a variety of misdirected treatments, including surgery for stenosis and immunomodulation for transverse myelitis. The radiologist is often the first to suggest the diagnosis based on its MR imaging appearance; the imager must then be familiar with imaging strategies to, first, conclusively identify the presence of a dural AVF and, second, locate the fistula site to guide selective angiography and intervention. This article reviews spinal vascular anatomy, imaging appearances of dural AVF, and imaging strategies for determining the fistula location.

Department of Radiology, Mayo Clinic, 200 First Street, SW, Rochester, MN 55905, USA
E-mail address: morris.jonathan@mayo.edu

Radiol Clin N Am 50 (2012) 823–839
doi:10.1016/j.rcl.2012.04.011

Table 1
Classification of spinal malformations

	Type	Cause	Feeding Artery	Draining Vein	Pathophysiology	Age of Onset (y)	Therapy
AVM	Perimedullary fistula (type I–III)	Inborn	Radiculomedullary	Intramedullary and superficial spinal cord veins draining to epidural venous plexus (orthograde)	Intraparenchymal or subarachnoid hemorrhage, chronic venous congestion, space occupying lesion	20–40	Type I: surgery Type II–III coil embolization
	Glomerular					<20	Particle or glue embolization
	Juvenile					<15	Embolization and/or surgery
Cavernoma	—	Inborn	N/A	N/A	Hemorrhage and progressive myelopathy	20–60	Surgery
Dural fistula	—	Acquired	Radiculomeningeal	Radicular vein draining to perimedullary veins (retrograde)	Chronic venous congestion	40–60	Glue embolization or surgery

SPINAL VASCULAR ANATOMY

A basic knowledge of spinal vascular anatomy is required to detect and interpret the appearance of SDAVF on MR imaging, MR angiography, computed tomography (CT) angiography, and spinal angiography. The spinal cord is supplied by a single anterior and paired posterior spinal arteries. These arteries arise from the segmental arteries, which also supply the vertebral bodies, paraspinal musculature, dura, and nerve roots. In the cervical spine, the anterior spinal artery originates from the vertebral arteries, but is reinforced at multiple levels by segmental arteries arising directly from the vertebral arteries as well as from branches of the ascending and deep cervical arteries. This anatomy is important to note, because the costovertebral and thyrocervical trunks should be angiographically evaluated in those patients in whom the origin of the fistula remains occult. There is often a large reinforcing artery, typically arising between C4 and C8, referred to as the artery of the cervical enlargement.

In the thoracolumbar region, the intercostal and lumbar arteries supply the radicular arteries. The dorsal branch of the intercostal artery gives rise to spinal radicular arteries supplying the dura (radiculomeningeal arteries) and the nerve root (**Fig. 1**). These arteries may continue as a radiculomedullary artery, which accompanies the dorsal and ventral rami of the nerve root into the thecal sac to supply the anterior and posterior spinal arteries. The primary supply to the thoracic cord and conus typically arises from 1 dominant radiculomedullary artery, possibly supplemented by 1 or 2 smaller contributors. Although, in any given patient, it cannot be known from which level this great radiculomedullary artery of Adamkiewicz (radiculomedullaris magna) originates, up to 75% of the time it arises on the left between T8 and L1. The anterior radiculomedullary artery branch continues along the course of the corresponding nerve root superiorly to the cord; in the midline the larger descending branch makes a characteristic hairpin turn inferiorly. In the sacral region, the radicular branches may arise from the middle or lateral sacral branches and iliolumbar arteries, which need to be investigated angiographically if the fistulous communication cannot be found (**Fig. 2**).

There is no similar organization for the venous system. The spinal cord drains through circumferential radial veins providing outflow to both the white and gray matter, which then drain into a pial venous network. This pial network drains into longitudinal anastomosing veins, then to medullary veins, and then radicular veins that follow the exiting nerve root, eventually piercing the dura on their way to the epidural plexus (see **Fig. 1**). Although these veins are valveless, there is anatomic narrowing at the dural penetration that some regard as a functional antireflux mechanism. At the conus medullaris and lower portion of the spinal cord, a drainage pattern similar to the arterial supply is seen, where a sulcal vein drains the gray matter and the anterior and posterior

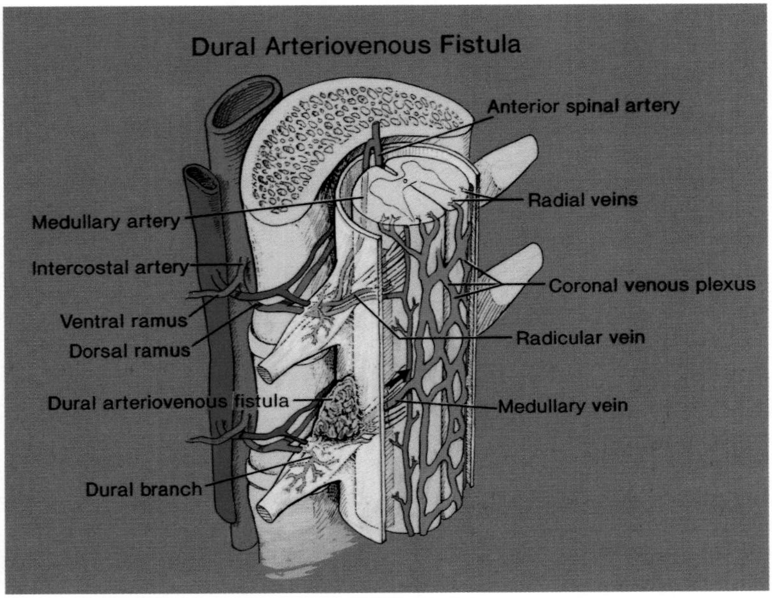

Fig. 1. Spinal vascular anatomy. The intercostal artery divides into ventral and dorsal branches. The dorsal branch gives rise to the radiculomedullary arteries that then give rise to the anterior and posterior spinal arteries. The intradural single point fistulous communication between the radicular branch and radicular vein is seen inferiorly.

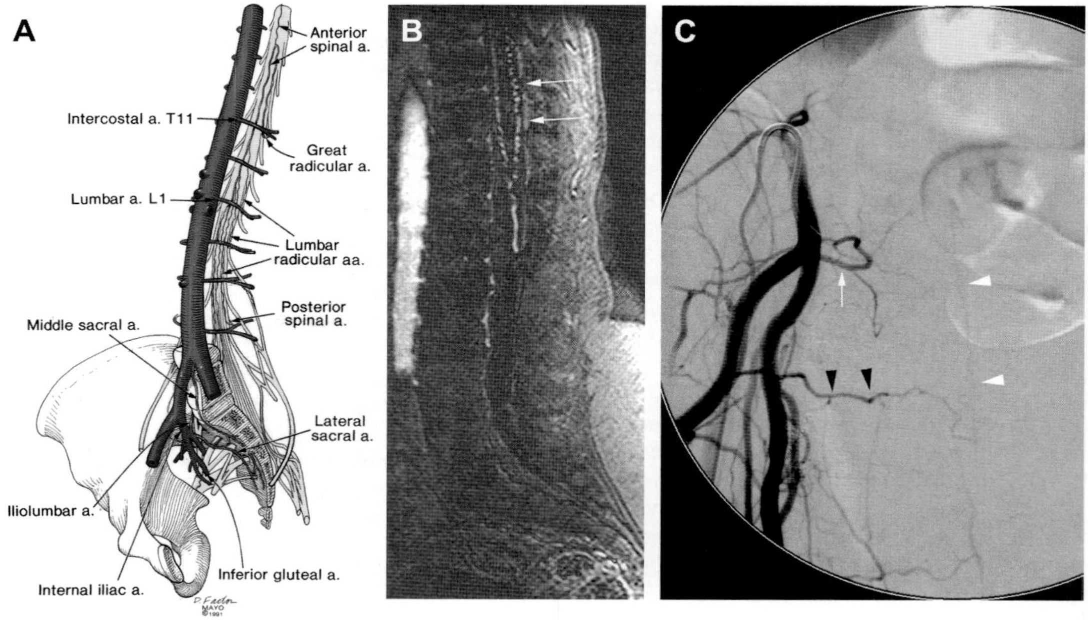

Fig. 2. Spinal vascular anatomy. (*A*) The middle sacral, lateral sacral, and iliolumbar arteries, which can supply SDAVF though the sacral foramen. (*B*) Gadolinium bolus MR angiography showing dilated tortuous perimedullary veins surrounding the conus (*white arrows*). (*C*) Digital subtraction angiography (DSA) of the internal iliac shows the lateral sacral branch (*black arrowheads*) supplying an SDAVF at the S4 level. Dilated perimedullary vein is seen ascending to the conus (*white arrowheads*). The iliolumbar artery is also seen (*white arrow*).

components encircle the conus like a basket, producing the normal venous prominence seen on contrast-enhanced T1-weighted imaging (T1WI) and MR angiography.

IMAGING EVALUATION

MR Imaging

MR imaging is the workhorse in dural fistula imaging. Given the nonspecific clinical findings, radiologists are often the first physicians who can suggest the diagnosis if they are aware of the imaging findings. Once the diagnosis is suggested on MR imaging, MR angiography is obtained to both substantiate the diagnosis and to determine the segmental level of the fistula to focus the spinal angiogram. At our institution, we also perform a heavily T2-weighted or myelographic sequence along with the MR angiography.

The MR imaging findings are a reflection of the pathophysiology of venous hypertension. Within the dural sleeve of the exiting nerve, the radiculomeningeal artery (no medullary component) fistulizes with the corresponding radicular vein (see **Fig. 1**), which arterializes the valveless perimedullary venous plexus with a loss of the arteriovenous gradient leading to decreased venous drainage, venous congestion, and intramedullary edema; if left unchecked, this results in chronic hypoxia and eventually ischemia and necrosis.[20]

MR imaging findings include enlargement of the cord primarily, in the lower thoracic region and conus, with associated central T2 hyperintensity and T1 hypointensity involving the gray and white matter of multiple segments of the thoracic and lumbar cord. Serpiginous, enlarged intradural vessels are seen along the dorsal and ventral aspect of the cord, sometimes scalloping it, and usually spanning more than 3 segments (**Fig. 3**).[21] If there is significant cord swelling, the veins can be compressed by the mass effect and not be detectable on imaging. Regardless of the location of the fistula, the T2 hyperintensity involves the conus up to 90% of the time[11,12,17] (**Fig. 4**) because of orthostasis; this is true even of the unusual lower cervical spine (C4–C8) dural AVF.[12,22] The upper cervical spinal (C1–C2) dural AVF (**Fig. 5**) often drains intracranially and presents more commonly with subarachnoid hemorrhage (SAH)[19,23–26] or radiculopathy.[10] The length of the T2 signal or enhancement does not correlate with weakness, sensory disturbances, or sphincter dysfunction, although holocord involvement and the presence of a thoracic fistula are associated with worsening weakness with

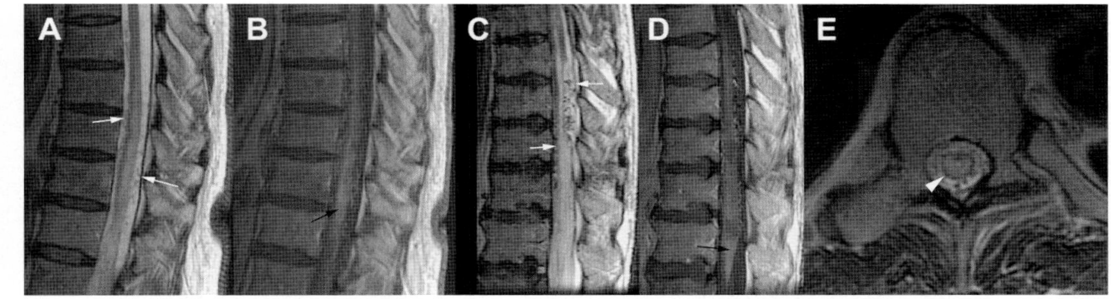

Fig. 3. Typical MR imaging findings for SDAVF in 2 patients. (*A, C*) Sagittal T2WI shows enlargement of the conus medullaris with diffuse infiltrative T2 hyperintensity extending over several levels. Enlarged perimedullary flow voids (*white arrows*) are seen along the ventral and dorsal aspect of the cord. In (*C*), these flow voids are seen scalloping the dorsal aspect of the cord. (*B, D*) Sagittal T1WI with gadolinium shows enlarged perimedullary veins as well as patchy intramedullary enhancement (*black arrows*). (*E*) Axial fast spin echo T2WI shows holocord involvement of the lower thoracic cord with peripheral T2 hypointensity (*arrowhead*).

exertion,[12] likely caused by the highly arterialized venous pressure.[27,28] Lack of T2 hyperintensity in the cord in the presence of a fistula is rare, although reported (**Fig. 6**).[11,12] If there is strong clinical suspicion and the initial MR imaging without contrast is unconvincing, the radiologist should proceed with gadolinium-enhanced and/or myelographic sequences (General Electric [GE], PC-FIESTA; Siemens, 3D-CISS; or Siemens, T2 SPACE). In this subset of patients, there typically are prominent vessels along the dorsal aspect of the cord that may be obscured on the sagittal T2-weighted imaging (T2WI). Our myelographic protocol is listed in **Table 2**. These myelographic or heavily weighted T2 sequences are obtained for the following reasons:

1. To aid in visualizing the flow voids along the dorsal aspect of the cord that might be obscured by pulsation artifact or mass effect.
2. As a dark blood angiogram to localize the fistula in concert with the gadolinium bolus MR angiography.
3. Problem solving in cases that are angiographically negative but MR imaging/A+.

These sequences are useful because they are volumetric, have high signal/noise ratios, and

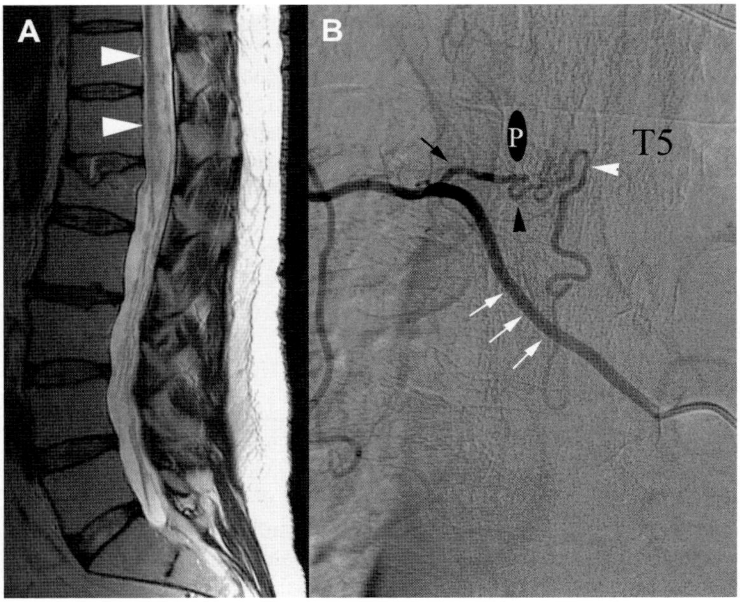

Fig. 4. SDAVF at T5 with most T2 hyperintensity and mass effect at the conus. (*A*) Sagittal T2 image shows T2 hyperintensity that was predominantly in the enlarged conus (*white arrowheads*). (*B*) DSA shows an SDAVF (*black arrowhead*) directly below the left T5 pedicle (*black oval*, P) fed by the dorsal branch (*black arrow*) of the fifth intercostal artery (*white arrows*). Arterialized serpiginous perimedullary draining veins can be seen (*white arrowhead*).

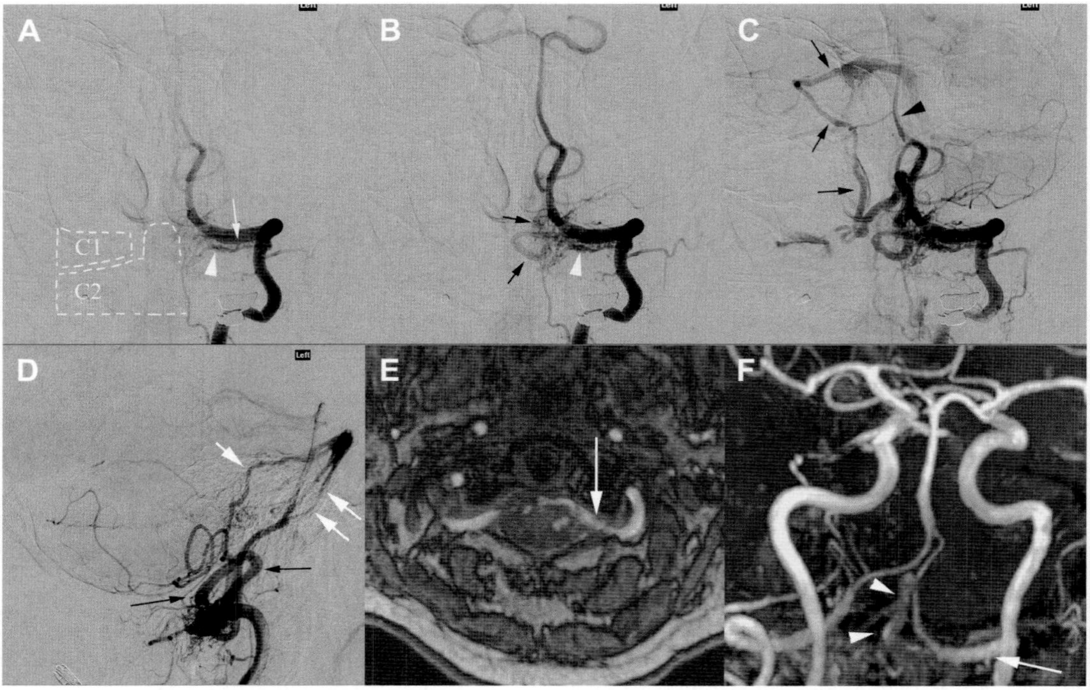

Fig. 5. High cervical SDAVF at C1 with intracranial drainage. (*A–C*) Progressive DSA images after injection of the left vertebral artery shows a branch of the vertebral artery at C1 (*white arrow*) supplying a dural fistula beneath the C1 pedicle (*white arrowhead*). Dilated arterialized veins extend superiorly through the foramen magnum to the level of the clivus (*black arrows*). The basilar artery can be seen (*black arrowhead*). (*D*) Lateral DSA shows the arterialized veins (*black arrows*) extending superiorly to the clivus (*white arrows*). (*E*) Axial time of flight (TOF) MR angiography shows the point of fistulization posterior to the C1 lateral mass (*white arrow*). (*F*) Maximal intensity projection (MIP) from the TOF MR angiography shows the branch of the vertebral artery feeding the fistula (*white arrow*) and dilated veins extending through foramen magnum (*white arrowheads*) correlating with the angiogram.

possess excellent spatial resolution (can be as small as 0.3 mm isotropic).[29] They are also not flow dependent; if there is poor cardiac output, poor bolus timing on the gadolinium bolus MR angiography, or increased venous pressure through the arterialized vein they are still diagnostic (**Fig. 7**).[29]

There have been reports of T2 hypointensity in the thin peripheral rim of the cord (see **Figs. 3**E and **7**C), thought to be related to slow flow of blood containing deoxyhemoglobin within a distended spinal cord capillary and venous system.[30–32] An alternative hypothesis states that this may be purely a visual phenomenon accentuated by the silhouetting of the periphery of the cord between the bright cerebrospinal fluid in the subarachnoid space and the high signal of the abnormal cord.[30]

At our institution, gadolinium is given during the initial examination in patients undergoing a workup for myelopathy. In patients with dural fistula, this is not only to identify enhancement within the cord itself but also to increase the conspicuity of the enlarged perimedullary venous plexus and serpiginous longitudinal veins that may be masked by pulsation or flow artifact on the sagittal T2WI (**Fig. 8**)[33,34] or by compression from the swollen cord (see **Fig. 7**A). Intramedullary enhancement is caused by the breakdown of the blood-cord barrier (see **Figs. 3** and **7**B).[35] Similar to the T2 hyperintensity, the segmental level of the enhancement does not correlate with the location of the fistula. Once the radiologist suggests the diagnosis of SDAVF, MR angiography becomes obligatory.

MR Angiography

Because the segmental level of T2 hyperintensity, enhancement, or cord enlargement are not predictors of the segmental level of the fistula, before the advent of MR angiography, the patient had to undergo selective catheterization of all of the arterial feeders to the spinal cord. This catheterization

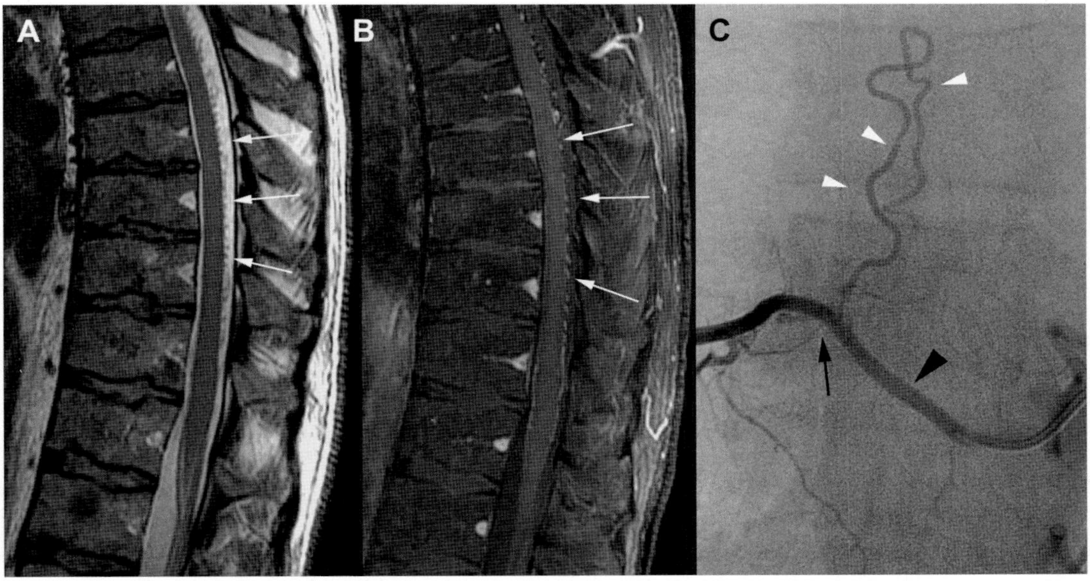

Fig. 6. SDAVF at T9 without intramedullary T2 signal or intramedullary enhancement; likely an early manifestation of the disease. (*A*) Sagittal T2WI showed perimedullary flow voids along the dorsal aspect of the cord (*white arrows*) without intramedullary T2 hyperintensity. (*B*) T1WI after gadolinium better shows the dilated perimedullary veins (*white arrows*). There is no intramedullary enhancement. (*C*) DSA of the T9 intercostal artery (*black arrowhead*) shows an SDAVF (*black arrow*) with arterialized ascending and descending dilated perimedullary veins (*white arrowheads*).

Table 2
Spine PC-FIESTA protocol

Variable	Data
Field strength (T)	1.5
Coil	Spine
Pulse sequence	PC-FIESTA
TR/TE/FA	6.2/3.15/70
BW	32
NEX	3
Directions	Frequency encoding: AP Phase encoding: SI
Matrix	256 × 256
FOV (cm)	26
Acquisition time (min)	5
Contrast	None
Slice thickness (mm)	1
Imaging plane	Sagittal
Reformats	Axial, coronal, and oblique coronal along the dorsal aspect of the cord

Abbreviations: AP, anterior posterior; BW, bandwidth; FA, flip angle; FOV, field of view; NEX, number of excitations; SI, superior inferior; TE, echo time; TR, recovery time.

sometimes required multiple procedures because of limits on contrast dose and radiation. The challenge with spine MR angiography is the trade-off between anatomic coverage and spatial resolution: because the fistula site is not predictable, a large field of view (FOV) covering skull base to the sacrum would be ideal, but this sacrifices needed spatial resolution. Early attempts at localizing the fistula or visualizing normal-sized spinal arterial vessels using blood flow techniques[36] and 3D contrast-enhanced time of flight (TOF)[33] were limited by spatial and temporal resolution, long acquisition times, and limited craniocaudal FOV. Fast contrast-enhanced MR angiography sequences[37] were then developed, but could not distinguish normal spinal arteries and suffered the same limitations as noted earlier. Later studies using a modified fast contrast-enhanced MR angiography technique detected the fistula level plus or minus 1 segment in up to 74% of patients.[21,38] We use a gadolinium bolus technique using 2 overlapping FOV acquired in the sagittal plane covering from C2 through the sacrum.[39] Maximal intensity projections (MIPs) in the sagittal, axial, and an oblique coronal plane along the posterior cord are reformatted at an independent workstation (**Fig. 9**). The use of an elliptical centric ordered 3D technique, rapid bolus injection, and a robust

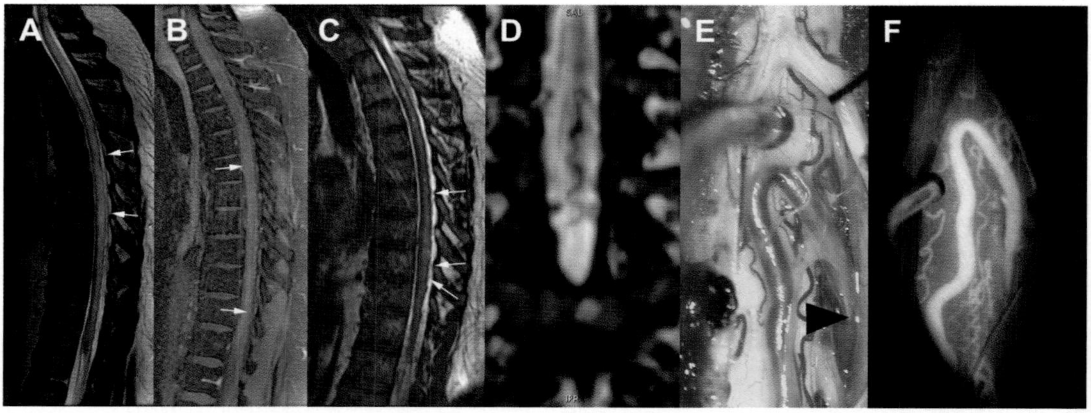

Fig. 7. 3D myelographic sequence for angiographically negative SDAVF at T6. (*A*) Sagittal T2WI shows diffuse intramedullary T2 hyperintensity from T3 to the conus. Pulsation artifact dorsal to the cord and cord swelling obscure visualization of the dorsal flow voids (*white arrows*) (*B*) Sagittal T1WI with gadolinium shows patchy linear enhancement from T3 to T12 (*white arrows*). There is no significant vascularity dorsal to the cord. (*C*) Myelographic sagittal PC-FIESTA images show flow voids (*white arrows*) posterior to the cord, better seen when reformatted in a volume viewer. (*D*) Oblique coronal reformats from the sagittal PC-FIESTA along the dorsal aspect of the cord show a hooked appearance to the superior aspect of the arterialized vein that extends to the lateral aspect of the dura. (*E*) Intraoperative photograph shows an arterialized vein emerging from the lateral dura (*black arrowhead*) taking a hairpin turn and extending inferiorly along the posterior aspect of the cord. (*F*) Intraoperative fluorescein angiography showing early and prominent filling of the vein resembling the sagittal PC-FIESTA myelographic picture.

timing mechanism allows us to complete the acquisition in 49 seconds, which is tolerable to most patients and limits motion artifact . Using this technique, we have reported a fistula detection rate, plus or minus 1 segmental level of 75%[39] and, more recently, plus or minus 2 segmental levels of 95%.[12] Our protocol is listed in **Table 3**. This protocol has resulted in a 50% reduction in radiation dose and contrast administered during confirmatory spinal angiograms. The

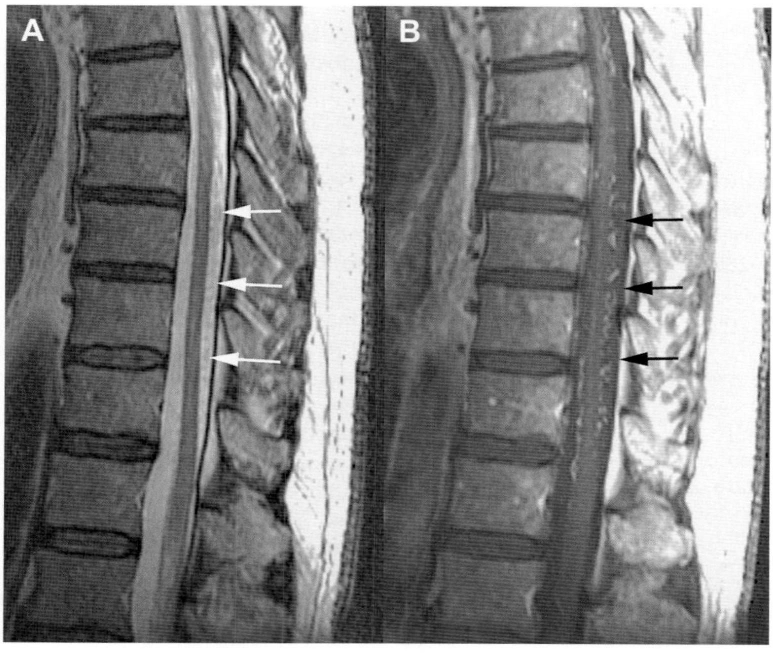

Fig. 8. Gadolinium-enhanced images documenting perimedullary vessels obscured on sagittal T2WI images. (*A*) Sagittal T2WI shows no intramedullary T2 hyperintensity. Pulsation artifact obscures visualization of dilated perimedullary veins (*white arrows*). (*B*) Sagittal T1WI with gadolinium shows the need for contrast in patients with high clinical suspicion for an SDAVF. Previously obscured veins on the T2WI are easily identified with gadolinium (*black arrows*).

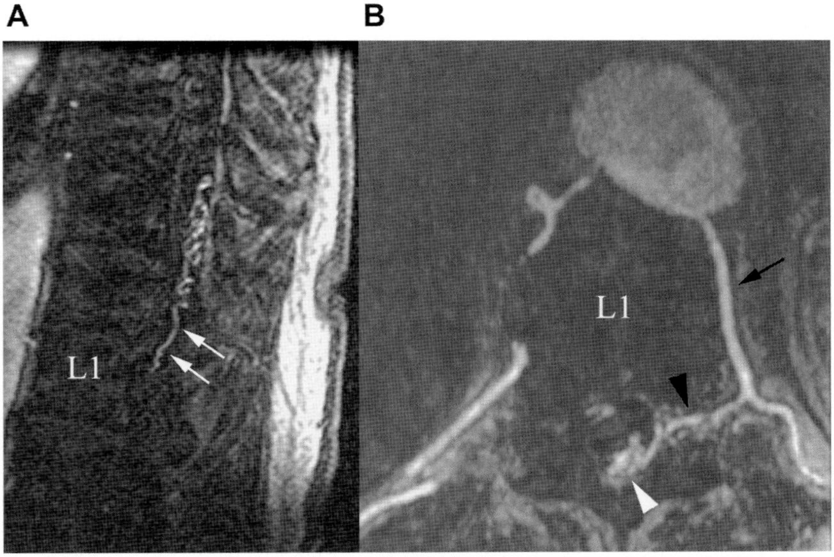

Fig. 9. Sagittal and axial MIP of an SDAVF at L1. (*A*) Sagittal MIP shows a radicular vein (*white arrows*) extending from the dilated perimedullary veins along the conus. (*B*) Axial MIP shows an SDAVF (*black arrowhead*) supplied by the dorsal branch of the left L1 lumbar artery (*black arrow*). Dilated perimedullary venous plexus is shown dorsal to the cord (*white arrowhead*).

technique has limitations in that the fistula is rarely seen, but the segmental level is inferred by tracing the draining medullary vein back to the radicular vein. Another limitation of this technique is the inability to distinguish the medullary veins from the anterior spinal artery, because this is a single-phase acquisition. More recently, dynamic multiphasic subtracted gadolinium bolus MR angiography techniques using a larger FOV (45 cm) have shown the fistula location plus or minus 1 segmental level in 100% of the thoracolumbar and sacral dural AVF. This technique demonstrated the normal artery of Adamkiewicz in all patients.[40] Other studies using this technique have shown the artery of Adamkiewicz in only 69% of patients.[41] A drawback of this study was the increased use of contrast (0.3 mmol/kg). Given recent awareness of the risks of nephrogenic systemic fibrosis (NSF), patient renal function should be evaluated, patients counseled about the increased dose of gadolinium, and gadolinium administrations separated in time.

Patients Incompatible with MR Imaging

There are several reasons a patient may not be able to complete an MR imaging, including pacemaker dependency, implanted defibrillators, hardware not compatible with MR imaging, severe claustrophobia, or severe back pain (which may be a contraindication to general anesthesia). In these patients, CT angiography of the spine may be performed (protocol **Table 4**).[42–44] Small series have shown successful localization of the fistula level by CT angiography in up to 75% of patients,[44] similar to MR angiography, thus guiding selective angiography. The limitations of CT angiography are the decrease in contrast resolution in the obese patient and in the upper thoracic spine, the use of iodinated contrast in a patient who may require an angiogram, and the dose of ionizing radiation. In addition, patients may undergo CT myelography; a 1995 article by Gilbertson and colleagues[11] noted tortuous vessels (extending 3–20 levels) on CT myelograms in all patients with SDAVF (**Fig. 10**). If CT myelography is to be performed, the patient should be scanned in the supine position. As with myelographic MR imaging and gadolinium bolus MR angiography, the goal is to localize the origin of the fistula to guide selective angiography. CT can also be useful during the angiogram once the feeding artery is found. At our institution, we obtain cone beam CT angiography during the injection of the feeding vessel, which improves visualization of the SDAVF vascular anatomy, aids in differentiation from a perimedullary fistula, and further defines the spatial relationships relative to adjacent osseous structures (**Fig. 11**).[45] These CT angiography images can be manipulated in real

Table 3
Spinal MR angiography protocol for GE scanner

Variable	Data
Field strength (T)	1.5
Coil	Spine
Pulse sequence	3D fast TOF SPGR
TR/TE/FA	6.7/min/45
BW	31.25
Slice thickness (mm)	0.7
Directions	Frequency encoding: SI Phase encoding: AP
Phase FOV (cm)	0.7
FOV (cm): Overlapping FOV Upper and lower	32 upper 32 lower
Acquisition time (min)	2.04
Contrast: 20 mL contrast at 3 mL/s followed by saline flush of 20 mL at 2 mL/s for upper FOV and then repeat for lower FOV	Multihance 20 mL, 529 mg/mL
Matrix	256 × 224
NEX	1
Imaging plane	Sagittal
Reformats	Coronal, axial, MIP sagittal and axial

Abbreviation: SPGR, spoiled gradient echo.

Table 4
Spinal CT angiography protocol for a Siemens 64-slice scanner

Variable	Data
Scan type	Spiral
Collimation	64 × 0.6
Pitch	1.1
kVp	140
Effective mAs	300
Start/end	Skull base/tip of sacrum
Kernel	B40
Contrast	100 mL Omnipaque 350 at 4 mL/s
Contrast trigger	Ascending aorta/ enhancement threshold 150
FOV (cm)	200
Reconstructed images: axial plane (mm)	Slice/recon increment 3.0/3.0 and 0.75/0.70
Reconstructed images: sagittal plane: entire spine, cervical, thoracic, and lumbar separated (mm)	2.5
Reconstructed images: coronal plane and curved coronal (mm)	2.5/2.0
Sagittal and curved coronal MIPs	—

time in the procedure room, helping to guide treatment.

TREATMENT

There are 2 treatment options in this patient population: endovascular or surgical occlusion of the shunt. Endovascular occlusion is performed with either glue or *N*-butyl-2-cyanoacrylate (Onyx) after superselective catheterization of the radiculomeningeal artery supplying the fistula.[46–48] This option has been proved to be more durable than embolization with particles,[49,50] with occlusion rates reported to be as high as 85%.[47,50–52] The goal in endovascular treatment is proximal occlusion of the draining vein as it exits the fistula, with embolic material entering and crossing the fistula site. Endovascular treatment is not performed in patients in whom the radicular artery also supplies the anterior spinal artery (**Fig. 12**). Embolization of a fistula that supplies a posterior spinal artery remains controversial, particularly given that surgical occlusion is a low-risk procedure. Endovascular treatment fails in approximately 15% to 20% of cases because of failure of selective catheterization of the radicular artery at the fistulous site.[47,48,50,51] If glue does not reach the fistula site, then early surgery is recommended.[3,53–55] Surgical occlusion consists of a targeted laminectomy and intradural exploration with coagulation or disconnection of the draining vein (**Fig. 13**). Surgical occlusion rates ranged up to 98% in a recent single-institution series and meta-analysis of the literature.[56] Intraoperative indocyanine green video angiography can be complimentary and provides real-time assessment of the local hemodynamics in cases in which the fistula was poorly seen on angiography, likely because of highly arterialized venous pressure (see **Fig. 7**F).[29] After treatment, this technique provides immediate confirmation of occlusion of the fistula site and can be repeated because it carries low risk[57] and requires no radiation or additional equipment in the operating room.[58]

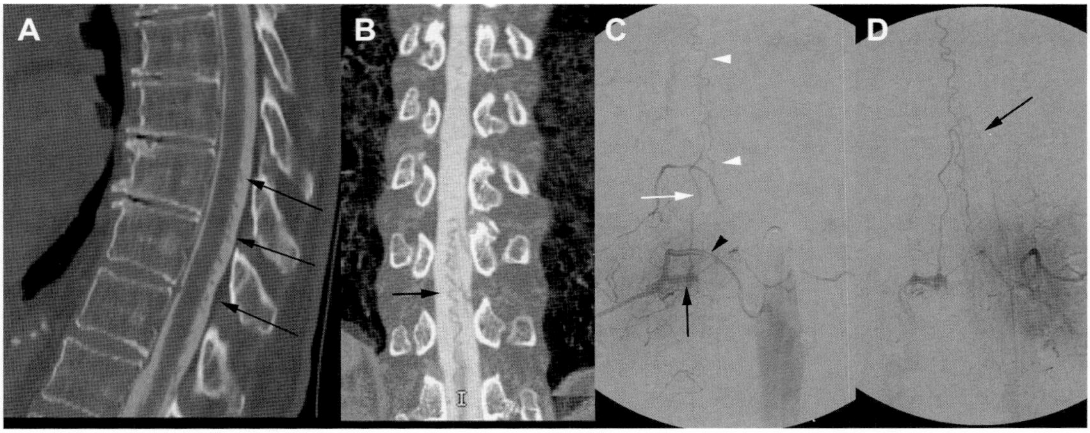

Fig. 10. CT myelogram appearance of L1 SDAVF. (*A*) Sagittal reformat and reconstructed coronal MIP (*B*) from CT myelogram showing dilated perimedullary veins along the dorsal aspect of the lower thoracic cord and conus (*black arrows*). (*C*) DSA of the L1 intercostal artery (*black arrowhead*) supplies an SDAVF beneath the right L1 pedicle (*black arrow*). Dilated radiculomedullary vein (*white arrow*) ascending to dilated perimedullary veins (*white arrowheads*). (*D*) Injection of the contralateral L1 intercostal artery shows the artery of Adamkiewicz (*black arrow*). Because the fistula originates from the contralateral intercostal, this is still amenable to embolization.

POSTTREATMENT CLINICAL RESPONSE AND IMAGING

Multiple factors need to be considered in defining realistic clinical outcomes for the patient, including duration of symptoms, rate of deterioration, pretreatment disability (motor and sensory deficit, bowel and bladder control), site of the fistula, and coexisting comorbidities.[18,19,52,59] Treatment goals are to halt the progression of the disease, improve the current disability, and prevent future decline. In long-term follow-up of patients in whom the fistula was successfully permanently occluded, either with embolic techniques or microsurgery, gait improvement was seen in 67% to 80%.[19,52,60] Worsening of motor symptoms has been shown to be an ominous sign and should lead to early reassessment of the fistula to determine whether there has been recanalization or development of a secondary feeder.[12,61] Hyperesthesias or dysesthesias improve in 50% to 60% and are unchanged in

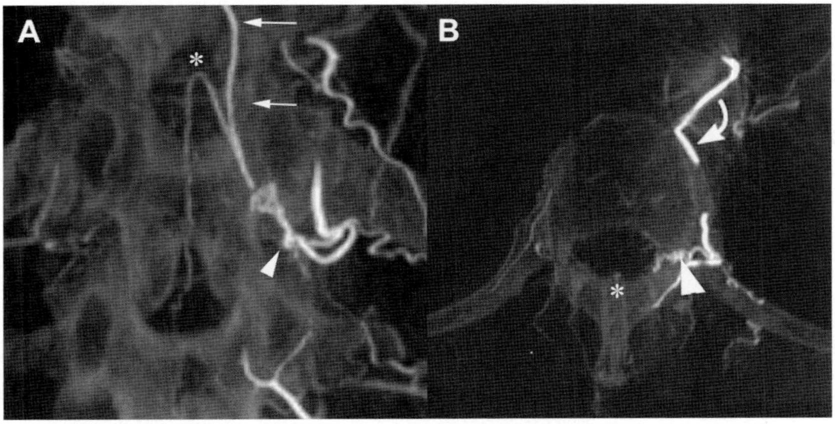

Fig. 11. Cone beam CT during angiogram of T12 SDAVF. (*A, B*) Coronal and axial MIP reconstructed from a T12 intercostal injection (*curved white arrow*) show the point of fistulization beneath the T12 pedicle (*white arrowheads*). Dilated radiculomedullary veins are seen ascending along the dorsal aspect of the spinal cord (*white arrows*). Radiculomedullary artery also supplied by the T12 injection is more definitively shown to be the posterior spinal artery (*white asterisks*) on CT.

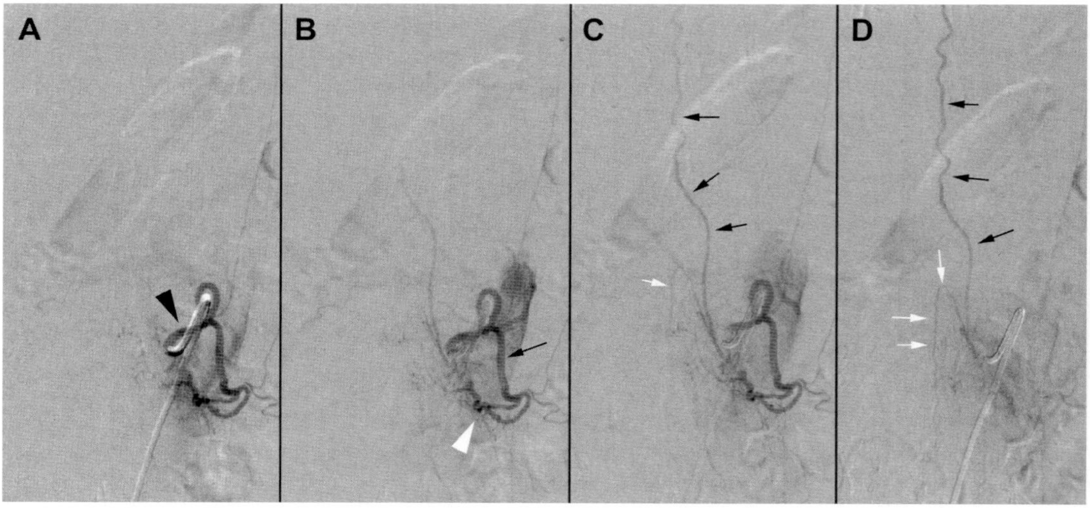

Fig. 12. T11 SDAVF with radiculomedullary artery also supplying the artery of Adamkiewicz. (*A*) DSA of the left T12 intercostal artery (*black arrowhead*). (*B*) The dorsal ramus (*black arrow*) supplies an SDAVF beneath the T11 pedicle (*white arrowhead*). (*C, D*) The dilated perimedullary veins are seen ascending (*black arrows*) and the artery of Adamkiewicz descending (*white arrows*). This case would be treated using microsurgical technique.

the remainder of patients.[19,52,60] If pain is a presenting symptom, it is relieved in a minority of patients (14%) and can even worsen.[19] Similarly, if the patient presents with bowel or bladder dysfunction, it is only reversed in a minority of patients.[16,18,46,50–52,56,62–64] Only 1 small study (n = 25) reporting long-term clinical outcomes after microsurgical occlusion of an SDAVF noted an overall deterioration in the clinical status of their patients.[64]

In patients with a successfully occluded fistula, the expected postoperative MR imaging appearance includes diminished cord enlargement, enhancement, and size and extent of perimedullary serpiginous flow voids (**Fig. 14**).[61,63,65,66] Persistent intramedullary T2 hyperintensity and

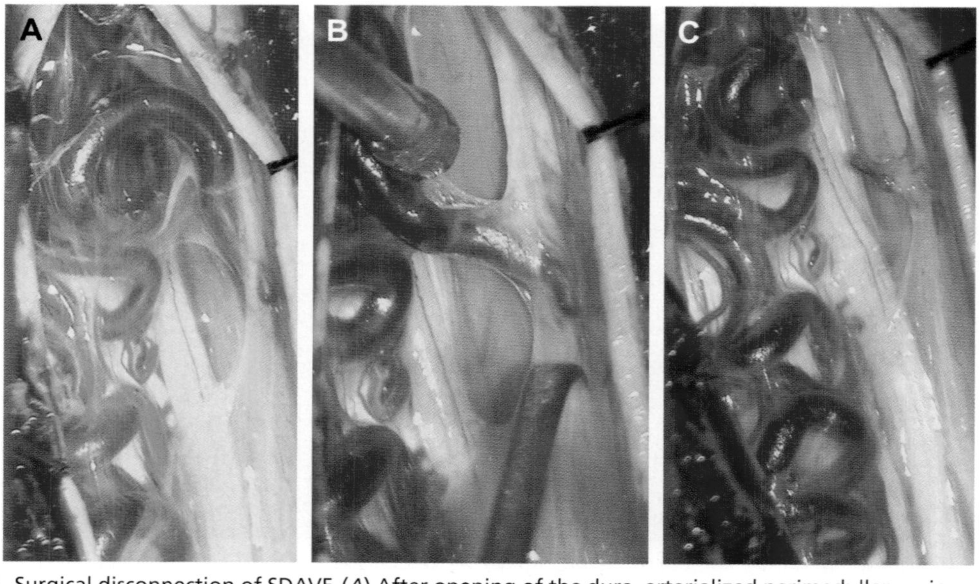

Fig. 13. Surgical disconnection of SDAVF. (*A*) After opening of the dura, arterialized perimedullary veins are seen along the dorsal aspect of the cord. (*B*) Proximal portion of the arterialized vein emerging from the dura in proximity with the corresponding nerve. (*C*) After coagulation of the intradural arterialized vein, the tortuous veins regain a bluish venous hue compared with (*A*).

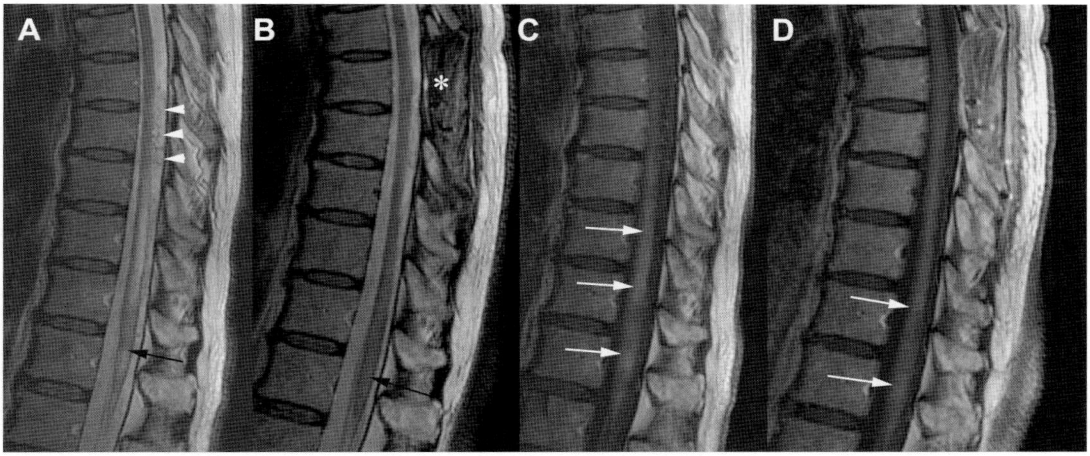

Fig. 14. Postoperative appearance of treated T7 SDAVF. (*A, B*) Pretreatment and 6-month posttreatment sagittal T2WI shows reduction in the intramedullary T2 hyperintensity (*black arrows*), resolution of the prominent dorsal perimedullary flow voids (*white arrowheads*), and resolution of the cord swelling. White asterisks shows laminectomy defect. (*C, D*) Pretreatment and 6-month posttreatment sagittal T1WI with gadolinium shows persistent but reduced intramedullary enhancement (*white arrows*).

enhancement can been seen at 1 year even in those patients who have undergone successful definitive treatment (**Fig. 15**).[61] These postoperative imaging features do not correlate with clinical outcomes and are not predictive of who will improve or deteriorate.[61,66] Conversely, spinal cord atrophy has negative prognostic significance and is associated with increased pain and decreased motor recovery.[19]

At our institution, MR imaging with and without gadolinium is obtained 3 months after treatment if the patient's clinical status stabilizes or improves. Persistent intramedullary T2 hyperintensity or enhancement without enlarged perimedullary vessels is not an indication for additional imaging unless there is clinical deterioration, in particular declining motor function. If there are persistent perimedullary vessels or the patient is clinically deteriorating, MR imaging is obtained with and without gadolinium, including a gadolinium bolus MR angiography, and heavily T2-weighted myelographic sequences. This method seeks to determine whether there has been recanalization of the arterial feeder or development of a second arterial feeder (**Fig. 16**). If the MR imaging findings are inconclusive, the patient proceeds to spinal

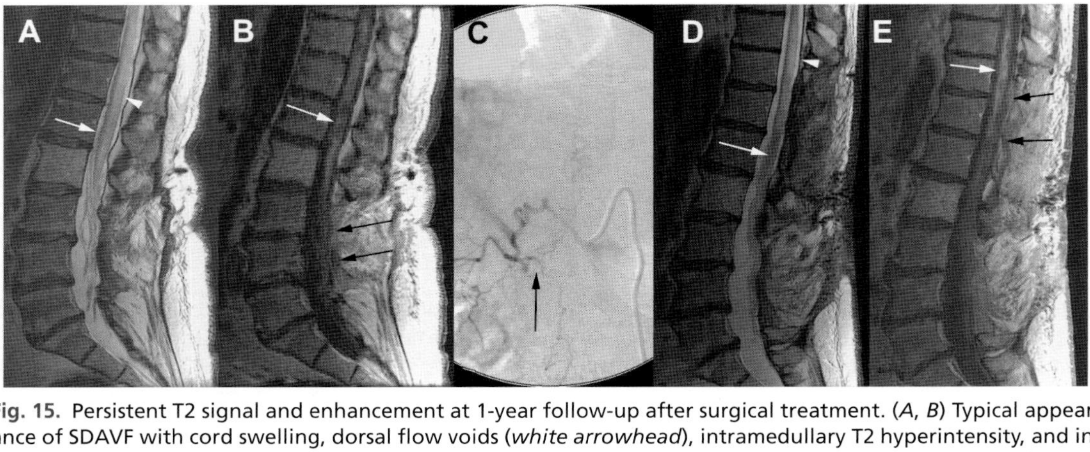

Fig. 15. Persistent T2 signal and enhancement at 1-year follow-up after surgical treatment. (*A, B*) Typical appearance of SDAVF with cord swelling, dorsal flow voids (*white arrowhead*), intramedullary T2 hyperintensity, and intramedullary enhancement (*white arrow*). *Black arrows* show previous laminectomy for spinal stenosis. (*C*) DSA shows SDAVF beneath the L1 pedicle (*black arrow*). (*D, E*) One-year postoperative follow-up in a stable patient shows a reduction but persistent T2 hyperintensity and enhancement (*white arrow*) despite treatment. There is reduction in cord swelling and resolution of dorsal flow voids (*white arrowhead*). No further imaging needed.

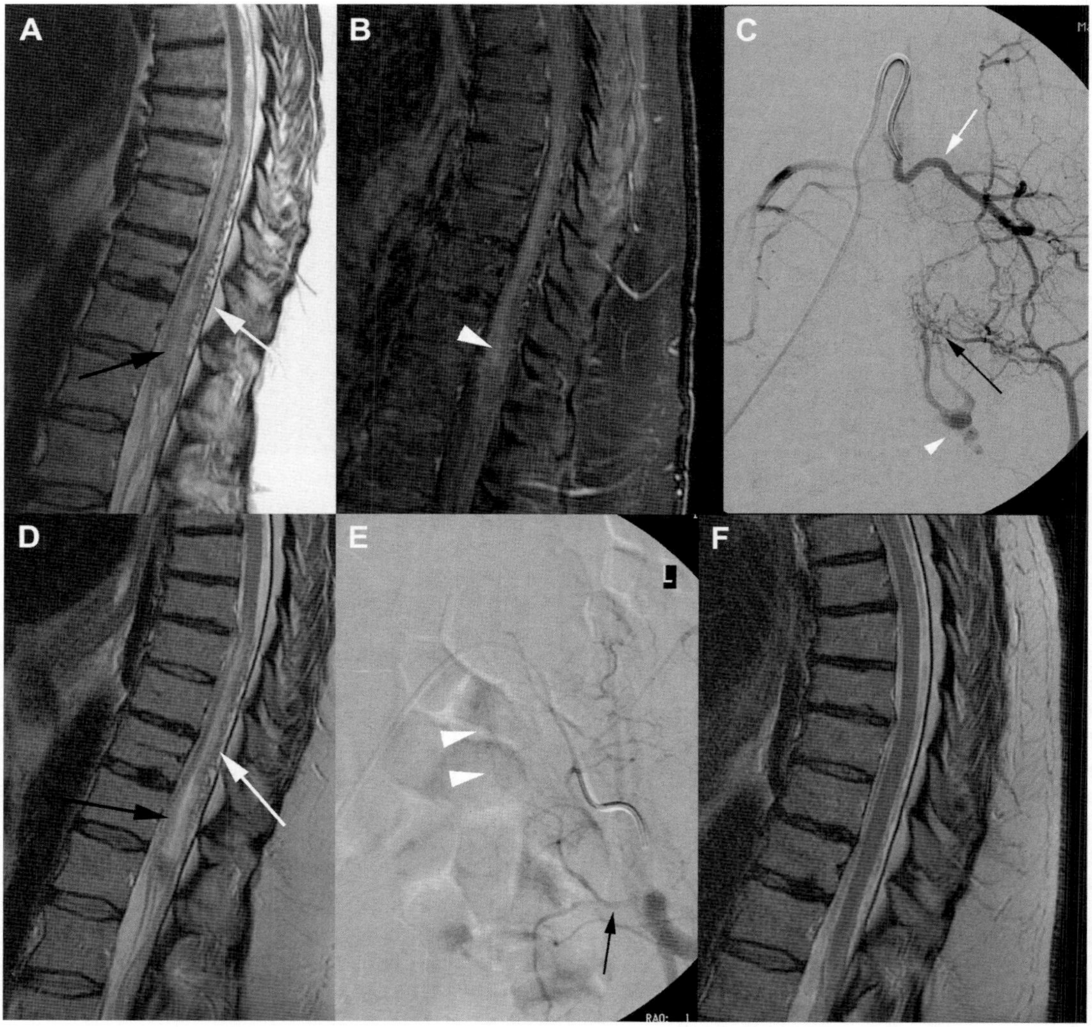

Fig. 16. SDAVF postoperative motor decline during the next year. Second arterial feeder. (*A, B*) Typical appearance of SDAVF with cord swelling, dorsal flow voids (*white arrow*), intramedullary T2 hyperintensity (*black arrow*), and intramedullary enhancement (*white arrowhead*). (*C*) DSA of the left L4 lumbar artery (*white arrow*) shows a dural fistula at the L5 foramen (*black arrow*). Dilated radicular vein extends inferiorly to a large varix (*white arrowhead*) that was surgically disconnected without complication and the patient's symptoms improved almost immediately. Four months after surgery the patient developed recurrent symptoms. (*D*) Follow-up MR imaging showed subtle increase in cord swelling with persistent intramedullary T2 hyperintensity (*black arrow*) and persistent flow voids (*white arrow*). (*E*) DSA showed obliteration of the L4 component. However, a tiny feeding artery from the lateral sacral artery (*black arrow*) was seen (*white arrowheads*). (*F*) MR imaging after surgical disconnection of the S1 component shows resolution of the cord swelling, T2 hyperintensity, and flow voids. The patient improved clinically.

angiogram for definitive evaluation. In patients who have been treated and have clinically stabilized or improved, we perform follow-up imaging in another 6 months.

SUMMARY

The diagnosis of SDAVF is often delayed because of its nonspecific clinical presentation, which may mimic more common entities. The radiologist is often the first physician who can suggest the diagnosis and thus should be familiar with the SDAVF imaging appearance of cord swelling, diffuse multilevel intramedullary T2 hyperintensity, patchy intramedullary enhancement, and perimedullary vascularity. MR angiography and myelographic sequences should guide selective spinal angiography; subsequent treatment options include catheter embolization if glue can be placed across the fistula into the draining vein, or microsurgical intervention through a targeted laminectomy. It is crucial to obtain a proper diagnosis in this patient population because, in most cases, motor and sensory function can be improved or at least stabilized if the process is recognized.

REFERENCES

1. Andersson T, van Dijk JM, Willinsky RA. Venous manifestations of spinal arteriovenous fistulas. Not Found In Database 2003;13(1):73–93.
2. Rodesch G, Hurth M, Alvarez H, et al. Classification of spinal cord arteriovenous shunts: proposal for a reappraisal–the Bicetre experience with 155 consecutive patients treated between 1981 and 1999. Neurosurgery 2002;51(2):374–9 [discussion: 379–80].
3. Krings T, Geibprasert S. Spinal dural arteriovenous fistulas. AJNR Am J Neuroradiol 2009;30(4):639–48.
4. Jahan R, Vinuela F. Vascular anatomy, pathophysiology, and classification of vascular malformations of the spinal cord. Semin Cerebrovasc Dis Stroke 2002;2(3):186–200.
5. Kim LJ, Spetzler RF. Classification and surgical management of spinal arteriovenous lesions: arteriovenous fistulae and arteriovenous malformations. Neurosurgery 2006;59(5 Suppl 3):S195–201 [discussion: S3–13].
6. Spetzler RF, Detwiler PW, Riina HA, et al. Modified classification of spinal cord vascular lesions. J Neurosurg 2002;96(Suppl 2):145–56.
7. Oldfield EH. Spinal vascular malformation. In: Wilkins RH, Rengachery SS, editors. Neurosurgery. New York: McGraw-Hill; 1996. p. 2541–58.
8. Muraszko KM, Oldfield EH. Vascular malformations of the spinal cord. Neurosurg Clin North Am 1990; 1:1631–52.
9. Thron A, Caplan LR. Vascular malformations and interventional neuroradiology of the spinal cord. Amsterdam: Academic; 2003.
10. Kawabori M, Hida K, Yano S, et al. Cervical epidural arteriovenous fistula with radiculopathy mimicking cervical spondylosis. Neurol Med Chir (Tokyo) 2009;49(3):108–13.
11. Gilbertson JR, Miller GM, Goldman MS, et al. Spinal dural arteriovenous fistulas: MR and myelographic findings. AJNR Am J Neuroradiol 1995;16(10):2049–57.
12. Muralidharan R, Saladino A, Lanzino G, et al. The clinical and radiological presentation of spinal dural arteriovenous fistula. Spine 2011;36(25):E1641–7.
13. Bao YH, Ling F. Classification and therapeutic modalities of spinal vascular malformations in 80 patients. Neurosurgery 1997;40(1):75–81.
14. Rosenblum B, Oldfield EH, Doppman JL, et al. Spinal arteriovenous malformations: a comparison of dural arteriovenous fistulas and intradural AVM's in 81 patients. J Neurosurg 1987;67(6):795–802.
15. Symon L, Kuyama H, Kendall B. Dural arteriovenous malformations of the spine. Clinical features and surgical results in 55 cases. J Neurosurg 1984; 60(2):238–47.
16. Van Dijk JM, TerBrugge KG, Willinsky RA, et al. Multidisciplinary management of spinal dural arteriovenous fistulas: clinical presentation and long-term follow-up in 49 patients. Stroke 2002;33(6):1578–83.
17. Koenig E, Thron A, Schrader V, et al. Spinal arteriovenous malformations and fistulae: clinical, neuroradiological and neurophysiological findings. J Neurol 1989;236(5):260–6.
18. Saladino A, Atkinson JL, Rabinstein AA, et al. Surgical treatment of spinal dural arteriovenous fistulae: a consecutive series of 154 patients. Neurosurgery 2010;67(5):1350–7 [discussion: 1357–8].
19. Shinoyama M, Endo T, Takahash T, et al. Long-term outcome of cervical and thoracolumbar dural arteriovenous fistulas with emphasis on sensory disturbance and neuropathic pain. World Neurosurg 2010;73(4):401–8.
20. Hurst RW, Kenyon LC, Lavi E, et al. Spinal dural arteriovenous fistula: the pathology of venous hypertensive myelopathy. Neurology 1995;45(7):1309–13.
21. Saraf-Lavi E, Bowen BC, Quencer RM, et al. Detection of spinal dural arteriovenous fistulae with MR imaging and contrast-enhanced MR angiography: sensitivity, specificity, and prediction of vertebral level. AJNR Am J Neuroradiol 2002;23(5):858–67.
22. Geibprasert S, Pongpech S, Jiarakongmun P, et al. Cervical spine dural arteriovenous fistula presenting with congestive myelopathy of the conus. Not Found In Database 2009;11(4):427–31.
23. Lucas JW, Jones J, Farin A, et al. Cervical spine dural arteriovenous fistula with coexisting spinal radiculopial artery aneurysm presenting as subarachnoid hemorrhage. Neurosurgery 2012;70(1): E259–63.
24. Do HM, Jensen ME, Cloft HJ, et al. Dural arteriovenous fistula of the cervical spine presenting with subarachnoid hemorrhage. AJNR Am J Neuroradiol 1999;20(2):348–50.
25. Hashimoto H, Iida J, Shin Y, et al. Spinal dural arteriovenous fistula with perimesencephalic subarachnoid haemorrhage. J Clin Neurosci 2000;7(1):64–6.
26. Kim DJ, Willinsky R, Geibprasert S, et al. Angiographic characteristics and treatment of cervical spinal dural arteriovenous shunts. AJNR Am J Neuroradiol 2010;31(8):1512–5.
27. Hassler W, Thron A. Flow velocity and pressure measurements in spinal dural arteriovenous fistulas. Neurosurg Rev 1994;17(1):29–36.
28. Hassler W, Thron A, Grote EH. Hemodynamics of spinal dural arteriovenous fistulas. An intraoperative study. J Neurosurg 1989;70(3):360–70.

29. Morris JM, Kaufmann TJ, Campeau NG, et al. Volumetric myelographic magnetic resonance imaging to localize difficult-to-find spinal dural arteriovenous fistulas. Not Found In Database 2011;14(3): 398–404.
30. Quencer RM. Is peripheral spinal cord hypointensity a sign of venous hypertensive myelopathy? AJNR Am J Neuroradiol 2000;21(4):617.
31. Hurst RW, Grossman RI. Peripheral spinal cord hypointensity on T2-weighted MR images: a reliable imaging sign of venous hypertensive myelopathy. AJNR Am J Neuroradiol 2000;21(4):781–6.
32. Schaat TJ, Salzman KL, Stevens EA. Sacral origin of a spinal dural arteriovenous fistula: case report and review. Spine 2002;27(8):893–7.
33. Bowen BC, Fraser K, Kochan JP, et al. Spinal dural arteriovenous fistulas: evaluation with MR angiography. AJNR Am J Neuroradiol 1995; 16(10):2029–43.
34. Minami S, Sagoh T, Nishimura K, et al. Spinal arteriovenous malformation: MR imaging. Radiology 1988; 169(1):109–15.
35. Terwey B, Becker H, Thron AK, et al. Gadolinium-DTPA enhanced MR imaging of spinal dural arteriovenous fistulas. J Comput Assist Tomogr 1989;13(1):30–7.
36. Mascalchi M, Quilici N, Ferrito G, et al. Identification of the feeding arteries of spinal vascular lesions via phase-contrast MR angiography with three-dimensional acquisition and phase display. AJNR Am J Neuroradiol 1997;18(2):351–8.
37. Binkert CA, Kollias SS, Valavanis A. Spinal cord vascular disease: characterization with fast three-dimensional contrast-enhanced MR angiography. AJNR Am J Neuroradiol 1999;20(10):1785–93.
38. Farb RI, Kim JK, Willinsky RA, et al. Spinal dural arteriovenous fistula localization with a technique of first-pass gadolinium-enhanced MR angiography: initial experience. Radiology 2002;222(3):843–50.
39. Luetmer PH, Lane JI, Gilbertson JR, et al. Preangiographic evaluation of spinal dural arteriovenous fistulas with elliptic centric contrast-enhanced MR angiography and effect on radiation dose and volume of iodinated contrast material. AJNR Am J Neuroradiol 2005;26(4):711–8.
40. Mull M, Nijenhuis RJ, Backes WH, et al. Value and limitations of contrast-enhanced MR angiography in spinal arteriovenous malformations and dural arteriovenous fistulas. AJNR Am J Neuroradiol 2007;28(7):1249–58.
41. Yamada N, Takamiya M, Kuribayashi S, et al. MRA of the Adamkiewicz artery: a preoperative study for thoracic aortic aneurysm. J Comput Assist Tomogr 2000;24(3):362–8.
42. Bertrand D, Douvrin F, Gerardin E, et al. Diagnosis of spinal dural arteriovenous fistula with multidetector row computed tomography: a case report. Neuroradiology 2004;46(10):851–4.
43. Lai PH, Weng MJ, Lee KW, et al. Multidetector CT angiography in diagnosing type I and type IVA spinal vascular malformations. AJNR Am J Neuroradiol 2006;27(4):813–7.
44. Si-jia G, Meng-wei Z, Xi-ping L, et al. The clinical application studies of CT spinal angiography with 64-detector row spiral CT in diagnosing spinal vascular malformations. Eur J Radiol 2009;71(1):22–8.
45. Aadland TD, Thielen KR, Kaufmann TJ, et al. 3D C-arm conebeam CT angiography as an adjunct in the precise anatomic characterization of spinal dural arteriovenous fistulas. AJNR Am J Neuroradiol 2010; 31(3):476–80.
46. Rodesch G, Hurth M, Alvarez H, et al. Spinal cord intradural arteriovenous fistulae: anatomic, clinical, and therapeutic considerations in a series of 32 consecutive patients seen between 1981 and 2000 with emphasis on endovascular therapy. Neurosurgery 2005;57(5):973–83 [discussion: 973–83].
47. Rodesch G, Lasjaunias P. Spinal cord arteriovenous shunts: from imaging to management. Eur J Radiol 2003;46(3):221–32.
48. Jellema K, Sluzewski M, van Rooij WJ, et al. Embolization of spinal dural arteriovenous fistulas: importance of occlusion of the draining vein. Not Found In Database 2005;2(5):580–3.
49. Nichols DA, Rufenacht DA, Jack CR Jr, et al. Embolization of spinal dural arteriovenous fistula with polyvinyl alcohol particles: experience in 14 patients. AJNR Am J Neuroradiol 1992;13(3):933–40.
50. Narvid J, Hetts SW, Larsen D, et al. Spinal dural arteriovenous fistulae: clinical features and long-term results. Neurosurgery 2008;62(1):159–66 [discussion: 166–7].
51. Niimi Y, Berenstein A, Setton A, et al. Embolization of spinal dural arteriovenous fistulae: results and follow-up. Neurosurgery 1997;40(4):675–82 [discussion: 682–3].
52. Sherif C, Gruber A, Bavinzski G, et al. Long-term outcome of a multidisciplinary concept of spinal dural arteriovenous fistulae treatment. Neuroradiology 2008;50(1):67–74.
53. Andres RH, Barth A, Guzman R, et al. Endovascular and surgical treatment of spinal dural arteriovenous fistulas. Neuroradiology 2008;50(10):869–76.
54. Dehdashti AR, Da Costa LB, terBrugge KG, et al. Overview of the current role of endovascular and surgical treatment in spinal dural arteriovenous fistulas. Neurosurg Focus 2009;26(1):E8.
55. Krings T, Thron AK, Geibprasert S, et al. Endovascular management of spinal vascular malformations. Neurosurg Rev 2010;33(1):1–9.
56. Steinmetz MP, Chow MM, Krishnaney AA, et al. Outcome after the treatment of spinal dural arteriovenous fistulae: a contemporary single-institution series and meta-analysis. Neurosurgery 2004; 55(1):77–87 [discussion: 87–8].

57. Raabe A, Nakaji P, Beck J, et al. Prospective evaluation of surgical microscope-integrated intraoperative near-infrared indocyanine green videoangiography during aneurysm surgery. J Neurosurg 2005;103(6): 982–9.
58. Oh JK, Shin HC, Kim TY, et al. Intraoperative indocyanine green video-angiography: spinal dural arteriovenous fistula. Spine 2011;36(24):E1578–80.
59. Cenzato M, Versari P, Righi C, et al. Spinal dural arteriovenous fistulae: analysis of outcome in relation to pretreatment indicators. Neurosurgery 2004; 55(4):815–22 [discussion: 822–3].
60. Behrens S, Thron A. Long-term follow-up and outcome in patients treated for spinal dural arteriovenous fistula. J Neurol 1999;246(3):181–5.
61. Kaufmann TJ, Morris JM, Saladino A, et al. Magnetic resonance imaging findings in treated spinal dural arteriovenous fistulas: lack of correlation with clinical outcomes. Not Found In Database 2011;14(4):548–54.
62. Lee TT, Gromelski EB, Bowen BC, et al. Diagnostic and surgical management of spinal dural arteriovenous fistulas. Neurosurgery 1998;43(2):242–6 [discussion: 246–7].
63. Song JK, Vinuela F, Gobin YP, et al. Surgical and endovascular treatment of spinal dural arteriovenous fistulas: long-term disability assessment and prognostic factors. J Neurosurg 2001;94(Suppl 2): 199–204.
64. Tacconi L, Lopez Izquierdo BC, Symon L. Outcome and prognostic factors in the surgical treatment of spinal dural arteriovenous fistulas. A long-term study. Br J Neurosurg 1997;11(4):298–305.
65. Willinsky RA, terBrugge K, Montanera W, et al. Posttreatment MR findings in spinal dural arteriovenous malformations. AJNR Am J Neuroradiol 1995; 16(10):2063–71.
66. Mascalchi M, Ferrito G, Quilici N, et al. Spinal vascular malformations: MR angiography after treatment. Radiology 2001;219(2):346–53.

Imaging of the Seronegative Spondyloarthopathies

Kimberly K. Amrami, MD

KEYWORDS

- Seronegative spondyloarthropathy • Sacroiliitis • Magnetic resonance imaging
- Inflammatory arthritis • Ankylosing spondylitis

KEY POINTS

- The seronegative spondyloarthropathies can be categorized based on imaging findings in association with clinical features and laboratory testing.
- Multiple modalities (radiography, computed tomography [CT] and magnetic resonance [MR] imaging) can be used to assess the axial and appendicular skeleton in patients suspected of seronegative spondyloarthopathies.
- MR imaging is the optimal modality for imaging the seronegative spondyloarthropathies, with improved sensitivity compared with radiography and CT.
- Contrast-enhanced MR imaging can distinguish between active and inactive disease and also assess response to treatment.

INTRODUCTION

Spondyloarthritis refers to a diverse group of diseases involving inflammation of the axial skeleton and peripheral joints.[1–3] The individual entities are distinguished by specific clinical and laboratory features with disease presentation often on a spectrum that is dynamic and progressive rather than static and unchanging. These diseases can be grouped based on common clinical and imaging features such as inflammatory back pain, sacroiliitis, spondylitis, and enthesitis. Laboratory studies, with the exception of the strong association with the genetically determined human leukocyte antigen B27 (HLA-B27), are generally nonspecific, with elevated inflammatory markers such as C-reactive protein and erythrocyte sedimentation rate sometimes present. Clinical features may allow some differentiation (such as urethritis in Reiter syndrome or reactive spondyloarthropathy), but there remains significant overlap.[1,3]

The original concept of a group of interrelated but distinctive disorders was developed by Moll and colleagues[4] in 1974 to describe a group of inflammatory diseases affecting the spine and sacroiliac joints. The term seronegative spondyloarthropathies was coined to indicate that rheumatoid factor was not present in these patients, with the individual forms of the disease including ankylosing spondylitis, psoriatic arthritis, reactive arthritis (formerly known as Reiter syndrome), arthritis related to inflammatory bowel disease, and a form of juvenile idiopathic arthritis distinguished only by the age of the patient.[5] Undifferentiated spondyloarthropathy and late-onset spondyloarthropathy are also sometimes included in this grouping.[6,7] In addition to the distinction by the absence of rheumatoid factor, the seronegative spondyloarthropathies uniquely affect entheses. The definition and subcategorization of the spondyloarthropathies has evolved over time, and multiple groups have attempted to characterize the symptoms and natural history of the spondyloarthropathies, including the New York criteria[8] for sacroiliitis and similar criteria for ankylosing spondylitis, in the 1960s and 1970s.[1,3] In the 1990s there was a move to reclassify the entire

Department of Radiology, Mayo Clinic, 200 First Street SW, Rochester, MN 55905, USA
E-mail address: amrami.kimberly@mayo.edu

Radiol Clin N Am 50 (2012) 841–854
doi:10.1016/j.rcl.2012.04.010

disease spectrum; this grouped all patients with inflammatory arthritis involving the axial skeletal as seronegative spondyloarthritis, despite a wide variety of clinical symptoms.[9] The Amor criteria addressed the difficulty in diagnosing these disorders through the creation of a scoring system.[9] A newer (2009) classification was proposed by the Assessment of Spondyloarthritis International Society (ASAS) after a large cross-sectional study.[10] Rather than focusing on specific subtypes such as ankylosing spondylitis, this classification depends on 2 important clinical features: axial symptoms and peripheral involvement. The investigators proposed the term "axial spondyloarthritis" for the entire spectrum of diseases whereby axial involvement predominates. This type can then be broken down into the more traditional subtypes based on clinical features, HLA-B27 positivity, and the presence or absence of sacroiliac involvement based on the detection of active inflammation by advanced imaging techniques such as magnetic resonance (MR) imaging. The ASAS criteria for axial spondyloarthritis consists of active sacroiliitis on imaging plus 1 or more features of spondyloarthritis or HLA-B27 positivity with 2 or more features of spondyloarthritis. In comparison, the criteria for peripheral spondyloarthritis are more complex and include such options as Crohn disease or ulcerative colitis, prior infection (as in Reiter syndrome), inflammatory back pain, or positive family history.[9] The diagnosis of a peripheral spondyloarthritis also can depend on the presence of sacroiliitis on imaging (ie, arthritis with sacroiliitis alone meets these criteria).[9] Although classification remains of interest for these complex disorders, the main challenge at the current time is the development of strategies for early diagnosis and treatment aimed at limiting disability and disease progression over time. The newer classifications all depend on advanced imaging techniques such as MR imaging, supplanting the prior use of radiography (and radiographic atlases) in assisting clinical decision making.

IMAGING TECHNIQUES

Although the spondyloarthropathies can involve the entire axial and appendicular skeleton, including central and peripheral entheses and joints, the hallmark for all types of spondyloarthritis remains sacroiliitis.[1–3] Inflammation of one or both sacroiliac joints is the most characteristic and consistent feature of these disorders. Involvement of the remainder of the axial skeleton is rare in the absence of sacroiliitis, as is peripheral involvement even when those symptoms, such as enthesitis at the heel, dominate the clinical picture. Inflammatory back pain is commonly associated with sacroiliitis, but is a nonspecific symptom and may be seen in other disorders unrelated to spondyloarthropathy. HLA-B27 positivity on its own is not an indication of spondyloarthritis in the absence of symptoms or positive imaging findings.[10,11] The unifying diagnostic tool for the seronegative spondyloarthropathies is imaging of the sacroiliac joints.

Conventional radiography remains the most common initial imaging study for patients suspected of having inflammatory arthritis of all kinds (**Fig. 1**).[3] Plain radiography of the pelvis for assessment of the sacroiliac joints has significant limitations, including the need for ionizing radiation in young patients as well as low sensitivity for detection of early disease.[2,3] Experience and knowledge of the clinical context may improve detection, but it is common for radiologists to miss advanced cases of sacroiliitis on radiography.[12] Five stages of radiographic changes in the sacroiliac joints have been described, ranging from 0 (normal) through 4.[8] The most difficult stages are 1 (unclear) and 2 (small erosions, sclerosis), with more advanced disease (3, definite erosions and 4, ankylosis) less problematic to detect, testifying to the poor specificity and moderate sensitivity of radiography in detecting sacroiliitis. The relatively low utility of radiography for sacroiliitis is exacerbated by poor interobserver and intraobserver reliability for subtle changes in early disease.[13–15] The detection of the structural changes of sacroiliitis is challenging enough, but the physiologic parameter of disease activity is beyond the capabilities of radiography, which precludes using radiography to monitor response to therapy.

The complexity of the sacroiliac joints themselves and the difficulty in seeing the entire joint in a 2-dimensional projection is part of the challenge, but studies comparing more specialized views such as the angled anteroposterior oblique Ferguson view have not shown significant improvement in accuracy.[1,3,16] Conventional views of the pelvis may actually have some added value over dedicated imaging of the sacroiliac joints, in that the hips are usually included in such images.[17] Despite these limitations, conventional radiographs are important, especially in distinguishing ankylosing spondylitis from other types of spondyloarthritis. Radiographic imaging of the entire spine and symptomatic individual peripheral joints can help to classify the various types of spondyloarthropathy and to visualize complications such as discovertebral fractures in ankylosing spondylitis, although with lower sensitivity than with computed tomography (CT).

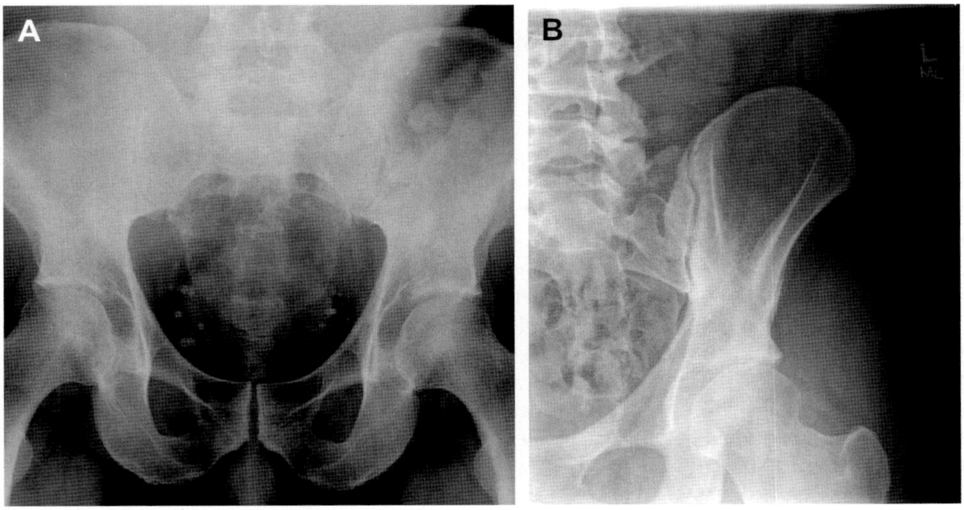

Fig. 1. Normal radiographs of the sacroiliac joints. (*A*) Normal anteroposterior (AP) radiograph of the sacroiliac joints. (*B*) Normal oblique radiograph of the left sacroiliac joint. Note resolution of some of the joint overlap seen in *A*.

Scintigraphy is another technique that has been traditionally used to evaluate the skeleton when spondyloarthritis is suspected. In the past, when radiography was the primary diagnostic tool, scintigraphy enhanced the sensitivity of plain radiographs for early-stage disease. Unfortunately, though sensitive, scintigraphy is too nonspecific to be used in isolation in the diagnosis of sacroiliitis.[18,19] In fact, mild activity at the sacroiliac joints can lead to overdiagnosis of sacroiliitis when only mild degenerative change is present.[20] Scintigraphy may be helpful in establishing bilateral disease whereby only unilateral disease has been seen on radiography, but it is inferior to more advanced cross-sectional imaging such as CT and especially MR imaging. The use of colloidal agents for joint imaging is similarly nonspecific when evaluating the spondyloarthropathies. Positron emission scanning (PET), with or without CT, has little role in the assessment of spondyloarthropathy at this time.

CT can be useful in assessing the spine and sacroiliac joints, having a higher degree of sensitivity than radiography and with better specificity than scintigraphy (**Fig. 2**).[20] Because of the high spatial resolution possible with CT, subtle erosions and subchondral sclerosis in the sacroiliac joints may be seen to better effect than with radiography; early syndesmophytes and "shiny corners" can be better seen in the spine. Unlike radiography the images may be obtained in any plane, so that visualization of the entire joint and individual disc spaces is optimized regardless of orientation. In fact, most modern CT acquisitions are essentially volumetric because of their isotropic nature, making multiplanar and even 3-dimensional reformatting easy to perform on a routine basis. CT is preferred for the detection of very early erosions of the sacroiliac joints and for early ankylosis.[21–23] CT requires the use of ionizing radiation in what are usually young patients; it is not an ideal method for following patients over time. Furthermore, active inflammation can be difficult to assess, as bone marrow edema is not generally visible on CT; burnt-out sclerosis without active disease may have a similar appearance to very active inflammation.[22,23] A final caveat is the normal progression of age-related subchondral sclerosis at the sacroiliac

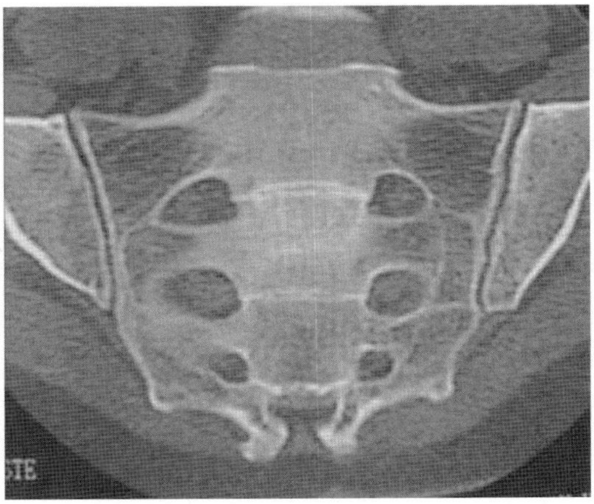

Fig. 2. Reconstructed oblique coronal CT image showing normal sacroiliac joints.

joints. Care must be taken not to confuse normal senescent changes or degenerative osteoarthritis with the erosions, irregularity, and subchondral sclerosis seen in sacroiliitis.[21]

Ultrasonography has some utility for the evaluation of sacroiliitis when it is very active, by using Doppler ultrasonography to assess blood flow and synovitis.[3,24] It may also be useful in some cases in young children as an initial study, but is limited to the evaluation of soft tissues surrounding the joint and not the joint itself.[17] Ultrasound guidance may be used for diagnostic and therapeutic injections into the sacroiliac joint as an alternative to fluoroscopy in some cases.[25]

MR imaging has become the gold standard for the imaging diagnosis of spondyloarthropathies of the spine and sacroiliac joints (**Fig. 3**).[1–3,13,21,26–30] MR imaging is highly sensitive and specific for the presence of inflammatory changes in and around the spine and sacroiliac joints.[31] As with CT, multiplanar acquisitions are routinely performed, which optimize visualization of the entire sacroiliac joint with the added benefit of improved soft-tissue and bone marrow contrast. Serial studies over time are not problematic in terms of radiation exposure. Subtle erosions may be difficult to see because of the relatively lower spatial resolution of MR imaging compared with CT, but T2-weighted sequences with fat suppression are exquisitely sensitive and specific in the detection of bone marrow edema, joint widening, and joint fluid and, thus, synovitis.[22,23] With contrast enhancement, MR imaging can distinguish active from inactive disease and can be used to monitor treatment response: a decrease in enhancement even in the presence of persistent bone marrow edema has been strongly correlated with clinical response to treatment.[32] Alternatively, a lack of response by imaging with no change in baseline enhancement suggests treatment failure and a need to alter the therapeutic regimen. Postcontrast imaging can be performed in a variety of ways using delayed enhancement, rapid imaging with dynamic enhancement, and with or without the use of image subtraction, which can be especially helpful when low-field (<1.5 T) imagers are used.[33] Enhancement can be measured in semiquantitative ways in addition to the qualitative visual assessment during image interpretation. All of these techniques can be very helpful when determining the value of drug regimens with significant side effects and high cost.[33]

MR imaging is also the preferred modality for imaging the remainder of the spine and for the peripheral joints (**Fig. 4**). The soft-tissue contrast is ideal for assessing the structures within the spinal canal (including the cord) and for assessing inflammatory or destructive changes in the joints. Dural ectasia and cauda equina syndrome seen in ankylosing spondylitis (AS) can be best evaluated with MR imaging.[34] Direct visualization of the atlantoaxial interval in the cervical spine can also be well seen on MR imaging; atlantoaxial subluxation can be evaluated in some upright MR imaging scanners, but is more typically assessed with radiography with flexion and extension.[6] CT may be used as an alternative to MR imaging when patients are unable to undergo MR imaging for any reason, and when rapid assessment is desired as in assessing discovertebral fractures after trauma.[28]

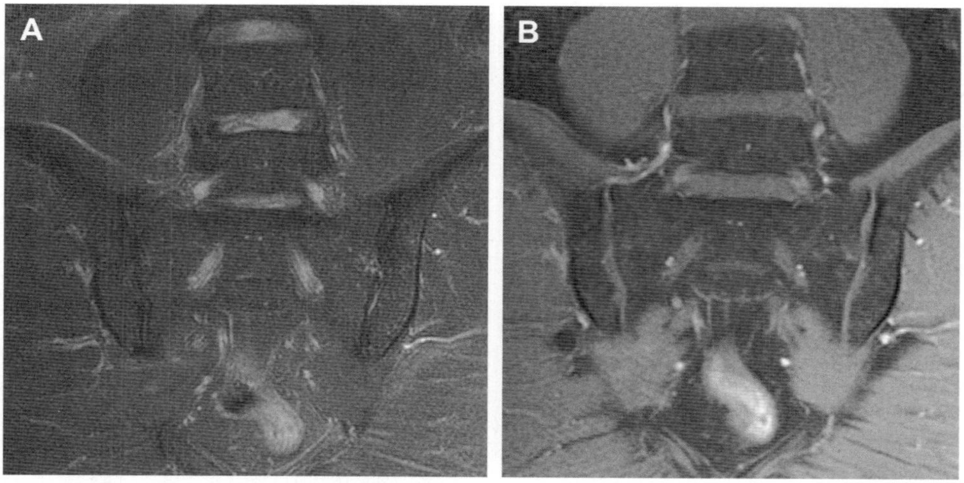

Fig. 3. Normal MR images of the sacroiliac joints. (*A*) Oblique coronal T2-weighted MR image of the sacroiliac joints with fat suppression showing no abnormal signal around the joint. (*B*) Coronal oblique T1-weighted MR image with fat suppression after contrast administration shows normal sacroiliac joints with no enhancement.

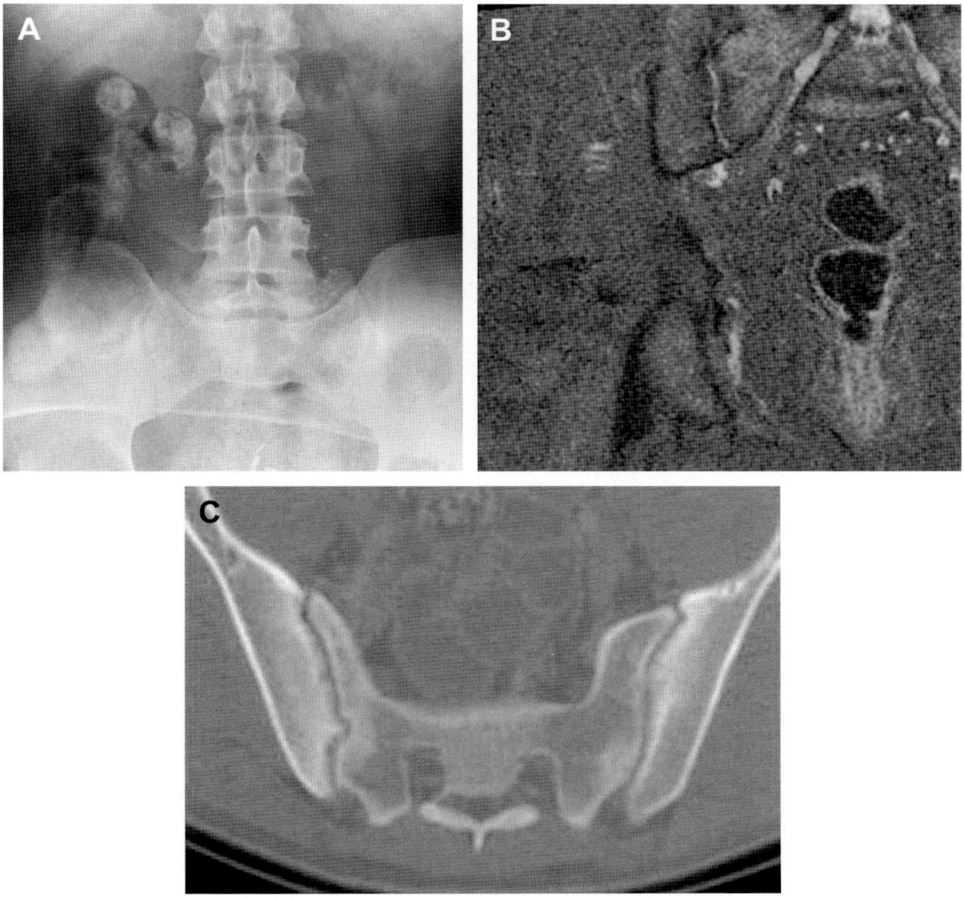

Fig. 4. Sacroiliitis. (*A*) AP radiograph of the pelvis showing bilateral sacroiliitis in a patient with inflammatory bowel disease. Note right lower quadrant ostomy and residual oral contrast. (*B*) Coronal short-tau inversion recovery (STIR) image of the right sacroiliac joint showing T2 hyperintensity on both sides of the joint consistent with sacroiliitis. Only the right side was imaged, owing to body habitus. This patient has undifferentiated spondyloarthropathy and is HLA-B27 positive. (*C*) Axial CT image showing irregularity and subchondral sclerosis at the sacroiliac joints bilaterally in a patient with ankylosing spondylitis.

IMAGING FINDINGS IN THE SERONEGATIVE SPONDYLOARTHROPATHIES

The seronegative arthropathies are a group of diverse disorders, which share some common features (such as an increased incidence of genetically determined HLA-B27 histocompatibility antigen and inflammation in the musculoskeletal system) but which can also be subclassified into specific entities based on imaging findings, clinical presentation, and natural history of the disease. Most of the entities described here have juvenile forms in addition to the usual presentation in young adulthood; rare patients present in old age with late-onset spondyloarthropathy, which may be difficult to characterize because of comorbid degenerative arthritis.[7] A small number of patients who cannot be categorized into one of the following subtypes are categorized as having undifferentiated spondyloarthropathy.[6]

Ankylosing Spondylitis

AS is the prototypical seronegative spondyloarthropathy. AS is primarily a disease of white males with the male to female ratio being between 4:1 and 10:1, with generally milder presentations in women. The normal prevalence of the HLA-B27 antigen in the North American population is 6% to 8%, but for patients with in AS it is more than 90%.[1,2] The disease commonly presents in late adolescence or early adulthood; presentation after age 40 years is very unusual. The most common presenting features of AS are morning stiffness and low back pain. Patients presenting at younger ages may experience peripheral symptoms such as heel pain rather than the usual inflammatory back pain. Because symptoms are nonspecific, the time to diagnosis from the first symptoms averages 7 years. About 20% of patients progress to severe debilitation primarily related to systemic manifestations of AS, such as lung fibrosis.[2,35]

AS is primarily a disease of the axial skeleton that affects the spine and sacroiliac joints. Sacroiliitis is a required element for diagnosis of AS.[2,3,8–10] The disease typically begins in the sacroiliac joints with small erosions resembling the serrated edges of a postage stamp, typically beginning on the iliac side of the joint, due to the thinner cartilage there compared with the sacrum. As the disease advances proliferative changes associated with the enthesitis dominate, with sclerosis seen in the subchondral areas progressing finally to complete ankylosis of the joint. When the fusion is complete the sclerosis resolves completely.[2] The sacroiliitis may appear asymmetric in the early stages, especially if MR imaging is used in early diagnosis, but the disease inevitably progresses to bilateral, symmetric involvement.

Spondylitis occurs in about 50% of AS patients, with females relatively less affected.[2,36] The changes in the spine occur first in thoracolumbar and lumbosacral regions with extension to the midlumbar, midthoracic, and cervical regions. Involvement of the cervical spine alone is very rare. The orderly progression of spine involvement is a unique feature of AS when compared with the other spondyloarthropathies, in which spine involvement tends to be more random. In AS the earliest changes in the spine are due to enthesitis at the insertion of the outer fibers of the annulus fibrosus on the ring apophysis of the vertebral endplate. This process results in subtle erosions with reactive sclerosis in the vertebral corners, known as shiny corners or Romanus lesions.[2,3] These phenomena are generally very short lived, with progression to the more commonly seen syndesmophytes, representing the ossification of the outer fibers of the annulus fibrosus.[2] These lesions are very fine and symmetric, bridging individual vertebral bodies from corner to corner. This same process results in the "squaring" of the vertebral bodies as the fusion progresses, and is best visualized in the lumbar spine where there is loss of the normal concave profile of the vertebrae. Other spinal elements are also ossified and fused as part of this progressive process, including the apophyseal joints, paraspinous ligaments, and spinous processes. When complete the appearance is very characteristic, and is termed the bamboo spine (**Fig. 5**).[2] The changes in the spine itself are very well visualized with conventional radiography but can also be seen on CT. MR imaging obtained in the active phase of enthesitis will show the inflammatory changes around the disc and at the apophyseal joints of the spine.

Pseudarthrosis in the spine may develop as a complication of erosions or because of trauma, resulting in fracture through the syndesmophytes in the fused spine.[37] Rarely a pseudarthrosis may develop at a level of lesser disease involvement between long fused segments.[2] The most common

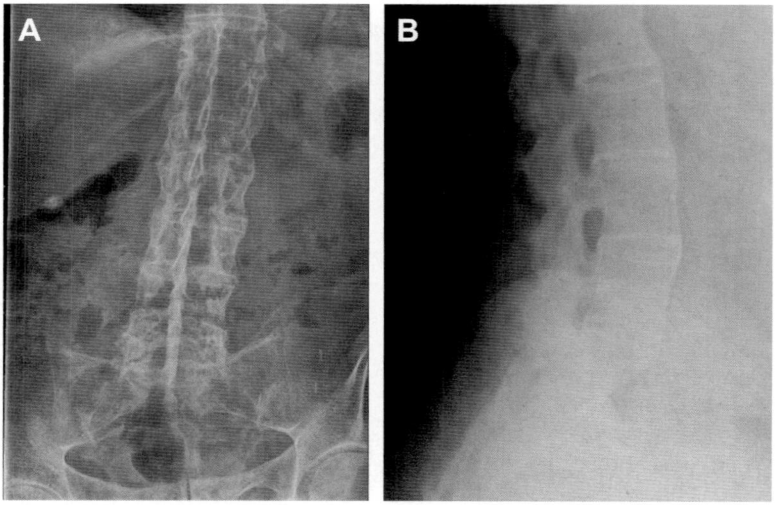

Fig. 5. Ankylosing spondylitis. (*A*) AP radiograph of the lumbar spine showing fusion of both sacroiliac joints and the typical bamboo spine of AS. (*B*) Lateral view in a different patient showing the fine, bridging osteophytes representing ossification of Sharpey fibers. Note also the loss of the normal concave contour (squaring) of the anterior aspect of the lumbar vertebrae.

site of traumatic lesions is at the thoracolumbar or cervicothoracic junctions, which commonly involve all 3 columns of the spine (**Fig. 6**). These lesions may be easily missed at the time of initial evaluation of trauma and may progress to a true pseudarthrosis with instability at the fracture site, potentially leading to cord injury and paralysis. AS patients suffering even modest trauma should be considered to harbor a spinal fracture until excluded by advanced imaging, preferably CT. Similarly, atlantoaxial subluxation may be seen in AS, but it is uncommon and is more likely to be present when patients have peripheral joint involvement.[38] Dural ectasia and leptomeningeal sacculations are common and may result in cauda equine syndrome, best evaluated with MR imaging (**Fig. 7**).[34,39] Large peripheral joints may be involved, but this is more likely when presenting symptoms occur before age 21 years. Small joint involvement is rare, but when present can lead to ankylosis and loss of mobility, especially in the hands.[2,3]

The most common extraskeletal manifestation of AS is progressive lung disease, including bullous emphysema and fibrosis, often complicated by unusual infections such as intracavitary aspergillosis.[2,3] Pulmonary changes occur late in the disease but may be the source of significant morbidity and mortality.[2] Inflammatory changes in the heart and aorta may result in conduction abnormalities and aortic insufficiency.[37] The association of inflammatory bowel disease and AS is tentative, but both are associated with HLA-B27 positivity.[11]

Psoriatic Arthritis

Psoriatic arthritis (PA) is an asymmetric, polyarticular disorder included in the spondyloarthropathies, as up to 40% of patients with PA will develop spondylitis or sacroiliitis. PA affects only about 7% of patients with cutaneous psoriasis.[40] The arthritis may antedate the skin changes by several years; the severity of the arthritis seems independent of the severity of the skin disease.[2,3] The presence of pitting nail changes correlates with the arthritis, especially when distal interphalangeal (DIP) joint involvement is severe.[2,41] Male/female involvement is nearly equal; the disease has a later onset than other spondyloarthropathies, with a typical onset between age 30 and 50 years.[2]

Sacroiliac involvement is not universal in PA. Only 5% of patients have exclusive spinal involvement without sacroiliitis.[2,3] The sacroiliac disease is generally asymmetric and ankylosis of the sacroiliac joints is very rare. MR imaging is most sensitive for the detection of subtle bilateral changes, which can be important in distinguishing PA from septic sacroiliitis in the early stages of the disease (**Fig. 8**).[13] The spondylitic changes in PA (and reactive spondyloarthritis) appear more randomly than those seen in AS,[2,3] and are usually but not always associated with sacroiliitis. Large, chunky-appearing paravertebral ossifications are commonly seen in the thoracolumbar junction.[2] These ossifications do not bridge the intervetebral discs as seen in AS but rather seem to attach

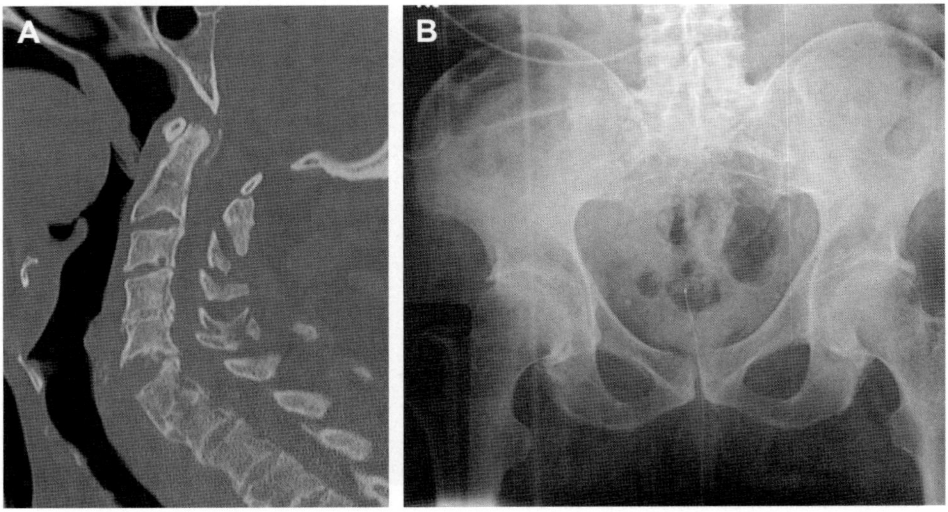

Fig. 6. Ankylosing spondylitis. (*A*) Sagittal reformatted CT image of the cervical spine showing a discovertebral fracture (Andersson lesion) at C5-C6 in this patient following a face-first fall. (*B*) AP radiograph in the same patient showing typical changes of AS with fusion of the sacroiliac joints and early changes of bamboo spine.

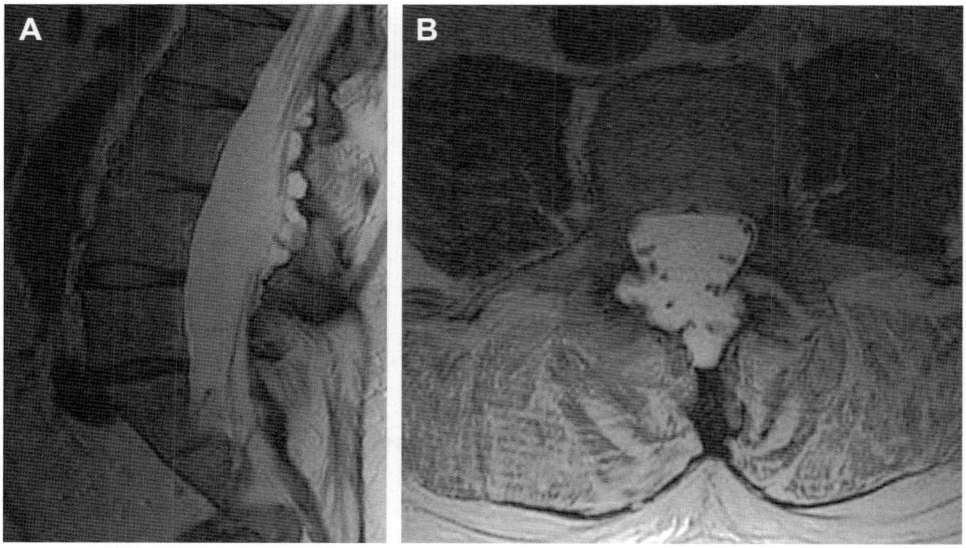

Fig. 7. Ankylosing spondylitis. Sagittal (*A*) and axial (*B*) T2-weighted MR images of the lumbar spine showing dural ectasia and sacculations in a patient with AS. This patient presented with cauda equina syndrome secondary to the tethering of the spinal nerve roots seen on these images.

to the lateral aspect of the vertebral bodies (**Fig. 9**A). Ankylosis of the apophyseal joints, squaring of the vertebral bodies, and spinal fusion are very rare in PA.

More distinctive in PA are the changes in the hands and feet. In the hands erosive changes develop within the interphalangeal joints, without the sparing seen in rheumatoid arthritis of the

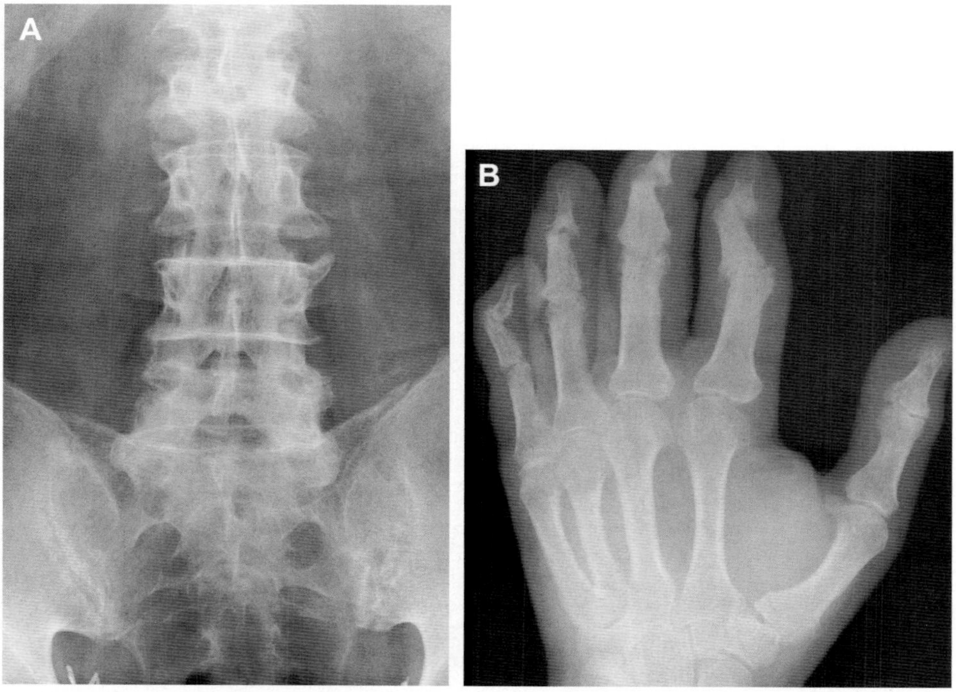

Fig. 8. Psoriatic arthritis. (*A*) AP view of the spine in a patient with psoriatic arthritis showing the large, chunky peripheral bridging osteophytes typical of psoriatic and reactive arthritis. Bilateral sacroiliitis is also present. (*B*) PA view of the hand in a different patient with psoriatic arthritis showing classic marginal erosions and proliferative periostitis in the digits. This patient does not have cutaneous psoriasis.

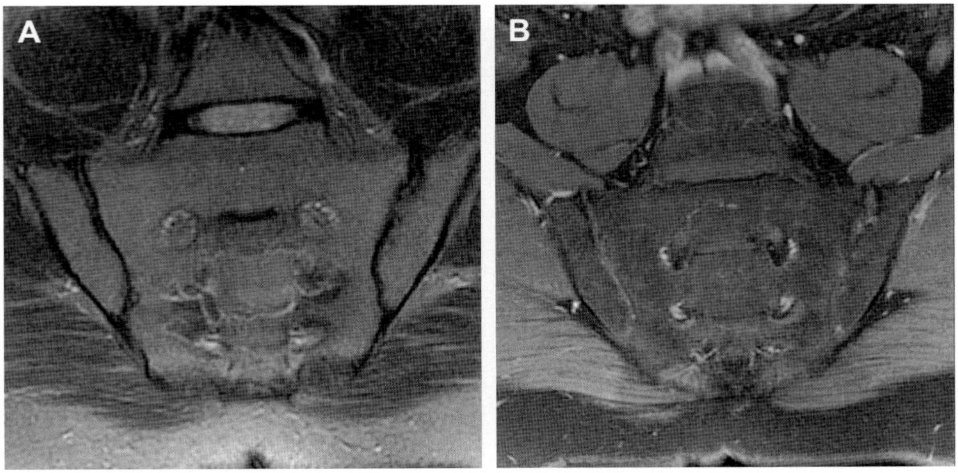

Fig. 9. (*A*) Coronal oblique T2-weighted MR image without fat suppression showing bilateral sacroiliitis, more prominent on the right. (*B*) Coronal oblique T1-weighted MR image with fat suppression after contrast shows patchy areas of enhancement consistent with active sacroiliitis in a patient with severe cutaneous psoriasis.

DIP joints (**Fig. 9**B).[2] The erosions are marginal and are often associated with marked soft-tissue swelling of the digits. Proliferative changes including fluffy periostitis are a common feature. Erosion of the distal portion of the phalanx with remodeling of the joint, the pencil-in-cup deformity, may be seen, as well as resorption or sometimes proliferation at the ungual tufts. The appearance is occasionally confused with erosive osteoarthritis (OA) but the presence of erosions at the marginal or bare areas of the phalanges in PA should be discernible from the central, subchondral erosions in erosive OA. Dense, circumferential periostitis may result in the so-called ivory phalanx on radiography. The interphalangeal joint of the great toe in the foot is the most common site for PA and may be confused with gout. If this is a serious concern, dual-energy CT may be helpful in this unique instance to determine whether the urate deposition of gout is present.[42]

Reactive Spondyloarthritis (Reiter Syndrome)

As with PA, reactive spondyloarthritis (RS) is a polyarticular, asymmetric arthritis. Unlike PA, RS preferentially affects the foot and large, peripheral joints.[2] If the hands are involved the interphalangeal joints are commonly involved, with relative sparing of the metacarpophalangeal and DIP joints. A common presenting symptom is heel pain caused by the fluffy enthesitis that can be seen with heel spurs in patients with RS (**Fig. 10**A).[43]

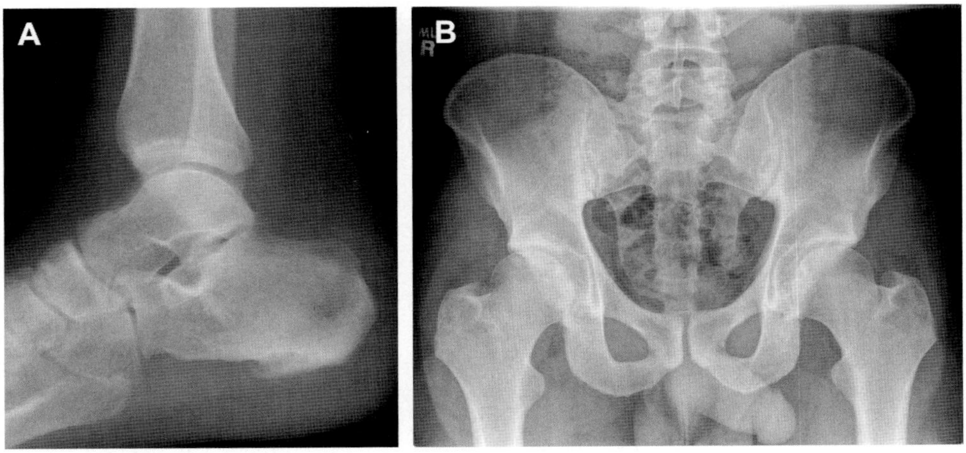

Fig. 10. Reactive arthritis. (*A*) Lateral radiograph of the hindfoot in a different patient with reactive arthritis showing enthesitis and periostitis at the plantar calcaneus. This patient presented with heel pain. (*B*) AP radiograph showing bilateral sacroiliitis, which is worse on the right in a patient with urethritis and uveitis. The patient had a history of *Chlamydia* infection.

Because of the historical association with venereal infection, this has sometimes been called lover's heel. Sacroiliitis and spondylitis are seen more commonly than in PA, with sacroiliitis present in up to 45% of patients.[2,3] The asymmetric and bilateral imaging appearance of sacroiliitis in RS is identical to that seen in PA, with ankylosis even less common than in PA (**Fig. 10**B). The radiographic appearance of the spinal changes is the same as in PA, with marginal, coarse syndesmophytes that appear to be randomly placed in the lower thoracic and lumbar spine.[2] Spine involvement is more common than in PA, seen in the lumbar spine in about 30% of patients with RS.[3] Upper thoracic and cervical spine involvement is very rare. It may sometimes be impossible to differentiate PA and RS on radiographs, but the clinical syndromes are usually distinct. Relatively few findings in the upper extremities, sparing of the DIP joints, and involvement of the sacroiliac joints and spine may tilt the diagnosis toward RS.

Classically RS has been diagnosed when the triad of urethritis, uveitis, and arthritis have been present, often in association with *Chlamydia* infection.[2,3] Patients with RS have a higher than average prevalence of HLA-B27 positivity, which may predispose them to develop the arthritis in the presence of a triggering event such as infection.[11] The term Reiter syndrome is only used when the specific triggering organism can be identified and when the arthritis appears within about a month of the original illness.[1] In addition to the classic association with venereal disease, RS can be seen in enteric infections from organisms such as *Shigella*, *Salmonella*, and *Yersinia*.[2] Human immunodeficiency virus (HIV) infection can of course coexist with both RS and PA, and the arthritis may be particularly severe in such cases. HIV can itself be associated with joint symptoms but without the typical radiographic findings seen in RS, and generally with more involvement of peripheral joints than the axial skeleton. HIV infection may exacerbate existing rheumatoid arthritis or PA; if severe, unexplained worsening is seen clinically, HIV testing may be warranted.[1]

Arthritis Associated with Inflammatory Bowel Disease (Enteropathic Arthritis)

Enteropathic arthritis may be seen equally in association with Crohn disease or ulcerative colitis.[2,3,44] The arthritis may have 1 of 2 forms that rarely coexist. Up to 20% of patients with inflammatory bowel disease may develop a nondestructive and often transient peripheral arthritis, the severity of which parallels the progress of the underlying bowel disease and which may actually resolve with surgery or other successful treatment.[2] This primarily involves joints such as the knees, ankles, elbows, and wrists, and is most often bilateral and symmetric.

The other form of enteropathic arthritis can involve the spine and/or sacroiliac joints. An isolated spondylitis that is radiographically identical to AS with the same fine, marginal syndesmophytes proceeding in orderly fashion from the thoracolumbar junction may be present in up to 6% of patients.[2,3,45] Shiny corners and squaring of the vertebral bodies may be present, although this is less common. Rarely this spondylitis may be present without sacroiliitis, an important distinction from AS. Sacroiliitis, when present, is similar to that seen in AS, with bilateral, symmetric findings and later ankylosis of the joints (**Fig. 11**).[2] Isolated sacroiliitis is more common than isolated spondylitis; it may be seen in up to 18% of patients with inflammatory bowel disease.[2,3,13] In contradistinction to the peripheral arthritis seen with inflammatory bowel disease, the severity of the spondylitis progresses independent of the course of disease or treatment of the primary intestinal problem.[2,3,46] The spondylitis may even precede the development of the bowel disease by months or years (**Fig. 12**). As with other forms of spondyloarthropathy, there is a predilection for HLA-B27 positivity but without the high prevalence seen with AS.[1,2,11]

Undifferentiated Spondyloarthropathy

Undifferentiated spondyloarthropathy is a term used when clinical symptoms are present such

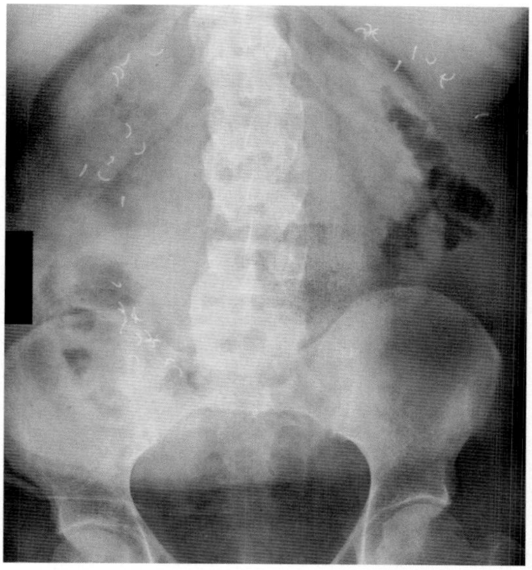

Fig. 11. Enteropathic arthritis. AP radiograph of the pelvis showing bilateral sacroiliitis and a right lower quadrant ostomy in a patient with Crohn disease.

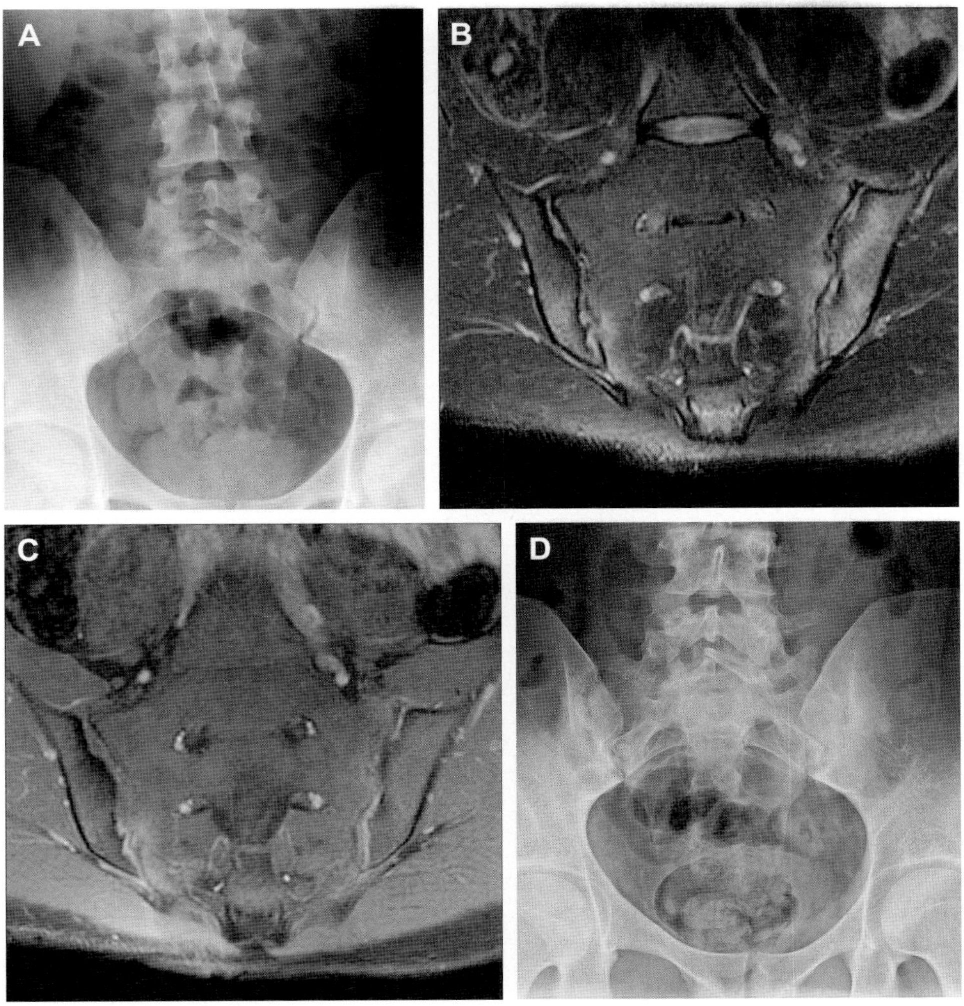

Fig. 12. Enteropathic arthritis. (*A*) AP radiograph showing asymmetric, bilateral sacroiliitis in a 21-year-old man with inflammatory back pain. (*B*) Oblique coronal T2-weighted MR image with fat suppression showing bilateral sacroiliitis. (*C*) Oblique coronal T1-weighted MR image with fat suppression showing enhancement consistent with active sacroiliitis. The patient is HLA-B27 negative. (*D*) Radiograph obtained 4 years after *A* shows worsening sacroiliitis. At this time the patient began experiencing bloody diarrhea and underwent endoscopy showing inflammatory bowel disease.

as peripheral arthritis, sacroiliitis, and enthesitis with inflammatory low back pain, but without distinguishing clinical or imaging features that would allow further subclassification.[6] Key features are sacroiliitis and increased HLA-B27 positivity, as in other forms of seronegative spondyloarthritis, but other stigmata such as inflammatory bowel disease or distinguishing patterns of peripheral joint involvement or inciting infection are absent. Atlantoaxial subluxation as an unusual manifestation of undifferentiated spondyloarthropathy was recently described in a case report in a young patient, reinforcing the need for a high degree of clinical suspicion when young patients present with inflammatory back or spinal pain (**Fig. 13**). Awareness of this syndrome may allow earlier diagnosis and treatment in the absence of classic findings of AS, PA, or RS.

Late-Onset Spondyloarthropathy

Although much more commonly seen in young patients, AS and other spondyloarthropathies may present in the elderly. The clinical presentations are sometimes confusing, often combining age-related degenerative osteoarthritis with imaging features more typical for spondyloarthropathy such as sacroiliitis.[7,31] HLA-B27 positivity is

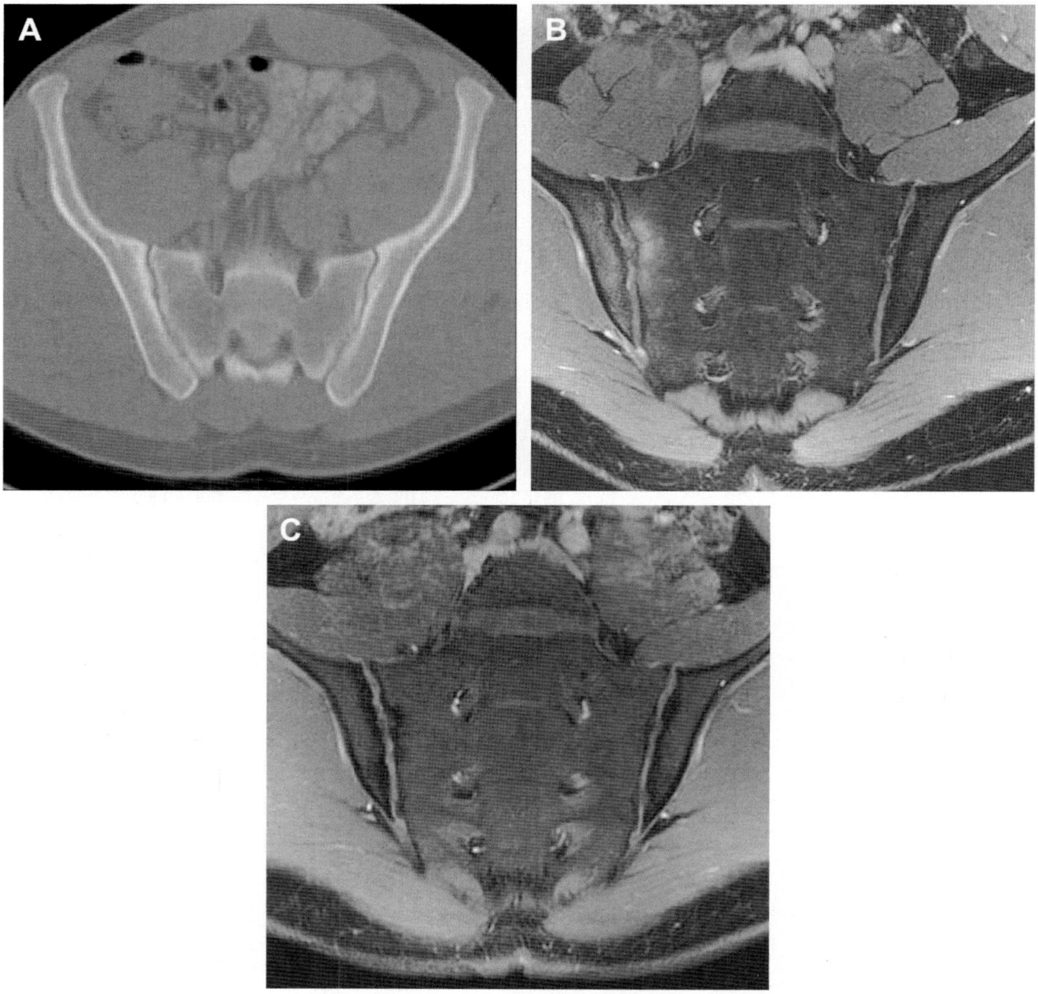

Fig. 13. Undifferentiated spondyloarthropathy. (*A*) Axial CT scan obtained without contrast shows bilateral changes of sacroiliitis in this 28-year-old man with inflammatory low back pain. He is HLA-B27 positive. (*B*) Oblique coronal T1-weighted MR image with fat suppression obtained after contrast administration. Note the florid enhancement on the right, representing active sacroiliitis. There were subtle positive findings present on the left as well. A fluoroscopic image from an injection of the right sacroiliac joint showed sacroiliitis in the same patient (not shown). (*C*) Oblique coronal T1-weighted MR image with fat suppression obtained after 1 year of treatment with enteracept (Enbrel). The enhancement has resolved, compatible with successful treatment. The patient's symptoms improved but did not completely resolve.

elevated in this group, as in the syndromes presenting in younger patients. The presenting disease is often more severe than in younger patients, and treatment options may be more limited because of the toxicity associated with treatments such as anti–tumor necrosis factor agents and comorbidities such as cardiovascular disease. In some older patients the new onset of symptoms of inflammatory back pain may be confused with diseases such polymyalgia rheumatica or even chronic pain syndromes such as fibromyalgia.[47] Awareness of this entity and the use of advanced cross-sectional imaging is increasing, allowing more accurate diagnosis and treatment in this unique group of patients.[31]

SUMMARY

The seronegative spondyloarthropathies are a diverse group of disorders affecting the axial skeleton and peripheral joints. Based on clinical presentation and imaging findings the individual entities have some unique features that can help to distinguish them, but all share inflammatory changes in the sacroiliac joints and spine and may present with back pain. Plain radiography is the mainstay of imaging, but MR imaging has significantly better sensitivity and specificity for detecting bone marrow edema and enhancement indicating inflammation. MR imaging may also be used to monitor therapy with disease-modifying drugs. Early MR imaging can help to establish the diagnosis in the early stages of disease, avoiding unnecessary delays and facilitating earlier treatment.

REFERENCES

1. Dougados M, Baeten D. Spondyloarthritis. Lancet 2011;377:2127–37.
2. El-Khoury GY, Kathol MH, Brandser EA. Seronegative spondyloarthropathies. Radiol Clin North Am 1996;34(2):343.
3. Luong AA, Salonen DC. Imaging of the seronegative spondyloarthropathies. Curr Rheumatol Rep 2000;2: 288–96.
4. Moll J, Haslock I, Macrae IF, et al. Associations between ankylosing spondylitis, psoriatic arthritis, Reiter's disease, the intestinal arthropathies, and Behcet's syndrome. Medicine (Baltimore) 1974;53:343–64.
5. Azouz E, Duffy C. Juvenile spondyloarthropathies: clinical manifestations and medical imaging. Skeletal Radiol 1995;24(6):399–408.
6. Muscal E, Satyan K, Jea A. Atlantoaxial subluxation as an early manifestation in an adolescent with undifferentiated spondyloarthritis: a case report and review of the literature. J Med Case Rep 2011;5(1):275.
7. Toussirot E. Late-onset ankylosing spondylitis and spondyloarthritis: and update on clinical manifestations, differential diagnosis and pharmacological therapies. Drugs Aging 2010;27(7):523–31.
8. Van Der Linden S, Valkenburg H, Cats A. Evaluation of diagnostic criteria for ankylosing spondylitis. A proposal for modification of the New York criteria. Arthritis Rheum 1984;27:361–8.
9. Amor B, Dougados M, Mijiyawa M. Criteria of the classification of spondyloarthropathies. Rev Rhum Mal Osteoartic 1991;57:85–9.
10. Rudwaleit M, Vand der Heijde D, Landewé R, et al. The development of Assessment of SpondyloArthritis international Society classification criteria for axial spondyloarthritis (part II): validation and final selection. Ann Rheum Dis 2009;68:777–83.
11. Fong K. The genetics of spondyloarthropathies. Ann Acad Med Singapore 2000;29(3):370–5.
12. Forrester D, Hollingsworth P, Dawkins RL. Difficulties in the radiographic diagnosis of sacroiliitis. Clin Rheum Dis 1983;9:323–32.
13. Braun J, Sieper J, Bollow M. Imaging of sacroiliitis. Clin Rheumatol 2000;19:51–7.
14. Hollingsworth P, Cheah P, Dawkins RL, et al. Observer variation in grading sacroiliac radiographs in HLA-B27 positive individuals. J Rheumatol 1983; 10:247–54.
15. Yacizi H, Turunc M, Ozdoğan H, et al. Observer variation in grading sacroiliac radiographs might be a cause of "sacroiliitis" reported in certain disease states. Ann Rheum Dis 1987;46:139–45.
16. Lawson T, Foley W, Carrera GF, et al. The sacroiliac joints: anatomic, plain roentgenographic, and computed tomographic analysis. J Comput Assist Tomogr 1982;6:307–14.
17. Battison M, Manaster B, Reda DJ, et al. Radiographic diagnosis of sacroiliitis: are sacroiliac views really better? J Rheumatol 1998;25:2395–401.
18. Chase W, Houk R, Winn RE, et al. The clinical usefulness of radionuclide scintigraphy in suspected sacro-iliitis: a prospective study. Br J Rheumatol 1983;22:67–72.
19. Ho GJ, Sadovnikoff N, Malhotra CM, et al. Quantitative sacroiliac joint scintigraphy: a critical assessment. Arthritis Rheum 1979;22:837–44.
20. Fam A, Rubenstein J, Chin-Sang H, et al. Computed tomography in the diagnosis of early ankylosing spondylitis. Arthritis Rheum 1985;28:930–7.
21. Carrera G, Foley W, Kozin F, et al. CT of sacroiliitis. AJR Am J Roentgenol 1981;136:41–6.
22. Wittram C, Whitehouse G, Bucknall RC. Fat suppressed contrast enhanced MR imaging in the assessment of sacroiliitis. Clin Radiol 1996;51:554–8.
23. Wittram C, Whitehouse G, Williams JW, et al. A comparison of MR and CT in suspected sacroiliitis. J Comput Assist Tomogr 1996;20:68–72.
24. Arslan H, Emin Sakarya M, Adak B, et al. Duplex and color Doppler sonographic findings in active sacroiliitis. AJR Am J Roentgenol 1999;173:677–80.
25. Klauser A, De Zordo T, Feuchtner G, et al. Feasibility of ultrasound-guided sacroiliac joint injection considering sonoanatomic landmarks at two different levels in cadavers and patients. Arthritis Rheum 2008;59(11):1618–24.
26. Braun J, Bollow M, Eggens U, et al. Use of dynamic magnetic resonance imaging with fast imaging in the detection of early and advanced sacroiliitis in spondyloarthropathy patients. Arthritis Rheum 1994;37:1039–45.
27. Kurugoglu S, Kanberoglu K, Kanberoglu A, et al. MRI appearances of inflammatory vertebral osteitis in early ankylosing spondylitis. Pediatr Radiol 2002;32:191–4.
28. Murphey M, Wetzel L, Bramble JM, et al. Sacroiliitis: MR imaging findings. Radiology 1991;180:239–44.
29. Weber U, Ostergaard M, Lambert RG, et al. The impact of MRI on the clinical management of inflammatory arthritides. Skeletal Radiol 2011; 40(9):1153–73.
30. Yu W, Feng F, Dion E, et al. Comparison of radiography, computed tomography and magnetic resonance imaging in the detection of sacroiliitis accompanying ankylosing spondylitis. Skeletal Radiol 1998;27:311–20.

31. Vanhoenacker F, Eyselbergs M, Cotten A. Spinal degeneration: beyond degenerative disc disease: how to discriminate degeneration from spondyloarthropathies? Neuroradiology 2011;53(Suppl 1):175–9.
32. Blum U, Buitrago-Tellez C, Mundinger A, et al. Magnetic resonance imaging (MRI) for detection of active sacroiliitis; a prospective study comparing conventional radiography, scintigraphy, and contrast enhanced MRI. J Rheumatol 1996;23:2107–15.
33. Xu M, Lin Z, Deng X, et al. The Ankylosing Spondylitis Disease Activating Score is a high discriminatory measure of disease activity and efficacy following tumour necrosis factor-a inhibitor therapies in ankylosing spondylitis and undifferentiated spondyloarthropathies in China. Rheumatology (Oxford) 2011;50(8):1466–72.
34. Fox M, Onofrio B, Kilgore JE. Neurological complications of ankylosing spondylitis. J Neurosurg 1993; 78:871–8.
35. Arnett F. Seronegative spondyloarthropathies. Bulletin on the Rheumatic Diseases, Arthritis Foundation 1987;37:1–12.
36. Braunstein E, Martel W, Moidel R. Ankylosing spondylitis in men and women: a clinical and radiographic comparison. Radiology 1982;144:91–4.
37. Fang D, Leong J, Ho EK, et al. Spinal pseudarthrosis in ankylosing spondylitis. J Bone Joint Surg 1988;70: 443–7.
38. Suarez-Almazor ME, Russell AS. Anterior atlantoaxial subluxation in patients with spondyloarthropathies: association with peripheral disease. J Rheumatol 1988;15(6):973–5.
39. Mitchell M, Sartoris D, Moody D, et al. Cauda equina syndrome complicating ankylosing spondylitis. Radiology 1990;175:521–5.
40. Leczinsky C. The incidence of arthropathy in a ten-year series of psoriasis cases. Acta Derm Venereol 1948;28:483–7.
41. Jones S, Armas J, Cohen MG, et al. Psoriatic arthritis: outcome of disease subsets and relationship of joint disease to nail and skin disease. Br J Rheumatol 1994;33:834–9.
42. Glazebrook K, Guimaraes L, Murthy NS, et al. Identification of intraarticular and periarticular uric acid crystals with dual-energy CT: initial evaluation. Radiology 2011;261(2):516–24.
43. Turlik M. Seronegative arthritis as a cause of heel pain. Clin Podiatr Med Surg 1990;7(2):369–75.
44. Grandbois L, Lomasney L, Demos TC, et al. Radiologic case study. Seronegative spondyloarthropathy associated with Crohn's disease. Orthopedics 2005; 28(11):1296, 1375–99.
45. McEwen C, DiTata D, Lingg C, et al. Ankylosing spondylitis and spondylitis accompanying ulcerative colitis, regional enteritis, psoriasis and Reiter's disease. Arthritis Rheum 1971;14:291–318.
46. Mielants H, Veys E. Enteropathic arthritis. In: Schumacher HJ, Klippel J, Koopman W, editors. Primer on the rheumatic diseases, vol. 10. Atlanta (GA): Arthritis Foundation; 1993. p. 163.
47. Aydeniz A, Altindag O, Oğüt E, et al. Late onset spondyloarthropathy mimicking polymyalgia rheumatica. Rheumatol Int 2012;32(5):1357–8.

Index

Note: Page numbers of article titles are in **boldface** type.

Radiol Clin N Am 50 (2012) 855–862
doi:10.1016/S0033-8389(12)00101-7